COGNITIVE ENHANCEMENT IN CNS DISORDERS AND BEYOND

COGNITIVE ENHANCEMENT IN CNS DISORDERS AND BEYOND

Edited by

Richard S.E. Keefe, PhD

Professor of Psychiatry, Psychology, & Neuroscience
Duke University Medical Center
Durham, North Carolina

Abraham Reichenberg, PhD

Professor, Departments of Psychiatry and Preventive Medicine
Icahn School of Medicine at Mount Sinai
New York, New York

Jeffrey Cummings, MD, ScD

Camille and Larry Ruvo Chair for Brain Health
Director, Cleveland Clinic Lou Ruvo Center for Brain Health
Director, Center for Neurodegeneration
and Translational Neuroscience
Professor, Cleveland Clinic Lerner College of Medicine
Las Vegas, Nevada

OXFORD
UNIVERSITY PRESS

OXFORD
UNIVERSITY PRESS

Oxford University Press is a department of the University of Oxford. It furthers the University's objective of excellence in research, scholarship, and education by publishing worldwide. Oxford is a registered trade mark of Oxford University Press in the UK and certain other countries.

Published in the United States of America by Oxford University Press
198 Madison Avenue, New York, NY 10016, United States of America.

© Oxford University Press 2018

CIP data is on file at the Library of Congress
ISBN 978–0–19–021440–1

This material is not intended to be, and should not be considered, a substitute for medical or other professional advice. Treatment for the conditions described in this material is highly dependent on the individual circumstances. And, while this material is designed to offer accurate information with respect to the subject matter covered and to be current as of the time it was written, research and knowledge about medical and health issues is constantly evolving and dose schedules for medications are being revised continually, with new side effects recognized and accounted for regularly. Readers must therefore always check the product information and clinical procedures with the most up-to-date published product information and data sheets provided by the manufacturers and the most recent codes of conduct and safety regulation. The publisher and the authors make no representations or warranties to readers, express or implied, as to the accuracy or completeness of this material. Without limiting the foregoing, the publisher and the authors make no representations or warranties as to the accuracy or efficacy of the drug dosages mentioned in the material. The authors and the publisher do not accept, and expressly disclaim, any responsibility for any liability, loss or risk that may be claimed or incurred as a consequence of the use and/or application of any of the contents of this material.

1 3 5 7 9 8 6 4 2
Printed by Sheridan Books, Inc., United States of America

Contents

Preface

There has never been a time that we knew more about cognition and never a time when cognition was more important to the functioning of human beings than right now. Psychological science and cognitive neuroscience have become the most popular endeavor of students worldwide (http://nces.ed.gov/programs/digest/d15/tables/dt15_322.10.asp?current=yes), are the focus of attention of our greatest scientific accomplishments (https://www.nobelprize.org/nobel_prizes/medicine/laureates/2014/press.html), and are the emphasis of many publications in the mainstream media.

Human activities that are dependent on intact cognitive functioning range from simply surviving to thoroughly thriving. Those who have lost cognitive capacities lose friends, lose jobs, and, in common cases of dementia and other CNS challenges, lose the ability to function independently. At the same time, those with superior cognitive ability have constructed the most beautiful works of art and science. And the importance of cognition in our lives increases yearly. Even rudimentary employment requires interaction with technology that depends on cognitive skills such as attention and speeded perceptual processing. Although social interactions have always involved the ability to keep pace with a flood of visual, auditory, and emotional stimuli, their complexity has increased with the ubiquitous presence of technology and social media, and these trends are expected to continue well into the future. Whereas previous generations depended more on human memory systems for the storage of information, the current global human cognitive environment dictates that the ability to obtain and process information quickly using the human–technology interface has become the currency of success and failure.

Given human dependence on cognitive abilities for survival, quality of life, and productivity, improving them has also never been more important. Those with impairments in key aspects of cognition suffer dearly, as they are unable to obtain and retain information, unable to make sound decisions based on the information at hand, and unable to plan future activities. The availability of pharmacological and behavioral interventions that can improve cognitive abilities and provide impaired individuals with the social, occupational, and functional quality of life that the rest of us enjoy has potential far-reaching implications. Such interventions can also benefit those who want to boost current cognitive abilities to higher levels, perhaps as a means to hone skills in providing products for others or to gain an edge on competition, for better or worse. This book is devoted to describing the latest cognitive science and neuroscience on the methods for enhancing cognition in healthy and unhealthy humans.

The first two chapters of the book provide background on cognitive enhancing treatment development and the basic neuroscience and pharmacology of cognition by two of the world's preeminent basic and clinical scientific leaders. These chapters are followed by a description of the cognitive impairment and treatment development for dementia and other neurological conditions, such as traumatic brain injury, Alzheimer's disease, mild cognitive impairment, Parkinson's disease, and epilepsy, by internationally acclaimed authors whose life work has been to study cognition in these disorders. For these conditions, clinicians have some understanding of the neurobiological underpinnings of the disease, and cognitive impairment is usually part of the definition of the disorder. In some cases, efforts to treat cognition have been ongoing for decades. These chapters include descriptions of the standard treatments that have provided benefit, as well as discussions of new strategies—some provocative—and the scientific methodologies to test their safety and efficacy.

The third section of the book includes chapters on the treatment of cognitive impairment in conditions such as schizophrenia, major depression, bipolar disorder, autism spectrum disorder, attention deficit hyperactivity disorder, and brain cancer, for which cognition has historically been a secondary concern. However, recent work suggests that the historical focus has been misguided, as the manifest components of these disorders—such as complaints of lethargy and sadness in depression or hallucinations and social isolation in schizophrenia—sit atop a larger and more destructive set of cognitive impairments that compromise functioning and quality of life in almost all people diagnosed with these conditions. Although few treatments are available for the cognitive components of these disorders, and to date none have received regulatory approval, a wealth of new treatments are being tested, and they are described in these pages by a set of innovative and forward-thinking authors who have been looking underneath the obvious presentations of these disorders for years.

The final section of the book grapples with a set of controversial issues in modern science. What are the current strategies for improving cognition in healthy aging? What are the ethical considerations of cognitive enhancement in general, particularly in healthy people, young and old? And finally, what are the regulatory processes for drug and device approval in the United States and Europe? These questions are addressed by authors who have a penchant for saying and writing what others have either ignored or felt more comfortable leaving alone.

We the editors have assembled these chapters from the leading cognitive and clinical scientists in the field to describe the latest research on cognitive impairments in a host of pathological conditions that affect CNS functioning, what treatments are available for these impairments, and how new treatments are being tested. Our expectation is that this volume will be of benefit to any investigators in cognitive science and clinical research, but we have also strived to make the chapters accessible to non-experts as well. Our intention was to advance the field toward the availability of cognitive enhancing drugs and devices that will benefit those who need them most and others who may believe that these techniques can help them to thrive. We hope that you feel we have achieved this goal.

Richard S.E. Keefe, PhD

Avi (Abraham) Reichenberg, PhD

Jeffrey Cummings, MD

Contributors

Gilberto S. Alves, MD, PhD
Universidade Federal do Ceará
Faculty of Medicine
Fortaleza, Ceará, Brazil

Jalayne J. Arias, JD, MA
Assistant Professor
Department of Neurology
Atlantic Fellow at the Global Brain
    Health Institute
University of California

Amy F. T. Arnsten, PhD
Department of Neurobiology
Yale University School of Medicine
New Haven, Connecticut

Sarah Banks, PhD
Neuropsychology Program
Cleveland Clinic Lou Ruvo Center for
    Brain Health
Las Vegas, Nevada

Louise Brennan, PhD
Tallagh Hospital
Dublin, Ireland

Karl Broich, MD
President
Federal Institute for Drugs and Medical
    Devices (BfArM)
Bonn, Germany

Helen J. Brooker, BsC
Wesnes Cognition Limited
Streatley, England, UK

André F. Carvalho, MD, PhD
Department of Clinical Medicine
    and Translational Psychiatry
    Research Group
Faculty of Medicine
Federal University of Ceará
Fortaleza, Brazil

Jeffrey Cummings, MD, ScD
Camille and Larry Ruvo Chair for
   Brain Health
Director, Cleveland Clinic Lou Ruvo
   Center for Brain Health
Director, Center for Neurodegeneration
   and Translational Neuroscience
Professor, Cleveland Clinic Lerner
   College of Medicine
Las Vegas, Nevada

Iulia Dud, MD
Royal College of Surgeons of Ireland
Beaumont Hospital
Dublin, Ireland

Paul J. Ford, PhD
NeuroEthics Program
Cleveland Clinic
Cleveland, Ohio

James Gilleen, PhD
King's College London
London, England, United Kingdom

Tessa Hart, PhD
Institute Scientist
Moss Rehabilitation Research Institute
Elkins Park, Pennsylvania
Research Professor
Department of Rehabilitation Medicine
Sidney Kimmel Medical College
Thomas Jefferson University
Philadelphia, Pennsylvania

Richard S.E. Keefe, PhD
Professor of Psychiatry, Psychology, &
   Neuroscience
Duke University Medical Center
Durham, North Carolina

Shelli R. Kesler, PhD
M.D. Anderson Cancer Center
University of Texas
Houston, Texas

Bryan Kibbe, PhD
Educator, Advisor, Researcher, Writer,
   Analyst
WellStar Health System
Loyola University Chicago
Greater Atlanta Area

Cristiano A. Köhler, MD, PhD
Brain Institute
Federal University of Rio Grande do
   Norte
Natal, Rio Grande do Norte, Brazil

Nicholas Kozauer, MD
Formerly, Senior Therapeutic
   Regulatory Lead, CNS
Quintiles IMS

Katie Mahon, PhD
Baptist Behavioral Health
Fleming Island, Florida

**Beth A. Leeman-Markowski, MD,
MA, MMSc**
Assistant Professor
Department of Neurology
New York University
NYU Langone Comprehensive
   Epilepsy-Sleep Institute
New York, NY

Roger S. McIntyre, MD, FRCP
Department of Psychiatry
University of Toronto
Toronto, Ontario, Canada

Kimford J. Meador, MD
Stanford University Medical Center
Palo Alto, California

Zara Melikyan, PhD
Associate Project Scientist
University of California Irvine

Constantinos D. Paspalas, PhD
Department of Neurobiology
Yale University School of Medicine
New Haven, Connecticut

Avi (Abraham) Reichenberg, PhD
Professor, Departments of Psychiatry
   and Preventive Medicine
Icahn School of Medicine at
   Mount Sinai
New York, New York

Dene Robertson, MD
Institute of Psychiatry
King's College London
London, England, United Kingdom

**M. Mercedes Perez-Rodriguez,
MD, PhD**
Department of Psychiatry
The Mount Sinai Hospital
New York, New York

Heather Romero, PhD
Clinical Psychology
Duke University
Durham, North Carolina

Manuela Russo, PhD
Icahn School of Medicine at
   Mount Sinai
New York, New York

Babak Tousi, MD, CMD, FACP
Geriatrics, Movement Disorders
Neurological Institute
Cleveland Clinic
Director, Senior Care Assessment
Lakewood Hospital
Lakewood, Ohio

Po-Heng Tsai, MD
Cleveland Clinic
Weston, Florida

Min J. Wang, PhD
Department of Neurobiology
Yale University School of Medicine
New Haven, Connecticut

Jeffrey S. Wefel, PhD, ABPP
Chief, Section of Neurophychology
Department of Neuro-Oncology
M.D. Anderson Cancer Center
Houston, Texas

**Kathleen A. Welsh-Bohmer, PhD,
ABPP**
Professor & Chief of Medical
   Psychology CPU, Department of
   Psychiatry
Director, Joseph & Kathleen Bryan
   Alzheimer's Disease Center
Department of Neurology

Keith A. Wesnes, PhD, Bsc

Head Honcho, Wesnes Cognition Ltd,
Streatley on Thames, RG8 9RD,
United Kingdom

Professor of Cognitive Neuroscience,
Medical School, University of
Exeter, United Kingdom

Visiting Professor, Department of
Psychology, Northumbria University,
Newcastle, United Kingdom

Adjunct Professor, Centre for Human
Psychopharmacology, Swinburne
University, Melbourne, Australia

Visiting Professor, Medicinal Plant
Research Group, Newcastle
University, United Kingdom

Kate Zhong, MD

Senior Director

Clinical Research and Development at
Cleveland Clinic

ONE

Promise and Challenges in Drug Development and Assessment for Cognitive Enhancers

JEFFREY CUMMINGS AND KATE ZHONG

COGNITIVE ENHANCERS: DRUG DEVELOPMENT AND CLINICAL TRIALS

Cognition is central to being human. Memory defines who we are and constructs a life-span biography; language is a specifically human enterprise that is developed to only the most rudimentary level in other animals; and insight and executive function allow us to plan, expect, judge, and play a role in communities. Cognition is affected in a variety of neuropsychiatric disorders and constitutes the principal disability in many. In all cases in which cognitive impairment occurs, it exaggerates the morbidity associated with the underlying condition, increases the challenges of mastering activities of daily living, amplifies dependence on others, complicates management of the principal illness, and undermines the autonomy and quality of life of the individual. Cognitive deficits exaggerate the challenges that these disorders present to the families of affected individuals and increase the affected person's dependency. The total global burden of cognitive disorders is enormous, comprising a portion of the disability associated with psychiatric illnesses (schizophrenia, depression, and obsessive–compulsive disorder); representing the defining deficit in developmental disorders and childhood disorders such as attention deficit hyperactivity disorder (ADHD), autism, and pervasive developmental disorder; accompanying many adult neurological disorders (multiple sclerosis and Parkinson's disease); comprising a major aspect of brain insults such as traumatic brain injury and stroke; and being the principal feature of late-onset neurodegenerative diseases such as Alzheimer's disease (AD) and frontotemporal dementia.

In all conditions in which cognitive deficits occur, the intellectual impairment is inadequately treated. There is no cognitive impairment syndrome that is currently optimally or even adequately managed by available medications. There is an urgent need to better understand the underlying mechanisms of cognitive impairment and to develop more effective medications. Disease-modifying therapies (DMTs) are likely to be specific to each condition, such as addressing tau or amyloid β protein in AD or α-synuclein in Parkinson's disease. Cognitive enhancement, however, implies improvement above baseline and may be subject to cross-disease extension, allowing lessons to be extrapolated from one condition to another. This chapter addresses principles of drug development and clinical trials for cognitive enhancing agents. It presents those principles that have wide application and can help scientists, clinicians, and industry sponsors to apply principles across disease states.

COGNITIVE DISORDERS

Treatment of cognitive disorders is a major unmet need in neuropsychiatry. Figure 1.1 presents disorders characterized by having cognitive impairment as one manifestation of the disorder. Developmental and early life disorders (e.g., autism and autistic spectrum disorders), midlife neurological conditions (e.g., multiple sclerosis), and late-life disorders (e.g., AD) all exhibit cognition impairment or decline as an important part of the disease phenotype. Cognitive disorders contribute in a major way to the disability of these conditions, and effective treatment with cognitive enhancers is urgently needed.

DEFINING COGNITIVE ENHANCEMENT

Cognitive enhancement is defined in this chapter as improvement above baseline (Figure 1.2). This contrasts with the observations in DMT drug development, in which the goal is the arrest or slowing of disease progression without the expectation of improvement (Figure 1.3). In this paradigm, cognitive enhancement occurs when there is a statistically significant improvement above baseline on a generally accepted measure of cognition relevant to the specific disorder. For example, in AD,

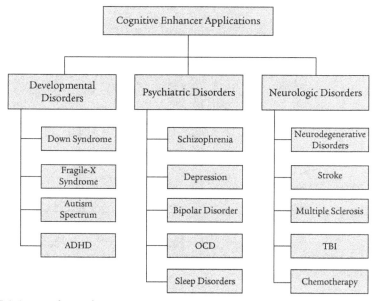

FIGURE 1.1 *Disorders with cognitive impairment.*

the commonly used measure of cognition is the Alzheimer's Disease Assessment Scale–Cognitive Subscale (ADAS-Cog);[1] in schizophrenia, the MATRICS Consensus Cognitive Battery (MCCB)[2] has become a standard.

The National Institutes of Health (NIH) has sponsored programs to advance cognitive measures that can be applied across disease states and across a broad age spectrum. The NIH Toolbox Cognitive Health Battery (NIHTB-CHB) is designed to measure neurological functions that span different disciplines, apply to diverse research questions, and measure a broad range of functions across the life span from age 3 to 85 years. The NIHTB-CHB is composed of four modules: cognition,

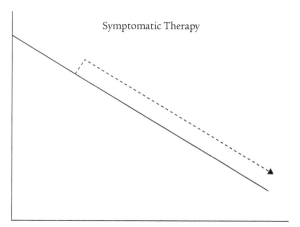

FIGURE 1.2 *Cognitive enhancement trajectories compared to baseline in static and progressive disorders.*

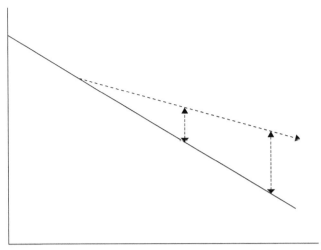

FIGURE 1.3 *Cognitive enhancement trajectories in patients with chronic progressive disorders treated with disease-modifying therapies.*

emotion, motor, and sensory.[3] Cognitive assessments of the NIHTB-CHB include measures of executive function, episodic memory, language, processing speed, working memory, and attention.[4] Similarly, the National Institute of Neurological Disease and Stroke funded a project to develop a tool for assessment of executive abilities called Executive Abilities: Measures and Instruments for Neurobehavioral Evaluation and Research (EXAMINER).[5] This tool is composed of measures of working memory, inhibition, set shifting, fluency, insight, planning, social cognition, and behavior relevant to assessment of executive and frontal lobe function. Neither of these instruments has yet found application in clinical trials, but the psychometric properties suggest that they may be sensitive to change over time, including changes induced by therapy. Use of the same tools across clinical trials in many types of disease would facilitate understanding of the common features and treatment responsiveness of cognitive domains across disease states.

CLINICAL TRIALS FOR COGNITIVE ENHANCERS

The general paradigm of cognitive enhancement trials is shown in Figure 1.4. Patients are defined as having a specific disorder using a syndromic definition such as those of the *Diagnostic and Statistical Manual of Mental Disorders*.[6] The severity of the target symptoms is established by an appropriate rating scale, and a baseline severity level for study participation is chosen to document that the patient has a sufficient symptom severity to warrant treatment and to allow demonstration of improvement by an effective intervention. A second symptom measure is typically chosen as an outcome measure that is administered at baseline and at the end of the trial to document any drug–placebo difference. Using

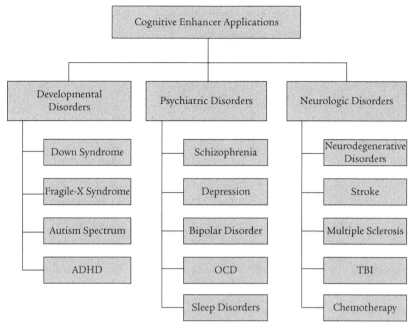

FIGURE 1.4 *General framework for testing cognitive enhancing agents in clinical trials.*

different scales for study participation and as an outcome minimizes the chance of regression to mean that occurs with many types of measurement. The outcomes are administered at intervals and at study end to document the effect of the test agent on the symptom severity.

Significant improvement on a cognitive measure documents cognitive enhancement but is not sufficient to establish that the intervention is clinically meaningful and will have an impact on the lives of the individuals affected. A global or functional measure is usually used as a key secondary or co-primary outcome to demonstrate the clinical meaningfulness of the therapy. Change on a cognitive measure by itself may not be viewed as clinically meaningful; when there is a corresponding change on a global measure or a measure of activities of daily living (ADLs), the treatment is regarded as more compellingly beneficial.[7] Proving clinical significance is a daunting challenge. Among the approaches used to show that there has been global improvement with drug therapy (cognitive, functional, and behavioral) are tools such as the Clinical Global Impression of Change (CGIC)[7] or ADL scales appropriate to the developmental stage of the individual and the disorder being treated.[8] Most clinical trials of cognitive enhancing agents use a dual-outcome strategy showing a cognitive benefit with a concomitant improvement on a global or ADL scale.

There is increasing interest from regulatory authorities, payers, and advocacy groups to include direct patient input in determining the value of treatment.[9] Patient-reported outcomes (PROs) are being developed across disease states and are being integrated into trials of cognitive enhancing agents. For example, patient global assessments and self-rated perceived deficits scales have been used in clinical trials of patients with mild cognitive impairment.[10]

A variety of secondary measures may be included in clinical trials of cognitive enhancing agents to collect data on the impact of drug administration. These data cannot be included in the package insert of an approved medication and cannot be used for marketing the agent. They can be published in the scientific literature and provide insight into the effects of an agent on multiple domains of patient function. For example, behavior is a critically important dimension of patient function, and identifying the effects on behavioral symptoms of cognitive enhancing agents is critical to understanding the universe of drug effects and the potential range of patient benefits. An apathy syndrome, for example, could be improved by cognitive enhancers in AD, Parkinson's disease, or schizophrenia and would comprise an important secondary outcome. If ADLs are not used as a primary outcome, then including them among secondary outcomes is an important aspect of study design.

Secondary outcome analysis also can be used to support the use of the agent with payers. For example, pharmacoeconomic analyses might establish that an agent reduces the use of emergency department services, decreases hospitalization rates, diminishes the need for in-home services, or delays nursing home care.[11] These observations translate into reduced costs and would help justify the reimbursement of an agent by a health care system or insurance company. Box 1.1 lists the general domains that might be assessed in trials of cognitive enhancing agents.

BOX 1.1
DOMAINS TO BE CONSIDERED AS SECONDARY OUTCOMES IN CLINICAL TRIALS OF COGNITIVE ENHANCING AGENTS

Special domains of cognition not assessed as the primary outcome (e.g., attention and executive function)

Global function (overall composite of cognition, function, and behavior)

Academic performance of school-age children

Social function and social cognition

Activities of daily living (instrumental and basic)

Behavior and neuropsychiatric symptoms

Quality of life (caregiver and patient)

Caregiver burden

Resource utilization

BIOMARKERS IN COGNITIVE ENHANCER TRIALS

Biomarkers are critical in trials of DMTs to support the biological effect of the treatment and establish the relationship between the biological effect and the clinical outcomes. In cognitive enhancer trials, there is no attempt to modify disease progression, and the role of biomarkers differs from their role in DMT drug development programs. In trials of symptomatic agents, biomarkers can be used to show blood–brain barrier penetration (e.g., induction of change on electroencephalography [EEG]),[12] receptor occupancy and dose relationships (ligand-labeled positron emission tomography [PET]),[13] metabolic effects (fluorodeoxyglucose [FDG]-PET), functional effects such as cerebral blood flow change or alterations in connectivity shown by functional magnetic resonance imaging (fMRI), or adverse events (electrocardiography and liver function tests). For example, increased cerebral metabolism demonstrated on FDG-PET correlates with cognitive improvement following treatment with cognitive enhancers in AD.[14,15] Box 1.2 provides examples of biomarkers used in cognitive enhancer drug development programs.

BOX 1.2
EXAMPLES OF BIOMARKERS USED IN COGNITIVE ENHANCER DRUG DEVELOPMENT PROGRAMS

BLOOD–BARRIER PENETRATION

Electroencephalography
Receptor occupancy with ligand-labeled positron emission tomography

DOSE EFFECTS

Receptor occupancy at different doses with ligand-labeled positron emission tomography

FUNCTIONAL AND METABOLIC EFFECTS

Fluorodeoxyglucose positron emission tomography
Cerebral blood flow
Functional magnetic resonance imaging

SAFETY

Electrocardiogram
Liver function tests
Complete blood counts
Serum chemistry profiles
Muscle enzymes

ADVANTAGES OF DEVELOPING COGNITIVE ENHANCERS COMPARED TO DISEASE-MODIFYING THERAPIES

There are few examples of successful development of DMTs. Treatment of multiple sclerosis with interferon and related agents is one example of disease modification with reduction in relapses, possible benefit in long-term disability, and reduced atrophy on MRI.[16,17] Among neurodegenerative disorders, cerebrovascular syndromes, or traumatic brain injury, however, no DMT has emerged despite substantial investment in the quest.

There are numerous advantages for development of symptomatic cognitive enhancers compared to DMTs (Box 1.3). There are successful development programs that can be modeled. For example, cognitive enhancers are approved for AD, the dementia of Parkinson's disease, and ADHD. These successes provide valuable insights into how to conduct development programs for cognitive enhancers. Regulatory agencies such as the US Food and Drug Administration and the European Medicine Agency are familiar with the cognitive enhancing strategies, and the approach to regulatory approval is relatively transparent. Similarly, past trials provide a guide to instrument performance in the trial setting, facilitating decisions about recruitment,

---

BOX 1.3
ADVANTAGES OF COGNITIVE ENHANCEMENT AS A DRUG DEVELOPMENT STRATEGY

Past success (e.g., in Alzheimer's disease) provides a model for the drug development approach.

Regulatory agencies such as the FDA and EMA are familiar with the strategy as some of the tools and measurement approaches.

Performance of instruments in trials is known for some of the disorders.

Biomarkers have a more limited role.

Improvement of above baseline is the desired outcome; this is aligned for patients, caregivers, and physicians.

Trials required are generally shorter than those required for DMT development.

Trials are generally smaller than required for DMT development.

Development programs are less expensive compared to DMT programs.

Targets of drug development are more conventional (receptors, transporters, channels, etc.) compared to the less well-known target of DMT development.

Agents may be applicable to multiple disorders with cognitive impairment and robust life cycle management programs.

DMT, disease-modifying therapy; EMA, European Medicines Agency; FDA, US Food and Drug Administration.

sites, sample sizes, and power. Although biomarkers such as PET receptor occupancy studies may have a role in cognitive enhancer drug development, the role of biomarkers is smaller in symptomatic than in DMT trials. Investment in development of new biomarkers and implementation in trials is often not required. Trials can be smaller and shorter than those required for DMTs, and this translates into lower development costs, shorter timelines, more residual patent life, longer market exclusivity, and greater revenue. Although the price and revenue generation of cognitive enhancers is likely to be less than that of DMTs, the income-generating difference is at least partially compensated by the smaller investment in the development program. The neurobiological targets of most cognitive enhancers—transmitters, receptors, and channels—are better understood than the protein targets of many DMTs, and the chances of technical success in a development program are greater. Finally, a successful cognitive enhancing agent may be approved for multiple disorders with cognitive impairment (e.g., AD, dementia or Parkinson's disease, and schizophrenia), leading to a robust life-cycle management approach.

FEATURES OF COGNITIVE ENHANCER DEVELOPMENT PATHWAYS

Cognitive enhancers may be developed for one indication only, as with any other agent class. The assumption, however, that the neurobiological basis of cognitive processes is similar across individuals and that cognitive enhancement can occur using similar mechanisms across a variety of disease states lends itself to dual (or more) development approaches. The cholinesterase inhibitor rivastigmine is approved for both AD and the dementia of Parkinson's disease.[18,19] EVP6124, an α_7 nicotinic agonist, was in development for both AD and the cognitive impairment of schizophrenia.[20] Down syndrome patients develop the pathology of AD and progressive cognitive deficits in later life and are another potential extended application of cognitive enhancers.[21] Table 1.1 provides examples of agents that are being developed for cognitive enhancement in multiple disorders. Cognitive enhancers lend themselves to orderly life-cycle management in which the agent's indications can be extended from one cognitive impairment syndrome to another.

Treatment of different disease stages or phases of severity represents another approach in cognitive enhancer development. Cholinesterase inhibitors, for example, began with indications for treatment of mild to moderate AD. Rivastigmine and donepezil later both extended their indications to include severe AD.[22,23] These extensions showed that patients with more severe disease could respond to therapy; formal approval helped ensure that health care plans would reimburse for use of

TABLE 1.1 Examples of Agents in Development for Cognitive Enhancement in More Than One Disorder

Agent/Class	AD	Fragile X Syndrome	Down Syndrome	Cognitive Impairment of Schizophrenia	Neurologic Impairment in Stroke	Dementia in Parkinson's Disease	ADHD
Memantine	X				X		
Cannabinoids	X	X	X				
GABA inhibitors			X				
α_7 nicotinic agonist	X			X			
Bryostatin (PKC activator)	X	X			X		
β_1-adrenergic receptor partial agonist	X		X			X	
Cholinesterase inhibitors	X		X	X		X	
Psychostimulants	X			X			X
AMPA potentiators	X			X			
PDE inhibitors	X			X			
H$_3$ antagonists	X						X
PAK dendritic spine modification	X	X		X			

AD, Alzheimer's disease; ADHD, attention deficit hyperactivity disorder; AMPA, α-amino-3-hydroxy-5-methyl-4-isoxazolepropionic acid receptor; H$_3$, histaminergic type 3 receptors; PAK, p21 activated kinase; PDE, phosphodiesterase; PKC, protein kinase C.

the therapies in more severely compromised patients. Attempts to extend therapy to more mildly affected patents—those with mild cognitive impairment—were also made but failed to show benefit or achieve regulatory approval.[24,25] Disease stage as well as illness type represent a critical strategy in cognitive enhancer drug development and life cycle management.

MECHANISMS OF COGNITIVE ENHANCERS

Enhancement of cholinergic function with cholinesterase inhibitors in AD and dementia of Parkinson's disease is the most successful example of cognitive enhancer drug development. The development approach was based on the observation of depleted presynaptic cholinergic neurons with relatively intact postsynaptic cholinergic architecture.[26–29] This provided a cogent anatomy for increasing presynaptic cholinergic function to allow improved postsynaptic stimulation. Several types of cholinergic agents—precursors, cholinesterase inhibitors, and receptor agonists—were tested. The class of agents that succeeded in producing cognitive improvement, cholinesterase inhibitors, increase synaptic residence time of acetylcholine, thus increasing receptor interactions and facilitating postsynaptic function.[26,30] Other attempts to stimulate specific aspects of the cholinergic system, such as with α_7 nicotinic agonists or muscarinic agonists, represent a continuing avenue of cognitive enhancer drug development.[20,31] Several cognitive enhancers currently being developed have as part of their mechanism the further increase in central nervous system acetylcholine (Table 1.2).[32–34]

Cholinergic deficits are found in other neurological diseases with cognitive decline providing a pathophysiological bridge for extension of cholinergic therapy to these disorders. Parkinson's disease dementia has a similar cholinergic pathology and responds to cholinesterase inhibitors; rivastigmine is approved for use in this disorder.[18] Dementia with Lewy bodies has a marked cholinergic deficit and represents a target therapeutic population for use of these agents.[35,36]

There are few other circumstances in which a presynaptic chemical deficit is combined with postsynaptic receptor integrity. The absence of this transmitter architecture in other transmitter systems may make it more difficult to identify agents that adequately stimulate remaining but compromised neuronal circuits.

A variety of other mechanisms are being explored in cognitive enhancement drug development programs. These emphasize cognitive enhancement in AD, ADHD, and the cognitive impairment of schizophrenia. Mechanisms being explored include histaminergic (H_3) antagonists, serotonergic (5-HT_6) antagonists, cannabinoid antagonists, glutamatergic (*N*-methyl-D-aspartate [NMDA] receptor) antagonists, and phosphodiesterase inhibitors.[37–47]

TABLE 1.2 Cognitive Enhancing Agents in Development That Increase Cholinergic Function as Part of Their Proposed Mechanism of Action

Class	Agent
Norepinephrine transporter inhibitor	Atomoxetine
Cannabinoid CB1 receptor antagonist	SR141716A
Dopamine D_1 receptor agonist	Dihydrexidine
Atypical antipsychotic	Clozapine
Benzodiazepine receptor partial inverse agonist	AC-3933
5 HT6 receptor antagonists	Intepirdine

Source: Tiraboschi P, Hansen LA, Alford M, et al. Early and widespread cholinergic losses differentiate dementia with Lewy bodies from Alzheimer disease. Arch Gen Psychiatry *2002;59(10):946–951.*

In AD drug development, agents beyond the usual transmitter approaches are being explored for their cognitive enhancing properties. Synaptic support and regeneration, insulin and insulin sensitizers, ketogenic agents, mitochondrial agents, psychotropic drugs with cognitive enhancing properties, and devices such as deep brain stimulation and repetitive transcranial magnetic stimulation are in clinical trials for cognitive enhancement in AD.[48–58] Success in this setting could lead to testing in other disorders with cognitive impairment.

Table 1.3 provides a list of mechanisms being explored for cognitive enhancement and some specific agents being assessed.

TABLE 1.3 Mechanisms and Examples of Cognitive Enhancers

System	Mechanism	Examples
Cholinergic	Cholinesterase inhibition	Rivastigmine, donepezil, galantamine, physostigmine
	α_7 agonist	EVP-6124
	Muscarinic receptor agonist	M1 allosteric modulators
Glutamatergic	NMDA receptor antagonist	Memantine
	Ampakines	CX717
Serotonergic	5-HT_6 antagonist	Idalopirdine
Phosphodiesterase	Inhibitor	PDE1, -3, -4, -10 inhibitors
Endocannabinoid	Cannabinoid antagonists	CB1 antagonists
Histaminergic	H_3 antagonists	GSK239512, ABT-288
Aminergic	Attention enhancers	Methylphenidate, atomoxetine, metadoxine
GABAergic	$GABA_A$ antagonists or inverse agonists	Experimental

GABA, γ-aminobutyric acid; NMDA, N-methyl-D-aspartate; PDE, phosphodiesterase.

OPPORTUNITIES IN COGNITIVE ENHANCEMENT DRUG DEVELOPMENT

In drug development, a research diagnostic approach to the phenotype such as the *International Classification of Diseases* (ICD) or the *Diagnostic and Statistical Manual of Mental Disorders* (DSM) is used. Patients are identified according to etiologic disorders—AD, ADHD, schizophrenia, and so on—and the diagnosis defines the treatment population. An alternative approach is to use a cognitive phenotype that may be present in many disorders and to determine if the phenotype responds to treatment. In this way, symptom complexes within many disorders might be identified as treatment targets (Table 1.4). Clinically, such a cognitive phenotype might include executive dysfunction with specific tests identifying this abnormality across multiple disease states such as AD, frontotemporal dementia, dementia with Lewy bodies, vascular dementia, depression, schizophrenia, autism, and ADHD. Alternatively, biomarkers such as fMRI might identify specific patterns of resting state or activated MRI (endophenotypes) that are present in patients responsive to a specific type of therapy. Over time, the fMRI finding could be matched to a drug mechanism. This would guide both drug development strategies and possibly patient selection after drug approval. Table 1.4 shows cognitive phenotypes that might guide therapeutic trials of cognitive enhancers across multiple diagnoses. Common cognitive phenotypes may be captured by tools such as the NIHTB-CHB[3,4] or EXAMINER.[5]

TABLE 1.4 Areas of Cognitive Impairment That Are Shared Across Disease States and That Might Be Targeted by Cognitive Enhancers (Cognitive Phenotypes)

Disorder	Apathy	Executive Dysfunction	Memory Impairment	Reduced Social Judgment
Schizophrenia	X	X		X
Mania		X		X
Depression	X	X	X	
Alzheimer's disease	X	X	X	
Frontotemporal dementia	X	X	X	X
Fragile X syndrome		X	X	X

CLINICAL TRIAL DESIGNS

Cognition studies are usually of short duration—typically 3–6 months. This duration of trial lends itself to some types of design and not to others. Adaptive designs, for example, may work best in longer term trials in which sufficient data have accumulated to allow adaptive conclusions to be drawn and adjustments implemented.

Parallel group designs are typically used in cognitive enhancer trials with comparison of change from baseline in the placebo group to change from baseline in the treatment group. If the placebo group experiences decline and the treatment group improves above baseline, then the total effect of treatment will be the sum of the positive change from baseline of the treatment group and the decline from baseline of the placebo group.[59] Placebo decline in short-term trials is typically negligible.

Crossover designs commonly use smaller populations and optimize the use of data from each patient because each is in both the treatment group and the placebo group in different phases of the trial. Crossover approaches may be more difficult to use in cognitive enhancer trials in patients with progressive degenerative disorders because the decline in cognition creates a different baseline for the active treatment and placebo periods. They have been used in schizophrenia[60] and in ADHD.[61]

Futility criteria may allow a trial to be interrupted in a timely manner if the analysis suggests that a treatment effect is missing and continuation of the trial is unwarranted.[41] The criterion used to terminate a study for futility must be cautiously prespecified to ensure that a potentially efficacious agent is not incorrectly identified as inactive. For example, in a recent AD trial terminated for futility, the termination rule was prespecified to assess the probability of rejecting the null hypothesis of a treatment difference versus placebo using a threshold of 10%.[62]

When the chances of a placebo response are high, the sequential parallel comparison design (SPCD) may be useful. In this approach, patients are assigned to a standard active treatment versus placebo period (Stage 1); then the placebo non-responders are re-randomized to drug or placebo, and a second trial period (Stage 2) is implemented after excluding those who responded to placebo in Stage 1.[63] The analysis from Stage 2 may provide useful insight into the activity of the agent. This design is most appropriate for a Phase II proof-of-concept trial to gain confidence in the test agent. The SPCD has been used most often with psychotropic agents.

NEXT STEPS

The need for cognitive enhancers is enormous (see Figure 1.1), and only a few have been developed. Some cognitive enhancers may be related to a specific disease mechanism and applicable to a particular disease; others may be applicable across a range of disorders. The general format for trials of cognitive enhancers has been worked out in a way that is acceptable to regulatory authorities, but much is left to be done in terms of refinement of population definitions, outcome measures, use of bio-markers, trial design, regulatory advances, and payer endorsement. Lessons learned from one disorder may be generalizable to others. Few things could be more exciting than expanding the intellectual function of individuals, restoring their insight into the world in which they live and allowing them to record their own history in the form of personal memory. The quest to develop effective cognitive enhancers is based on this need to help patients engage the world with optimized cognitive resources.

DISCLOSURES

Dr. Cummings has provided consultation to Abbott, Acadia, Adamas, Anavex, Astellas, Avanir, Bayer, BMS, Eisai, EnVivo, Forest, Genentech, GSK, Lundbeck, Neuronetrix, Novartis, Otsuka, Pfizer, Prana, QR, Sanofi-Aventis, Signum, Takeda, and Toyama pharmaceutical companies. Dr. Cummings has provided consultation to MedAvante, Neurotrax, Avid, ExonHit, GE Healthcare, and UBC assessment companies. Dr. Cummings owns the copyright of the Neuropsychiatric Inventory. Dr. Cummings has stock options in Prana, Neurokos, ADAMAS, MedAvante, and QR pharma. Dr. Cummings discusses the use of drugs in development and not approved by the US Food and Drug Administration.

REFERENCES

1. Rosen WG, Mohs RC, Davis KL. A new rating scale for Alzheimer's disease. *Am J Psychiatry* 1984;141(11):1356–1364.
2. Buchanan RW, Keefe RS, Umbricht D, et al. The FDA–NIMH–MATRICS guidelines for clinical trial design of cognitive-enhancing drugs: What do we know 5 years later? *Schizophr Bull* 2011;37(6):1209–1217.
3. Weintraub S, Dikmen SS, Heaton RK, et al. The cognition battery of the NIH toolbox for assessment of neurological and behavioral function: Validation in an adult sample. *J Int Neuropsychol Soc* 2014;20(6):567–578.
4. Weintraub S, Dikmen SS, Heaton RK, et al. Cognition assessment using the NIH toolbox. *Neurology* 2013;80(11 Suppl 3):S54–S64.
5. Kramer JH, Mungas D, Possin KL, et al. NIH EXAMINER: Conceptualization and development of an executive function battery. *J Int Neuropsychol Soc* 2014;20(1):11–19.
6. American Psychiatric Association. *Diagnostic and statistical manual of mental disorders.* 5 ed. Arlington, VA: American Psychiatric Publishing; 2013.
7. Reisberg B. Global measures: Utility in defining and measuring treatment response in dementia. *Int Psychogeriatr* 2007;19(3):421–456.
8. Harrison JK, McArthur KS, Quinn TJ. Assessment scales in stroke: Clinimetric and clinical considerations. *Clin Interv Aging* 2013;8:201–211.

9. Basch E. Beyond the FDA PRO guidance: Steps toward integrating meaningful patient-reported outcomes into regulatory trials and US drug labels. *Value Health* 2012;15(3):401–403.

10. Doody RS, Ferris SH, Salloway S, et al. Donepezil treatment of patients with MCI: A 48-week randomized, placebo-controlled trial. *Neurology* 2009;72(18):1555–1561.

11. Nagy B, Brennan A, Brandtmuller A, et al. Assessing the cost-effectiveness of the rivastigmine transdermal patch for Alzheimer's disease in the UK using MMSE- and ADL-based models. *Int J Geriatr Psychiatry* 2011;26(5):483–494.

12. Jobert M, Wilson FJ, Ruigt GS, et al. Guidelines for the recording and evaluation of pharmaco-EEG data in man: The International Pharmaco-EEG Society (IPEG). *Neuropsychobiology* 2012;66(4):201–220.

13. Van Laere KJ, Sanabria-Bohorquez SM, Mozley DP, et al. (11)C-MK-8278 PET as a tool for pharmacodynamic brain occupancy of histamine 3 receptor inverse agonists. *J Nucl Med* 2014;55(1):65–72.

14. Potkin SG, Anand R, Fleming K, et al. Brain metabolic and clinical effects of rivastigmine in Alzheimer's disease. *Int J Neuropsychopharmacol* 2001;4(3):223–230.

15. Cummings J, Zhong K. Biomarker-driven therapeutic management of Alzheimer's disease: Establishing the foundations. *Clin Pharmacol Ther* 2014;95(1):67–77.

16. Marta M, Giovannoni G. Disease modifying drugs in multiple sclerosis: Mechanisms of action and new drugs in the horizon. *CNS Neurol Disord Drug Targets* 2012;11(5):610–623.

17. De SN, Airas L, Grigoriadis N, et al. Clinical relevance of brain volume measures in multiple sclerosis. *CNS Drugs* 2014;28(2):147–156.

18. Emre M, Aarsland D, Albanese A, et al. Rivastigmine for dementia associated with Parkinson's disease. *N Engl J Med* 2004;351(24):2509–2518.

19. Emre M, Cummings JL, Lane RM. Rivastigmine in dementia associated with Parkinson's disease and Alzheimer's disease: Similarities and differences. *J Alzheimers Dis* 2007;11(4):509–519.

20. Deardorff WJ, Shobassy A, Grossberg GT. Safety and clinical effects of EVP-6124 in subjects with Alzheimer's disease currently or previously receiving an acetylcholinesterase inhibitor medication. *Expert Rev Neurother* 2015;15(1):7–17.

21. Das D, Phillips C, Hsieh W, et al. Neurotransmitter-based strategies for the treatment of cognitive dysfunction in Down syndrome. *Prog Neuropsychopharmacol Biol Psychiatry* 2014;54:140–148.

22. Cummings JL, Froelich L, Black SE, et al. Randomized, double-blind, parallel-group, 48-week study for efficacy and safety of a higher-dose rivastigmine patch (15 vs. 10 cm(2)) in Alzheimer's disease. *Dement Geriatr Cogn Disord* 2012;33(5):341–353.

23. Farlow MR, Salloway S, Tariot PN, et al. Effectiveness and tolerability of high-dose (23 mg/d) versus standard-dose (10 mg/d) donepezil in moderate to severe Alzheimer's disease: A 24-week, randomized, double-blind study. *Clin Ther* 2010;32(7):1234–1251.

24. Jelic V, Kivipelto M, Winblad B. Clinical trials in mild cognitive impairment: Lessons for the future. *J Neurol Neurosurg Psychiatry* 2006;77(4):429–438.

25. Raschetti R, Albanese E, Vanacore N, et al. Cholinesterase inhibitors in mild cognitive impairment: A systematic review of randomised trials. *PLoS Med* 2007;4(11):e338.

26. Francis PT, Palmer AM, Snape M, et al. The cholinergic hypothesis of Alzheimer's disease: A review of progress. *J Neurol Neurosurg Psychiatry* 1999;66(2):137–147.

27. Jiang S, Li Y, Zhang C, et al. M1 muscarinic acetylcholine receptor in Alzheimer's disease. *Neurosci Bull* 2014;30(2):295–307.

28. Mufson EJ, Counts SE, Perez SE, et al. Cholinergic system during the progression of Alzheimer's disease: Therapeutic implications. *Expert Rev Neurother* 2008;8(11):1703–1718.

29. Schliebs R, Arendt T. The significance of the cholinergic system in the brain during aging and in Alzheimer's disease. *J Neural Transm* 2006;113(11):1625–1644.

30. Sirvio J. Strategies that support declining cholinergic neurotransmission in Alzheimer's disease patients. *Gerontology* 1999;45(Suppl 1):3–14.

31. Umbricht D, Keefe RS, Murray S, et al. A randomized, placebo-controlled study investigating the nicotinic alpha7 agonist, RG3487, for cognitive deficits in schizophrenia. *Neuropsychopharmacology* 2014;39(7):1568–1577.

32. Hashimoto T, Hatayama Y, Nakamichi K, et al. Procognitive effect of AC-3933 in aged mice, and synergistic effect of combination with donepezil in scopolamine-treated mice. *Eur J Pharmacol* 2014;745:123–128.

33. Melancon BJ, Tarr JC, Panarese JD, et al. Allosteric modulation of the M1 muscarinic acetylcholine receptor: Improving cognition and a potential treatment for schizophrenia and Alzheimer's disease. *Drug Discov Today* 2013;18(23–24):1185–1199.

34. Tzavara ET, Wade MR, Davis RJ, et al. Role of metabotropic glutamate receptor 5 in the procholinergic effects of neuropsychotherapeutic compounds. *Synapse* 2008;62(12):940–943.

35. Tiraboschi P, Hansen LA, Alford M, et al. Cholinergic dysfunction in diseases with Lewy bodies. *Neurology* 2000;54(2):407–411.

36. Tiraboschi P, Hansen LA, Alford M, et al. Early and widespread cholinergic losses differentiate dementia with Lewy bodies from Alzheimer disease. *Arch Gen Psychiatry* 2002;59(10):946–951.

37. Black MD, Stevens RJ, Rogacki N, et al. AVE1625, a cannabinoid CB1 receptor antagonist, as a co-treatment with antipsychotics for schizophrenia: Improvement in cognitive function and reduction of antipsychotic side effects in rodents. *Psychopharmacology (Berl)* 2011;215(1):149–163.

38. Busquets-Garcia A, Gomis-Gonzalez M, Guegan T, et al. Targeting the endocannabinoid system in the treatment of fragile X syndrome. *Nat Med* 2013;19(5):603–607.

39. Francis PT. Glutamatergic approaches to the treatment of cognitive and behavioural symptoms of Alzheimer's disease. *Neurodegener Dis* 2008;5(3–4):241–243.

40. Grove RA, Harrington CM, Mahler A, et al. A randomized, double-blind, placebo-controlled, 16-week study of the H3 receptor antagonist, GSK239512 as a monotherapy in subjects with mild-to-moderate Alzheimer's disease. *Curr Alzheimer Res* 2014;11(1):47–58.

41. Haig GM, Pritchett Y, Meier A, et al. A randomized study of H3 antagonist ABT-288 in mild-to-moderate Alzheimer's dementia. *J Alzheimers Dis* 2014;42(3):959–971.

42. Heckman PR, Wouters C, Prickaerts J. Phosphodiesterase inhibitors as a target for cognition enhancement in aging and Alzheimer's disease: A translational overview. *Curr Pharm Des* 2014;21(3):317–331.

43. Meltzer HY, Rajagopal L, Huang M, et al. Translating the *N*-methyl-D-aspartate receptor antagonist model of schizophrenia to treatments for cognitive impairment in schizophrenia. *Int J Neuropsychopharmacol* 2013;16(10):2181–2194.

44. Partin KM. AMPA receptor potentiators: From drug design to cognitive enhancement. *Curr Opin Pharmacol* 2014;20C:46–53.

45. Smith SM, Uslaner JM, Cox CD, et al. The novel phosphodiesterase 10A inhibitor THPP-1 has antipsychotic-like effects in rat and improves cognition in rat and rhesus monkey. *Neuropharmacology* 2013;64:215–223.

46. Upton N, Chuang TT, Hunter AJ, et al. 5-HT6 receptor antagonists as novel cognitive enhancing agents for Alzheimer's disease. *Neurotherapeutics* 2008;5(3):458–469.

47. Wilkinson D, Windfeld K, Colding-Jorgensen E. Safety and efficacy of idalopirdine, a 5-HT6 receptor antagonist, in patients with moderate Alzheimer's disease (LADDER): A randomised, double-blind, placebo-controlled phase 2 trial. *Lancet Neurol* 2014;13(11):1092–1099.

48. Bentwich J, Dobronevsky E, Aichenbaum S, et al. Beneficial effect of repetitive transcranial magnetic stimulation combined with cognitive training for the treatment of Alzheimer's disease: A proof of concept study. *J Neural Transm* 2011;118(3):463–471.

49. Freiherr J, Hallschmid M, Frey WH, et al. Intranasal insulin as a treatment for Alzheimer's disease: A review of basic research and clinical evidence. *CNS Drugs* 2013;27(7):505–514.

50. Gonzalez-Lima F, Barksdale BR, Rojas JC. Mitochondrial respiration as a target for neuroprotection and cognitive enhancement. *Biochem Pharmacol* 2014;88(4):584–593.

51. Hescham S, Lim LW, Jahanshahi A, et al. Deep brain stimulation in dementia-related disorders. *Neurosci Biobehav Rev* 2013;37(10 Pt 2):2666–2675.

52. Hongpaisan J, Sun MK, Alkon DL. PKC epsilon activation prevents synaptic loss, Abeta elevation, and cognitive deficits in Alzheimer's disease transgenic mice. *J Neurosci* 2011;31(2):630–643.

53. Nardone R, Tezzon F, Holler Y, et al. Transcranial magnetic stimulation (TMS)/repetitive TMS in mild cognitive impairment and Alzheimer's disease. *Acta Neurol Scand* 2014;129(6):351–366.
54. Olde Rikkert MG, Verhey FR, Blesa R, et al. Tolerability and safety of Souvenaid in patients with mild Alzheimer's disease: Results of multi-center, 24-week, open-label extension study. *J Alzheimers Dis* 2015;44(2):471–480.
55. Scheltens P, Twisk JW, Blesa R, et al. Efficacy of Souvenaid in mild Alzheimer's disease: Results from a randomized, controlled trial. *J Alzheimers Dis* 2012;31(1):225–236.
56. Shevtsova EF, Vinogradova DV, Kireeva EG, et al. Dimebon attenuates the Abeta-induced mitochondrial permeabilization. *Curr Alzheimer Res* 2014;11(5):422–429.
57. Xiang GQ, Tang SS, Jiang LY, et al. PPARgamma agonist pioglitazone improves scopolamine-induced memory impairment in mice. *J Pharm Pharmacol* 2012;64(4):589–596.
58. Yarchoan M, Arnold SE. Repurposing diabetes drugs for brain insulin resistance in Alzheimer disease. *Diabetes* 2014;63(7):2253–2261.
59. Winblad B, Cummings J, Andreasen N, et al. A six-month double-blind, randomized, placebo-controlled study of a transdermal patch in Alzheimer's disease—Rivastigmine patch versus capsule. *Int J Geriatr Psychiatry* 2007;22(5):456–467.
60. Roh S, Hoeppner SS, Schoenfeld D, et al. Acute effects of mecamylamine and varenicline on cognitive performance in non-smokers with and without schizophrenia. *Psychopharmacology (Berl)* 2014;231(4):765–775.
61. Adler LA, Alperin S, Leon T, et al. Clinical effects of lisdexamfetamine and mixed amphetamine salts immediate release in adult ADHD: Results of a crossover design clinical trial. *Postgrad Med* 2014;126(5):17–24.
62. Galasko D, Bell J, Mancuso JY, et al. Clinical trial of an inhibitor of RAGE-Abeta interactions in Alzheimer disease. *Neurology* 2014;82(17):1536–1542.
63. Doros G, Pencina M, Rybin D, et al. A repeated measures model for analysis of continuous outcomes in sequential parallel comparison design studies. *Stat Med* 2013;32(16):2767–2789.

TWO

The Neuroscience of Cognition and Cognitive Enhancing Compounds

AMY F. T. ARNSTEN, MIN J. WANG,

AND CONSTANTINOS D. PASPALAS

HIGHER COGNITIVE ABILITIES IN HUMANS DEPEND ON THE INTEGRITY of the newly evolved association cortices. Thus, the development of effective cognitive enhancers requires strategies that optimize the functioning of these higher cortical circuits. This chapter briefly reviews the neuroscience of the primate association cortex, with particular focus on the prefrontal cortex (PFC). The review describes the unique molecular regulation of PFC circuits needed for optimal cognitive function and the challenges posed in developing effective therapeutics for higher cognitive disorders in humans.

ASSOCIATION CORTEX CIRCUITS MEDIATING COGNITIVE FUNCTION

Higher cognitive abilities arise from an intricate web of network connections among the association cortices (schematically illustrated in Figure 2.1). Incoming sensory information is processed by parallel but interconnecting circuits, whereby spatial position and the movement of sensory stimuli are processed separately from sensory

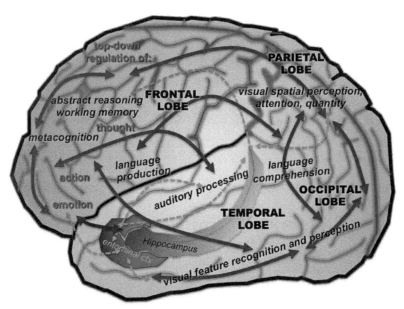

FIGURE 2.1 *Functions of the primate association cortices. A highly schematized summary of the functions of the association cortices in human brain (see text for details). Projections into the hippocampal formation are shown by dashed lines.*

features. This parallel processing is maintained into the PFC, where there are separate domains for the representation of spatial versus feature information. This section provides a brief review of the contributions of the parietal (PAC), temporal (TAC), and PFC association cortices to cognitive functioning. Although described separately, the PFC, PAC, and TAC areas are intricately interconnected, creating both feedforward and feedback loops that work together to provide a unified cognitive experience. These higher cortical circuits additionally project via the entorhinal cortex into the hippocampal formation for long-term memory consolidation (Figure 2.1, dashed lines) and in parallel loops through the basal ganglia and cerebellum for automated cognitive habits (see Figure 2.2).

Posterior Parietal Cortex

The anterior PAC analyzes somatosensory information, whereas the posterior PAC is specialized for the analysis of visual movement and visual–spatial relationships, for analyzing quantity and constructing spatial maps, and for orienting attention in time and space.[1,2] Some researchers have proposed that the PAC is responsible for binding features with spatial position to allow perception itself. The PAC is important for "paying attention"—that is, allocating attentional resources in time and space.[3] Much of the research on the neural bases of attention has been motivated by the phenomenon of contralateral neglect—the loss of perception for the left side of visual

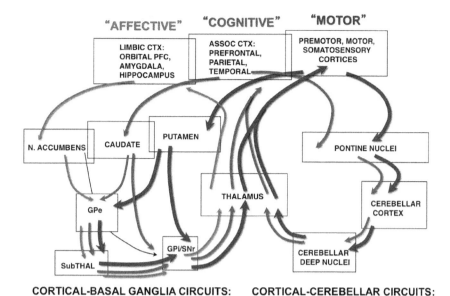

FIGURE 2.2 *Parallel basal ganglia and cerebellar cortical circuits. The basal ganglia and cerebellar circuits provide parallel loops for the planning and/or execution of movement (thick arrows), cognition (medium arrows), and emotion (thin arrows, basal ganglia only). The association cortices especially contribute to the cognitive and affective loops. Basal ganglia structures are densely innervated by dopamine, cerebellar structures are innervated by norepinephrine, and cortical structures are innervated by both catecholamines. ASSOC., association; CTX, cortex; GPe, globus pallidus external segment; GPi, globus pallidus internal segment; N. ACCUMBENS, nucleus accumbens; PFC, prefrontal cortex; SNr, substantia nigra pars reticulata; SubTHAL, subthalamic nucleus.* SOURCE: BASED ON THE WORK OF PETER STRICK.

space in patients with right-sided PAC brain lesions (with large lesions, neglect can extend to extravisual modalities as well).[4] The PAC also controls the covert movement of attention—that is, the orienting of attention without overt movement (e.g., as tested using the Posner paradigm, in which attention is captured by a valid vs. invalid cue).[5] Interestingly, imaging research in humans has shown that *left* PAC is activated when attention is oriented to an interval in *time* rather than space, whereas PAC activates bilaterally when one attends to both time and space.[1]

Physiological recordings from monkeys have provided the cellular basis for the imaging and lesion data from humans. For example, recordings from area MT have found columns of neurons that respond to visual stimuli moving in a specific direction in three dimensions,[6] and lesions to this area produce deficits in perceiving visual movement.[7] Farther forward in the parietal cortex, recordings show neurons responding based on attentional state. For example, the link between PAC and visuospatial attention has been confirmed by recordings in monkeys performing the Posner task,[8] in which neurons in area 7a increased their firing dependent on whether the animal attended to the region of space where the stimulus occurred. Neurons in area 7A have also been shown to create world-referenced maps of visual space,[9] and they project this information to the dorsolateral PFC, which uses this information to effectively guide behavior,[10,11] and to the parahippocampal cortex for memory consolidation via the entorhinal–hippocampal system.[10] The parietal association cortex also integrates visual and somatosensory maps of the body and uses body-referenced maps to guide movement.[9] Recently, neurons have been found in the monkey PAC that represent numbers (quantity),[12] similar to what is seen in imaging studies of humans.[13] Thus, there is a good correspondence between data from monkey research and data from human research.

Temporal Association Cortex

The temporal lobe is the site of parallel processing of olfactory, auditory, and visual feature information. Olfactory information is relayed from the olfactory bulbs to the olfactory cortices on the anterior medial aspects of the temporal cortex, which then project onto the insular and orbital cortices.[14] In contrast, the superior TAC mediates auditory processing, with separate "belts" for processing of feature versus spatial aspects, whereas the ventral (inferior) TAC mediates visual feature analysis.[15] Because rhesus monkeys often perform poorly on auditory tasks, less is known about this modality. In contrast, a great deal is known about the roles of the inferior TAC in visual feature processing. Electrophysiological studies in monkeys and imaging studies in humans indicate that attention usually has little effect on processing very early in the processing streams, but it plays an increasing role as one moves higher up these cortical pathways.[16,17] Attentional relevance increases processing in area V4 (e.g., based on color); farther forward, there are areas specialized for the processing of faces, and more laterally, there are areas specialized for more generalized visual feature processing.

Farther forward in the visual feature processing stream, there are subregions of the inferior TAC where neurons selectively respond to faces,[18] whereas most of this region performs more general processing of visual features, where a column of neurons all respond to a similar feature, likely related to fundamental shapes called "geons."[19] Highly processed sensory information feeds into medial temporal cortex memory, as described later. The activity of inferior TAC neurons is reduced by repeated experience with the same visual stimulus, a phenomenon known as repetition suppression that is a clue to familiarity.[16] Processing of visual stimuli is also diminished by competition from nearby stimuli in the same visual field.[20] Both of these suppressive effects result from intrinsic properties of inferior temporal cortex (ITC) neurons. (In contrast, processing can be inhibited more thoughtfully by extrinsic projections from the PFC that serve to gate irrelevant stimuli, as discussed later.) "Top-down" inputs from the PFC and PAC can also enhance stimulus processing in the ITC. For example, directing attention to a region of space reduces the suppressive interactions between multiple stimuli, particularly for low-contrast stimuli. Responses can also be enhanced due to learned relevance; for example, attending to a color (red vs. green) that signals reward increases firing of V4 cells, whereas the irrelevant color reduces firing.[21] Inferior TAC neurons can also hold information "on line" over a short delay if there are no distracters.[22] However, the PFC is needed to maintain information under conditions of interference.

Farthest forward is the temporal pole, an area that expands in primate evolution[23] and whose complex functions remain somewhat of a mystery.[24] The temporal pole is tightly interconnected with the PFC and with limbic structures such as the amygdala, in addition to receiving parallel streams of olfactory/gustatory (medial), auditory (dorsal), and visual (ventral) information. Data from both humans and nonhuman primates indicate that the temporal pole has a role in social and emotional processing and may bind complex, highly processed, but still parallel, perceptual inputs to visceral emotional responses in a channel-specific manner.[24] Lesions to the temporal pole produce the symptoms of Kluver–Bucy syndrome—for example, abnormal social behavior, eating inappropriate objects, lack of empathy and impaired understanding of others, and mood changes that can resemble bipolar disorder. Lesions to this area in humans can produce preserved perception but impaired recognition, in which the right hemisphere is specialized for objects and faces and the left hemisphere for names.[25,26] Olson et al.[24] describe the possibility that the memory functions of the temporal pole allow storage of perception–emotion linkages that form the basis of personal semantic memory. Some of these functions likely involve interactions with the PFC.

Prefrontal Cortex

The PFC generates mental representations (i.e., working memory) to maintain information in the absence of sensory stimulation, the foundation of abstract thought. This fundamental property underlies the PFC's involvement in higher reasoning; decision-making; insight; and a variety of so-called executive functions, including regulation of attention, planning, and organizing for the future.[27–30] The PFC provides top-down guidance of thought/attention, action, and emotion. It does so in a topographically organized manner (see Figure 2.1), whereby the lateral surface represents the external world, and the medial or ventral areas represent the internal, visceral world and emotion.[31,32] The PFC also appears to be organized in a caudal to rostral manner, where more rostral areas of the PFC process increasingly more abstract information;[33] for example, the most rostral areas are involved in metacognition—insight about oneself and "thinking about thinking."[34,35] The rostral and dorsomedial aspects of the PFC also play important roles in social cognition, including so-called theory of mind, the ability to think about what another person must be thinking.[36,37] Finally, the PFC in humans also appears to be lateralized, where the left hemisphere specializes in generative processes,[38] and the right hemisphere is specialized for inhibiting inappropriate actions, thoughts, and emotions.[39]

The topographic organization of the PFC is reflected in its connections, whereby the lateral areas have reciprocal projections with visual, auditory, and somatosensory association cortices, whereas the ventral and medial PFC regions interconnect with olfactory–taste circuitry, insular cortex, and limbic brain areas.[31,32] Through all these connections, the PFC is positioned to provide top-down regulation, promoting or arresting inappropriate thoughts, actions, and emotions. This topography extends to basal ganglia circuits, whereby the dorsolateral PFC projects to the dorsal striatum (caudate), and the ventromedial PFC projects to the ventral striatum. This topographic organization also can be observed at the cellular level in recordings from cognitively engaged monkeys. For example, there are neurons in the dorsolateral PFC that generate persistent representations of visual space,[40] whereas neurons in dorsomedial PFC generate persistent representations of punishment.[41] The microcircuitry underlying persistent representations of visual space in the dorsolateral PFC is described in more detail later.

Circuits Mediating Language

In humans, the association cortices also mediate language. The neurobiology of language has been challenging to study because it requires human subjects, and much of the key research has arisen from neurosurgical investigations. The classic view is that language is produced in the inferior PFC of the dominant hemisphere (usually the left)—that is, Broca's area—whereas the comprehension of language (semantics) is performed in Wernicke's area, which sits posterior to the left (dominant) auditory cortices. (In contrast, the right (nondominant) hemisphere mediates emotion in language, with the frontal area producing and the posterior area comprehending emotional expression, also called prosody.) However, recent research indicates that the neurobiology of language is far more complex than this simple scheme, with production and comprehension more widely distributed. Some current theories propose a bilateral, ventral stream emanating from the auditory cortex into the middle and anterior temporal cortices that is involved in speech recognition and the representation of lexical concepts and also more dorsal pathways focused in the dominant hemisphere (including Broca's and Wernicke's areas) that integrate sensorimotor aspects of language by mapping phonological information onto motor representations needed for articulation.[42]

Subcortical Pathways

As illustrated in Figure 2.2, the PFC, PAC, and TAC all project to the dorsal striatum (e.g., caudate nucleus) as part of the "cognitive circuit" through the basal ganglia, which in turn projects via the thalamus back to the PFC.[43] These circuits are thought to mediate cognitive habits such as reading. In contrast, the "motor" circuit involves cortical projections to the region of the putamen, which in turn projects back onto the premotor cortices (see Figure 2.2). This pathway is important for the planning, selection, initiation, and execution of movements. The "affective" circuit mediates emotional habits and involves ventral and medial aspects of PFC and the amygdala projections to the ventral striatum (see Figure 2.2). The PFC and PAC also project via the pons to the cerebellar cortex, which ultimately projects back to the primary motor cortex.[43,44] This pathway may serve as a "biological gyroscope," providing online correction of movements and possibly providing the same refinement for cognitive operations.

The association cortices also interconnect with the hippocampal formation for the long-term consolidation and recall of memories (schematically illustrated in Figure 2.1). Thus, damage to this area causes amnesia, as in the famous case of H.M.[45] In humans, lesions limited to the hippocampus impair memory without altering spatial abilities,[46] and recordings from the human hippocampus identify neuronal firing patterns that correlate with performance of a test of episodic memory.[47] The entorhinal cortex (ERC) is the gateway in and out of the hippocampus. Circuits processing visual space (dorsolateral PFC and PAC) project in and out of the ERC–hippocampus via the parahippocampal cortex/caudomedial lobule,[10] whereas the ventromedial PFC and TAC project in and out of the ERC directly or via the perirhinal cortex, respectively.[48] Damage to the parahippocampal cortex markedly impairs spatial memory,[49] whereas the perirhinal cortex is important for visual feature memory, as observed in both physiological[50,51] and lesion[52] studies. In rodents, lesions to entorhinal and hippocampus impair recollection of both feature and space.[53] However, the hippocampus is also a center of spatial cognition in rodents, whereas humans do not need the hippocampus for spatial processing—just for memory.[54]

THE MICROCIRCUITRY IN DORSOLATERAL PREFRONTAL CORTEX SUBSERVING MENTAL REPRESENTATION

The dorsolateral aspects of the PFC (dlPFC) in primates subserve working memory, where even small lesions produce permanent deficits in a domain-specific manner.[55] Examination of the neural circuitry within the dlPFC has found that deep layer III pyramidal cells are key for the mental representations that subserve higher cognitive processing[56] (Figure 2.3). Importantly, these are the neurons that expand most in brain evolution.[57,58] Rodents not only have a small PFC but also have a very sparse layer III.[32,58] The expansion in the number of basal dendrites and spines on layer III pyramidal cells permits the immense increase in network connections needed for higher cognition.[57,59,60] These connections are made onto long, thin spines, with a mature morphology (e.g., a well-developed synapse and spine apparatus,[61,62] which contrasts with the thin, "learning spines" in hippocampus that do not have these features until they enlarge into mushroom spines[63]). The long, thin geometry of many dlPFC layer III spines may optimize the ability to rapidly gate connections, as described later.[61]

Goldman-Rakic and colleagues revealed the physiology and microcircuitry in the primate dlPFC that underlie visual–spatial working memory and likely apply to other processing domains.[64] They recorded monkeys performing an oculomotor version of the spatial working memory task (Figure 2.3A) and discovered neurons in the dlPFC that are able to generate neural representations of visual space in the absence of sensory stimulation—for example, maintaining firing to the memory of a visual cue at 270 degrees (the preferred direction of the neuron) but not to other spatial locations (nonpreferred directions)[40] (Figure 2.3B). These neurons are termed delay cells because they are able to maintain persistent, spatially tuned firing across the delay epoch in a spatial working memory task. Delay cell persistent firing is generated by the recurrent excitation of pyramidal cells with similar spatial tuning.[64] These microcircuits are localized in deep layer III, and possibly superficial layer V, of the primate dlPFC (Figure 2.3D). Delay cells excite each other through NMDA receptor (NMDAR) glutamatergic synapses on dendritic spines.[65] Both NMDAR with the NR2A subunit and NMDAR with the NR2B subunit are needed for persistent firing, with only minor reliance on AMPAR stimulation.[65] These findings contrast with classic synapses, such as in the hippocampus or primary visual cortex (V1), in which NMDAR–NR2B are extra-synaptic in the adult, and AMPAR stimulation is essential for permitting NMDAR actions.[66] The spatial tuning of dlPFC delay cells is refined through lateral inhibition from parvalbumin-containing (i.e., fast-spiking) GABA interneurons.[64] This also differs from more classic circuits, in which there is feedforward rather than lateral inhibition.[67]

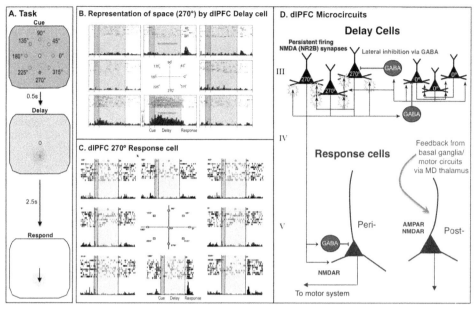

FIGURE 2.3 *The microcircuits in the dlPFC underlying spatial working memory. (A) Schematic illustration of the oculomotor delayed-response (ODR) version of a spatial working memory task, in which a cue briefly (0.5 s) appears at one of eight locations (e.g., 270 degrees) while the monkey fixates on a central spot. The location must be remembered over a delay period of several seconds until the fixation spot disappears and the monkey can move its eyes to the remembered location for juice reward. The cued location constantly changes over hundreds of trials, requiring the constant updating of working memory. (B) An example of the firing patterns of a dlPFC delay cell representing the 270 degrees location, the neuron's preferred direction. This delay cell maintains firing across the delay epoch if the cue had appeared at 270 degrees but not other locations. (C) An example of the firing patterns of a dlPFC response cell that is providing feedback during the eye movement to 270 degrees. (D) The microcircuitry in the primate dlPFC thought to underlie working memory. Microcircuits underlying delay cell firing are thought to reside in deep layer III, the layer that expands most in primate evolution. Clusters of pyramidal cells with similar preferred directions excite each other to maintain persistent firing across the delay period in the absence of sensory stimulation. This requires glutamate stimulation of NMDAR with NR2B subunits, which are localized exclusively within the PSD. The spatial specificity is refined by lateral inhibition from GABAergic interneurons. In contrast, response cells are thought to reside in layer V. There are response cells that fire leading up to the motor response (peri-saccadic) and response cells that are thought to carry the corollary discharge feedback that a response has occurred (post-saccadic). The post-saccadic response cells are influenced by both NMDAR and AMPAR stimulation. Delay cells likely inhibit response cells during the delay epoch via an inhibitory interneuron.*

The dlPFC also contains neurons that fire in relationship to the saccadic response—that is, so-called response cells (Figure 2.3C). These include neurons that fire immediately prior to the saccade and are likely carrying commands to the motor system, as well as neurons that fire during or after the movement and are likely conveying feedback that the response has occurred (corollary discharge and efference copy).[68] These latter cells may be especially relevant to the symptoms of hallucinations and delusions in schizophrenia, which have been associated with altered corollary discharge.[69] Response cells are likely concentrated in layer V of the dlPFC[65] and appear to be the most common type of neuron in rodent PFC[70] (see Figure 2.3D). Both types of response cells depend on NMDAR stimulation in primate dlPFC, but feedback response cells are also sensitive to AMPAR blockade, perhaps because they are part of a proprioceptive sensory circuit.[65]

INSULTS TO THE ASSOCIATION CORTICES IN COGNITIVE DISORDERS

Higher cognitive disorders in humans particularly afflict the association cortices, especially targeting the most highly evolved pyramidal cell circuits with the most extensive network connections. The PFC is a focus of pathology in neuropsychiatric disorders, in which dysfunction of the lateral PFC results in cognitive disorders such as schizophrenia,[71] whereas dysfunction of the ventral and/or medial PFC is associated with mood disorders such as depression[72,73] or obsessive–compulsive disorder.[74] Disorders of impulse control have impaired function of the right hemisphere in particular: The right, inferior lateral PFC develops abnormally in attention deficit hyperactivity disorder (ADHD),[75,76] and this same area is underactive during the manic phase of bipolar disorder.[77] Dysfunction of the PFC has also been related to the deficits in social cognition that typify autism spectrum disorders, including theory of mind,[78] although genetic insults in this spectrum of disorders produce more fundamental changes in cortical development.[79]

Postmortem studies of patients with schizophrenia have found profound insults in the layer III dlPFC microcircuits that generate mental representations. These studies have found reduced neuropil,[80,81] as well as loss of dendrites and spines from deep layer III pyramidal cells.[82] Layer V pyramidal cells appear to be impacted as well.[83] GABAergic parvalbumin interneurons are also weakened, but these changes are now thought to be compensatory rather than a primary insult.[84] Although previous findings have suggested that pyramidal cells might be disinhibited in schizophrenia producing a hyperglutamatergic state, recent transcriptome analyses from actual layer III and layer V pyramidal cells in the dlPFC of patients with schizophrenia show that layer III and layer V dlPFC pyramidal cells are profoundly underactive, as indicated by a marked loss of mitochondrial markers.[71] These new data emphasize that the goal of treatment should not be to reduce PFC glutamate release but, rather, to try to boost the information-processing abilities of NMDAR circuits.

The pattern of neurofibrillary degeneration in Alzheimer's disease (AD) is consistent with the known connections of the association cortices. Neurofibrillary tangles (NFTs) specifically afflict pyramidal cells in the association cortex and stellate cells in entorhinal cortex, but they do not afflict those in the primary sensory cortices.[85,86] Indeed, the neurons most affected are those with the most excitatory, cortical–cortical connections.[87] The cognitive deficits of AD correlate with the number of NFTs and degenerating cells but not with plaques.[88] The sequence of cognitive symptoms generally fits with the progression of NFT pathology,[89,90] in which degeneration begins in the entorhinal cortex, creating recent memory deficits as the hippocampus is disconnected from the association cortex.[91] Degeneration then spreads to the association cortices, leading to the global cognitive deficits of dementia, including impaired spatial abilities and wandering (degeneration of the PAC); loss of recognition of loved ones (degeneration of the TAC); and impaired abstract reasoning, loss of insight, and inappropriate behaviors (degeneration in PFC). Evidence from animal models indicates that phosphorylated tau can spread within excitatory cortical circuits,[62,92,93] and in the dlPFC it may relate to age-related dysregulation of calcium–cAMP signaling in highly evolved cortical circuits.[62]

THE UNIQUE MODULATION OF DLPFC CIRCUITS GENERATING MENTAL REPRESENTATIONS

A major goal of cognitive optimization should be to strengthen and protect the layer III dlPFC microcircuits that generate the mental representations that are the foundation of higher cognition. Data from nonhuman primates indicate that these circuits are modulated very differently than sensory cortex and subcortical structures and that these differences must be respected if we are to develop effective cognitive treatments.[61] Research is uncovering a variety of molecular mechanisms in layer III pyramidal cells that can rapidly and reversibly alter the strength of synaptic connections—a process termed dynamic network connectivity (DNC).[61] DNC mechanisms promote mental flexibility and coordinate arousal state with cognitive state—for example, allowing conscious cognitive experience when we are awake but not in deep sleep and switching control of behavior to more primitive brain circuits when we are stressed and feel out of control.

One important example of unique modulatory control is the effect of cholinergic stimulation of α_7 nicotinic receptors (α_7-nAChRs) on layer III dlPFC delay cell firing (Figure 2.4). As described previously, AMPAR blockade has very subtle effects on delay cell firing, in contrast to their prominent role in sensory and hippocampal circuits.[65] These data suggest that additional mechanisms must provide the permissive, membrane depolarization needed to relieve the magnesium block of NMDAR and allow them to conduct sodium and calcium in response to glutamate stimulation. As schematically illustrated in Figure 2.5B, ultrastructural analyses showed that

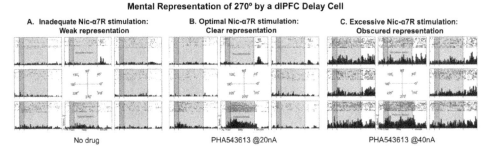

FIGURE 2.4 *Low, but not high, doses of a α_7-nAChR agonist enhance the neural representation of visual space by dlPFC delay cells. (A) A dlPFC delay cell has weak delay-related firing under control conditions, with subtle representation of 270 degrees. In other words, the neuron shows weak delay-related firing following cues at 270 degrees but not other directions. (B) Iontophoresis of a low dose of the α_7-nAChR agonist PHA543613 (20 nA) enhanced the representation of 270 degrees by increasing persistent firing across the delay period only on trials in which the monkey was remembering 270 degrees. (C) A higher dose of PHA543613 (40 nA) increased persistent firing for all directions, thus eroding the information held in working memory stores. These data emphasize why cognitive enhancement can disappear at higher doses.*

α_7-nAChRs are positioned to perform this function because they are localized within and next to the post-synaptic density (PSD) of glutamate synapses in layer III of the dlPFC, often with a cholinergic synapse nearby.[94] Physiological recordings indicate that α_7-nAChRs are necessary for NMDAR actions and delay cell firing, and indeed produce the permissive actions on NMDAR normally associated with AMPAR in sensory circuits.[94] Thus, α_7-nAChR stimulation allows dlPFC neurons to connect under conditions when we are awake and acetylcholine is released but not when we are in deep sleep when there is no acetylcholine release.[95] In other words, our conscious cognitive experience may be partly a function of cholinergic stimulation of α_7-nAChRs in the dlPFC.[94] Importantly for the development of cognitive enhancers, the effects of α_7-nAChR agonists are highly dose dependent: Low doses of a nic-α_{7R} agonist enhance the spatially tuned, persistent firing of delay cells, increasing firing for the neuron's preferred direction but not altering firing for its nonpreferred directions (Figures 2.4A and 2.4B). However, higher doses of α_7-nAChR agonist produce nonspecific increases in neuronal firing, where the neuron increases its firing to both preferred and nonpreferred directions, thus obscuring the pattern of information (Figure 2.4C). As described later, this inverted U-shaped dose response makes it especially difficult to identify effective low doses for human use.

DNC mechanisms also include powerful, feedforward cAMP–calcium signaling actions localized in spines near the NMDAR synapse. These cAMP–calcium actions rapidly *weaken* connectivity—actions that are opposite the traditional effects of cAMP signaling in classic circuits.[61] Research on hippocampal and sensory circuits has found that high levels of cAMP activation of protein kinase A (PKA) signaling and calcium activation protein kinase C (PKC) signaling enhance long-term plasticity—for example, increasing long-term potentiation (LTP) or enlarging a mushroom-shaped spine[96,97] (Figure 2.5A). These signaling pathways also increase glutamate release from presynaptic terminals—for example, by priming vesicles for release[98] (see Figure 2.5A). Thus, traditional research on phylogenetically older neural circuits has generally found enhancing effects of calcium–cAMP signaling.

In contrast to classical synapses, feedforward calcium–cAMP signaling in newly evolved layer III dlPFC circuits rapidly weakens connections by opening nearby potassium (K+) channels in spines (schematically summarized in Figure 2.5). For example, the open state of HCN and KCNQ channels is increased by cAMP[99] and PKA,[100] respectively, and both channels are concentrated in layer III spines near the synapse and in the spine neck.[61,101] Many thin spines in layer III of the dlPFC contain a spine apparatus, the extension of the smooth endoplasmic reticulum into the spine, which stores and releases calcium.[61] cAMP–PKA signaling proteins are anchored near the spine apparatus, where they are positioned to enhance IP3 receptor-gated calcium release.[62] As calcium increases the production of cAMP, feedforward signaling can rapidly build levels to open nearby K+ channels and functionally disconnect the circuit. Conversely, the phosphodiesterase PDE4A catabolizes cAMP and is anchored near the spine apparatus by DISC1 (disrupted in schizophrenia),[61,62,101] positioned to hold feedforward cAMP–calcium signaling in check.

Calcium–cAMP–PKA opening of K+ channels near the synapse appears to contribute to a number of important cellular functions. They can provide negative feedback to prevent seizures within recurrent excitatory networks—for example, by opening KCNQ channels—as loss of this ability leads to epilepsy.[100] Interestingly, mGluR1a and mGluR5 are localized near the synapse,[102] where they are positioned to activate feedforward calcium–cAMP–K+ channel signaling when glutamate overflow spills beyond the synapse. Calcium–cAMP opening of K+ channels on a discreet set of spines can also serve to sculpt the contents of working memory, gating out nonpreferred inputs or, with very high levels of cAMP–calcium signaling (e.g., during uncontrollable stress), totally suppress all delay cell firing. For example, dopamine (DA) D1 receptors (D1Rs) are localized in layer III spines, both in the synapse itself, where they may enhance NMDAR insertion into the PSD, and next to the synapse, where they are co-localized with HCN channels.[103] D1R generation of cAMP increases the open state of HCN channels, weakening a synaptic connection.[103,104] During optimal levels of DA release, D1R–HCN channel actions sculpt away "noise," preferentially weakening the effects of nonpreferred inputs. However, at higher levels of D1R stimulation during uncontrollable stress, all inputs are weakened and the delay cells stop firing,[105] thus creating an inverted U-shaped

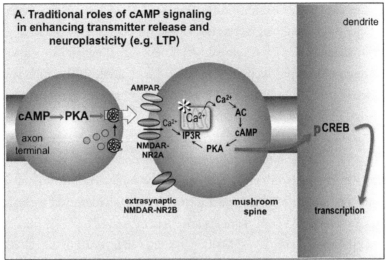

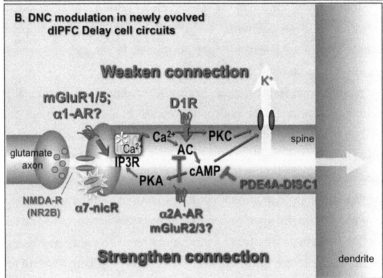

FIGURE 2.5 *Roles of cAMP–PKA signaling in traditional versus dlPFC DNC synapses. (A) In classical synapses, cAMP–PKA signaling can enhance transmitter release (e.g., glutamate release) from the presynaptic terminal by priming vesicles for release, and it can drive late-stage LTP, which can lead to architectural changes that strengthen the synapse. Sufficient activation of PKA can lead to phosphorylation of CREB and transcriptional changes (e.g., an immature thin "learning" spine becomes a mushroom spine). (B) Dynamic network connectivity (DNC) in a mature, long thin spine in layer III of the primate dlPFC rapidly and reversibly alters synapse strength to coordinate cognitive and arousal states. These synapses have only a subtle AMPAR component, and the permissive excitation needed for NMDAR opening is mediated by cholinergic stimulation of α_7-nAChR. Mechanisms that increase feedforward calcium–cAMP–PKA signaling (shown in red, many engaged by stress) weaken synaptic connections by opening nearby K$^+$ channels (HCN and KCNQ) on the spine head and/or neck. In contrast, inhibiting feedforward calcium–cAMP–PKA signaling (green) strengthens connectivity and enhances delay cell firing. Loss of inhibition—for example, through genetic insults to DISC1 that would unanchor key proteins—may contribute to spine loss and impaired dlPFC function. The unique modulation of layer III dlPFC pyramidal cell synapses provides therapeutic strategies for cognitive disorders.*

dose response. High levels of noradrenergic (NE) α_1-adrenoceptor stimulation also contribute to loss of delay cell firing, via increased calcium–PKC mechanisms.[106] Thus, feedforward calcium–cAMP opening of K^+ channels can rapidly take the PFC "offline" during stress exposure, a mechanism that may have survival value during danger to switch control of behavior to more primitive, reflexive circuitry. These built-in mechanisms to purposefully impair dlPFC function likely help explain why this cortex dysfunctions so readily in many different disorders, especially those that are exacerbated by stress exposure.

Importantly, inhibition of feedforward cAMP–calcium signaling strengthens connectivity, enhances delay cell firing, and improves dlPFC cognitive abilities in primates. For example, NE α_{2A}-adrenoceptors (α_{2A}-ARs) inhibit cAMP production and are co-localized with HCN channels in layer III spines near the synapse and in the spine neck (Figure 2.6A).[107] Stimulation of α_{2A}-ARs (e.g., with the α_{2A}-AR agonist guanfacine) selectively increases firing for the neuron's preferred direction, thus enhancing mental representations[107] (Figure 2.6B). In contrast, blockade of α_{2A}-ARs with yohimbine causes a complete collapse of dlPFC network firing[108] that can be restored by blocking HCN channels.[107] Parallel effects are seen on cognitive behavior in monkeys, in which intra-dlPFC infusion of guanfacine improves working memory,[109] and systemic administration of guanfacine improves a variety of PFC cognitive functions, including working memory, reversal learning, behavioral inhibition, regulation of attention, and rapid associative learning.[110] Importantly, guanfacine improves impulse control, allowing monkeys to inhibit responses to immediate, small rewards and instead be able to wait for a larger reward—a cognitive ability that is especially important for success in life.[111] Conversely, infusion of the α_{2A}-AR antagonist yohimbine into the dlPFC impairs working memory[112] and impulse control,[113] and it induces locomotor hyperactivity.[114] Thus, α_{2A}-AR stimulation strengthens the efficacy of dlPFC connections, enhances delay cell representations, and strengthens top-down regulation of behavior.

Some studies in rodents have also shown beneficial actions of guanfacine. In vitro recordings from layer II/III pyramidal cells in PFC slices have provided results similar to those of monkeys, in which α_{2A}-AR stimulation enhances persistent firing via HCN channel closure.[115] (However, recordings of layer V neurons show reduced presynaptic glutamate release;[116] see the discussion on the important laminar differences in PFC.) Studies in mice found that mutation of α_{2A}-AR prevented guanfacine's cognitive enhancing effects.[117] However, the drug effects on working memory in wild-type mice were much less robust than those in monkeys, consistent with the very small number of layer II/III PFC neurons in mice. Recent studies on rats indicate that systemic administration of guanfacine can protect PFC layer II/III dendritic

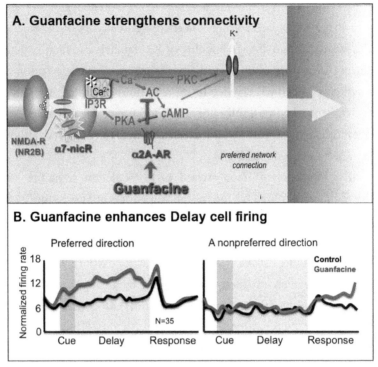

FIGURE 2.6 *The α_{2A}-AR agonist, guanfacine, strengthens dlPFC network connections and enhances dlPFC network firing. (A) A schematic illustration of guanfacine's actions in the primate dlPFC, stimulating post-synaptic α_{2A}-AR on spines to inhibit feedforward cAMP–calcium–K^+ channel signaling and strengthen NMDAR connections. (B) Guanfacine increases the firing of delay cells for their preferred direction. The figure demonstrates the normalized mean firing rate of 35 delay cells under control conditions (black) and following iontophoresis of guanfacine (green). The figure shows the neurons' preferred direction and the nonpreferred direction opposite to the preferred direction. Guanfacine has been shown to improve a variety of PFC cognitive functions, and it is currently in clinical use to treat PFC disorders.*

spines and cognitive abilities from the detrimental effects of oxygen deprivation[118] or chronic restraint stress.[119] Repeated guanfacine administration may actually increase the number of spines on layer II/III neurons under basal conditions[119] and enhance PFC spine maturation in vitro.[120] Guanfacine's protection of spines from chronic stressors may involve a number of mechanisms, including reducing stress-induced catecholamine release, strengthening PFC connections, and reducing inflammation by deactivating activated microglia.[121] The beneficial effects of guanfacine in animals have translated successfully to humans with PFC dysfunction (discussed later), suggesting that focus on delay cell needs is a useful strategy for treating cognitive disorders.

Finally, dlPFC response cells are regulated very differently than dlPFC delay cells. For example, response cells are not altered by DA D1R stimulation but are altered by D2R actions, which is the opposite profile of delay cells.[122] Response cells also appear to be regulated in a more classic manner than delay cells. Post-saccadic response cells are very sensitive to AMPAR blockade, whereas delay cells show only subtle changes when AMPARs are blocked.[65] These findings in response cells are similar to those for rodent PFC, in which neurons are very sensitive to AMPAR blockade.[123,124] Studies of the rodent PFC often focus on layer V pyramidal cells because they are numerous (layer V is more than twice the size of layer III in rodents, whereas layer III is more than twice the size of layer V in primates[125]), and the large size of layer V pyramidal cells enables recordings. However, we caution that theories based solely on data from layer V in rodent PFC may be misleading because these neurons are often modulated very differently from the delay cells that generate mental representations in primates.

SUCCESSFUL TRANSLATIONS FROM MONKEY TO HUMAN

A number of findings from nonhuman primate studies of the dlPFC have translated successfully to human subjects. The DA "D1 inverted U-shaped" dose response first discovered in monkeys can be seen in humans in regard to catechol-O-methyltransferase (COMT) genotype as well as in drug studies. COMT is an enzyme that catabolizes catecholamines, but it is weakened by a methionine–valine substitution.[126–129] Weaker enzymatic activity can be helpful to cognition under basal conditions, but it worsens working memory abilities under conditions of stress exposure, consistent with the inverted U-shaped dose response.[130] Although there are currently no US Food and Drug Administration-approved D1R/D5R selective compounds that can be used to conduct studies in humans, research utilizing nonselective compounds[131,132] suggests an inverted U-shaped dose response in humans as well. The selective D1R/D5R agonist dihydrexidine (referred to as DAR-0100A) is currently being tested as a potential treatment for schizophrenia, and it has recently been tested in schizotypal patients who have cognitive deficits resembling those in schizophrenia.[133] The mixed effects of this compound may be due to the challenging aspects of the inverted U-shaped dose response.[133]

The α_{2A}-AR agonist guanfacine is as an example of successful translation from research in animals to cognitive disorders in humans. As described previously, studies in animals showed that guanfacine can strengthen dlPFC network connectivity, enhance delay cell firing, and improve performance of a variety of cognitive tasks that depend on the PFC. Based on results in animals,[134] guanfacine was developed for use in human PFC disorders. Although guanfacine has a long half-life in older adults, it is metabolized very quickly in the young; thus, an extended-release formulation was created for the treatment of pediatric ADHD (Intuniv).[135] Guanfacine is also commonly used for additional pediatric disorders that benefit from stronger PFC regulation of behavior, including Tourette's syndrome,[136] autism spectrum illness,[137] and emotional trauma such as physical abuse and neglect.[138,139] In adults, guanfacine is being tested or used to treat traumatic brain injury that involves the frontal lobe[140] and to aid top-down control in the treatment of substance abuse.[141,142] It has been shown to help patients with strokes or infections affecting the association cortex.[143,144] Guanfacine is also beginning to be tested in prodromal schizophrenia, with the hope that it may protect the PFC from the wave of gray matter loss and inflammation that heralds the descent into illness.[145]

As described earlier, studies in animals have shown that high levels of NE release during stress exposure stimulate α_1-AR, which reduces dlPFC delay cell firing and impairs PFC function through calcium–PKC signaling.[106,146] Based in part on this research, the α_1-AR antagonist prazosin is now in widespread use for the treatment of post-traumatic stress disorder in veterans, active-duty soldiers, and civilians.[139,147,148] Because the NE system appears to grow stronger with repeated stress,[149–151] this may be an especially effective strategy in chronic stress disorders.

It is hoped that additional strategies will successfully translate to human subjects with cognitive disorders. For example, the α_7-nAChR seems to be an important therapeutic target, given its ability to strengthen NMDAR synapses in dlPFC. Agonists and modulators of the α_7-nAChR are currently in development for the treatment of schizophrenia.[152] Some of the many challenges facing the successful translation to human cognition are discussed next.

CHALLENGES IN DEVELOPING THERAPEUTICS FOR COGNITIVE DISORDERS

There are multiple challenges in successfully translating cognitive enhancing drug actions from animal models to human treatments. Although this chapter has used the term cognitive enhancement, we are truly discussing the goal of *cognitive optimization*, not enhancement, because unlike steroids in sports, "cognitive enhancers" do not make one smarter than one originally was but, rather, optimize one's own (limited) capabilities. Intelligence is determined by genetics (i.e., brain development creating neurons and their connections), which is then acted upon by experience (e.g., learning creating an enriched pattern of connections vs. chronic stress and toxins removing connections). A drug can enhance existing connections, but it cannot substitute for actual experience.

The overarching goal for a cognitive treatment is to enhance the precise pattern of cortical network connections that generate and sustain a mental representation. It is easy to obscure this precise pattern—for example, with higher doses producing nonspecific increases in excitability (e.g., α_7-nAChR agonists) or nonspecific suppression of firing (e.g., D1R/D5R agonists) that brings the drug over the top of the inverted U-shaped dose response and erodes information. This often occurs at doses that have no overt side effects, increasing the difficulty of dose identification. Thus, cognitive enhancement is a delicate process that requires a precise, and usually low, dose range. This is a very different approach than the classic pharmacological goal of maximizing receptor occupancy. The challenge is further complicated by the frequent individual variability in patients—for example, in regard to endogenous brain state. It is hoped that drug assessments in monkeys can be a helpful bridge for identifying a ballpark dose range (as was very useful in the translation of guanfacine to the clinic). It will also be important to allow for increased Phase 1 and 2 exploration of doses, and perhaps even open-label explorations, prior to large commitments in Phase 3 trials.

Another challenge is recognizing the limits of rodent research, even though rodents are the traditional, affordable animal models for pharmacological screening and research. Rodents have very limited association cortex,[153] and even within PFC, they have a small layer III and very large layer V, which is opposite that in primates.[58] Rodents have evolved to use the hippocampus as a major cognitive organ—for example, spatial cognition requires the hippocampus in rodents but not in primates.[54] Thus, overreliance on rodent models can be misleading when developing compounds for higher cognitive disorders in humans, especially because compounds that strengthen hippocampal function often weaken dlPFC abilities.

Finally, a remaining challenge for the creation of cognitive enhancers is our ignorance regarding the molecular needs of most of the primate association cortex. We cannot assume that the mechanisms modulating layer III circuits in the dlPFC necessarily extend to other cortical regions. Indeed, we have already learned that the orbital PFC has different needs from the dlPFC—for example, with regard to reliance on serotonin.[154–156] There are also conditions in which one may want to alter the function of one cortical area without altering those of another. For example, mechanisms that improve dlPFC cognition may also increase the activity of visceromotor PFC (Brodmann's area 25) and aggravate symptoms of depression. Thus, we need to determine whether there might be mechanisms unique to specific cortical areas that may allow more refined manipulations. This is one of many important areas for future research.

ACKNOWLEDGMENTS

The authors are funded by PHS Pioneer Award DP1AG047744-01, R01AG043430-01A1, RO1 MH100064-01A1, and R01 MH 09335401A1.

DISCLOSURE

Yale University and Amy F. T. Arnsten receive royalties from the sales of Intuniv (extended-release guanfacine) from Shire Pharmaceuticals but do not receive funds from the sales of generic Intuniv or immediate-release guanfacine.

REFERENCES

1. Coull JT, Nobre AC. Where and when to pay attention: The neural systems for directing attention to spatial locations and to time intervals as revealed by both PET and fMRI. *J Neurosci* 1998;18:7426–7435.
2. Mesulam M-M. *Principles of behavioral and cognitive neurology.* 2nd ed. New York, NY: Oxford University Press; 2000.
3. Friedman-Hill SR, Robertson LC, Treisman A. Parietal contributions to visual feature binding: Evidence from a patient with bilateral lesions. *Science* 1995;269:853–855.
4. Mesulam MM. A cortical network for directed attention and unilateral neglect. *Ann Neurol* 1981;10:309–325.
5. Posner MI, Walker JA, Friedrich FJ, et al. Effects of parietal injury on covert orienting of visual attention. *J Neurosci* 1984;4:1863–1874.
6. Sanada TM, DeAngelis GC. Neural representation of motion-in-depth in area MT. *J Neurosci* 2014;34:15508–15521.
7. Rudolph K, Pasternak T. Transient and permanent deficits in motion perception after lesions of cortical areas MT and MST in the macaque monkey. *Cereb Cortex* 1999;9:90–100.
8. Robinson DL, Bowman EM, Kertzman C. Covert orienting of attention in macaques: II. Contributions of parietal cortex. *J Neurophysiol* 1995;74:698–712.
9. Snyder LH, Grieve KL, Brotchie P, et al. Separate body- and world-referenced representations of visual space in parietal cortex. *Nature* 1998;394:887–891.
10. Selemon LD, Goldman-Rakic PS. Common cortical and subcortical targets of the dorsolateral prefrontal and posterior parietal cortices in the rhesus monkey: Evidence for a distributed neural network subserving spatially guided behavior. *J Neurosci* 1988;8(11):4049–4068.
11. Chafee MV, Goldman-Rakic PS. Matching patterns of activity in primate prefrontal area 8a and parietal area 7ip neurons during a spatial working memory task. *J Neurophysiol* 1998;79:2919–2940.
12. Viswanathan P, Nieder A. Neuronal correlates of a visual "sense of number" in primate parietal and prefrontal cortices. *Proc Natl Acad Sci USA* 2013;110:11187–11192.
13. Dehaene S, Spelke E, Pinel P, et al. Sources of mathematical thinking: Behavioral and brain-imaging evidence. *Science* 1999;284:970–974.
14. Carmichael ST, Clugnet MC, Price JL. Central olfactory connections in the macaque monkey. *J Comp Neurol* 1994;346:403–434.
15. Rauschecker JP, Tian B. Mechanisms and streams for processing of "what" and "where" in auditory cortex. *Proc Natl Acad Sci USA* 2000;97:11800–11806.
16. Desimone R. Neural mechanisms for visual memory and their role in attention. *Proc Natl Acad Sci USA* 1996;93:13494–13499.

17. Kastner S, De Weerd P, Desimone R, et al. Mechanisms of directed attention in the human extrastriate cortex as revealed by functional MRI. *Science* 1998;282:108–111.
18. Desimone R, Albright TD, Gross CG, et al. Stimulus-selective properties of inferior temporal neurons in the macaque. *J Neurosci* 1984;4:2051–2062.
19. Fujita I, Tanaka K, Ito M, et al. Columns for visual features of objects in monkey inferotemporal cortex. *Nature* 1992;360:343–346.
20. Desimone R. Visual attention mediated by biased competition in extrastriate visual cortex. *Philos Trans R Soc London B Biol Sci* 1998;353:1245–1255.
21. Moran J, Desimone R. Selective attention gates visual processing in the extrastriate cortex. *Science* 1985;229:782–784.
22. Miller EK, Li L, Desimone R. Activity of neurons in anterior inferior temporal cortex during a short-term memory task. *J Neurosci* 1993;13:1460–1478.
23. Pascual B, Masdeu JC, Hollenbeck M, et al. Large-scale brain networks of the human left temporal pole: A functional connectivity MRI study. *Cereb Cortex* 2015;25:680–702.
24. Olson IR, Plotzker A, Ezzyat Y. The enigmatic temporal pole: A review of findings on social and emotional processing. *Brain* 2007;130:1718–1731.
25. Glosser G, Salvucci AE, Chiaravalloti ND. Naming and recognizing famous faces in temporal lobe epilepsy. *Neurology* 2003;61:81–86.
26. Tranel D. The left temporal pole is important for retrieving words for unique concrete entities. *Aphasiology* 2009;23:867.
27. Robbins TW. Dissociating executive functions of the prefrontal cortex. *Philos Trans R Soc London* 1996;351:1463–1471.
28. Stuss DT, Knight RT, eds. *Principles of frontal lobe function.* New York, NY: Oxford University Press; 2002.
29. Thompson-Schill SL, Jonides J, Marshuetz C, et al. Effects of frontal lobe damage on interference effects in working memory. *Cogn Affect Behav Neurosci* 2002;2:109–120.
30. Fuster JM. *The prefrontal cortex.* 4th ed. San Diego, CA: Academic Press; 2008.
31. Goldman-Rakic PS. Circuitry of the primate prefrontal cortex and the regulation of behavior by representational memory. In Plum F (Ed.), *Handbook of physiology: The nervous system: Higher functions of the brain* (Vol. 5). Bethesda, MD: American Physiological Society; 1987:373–417.
32. Ongür D, Price JL. The organization of networks within the orbital and medial prefrontal cortex of rats, monkeys and humans. *Cereb Cortex* 2000;10(3):206–219.
33. Badre D, D'Esposito M. Functional magnetic resonance imaging evidence for a hierarchical organization of the prefrontal cortex. *J Cogn Neurosci* 2007;19:2082–2099.
34. Hilgenstock R, Weiss T, Witte OW. You'd better think twice: Post-decision perceptual confidence. *Neuroimage* 2014;99:323–331.
35. Fleming SM, Huijgen J, Dolan RJ. Prefrontal contributions to metacognition in perceptual decision making. *J Neurosci* 2012;32:6117–6125.
36. Amodio DM, Frith CD. Meeting of minds: The medial frontal cortex and social cognition. *Nat Rev Neurosci* 2006;7(4):268–277.
37. Seo H, Cai X, Donahue CH, et al. Neural correlates of strategic reasoning during competitive games. *Science* 2014;346:340–343.
38. Robinson RG, Lipsey JR. Cerebral localization of emotion based on clinical–neuropathological correlations: Methodological issues. *Psychiatric Dev* 1985;3:335–347.
39. Aron AR. From reactive to proactive and selective control: Developing a richer model for stopping inappropriate responses. *Biol Psychiatry* 2011;69(12):e55–e68.
40. Funahashi S, Bruce CJ, Goldman-Rakic PS. Mnemonic coding of visual space in the monkey's dorsolateral prefrontal cortex. *J Neurophysiol* 1989;61:331–349.
41. Seo H, Lee D. Behavioral and neural changes after gains and losses of conditioned reinforcers. *J Neurosci* 2009;29(11):3627–3641.
42. Chang EF, Raygor KP, Berger MS. Contemporary model of language organization: An overview for neurosurgeons. *J Neurosurg* 2015;122:250–261.

43. Middleton FA, Strick PL. Basal ganglia and cerebellar loops: Motor and cognitive circuits. *Brain Res Brain Res Rev* 2000;31:236–250.
44. Dum RP, Li C, Strick PL. Motor and nonmotor domains in the monkey dentate. *Ann N Y Acad Sci* 2002;978:289–301.
45. Milner B. The medial temporal-lobe amnesic syndrome. *Psychiatr Clin North Am* 2005;28:599–611.
46. Kim S, Dede AJ, Hopkins RO, et al. Memory, scene construction, and the human hippocampus. *Proc Natl Acad Sci USA* 2015;112:4767–4772.
47. Wixted JT, Squire LR, Jang Y, et al. Sparse and distributed coding of episodic memory in neurons of the human hippocampus. *Proc Natl Acad Sci USA* 2014;111:9621–9626.
48. Price JL. Definition of the orbital cortex in relation to specific connections with limbic and visceral structures and other cortical regions. *Ann N Y Acad Sci* 2007;1121:54–71.
49. Malkova L, Mishkin M. One-trial memory for object–place associations after separate lesions of hippocampus and posterior parahippocampal region in the monkey. *J Neurosci* 2003;23:1956–1965.
50. Davachi L, Goldman-Rakic PS. Primate rhinal cortex participates in both visual recognition and working memory tasks: Functional mapping with 2-DG. *J Neurophysiol* 2001;85:2590–2601.
51. Takeuchi D, Hirabayashi T, Tamura K, et al. Reversal of interlaminar signal between sensory and memory processing in monkey temporal cortex. *Science* 2011;331:1443–1447.
52. Baxter MG, Murray EA. Impairments in visual discrimination learning and recognition memory produced by neurotoxic lesions of rhinal cortex in rhesus monkeys. *Eur J Neurosci* 2001;13(6):1228–1238.
53. Eichenbaum H, Sauvage M, Fortin N, et al. Towards a functional organization of episodic memory in the medial temporal lobe. *Neurosci Biobehav Rev* 2012;36:1597–1608.
54. Kim S, Sapiurka M, Clark RE, et al. Contrasting effects on path integration after hippocampal damage in humans and rats. *Proc Natl Acad Sci USA* 2013;110:4732–4737.
55. Goldman PS, Rosvold HE, Vest B, et al. Analysis of the delayed-alternation deficit produced by dorsolateral prefrontal lesions in the rhesus monkey. *J Comp Phys Psych* 1971;77:212–220.
56. Kritzer MF, Goldman-Rakic PS. Intrinsic circuit organization of the major layers and sublayers of the dorsolateral prefrontal cortex in the rhesus monkey. *J Comp Neurol* 1995;359:131–143.
57. Elston GN, Benavides-Piccione R, Elston A, et al. Specializations of the granular prefrontal cortex of primates: Implications for cognitive processing. *Anat Rec A Discov Mol Cell Evol Biol* 2006;288:26–35.
58. DeFelipe J. The evolution of the brain, the human nature of cortical circuits, and intellectual creativity. *Front Neuroanat* 2011;5:29.
59. Elston GN. Pyramidal cells of the frontal lobe: All the more spinous to think with. *J Neurosci* 2000;20:RC95.
60. Elston GN. Cortex, cognition and the cell: New insights into the pyramidal neuron and prefrontal function. *Cereb Cortex* 2003;13:1124–1138.
61. Arnsten AFT, Wang M, Paspalas CD. Neuromodulation of thought: Flexibilities and vulnerabilities in prefrontal cortical network synapses. *Neuron* 2012;76(1):223–239.
62. Carlyle BC, Nairn AC, Wang M, et al. cAMP-PKA phosphorylation of tau confers risk for degeneration in aging association cortex. *Proc Natl Acad Sci USA* 2014;111:5036–5041.
63. Bourne J, Harris KM. Do thin spines learn to be mushroom spines that remember? *Curr Opin Neurobiol* 2007;17:381–386.
64. Goldman-Rakic PS. Cellular basis of working memory. *Neuron* 1995;14(3):477–485.
65. Wang M, Yang Y, Wang CJ, et al. NMDA receptors subserve persistent working memory during neuronal firing in dorsolateral prefrontal cortex. *Neuron* 2013;77(4):736–749.
66. Liu XB, Murray KD, Jones EG. Switching of NMDA receptor 2A and 2B subunits at thalamic and cortical synapses during early postnatal development. *J Neurosci* 2004;24:8885–8895.
67. Gabernet L, Jadhav SP, Feldman DE, et al. Somatosensory integration controlled by dynamic thalamocortical feed-forward inhibition. *Neuron* 2005;48:315–327.

68. Funahashi S, Bruce CJ, Goldman-Rakic PS. Neuronal activity related to saccadic eye movements in the monkey's dorsolateral prefrontal cortex. *J Neurophysiol* 1991;65:1464–1483.

69. Ford JM, Mathalon DH, Whitfield S, et al. Reduced communication between frontal and temporal lobes during talking in schizophrenia. *Biol Psychiatry* 2002;51(6):485–492.

70. Caetano MS, Horst NK, Harenberg L, et al. Lost in transition: Aging-related changes in executive control by the medial prefrontal cortex. *J Neurosci* 2012;32(11):3765–3777.

71. Arion D, Corradi JP, Tang S, et al. Distinctive transcriptome alterations of prefrontal pyramidal neurons in schizophrenia and schizoaffective disorder. *Mol Psychiatry* 2015;20(11):1397–1405.

72. Drevets WC, Price JL, Simpson JRJ, et al. Subgenual prefrontal cortex abnormalities in mood disorders. *Nature* 1997;386:824–827.

73. Mayberg HS, Lozano AM, Voon V, et al. Deep brain stimulation for treatment-resistant depression. *Neuron* 2005;45(5):651–660.

74. Insel TR, Winslow JT. Neurobiology of obsessive compulsive disorder. *Psychiatr Clin North Am* 1992;15:813–824.

75. Shaw P, Lalonde FM, Lepage C, et al. Development of cortical asymmetry in typically developing children and its disruption in attention-deficit/hyperactivity disorder. *Arch Gen Psychiatry* 2009;66:888–896.

76. Shaw P, Gogtay N, Rapoport J. Childhood psychiatric disorders as anomalies in neurodevelopmental trajectories. *Hum Brain Mapp* 2010;31:917–925.

77. Blumberg HP, Stern E, Ricketts S, et al. Rostral and orbital prefrontal cortex dysfunction in the manic state of bipolar disorder. *Am J Psychiatry* 1999;156(12):1986–1988.

78. Sugranyes G, Kyriakopoulos M, Corrigall R, et al. Autism spectrum disorders and schizophrenia: Meta-analysis of the neural correlates of social cognition. *PLoS One* 2011;6(10):e25322.

79. Tebbenkamp AT, Willsey AJ, State MW, et al. The developmental transcriptome of the human brain: Implications for neurodevelopmental disorders. *Curr Opin Neurol* 2014;27:149–156.

80. Selemon LD, Rajkowska G, Goldman-Rakic PS. Abnormally high neuronal density in the schizophrenic cortex: A morphometric analysis of prefrontal area 9 and occipital area 17. *Arch Gen Psychiatry* 1995;52:805–818.

81. Selemon LD, Goldman-Rakic PS. The reduced neuropil hypothesis: A circuit based model of schizophrenia. *Biol Psychiatry* 1999;45:17–25.

82. Glantz LA, Lewis DA. Decreased dendritic spine density on prefrontal cortical pyramidal neurons in schizophrenia. *Arch Gen Psychiatry* 2000;57:65–73.

83. Black JE, Kodish IM, Grossman AW, et al. Pathology of layer V pyramidal neurons in the prefrontal cortex of patients with schizophrenia. *Am J Psychiatry* 2004;161:742–744.

84. Curley AA, Eggan SM, Lazarus MS, et al. Role of glutamic acid decarboxylase 67 in regulating cortical parvalbumin and GABA membrane transporter 1 expression: Implications for schizophrenia. *Neurobiol Dis* 2013;50:179–186.

85. Pearson RCA, Esiri MM, Hiorns RW, et al. Anatomical correlates of the distribution of the pathological changes in the neocortex in Alzheimer disease. *Proc Natl Acad Sci USA* 1985;82:4531–4534.

86. Lewis DA, Campbell MJ, Terry RD, et al. Laminar and regional distributions of neurofibrillary tangles and neuritic plaques in Alzheimer's disease: A quantitative study of visual and auditory cortices. *J Neurosci* 1987;7:1799–1808.

87. Bussière T, Giannakopoulos P, Bouras C, et al. Progressive degeneration of nonphosphorylated neurofilament protein-enriched pyramidal neurons predicts cognitive impairment in Alzheimer's disease: Stereologic analysis of prefrontal cortex area 9. *J Comp Neurol* 2003;463:281–302.

88. Giannakopoulos P, Herrmann FR, Bussière T, et al. Tangle and neuron numbers, but not amyloid load, predict cognitive status in Alzheimer's disease. *Neurology* 2003;60:1495–1500.

89. Braak H, Braak E. Staging of Alzheimer's disease-related neurofibrillary changes. *Neurobiol Aging* 1995;16:271–278.

90. Braak H, Thal DR, Ghebremedhin E, et al. Stages of the pathologic process in Alzheimer disease: Age categories from 1 to 100 years. *J Neuropathol Exp Neurol* 2011;70:960–969.

91. Hyman BT, Van Hoesen GW, Damasio AR, et al. Alzheimer's disease: Cell-specific pathology isolates the hippocampal formation. *Science* 1984;225:1168–1170.

92. Liu L, Drouet V, Wu JW, et al. Trans-synaptic spread of tau pathology in vivo. *PLoS One* 2012;7:e31302.

93. Walker LC, Diamond MI, Duff KE, et al. Mechanisms of protein seeding in neurodegenerative diseases. *JAMA Neurol* 2013;70:304–310.

94. Yang Y, Paspalas CD, Jin LE, et al. Nicotinic α_7 receptors enhance NMDA cognitive circuits in dorsolateral prefrontal cortex. *Proc Natl Acad Sci USA* 2013;110(29):12078–12083.

95. Hobson JA. Sleep and dreaming: Induction and mediation of REM sleep by cholinergic mechanisms. *Curr Opin Neurobiol* 1992;2:759–763.

96. Abel T, Nguyen PV, Barad M, et al. Genetic demonstration of a role for PKA in the late phase of LTP and in hippocampus-based long-term memory. *Cell* 1997;88:615–626.

97. Hongpaisan J, Alkon DL. A structural basis for enhancement of long-term associative memory in single dendritic spines regulated by PKC. *Proc Natl Acad Sci USA* 2007;104:19571–19576.

98. Nagy G, Reim K, Matti U, et al. Regulation of releasable vesicle pool sizes by protein kinase A-dependent phosphorylation of SNAP-25. *Neuron* 2004;41(3):417–429.

99. Chen S, Wang J, Siegelbaum SA. Properties of hyperpolarization-activated pacemaker current defined by coassembly of HCN1 and HCN2 subunits and basal modulation by cyclic nucleotide. *J Gen Physiol* 2001;117:491–504.

100. Jentsch TJ. Neuronal KCNQ potassium channels: Physiology and role in disease. *Nat Rev Neurosci* 2000;1:21–30.

101. Paspalas CD, Min Wang M, Arnsten AFT. Constellation of HCN channels and cAMP regulating proteins in dendritic spines of the primate prefrontal cortex: Potential substrate for working memory deficits in schizophrenia. *Cereb Cortex* 2013; 23:1643–1654.

102. Muly EC, Maddox M, Smith Y. Distribution of mGluR1alpha and mGluR5 immunolabeling in primate prefrontal cortex. *J Comp Neurol* 2003;467:521–535.

103. Gamo NJ, Lur G, Higley MJ, et al. Stress impairs prefrontal cortical function via D1 dopamine receptor interactions with HCN channels. *Biol Psychiatry* 2015;78(12):860–870.

104. Vijayraghavan S, Wang M, Birnbaum SG, et al. Inverted-U dopamine D1 receptor actions on prefrontal neurons engaged in working memory. *Nat Neurosci* 2007;10:376–384.

105. Arnsten AFT, Wang M, Paspalas CD. Dopamine's actions in primate prefrontal cortex: Challenges for treating cognitive disorders. *Pharmacol Rev* 2015;67(3):681–696.

106. Birnbaum SB, Yuan P, Wang M, et al. Protein kinase C overactivity impairs prefrontal cortical regulation of working memory. *Science* 2004;306:882–884.

107. Wang M, Ramos B, Paspalas C, et al. Alpha2A-adrenoceptor stimulation strengthens working memory networks by inhibiting cAMP-HCN channel signaling in prefrontal cortex. *Cell* 2007;129:397–410.

108. Li B-M, Mao Z-M, Wang M, et al. Alpha-2 adrenergic modulation of prefrontal cortical neuronal activity related to spatial working memory in monkeys. *Neuropsychopharmacology* 1999;21:601–610.

109. Mao Z-M, Arnsten AFT, Li B-M. Local infusion of alpha-1 adrenergic agonist into the prefrontal cortex impairs spatial working memory performance in monkeys. *Biol Psychiatry* 1999;46:1259–1265.

110. Arnsten AF. The use of alpha2A adrenergic agonists for the treatment of attention-deficit/hyperactivity disorder. *Expert Rev Neurother* 2010;10:1595–1605.

111. Kim S, Bobeica I, Gamo NJ, et al. Effects of α-2A adrenergic receptor agonist on time and risk preference in primates. *Psychopharmacology* 2012;219:363–375.

112. Li B-M, Mei Z-T. Delayed response deficit induced by local injection of the alpha-2 adrenergic antagonist yohimbine into the dorsolateral prefrontal cortex in young adult monkeys. *Behav Neural Biol* 1994;62:134–139.

113. Ma C-L, Qi X-L, Peng J-Y, et al. Selective deficit in no-go performance induced by blockade of prefrontal cortical alpha2-adrenoceptors in monkeys. *Neuroreport* 2003;14:1013–1016.

114. Ma C-L, Arnsten AFT, Li B-M. Locomotor hyperactivity induced by blockade of prefrontal cortical alpha-2-adrenoceptors in monkeys. *Biol Psychiatry* 2005;57:192–195.

115. Zhang Z, Cordeiro Matos S, Jego S, et al. Norepinephrine drives persistent activity in prefrontal cortex via synergistic α₁ and α₂ adrenoceptors. *PLoS One* 2013;8:e66122.

116. Yi F, Liu SS, Luo F, et al. Signaling mechanism underlying α2A-adrenergic suppression of excitatory synaptic transmission in the medial prefrontal cortex of rats. *Eur J Neurosci* 2013;38:2364–2373.

117. Franowicz JS, Kessler L, Dailey-Borja CM, et al. Mutation of the alpha2A-adrenoceptor impairs working memory performance and annuls cognitive enhancement by guanfacine. *J Neurosci* 2002;22:8771–8777.

118. Kauser H, Sahu S, Kumar S, et al. Guanfacine is an effective countermeasure for hypobaric hypoxia-induced cognitive decline. *Neuroscience* 2013;254:110–119.

119. Hains AB, Yabe Y, Arnsten AFT. Chronic stimulation of alpha-2A-adrenoceptors with guanfacine protects rodent prefrontal cortex dendritic spines and cognition from the effects of chronic stress. *Neurobiol Stress* 2015;2:1–9.

120. Ren WW, Liu Y, Li BM. Stimulation of α(2A)-adrenoceptors promotes the maturation of dendritic spines in cultured neurons of the medial prefrontal cortex. *Mol Cell Neurosci* 2011;49:205–216.

121. Gyoneva S, Traynelis SF. Norepinephrine modulates the motility of resting and activated microglia via different adrenergic receptors. *J Biol Chem* 2013;288:15291–15302.

122. Wang M, Vijayraghavan S, Goldman-Rakic PS. Selective D2 receptor actions on the functional circuitry of working memory. *Science* 2004;303:853–856.

123. Moghaddam B, Adams BW, Verma A, et al. Activation of glutamatergic neurotransmission by ketamine: A novel step in the pathway from NMDA receptor blockade to dopaminergic and cognitive disruptions associated with the prefrontal cortex. *J Neurosci* 1997;17(8):2921–2927.

124. Shi WX, Zhang XX. Dendritic glutamate-induced bursting in the prefrontal cortex: Further characterization and effects of phencyclidine. *J Pharmacol Exp Ther* 2003;305:680–687.

125. Defelipe J. The evolution of the brain, the human nature of cortical circuits, and intellectual creativity. *Front Neuroanat* 2011;5:29.

126. Bellgrove MA, Domschke K, Hawi Z, et al. The methionine allele of the COMT polymorphism impairs prefrontal cognition in children and adolescents with ADHD. *Exp Brain Res* 2005;163:352–360.

127. Bertolino A, Blasi G, Latorre V, et al. Additive effects of genetic variation in dopamine regulating genes on working memory cortical activity in human brain. *J Neurosci* 2006;26:3918–3922.

128. Williams-Gray CH, Hampshire A, Robbins TW, et al. Catechol *O*-methyltransferase Val158Met genotype influences frontoparietal activity during planning in patients with Parkinson's disease. *J Neurosci* 2007;27:4832–4838.

129. Jacobs E, D'Esposito M. Estrogen shapes dopamine-dependent cognitive processes: Implications for women's health. *J Neurosci* 2011;31:5286–5293.

130. Qin S, Cousijn H, Rijpkema M, et al. The effect of moderate acute psychological stress on working memory-related neural activity is modulated by a genetic variation in catecholaminergic function in humans. *Front Integr Neurosci* 2012;6:16.

131. Gibbs SE, D'Esposito M. A functional magnetic resonance imaging study of the effects of pergolide, a dopamine receptor agonist, on component processes of working memory. *Neuroscience* 2006;139:359–371.

132. Cools R, D'Esposito M. Inverted U-shaped dopamine actions on human working memory and cognitive control. *Biol Psychiatry* 2011;69:e113–e125.

133. Rosell DR, Zaluda LC, McClure MM, et al. Effects of the D1 dopamine receptor agonist dihydrexidine (DAR-0100A) on working memory in schizotypal personality disorder. *Neuropsychopharmacology* 2015;40:446–453.

134. Arnsten AFT, Steere JC, Hunt RD. The contribution of alpha-2 noradrenergic mechanisms to prefrontal cortical cognitive function: Potential significance to attention deficit hyperactivity disorder. *Arch Gen Psychiatry* 1996;53:448–455.

135. Biederman J, Melmed RD, Patel A, et al. A randomized, double-blind, placebo-controlled study of guanfacine extended release in children and adolescents with attention-deficit/hyperactivity disorder. *Pediatrics* 2008;121:e73–e84.

136. Scahill L, Chappell PB, Kim YS, et al. A placebo-controlled study of guanfacine in the treatment of children with tic disorders and attention deficit hyperactivity disorder. *Am J Psychiatry* 2001;158:1067–1074.

137. McCracken JT, Aman MG, McDougle CJ, et al. Possible influence of variant of the P-glycoprotein gene (MDR1/ABCB1) on clinical response to guanfacine in children with pervasive developmental disorders and hyperactivity. *J Child Adolesc Psychopharmacol* 2010;20:1–5.

138. Connor DF, Grasso DJ, Slivinsky MD, et al. An open-label study of guanfacine extended release for traumatic stress related symptoms in children and adolescents. *J Child Adolescent Psychopharmacol* 2013;23:244–251.

139. Arnsten AFT, Raskind M, Taylor FB, et al. The effects of stress exposure on prefrontal cortex: Translating basic research into successful treatments for post-traumatic stress disorder. *Neurobiol Stress* 2015;1:89–99.

140. McAllister TW, McDonald BC, Flashman LA, et al. Alpha-2 adrenergic challenge with guanfacine one month after mild traumatic brain injury: Altered working memory and BOLD response. *Int J Psychophysiol* 2011;82:107–114.

141. Fox HC, Seo D, Tuit K, et al. Guanfacine effects on stress, drug craving and prefrontal activation in cocaine dependent individuals: Preliminary findings. *J Psychopharmacol* 2012;26:958–972.

142. McKee S, Potenza M, Kober H, et al. α2A-AR agonist shows promise for nicotine dependence: Enhancing self control during stress. *J Psychopharmacol* 2014.

143. Malhotra PA, Parton AD, Greenwood R, et al. Noradrenergic modulation of space exploration in visual neglect. *Ann Neurol* 2006;59:186–190.

144. Singh-Curry V, Malhotra P, Farmer SF, et al. Attention deficits following ADEM ameliorated by guanfacine. *J Neurol Neurosurg Psychiatry* 2011;82:688–690.

145. Cannon TD, Chung Y, He G, et al. Progressive reduction in cortical thickness as psychosis develops: A multisite longitudinal neuroimaging study of youth at elevated clinical risk. *Biol Psychiatry* 2015;77(2):147–157.

146. Birnbaum SG, Gobeske KT, Auerbach J, et al. A role for norepinephrine in stress-induced cognitive deficits: Alpha-1-adrenoceptor mediation in prefrontal cortex. *Biol Psychiatry* 1999;46:1266–1274.

147. Raskind MA, Peskind ER, Kanter ED, et al. Reduction in nightmares and other PTSD symptoms in combat veterans by prazosin: A placebo-controlled study. *Am J Psychiatry* 2003;160:371–373.

148. Taylor FB, Lowe K, Thompson C, et al. Daytime prazosin reduces psychological distress to trauma-specific cues in civilian trauma posttraumatic stress disorder. *Biol Psychiatry* 2006;59:577–581.

149. Nestler EJ, Alreja M, Aghajanian GK. Molecular control of locus coeruleus neurotransmission. *Biol Psychiatry* 1999;46(9):1131–1139.

150. Miner LH, Jedema HP, Moore FW, et al. Chronic stress increases the plasmalemmal distribution of the norepinephrine transporter and the coexpression of tyrosine hydroxylase in norepinephrine axons in the prefrontal cortex. *J Neurosci* 2006;26:1571–1578.

151. Bangasser DA, Valentino RJ. Sex differences in molecular and cellular substrates of stress. *Cell Mol Neurobiol* 2012;32:709–723.

152. Preskorn SH, Gawryl M, Dgetluck N, et al. Normalizing effects of EVP-6124, an α-7 nicotinic partial agonist, on event-related potentials and cognition: A proof of concept, randomized trial in patients with schizophrenia. *J Psychiatr Pract* 2014;20:12–24.

153. Preuss T. Do rats have prefrontal cortex? The Rose–Woolsey–Akert program reconsidered. *J Cognit Neurosci* 1995;7:1–26.

154. Brozoski T, Brown RM, Rosvold HE, et al. Cognitive deficit caused by regional depletion of dopamine in prefrontal cortex of rhesus monkey. *Science* 1979;205:929–931.

155. Clarke HF, Walker SC, Dalley JW, et al. Cognitive inflexibility after prefrontal serotonin depletion is behaviorally and neurochemically specific. *Cereb Cortex* 2007;17:18–27.

156. Roberts AC. The importance of serotonin for orbitofrontal function. *Biol Psychiatry* 2011;69:1185–1191.

THREE

Cognitive Enhancers for Alzheimer's Disease

PO-HENG TSAI

DEMENTIA DESCRIBES A DECLINE IN COGNITION THAT IS SEVERE ENOUGH to interfere with a person's ability to work or perform usual everyday activities.[1] Alzheimer's disease (AD) is the most common cause of dementia. In the United States, an estimated 5.3 million people had AD dementia in 2015, including 200,000 individuals who were younger than age 65 years. The number of people who are affected by AD is projected to reach 16 million by 2050. There is a tremendous cost associated with caring for people with AD. In 2015, the direct cost to US society of caring for those with AD totaled an estimated $226 billion, and if no effective disease-modifying treatments become available, this cost could increase to $1.1 trillion by 2050. In addition to medical costs, in 2014, caregivers of people with AD and other dementias provided an estimated 17.9 billion hours of unpaid assistance, which translates to a value of $217.7 billion. Furthermore, a large percentage of caregivers report a high rate of emotional stress associated with caregiving.[2] Therefore, cognitive enhancers for AD could address symptoms associated with AD, reduce caregiver burden, and limit health care costs.

PHARMACOLOGICAL INTERVENTIONS

Currently, two classes of medication are approved by the US Food and Drug Administration (FDA) for the treatment of cognitive symptoms in AD: (1) cholinesterase inhibitors, including donepezil, galantamine, and rivastigmine; and (2) memantine, an N-methyl-D-aspartate (NMDA) receptor antagonist. In addition, medical foods, such as Axona, CerefolinNAC, and Souvenaid, are available for dietary management of AD.

Cholinesterase Inhibitors

Three cholinesterase inhibitors are currently available for the treatment of AD: donepezil, galantamine, and rivastigmine. Tacrine, the first cholinesterase inhibitor approved by the FDA, was withdrawn from the US market in 2012 due to concern regarding its hepatotoxicity. Cholinesterase inhibitors reversibly bind to and inactivate acetylcholinesterase, which is a postsynaptic enzyme that breaks down the neurotransmitter acetylcholine. As a result, more acetylcholine molecules are available for cholinergic transmission. The rationale for their use is based on biochemical and pathological studies of AD demonstrating acetylcholine deficiency associated with degeneration of cholinergic neurons of nucleus basalis of Meynert in the basal forebrain.[3,4] Additional mechanisms of action that enhance acetylcholine action have been proposed for rivastigmine and galantamine. Rivastigmine inhibits butyrylcholinesterase, a nonspecific cholinesterase, and galantamine acts as an allosteric potentiating ligand of neuronal nicotinic receptors for acetylcholine[5] (Table 3.1).

Randomized, double-blind, placebo-controlled trials (RCTs) have been conducted to demonstrate the efficacy of the three medications. The cholinesterase inhibitors with modest effect have been shown to improve cognition, activities of daily living (ADLs), global change, and possibly behavior compared to placebo.[6,7] A small percentage of subjects have an immediate improvement in cognition, and a larger percentage of patients are temporarily stabilized. Observational and open-label extension studies suggest that the benefits of cholinesterase inhibitors could persist for several years.[8]

The most common adverse reactions are gastrointestinal symptoms related to cholinergic effect on the parasympathetic nervous system, including nausea, vomiting, and diarrhea. These side effects can be reduced by increasing the dose titration duration, giving the medication with food, or reducing the dose.

TABLE 3.1   Administration, Pharmacology, and Common Adverse Reactions of Cholinesterase Inhibitors

	Donepezil	Galantamine	Rivastigmine Oral Formulation	Rivastigmine Transdermal System
Dosage and titration	Start at 5 mg daily and increase to 10 mg after 4–6 weeks. The dosage can then be increased to 23 mg daily for severe AD after at least 3 months.	Start at 4 mg twice daily (or 8 mg daily for ER formulation) and increase by 4 mg twice daily (or 8 mg ER daily) every 4 weeks at the minimum to maximum dosage of 12 mg twice daily (or 24 mg ER daily).	Start at 1.5 mg twice daily and increase by 1.5 mg twice daily every 2 weeks at the minimum to a maximum dosage of 6 mg twice daily.	Start at 4.6 mg daily and increase to 9.5 mg after a minimum of 4 weeks. The dosage can then be increased to 13.3 mg for severe AD after at least 4 weeks.
Conversion between formulations	Not applicable	Conversion from immediate-release to ER formulation occurs on the same total daily dosage (e.g., 8 mg twice daily to 16 mg ER daily).	A total daily dose of <6 mg of oral rivastigmine can be switched to the 4.6 mg/24 hours rivastigmine patch, and a total daily dose of 6 mg to 12 mg of oral rivastigmine can be switched to the 9.5 mg/24 hours patch.	
Elimination half-life	70 hours	7 hours	1.5 hours	3 hours (peripheral); 8 hours in CNS; 24 hours for patch formulation
Absorption	Can be given with or without food	Give with food	Give with food	Highest when applied to upper back, chest, or upper arm
Most common adverse reactions	Nausea, diarrhea, insomnia, vomiting, muscle cramps, fatigue, and anorexia	Nausea, vomiting, diarrhea, anorexia, and weight decrease	Nausea, vomiting, anorexia, dyspepsia, and asthenia	Nausea, vomiting, diarrhea, depression, headache, anxiety, and application site reaction

AD, Alzheimer's disease; CNS, central nervous system; ER, extended release.

Donepezil

Donepezil is available in tablets in three strengths (5, 10, and 23 mg) and in orally disintegrating tablets in two strengths (5 and 10 mg). It is approved by the FDA for treatment of mild, moderate, and severe AD dementia.

Galantamine

Galantamine is available in immediate-release tablets in three strengths (4, 8, and 12 mg) and as extended-release capsules in three strengths (8, 16, and 24 mg). It is also available as a 4 mg/ml oral solution. It is approved for the treatment of mild to moderate AD dementia.

Rivastigmine

Rivastigmine is available in capsules in four strengths (1.5, 3, 4.5, and 6 mg), as a 240-hour transdermal system ("patch") in three strengths (4.6, 9.5, and 13.3 mg), and as a 2 mg/ml oral solution. It is approved for the treatment of mild, moderate, and severe AD dementia.

Management of Cholinesterase Inhibitors

Studies comparing the three cholinesterase inhibitors and meta-analyses have generally demonstrated similar levels of efficacy and adverse reactions among the three medications.[6,7,9] If therapy with one agent is ineffective or there is loss of efficacy or intolerable side effects, it is reasonable to switch to an alternative agent. It is recommended that a minimum of 6 months should be allowed after reaching optimal dosage of the initial therapy before contemplating a switch in medication. A prolonged washout period is not necessary unless the initial agent resulted in significant adverse reactions. The new medication should be started at the lowest dosage and titrated up as tolerated.[10,11]

Memantine

Excitotoxicity refers to the pathological process in which neurons are damaged or killed via excessive stimulation by excitatory neurotransmitters such as glutamate. This overstimulation leads to persistent activation of NMDA receptors and an influx of calcium ions that triggers a cascade of events such as lipid peroxidation, nucleic acid damage, and mitochondrial disruption, which result in cell death. It has been hypothesized to be involved in neurodegenerative disorders such as AD. Memantine is a low- to moderate-affinity, noncompetitive NMDA receptor antagonist that binds preferentially to the NMDA receptor-operated cation channels and blocks excessive NDMA receptor activity.[12,13]

Memantine is approved by the FDA for the treatment of moderate to severe AD dementia. Its efficacy has been demonstrated through RCTs, with beneficial effects seen in cognition, ADLs, and behaviors in patients with AD.[14,15]

Memantine is available in tablets in two strengths (5 and 10 mg), in extended-release capsule formulation in four strengths (7, 14, 21, and 28 mg), and as a 2 mg/ml oral solution (Table 3.2).

The principal adverse reactions of memantine are dizziness, headaches, and somnolence.

Combination Therapy

Combination therapy of cholinesterase inhibitors and memantine has been advocated due to their different and potentially complementary mechanisms of action. Randomized controlled trials and meta-analysis have demonstrated benefits of combination therapy in cognition, ADLs, behavior, and global change in patients with moderate to severe AD dementia. Safety profile and tolerability are generally good.[16–19] Memantine is usually added to a cholinesterase inhibitor after the patient has been on treatment with a cholinesterase inhibitor for at least 6 months with a

TABLE 3.2 Administration, Pharmacology, and Common Adverse Reactions of Memantine

	Tablet and Oral Solution	Extended-Release Capsule Formulation
Dosage and titration	Start at 5 mg once daily and increase by 5 mg daily every week at the minimum to maximum dosage of 10 mg twice daily (5 mg daily to 5 mg twice daily to 5 mg and 10 mg separately to 10 mg twice daily).	Start at 7 mg ER once daily and increase by 7 mg daily every week at the minimum to maximum dosage of 28 mg ER daily.
Conversion between formulations	Patients taking 10 mg twice daily of memantine tablet can be converted to 28 mg ER formulation once daily after the last tablet dose.	
Elimination half-life	60–80 hours	
Absorption	Can be given with or without food	
Most common adverse reactions	Dizziness, confusion, headache, and constipation	Headache, diarrhea, and dizziness

ER, extended release.

stable dosing regimen for at least 3 months. Combination therapy is usually initiated due to decline of a patient's status while on monotherapy. Donepezil and memantine are available in a single-capsule fix combination (Namzaric).

Medical Foods

The term *medical food* is defined in the FDA's Orphan Drug Act (21 U.S.C. 360ee (b) (3)) section 5(b) as

> a food which is formulated to be consumed or administered enterally under the supervision of a physician and which is intended for the specific dietary man-agement of a disease or condition for which distinctive nutritional requirements, based on recognized scientific principles, are established by medical evaluation.

Medical foods must have constituents generally recognized as safe (GRAS) and suitable and must comply with all applicable FDA provisions, but they do not have to undergo approval by the FDA. Medical foods are also exempted from the labeling requirements for health claims and nutrient content claims under the Nutrition Labeling and Education Act of 1990 (see 21 U.S.C. 343 (q) (5) (A) (iv)). Currently, there are three medical foods available to address the metabolic and nutritional needs of AD: Axona, CerefolinNAC, and Souvenaid. Souvenaid is available in Europe but not in the United States (Table 3.3).

Axona (Caprylic Triglyceride)

One of the metabolic signatures of AD is the progressive reduction of cerebral glu-cose metabolism in posterior cingulate, parietal, and temporal regions as measured by ^{18}F-fluorodeoxyglucose positron emission tomography studies.[20] Axona is a propri-etary formulation of caprylic triglyceride, a medium-chain fatty acid. It is converted by the liver into ketone bodies, which are theorized to provide an alternative energy source for the brains of AD patients that are not able to utilize glucose efficiently.[21]

A 90-day Phase II RCT was carried out to assess the efficacy of Axona in patients with mild to moderate AD.[22] The study demonstrated statistically significant improve-ment in cognition on day 45 but not on day 90. After the results were stratified by APOE4 (epsilon 4 variant of the apolipoprotein E gene) status, statistically significant differences in cognition were observed on both day 45 and day 90 for those patients who did not possess APOE4. No significant difference in global change was observed. The most common adverse reaction was gastrointestinal side effects such as diarrhea, flatulence, and dyspepsia, which could be reduced by slow titration of the dosage.

TABLE 3.3 Formulation, Administration, and Common Adverse Reactions of Medical Foods

	Axona	CerefolinNAC	Souvenaid
Dosage and formulation	Powder supplied in 40-g packet with each packet containing 20 g of caprylic triglyceride. A titration kit is also available.	Caplet containing 6 mg of L-methylfolate calcium, 2 mg of methylcobalamin, and 600 mg of N-acetyl-L-cysteine.	Bottle of 125 ml of nutrition drink containing 300 mg of EPA, 1200 mg of DHA, 106 mg of phospholipids, 400 mg of choline, 625 mg of UMP, 40 mg of vitamin E, 80 mg of vitamin C, 60 μg of selenium, 3 μg of vitamin B_{12}, 1 mg of vitamin B_6, and 400 μg of folic acid.
Administration	Fully mix powder in cold water or other liquids and take after a full meal once daily.	One caplet once daily	One bottle once daily
Titration	1 tbsp for 2 days, 2 tbsp for 2 days, 3 tbsp for 2 days, 4 tbsp on day 7, and then one 40-g packet daily	Not applicable	Not applicable
Most common adverse reactions	Diarrhea, flatulence, and dyspepsia	Mild transient diarrhea, polycythemia vera, itching, transitory exanthema, and the feeling of swelling of the entire body have been associated with methylcobalamin. Nausea, vomiting, diarrhea, transient skin rash, flushing, epigastric pain, and constipation have been associated with N-acetyl-L-cysteine.	Gastrointestinal: constipation, diarrhea, flatulence, and nausea

DHA, docosahexaenoic acid; EPA, eicosapentaenoic acid; tbsp, tablespoon; UMP, uridine monophosphate.

CerefolinNAC

The active ingredients of CerefolinNAC consist of methylcobalamine, L-methylfolate, and N-acetylcysteine. Methylcobalamine and L-methylfolate are proposed to decrease the level of homocysteine, whereas N-acetylcysteine increases the level of glutathione.

An elevated level of homocysteine has been associated with the development of AD and memory impairment in observational studies.[23] In addition, hyperhomocysteinemia has been shown to impair DNA repair in hippocampal neurons, to sensitize them to amyloid toxicity, and to increases β-amyloid by enhancing expression of γ-secretase in animal models of AD.[24,25]

Oxidative stress reflects an imbalance between the production of reactive oxidative species (ROS) and the antioxidant system that detoxifies ROS. Oxidative imbalance has been implicated in the pathogenesis of AD.[26] Levels of glutathione, which is part of the antioxidant system, have been observed to be decreased in AD.[27]

The efficacy of CerefolinNAC has not been demonstrated by RCTs. There are open-label and case studies that have shown ingredients of CerefolinNAC to be beneficial in AD.[28] A recent RCT demonstrated clinical benefits and slowing of the rate of cerebral atrophy in patients with mild cognitive impairment treated with B vitamins during a 2-year period.[29,30]

Souvenaid

Synaptic loss is considered to be one of the important pathological features of AD because of its close correlation with onset of memory loss.[31] Souvenaid contains a patented combination of nutrients that includes omega-3 fatty acids, choline, uridine monophosphate, and a mixture of antioxidants and B vitamins. This mixture is theorized to restore synaptic function by providing rate-limiting precursors for membrane phospholipid synthesis, increasing levels of synaptic proteins, and promoting formation of dendritic spines.[32,33]

The results of two RCTs designed to assess the efficacy of Souvenaid in patients with mild AD have been published.[34,35] The first trial was a 12-week trial with optional 12-week extension. The study demonstrated statistically significant improvement in delayed recall of verbal memory but no differences in ADL, behavior, or global change (the trial was not powered to show differences in these outcomes). The second trial was 24 weeks long and demonstrated a significant increase in memory domain score of a neuropsychologist test battery. The study also included functional status and electroencephalogram (EEG), which was used as a marker of synaptic connectivity, as secondary outcomes. There was no difference in functional status, but EEG delta bands were significantly different, suggesting that the treatment group had improved connectivity.

Implementing Treatment with Medical Foods

Medical foods represent an alternative to standard therapy with cholinesterase inhibitors and memantine. They are usually used as an "add-on" therapy in patients who are declining on standard pharmacotherapy. Side effect monitoring is important to enhance treatment adherence and patient safety.

NONPHARMACOLOGICAL INTERVENTIONS

Given the fact that currently available pharmacotherapies offer only modest improvement of cognitive symptoms associated with AD, there has been an increased interest in using nonpharmacological techniques such as physical activities, cognitive interventions, and noninvasive brain stimulations as therapy options.

Physical Activities

Various mechanisms have been proposed to explain the role of physical activity in brain health enhancement. One theory is that regular exercise improves cerebrovascular perfusion via decreases in blood pressure and oxidative stress and an increase in antioxidant activity. In addition, physical activity is associated with elevated levels of brain-derived neurotrophic factor and nitric oxide, which promote neurogenesis, angiogenesis, and synaptogenesis.[36] Neuroimaging studies have also demonstrated that physical activity leads to an increase in the size of the hippocampus and other brain regions, such as the prefrontal cortex.[37]

A recent systematic review was published by the Cochrane Collaboration on the topic of exercise programs for people with dementia.[38] The review examined 17 RCTs with 1067 participants and concluded that there was no clear evidence of benefit from exercise on cognitive functioning. However, there is promising evidence that exercise programs may improve the ability to perform ADLs in people with dementia. It was noted that the included trials were highly heterogeneous in the dementia subtype and severity and also in the type, duration, and frequency of the exercises.

Another recent systemic review was performed that focused specifically on AD dementia.[39] It identified six RCTs with exercise intervention for at least 4 weeks' duration and concluded that there is preliminary evidence of the beneficial effects of exercise on cognition for people with AD. Meta-analysis was carried out on four of the six trials with objective cognitive outcomes assessment, which revealed a positive effect on global cognitive function. Again, there was heterogeneity regarding the type, duration, and frequency of exercises. Multiple-dimensional interventions including physical exercise and diet optimization have been shown to be associated with better cognition in individuals with normal cognition or mild impairment.[40]

Cognitive Interventions

Three approaches in cognitive intervention have been described in AD: cognitive stimulation, cognitive training, and cognitive rehabilitation.[41] Proposed mechanisms of cognitive enhancement include increase of cognitive reserve, which is defined as the brain's ability to perform cognitive tasks adequately despite neuropathological damage, and increase of central nervous system plasticity via regular activation of various brain networks from cognitive interventions[42] (Table 3.4).

A Cochrane meta-analysis identified 11 RCTs with cognitive training and 1 RCT with cognitive rehabilitation as active treatment for mild to moderate AD and vascular dementia.[41] The authors concluded that no significant benefit was derived from cognitive training, but the sole cognitive rehabilitation trial showed promise. Another Cochrane review analyzed 15 RCTs that utilized cognitive stimulation in people with dementia.[43] The meta-analysis demonstrated evidence that cognitive stimulation had beneficial effect on cognition in people with mild to moderate dementia over and above any medication effects. However, the authors had concerns regarding quality variability, small sample sizes, and lack of randomization method transparency in the trials.

Another recent meta-analysis investigating cognitive interventions in dementia reaffirmed that cognitive stimulation improves scores on cognitive measures of Mini-Mental State Examination (MMSE) and Alzheimer's Disease Assessment Scale-Cognition (ADAS-Cog), although clinical significance of ADAS-Cog change is weak.[44] In addition, the analysis highlighted the difficulty of blinding of patients and use of appropriate placebo controls in cognitive intervention trials.

TABLE 3.4 Definitions of Cognitive Interventions

Cognitive Stimulation	Cognitive Training	Cognitive Rehabilitation
Engagement in a range of activities and discussions, usually taken place in a group setting, that aim to enhance general cognitive and social functioning	Involvement in repeated guided practice on a set of standardized tasks designed to reflect particular cognitive functions, such as memory, attention, or problem-solving	Implementation of individualized approach on personally relevant compensatory strategies to improve daily functioning

There are also studies that have demonstrated benefits with combined physical activity and cognitive intervention.[45]

Noninvasive Brain Stimulation

The two most commonly employed methods of noninvasive brain stimulations are transcranial magnetic stimulation (TMS) and transcranial direct current stimulation (tDCS).[46] TMS is administered via a coiled wire placed on the scalp, through which a brief electric current is delivered. It is believed to modulate cortical plasticity from altered neuronal activity induced by the time-varying magnetic field generated by the stimulation. On the other hand, in tDCS, a weak electrical current is delivered through two scalp electrodes placed in accordance with the international 10–20 system. tDCS is speculated to exert its effect by modulating cortical excitability by changing spontaneous neuronal activity in a polarity-specific manner.

The effects of TMS and tDCS on cognitive and neuropsychiatric symptoms in dementias were evaluated in a recent systemic review.[46] The authors identified 13 trials that investigated noninvasive brain stimulations in AD and concluded that there was a general trend for improvements across a wide range of cognitive outcome measures following treatment with TMS and tDCS. However, the majority of the trials were open label in design, had small sample sizes, and varied in stimulation protocols.

CONCLUSION

Current pharmacological therapies for AD offer modest cognitive improvement. New treatment options such as disease-modifying agents and new symptomatic drugs are being developed, and some are in clinical trials. There is optimism regarding nonpharmacological interventions, but the lack of consensus regarding the specifics of methodology makes implementation of these strategies difficult. Optimal disease management will evolve as successful new medications emerge and the practice of nonpharmacological treatments is better defined.

REFERENCES

1. McKhann GM, Knopman DS, Chertkow H, et al. The diagnosis of dementia due to Alzheimer's disease: Recommendations from the National Institute on Aging–Alzheimer's Association workgroups on diagnostic guidelines for Alzheimer's disease. *Alzheimers Dement* 2011;7(3):263–269.
2. Alzheimer's Association. 2015 Alzheimer's disease facts and figures. *Alzheimers Dement* 2015;11(3):332–384.
3. Mesulam M, Shaw P, Mash D, et al. Cholinergic nucleus basalis tauopathy emerges early in the aging–MCI–AD continuum. *Ann Neurol* 2004;55(6):815–828.

4. Whitehouse PJ, Price DL, Clark AW, et al. Alzheimer disease: Evidence for selective loss of cholinergic neurons in the nucleus basalis. *Ann Neurol* 1981;10:122–126.

5. Villarroya M, García AG, Marco JL. New classes of AChE inhibitors with additional pharmacological effects of interest for the treatment of Alzheimer's disease. *Curr Pharm Des* 2004;10(25):3177–3184.

6. Birks J. Cholinesterase inhibitors for Alzheimer's disease. *Cochrane Database Syst Rev* 2006;2006(1):CD005593.

7. Hansen RA, Gartlehner G, Webb AP, et al. Efficacy and safety of donepezil, galantamine, and rivastigmine for the treatment of Alzheimer's disease: A systematic review and meta-analysis. *Clin Interv Aging* 2008;3(2):211–225.

8. Zhu CW, Livote EE, Scarmeas N, et al. Long-term associations between cholinesterase inhibitors and memantine use and health outcomes among patients with Alzheimer's disease. *Alzheimers Dement* 2013;9(6):733–740.

9. Alva G, Cummings JL. Relative tolerability of Alzheimer's disease treatments. *Psychiatry (Edgmont)* 2008;5(11):27–36.

10. Gauthier S, Emre M, Farlow MR, et al. Strategies for continued successful treatment of Alzheimer's disease: Switching cholinesterase inhibitors. *Curr Med Res Opin* 2003;19(8):707–714.

11. Bartorelli L, Giraldi C, Saccardo M, et al. Effects of switching from an AChE inhibitor to a dual AchE–BuChE inhibitor in patients with Alzheimer's disease. *Curr Med Res Opin* 2005;21(11):1809–1818.

12. Rogawski MA, Wenk GL. The neuropharmacological basis for the use of memantine in the treatment of Alzheimer's disease. *CNS Drug Rev* 2003;9(3): 275–308.

13. Lipton SA. Paradigm shift in NMDA receptor antagonist drug development: Molecular mechanism of uncompetitive inhibition by memantine in the treatment of Alzheimer's disease and other neurologic disorders. *J Alzheimers Dis* 2004;6(6 Suppl):S61–S74.

14. McShane R, Areosa Sastre A, Minakaran N. Memantine for dementia. *Cochrane Database Syst Rev* 2006;2006(2):CD003154.

15. Maidment ID, Fox CG, Boustani M, et al. Efficacy of memantine on behavioral and psychological symptoms related to dementia: A systematic meta-analysis. *Ann Pharmacother* 2008;42(1):32–38.

16. Tariot PN, Farlow MR, Grossberg GT, et al.; Memantine Study Group. Memantine treatment in patients with moderate to severe Alzheimer disease already receiving donepezil: A randomized controlled trial. *JAMA* 2004;291:317–324.

17. Feldman HH, Schmitt FA, Olin JT. Activities of daily living in moderate-to-severe Alzheimer disease: An analysis of the treatment effects of memantine in patients receiving stable donepezil treatment. *Alzheimer Dis Assoc Disord* 2006;20(4):263–268.

18. Porsteinsson AP, Grossberg GT, Mintzer J, et al; Memantine MEM–MD-12 Study Group. Memantine treatment in patients with mild to moderate Alzheimer's disease already receiving a cholinesterase inhibitor: A randomized, double-blind, placebo-controlled trial. *Curr Alzheimer Res* 2008;5:83–89.

19. Atri A, Molinuevo JL, Lemming O, et al. Memantine in patients with Alzheimer's disease receiving donepezil: New analyses of efficacy and safety for combination therapy. *Alzheimers Res Ther* 2013;5(1):6.

20. Minoshima S, Giordani B, Berent S, et al. Metabolic reduction in the posterior cingulate cortex in very early Alzheimer's disease. *Ann Neurol* 1997;42(1):85–94.

21. Henderson ST. Ketone bodies as a therapeutic for Alzheimer's disease. *Neurotherapeutics* 2008;5(3):470–480.

22. Henderson ST, Vogel JL, Barr LJ, et al. Study of the ketogenic agent AC-1202 in mild to moderate Alzheimer's disease: A randomized, double-blind, placebo-controlled, multicenter trial. *Nutr Metab (Lond)* 2009;6:31. (Published online August 10, 2009; doi:10.1186/1743-7075-6-31)

23. Seshadri S, Beiser A, Selhub J, et al. Plasma homocysteine as a risk factor for dementia and Alzheimer's disease. *N Engl J Med* 2002;346(7):476–483.

24. Kruman II, Kumartavel TS, Lohani A, et al. Folic acid deficiency and homocysteine impair DNA repair in hippocampal neurons and sensitize them to amyloid toxicity in experimental models of Alzheimer's disease. *J Neurosci* 2002;70:694–702

25. Zhang CE, Wei W, Liu YH, et al. Hyperhomocysteinemia increases β-amyloid by enhancing expression of γ-secretase on phosphorylation of amyloid precursor protein in rat brain. *Am J Pathol* 2009;174:1481–1491.

26. Guidi I, Galimberti D, Lonarti S, et al. Oxidative imbalance in patients with mild cognitive impairment and Alzheimer's disease. *Neurobiol Aging* 2006;27(2):262–269.

27. Puertas MC, Martínez-Martos JM, Cobo MP, et al. Plasma oxidative stress parameters in men and women with early stage Alzheimer type dementia. *Exp Gerontol* 2012;47:625–630.

28. McCaddon A, Hudson PR. L-Methylfolate, methylcobalamin, and N-acetylcysteine in the treatment of Alzheimer's disease-related cognitive decline. *CNS Spectr* 2010;15(Suppl 11):2–5.

29. de Jager CA, Oulhaj A, Jacoby R, et al. Cognitive and clinical outcomes of homocysteine-lowering B-vitamin treatment in mild cognitive impairment: A randomized controlled trial. *Int J Geriatr Psychiatry* 2012;27(6):592–600.

30. Douaud G, Refsum H, de Jager CA, et al. Preventing Alzheimer's disease-related gray matter atrophy by B-vitamin treatment. *Proc Natl Acad Sci USA* 2013;110(23):9523–9528.

31. Selkoe DJ. Alzheimer's disease is a synaptic failure. *Science* 2002;298(5594): 789–791.

32. Cansev M, Wurtman RJ. Chronic administration of docosahexaenoic acid or eicosapentaenoic acid, but not arachidonic acid, alone or in combination with uridine, increases brain phosphatide and synaptic protein levels in gerbils. *Neuroscience* 2007;148(2):421–431.

33. Sakamoto T, Cansev M, Wurtman RJ. Oral supplementation with docosahexaenoic acid and uridine-5′-monophosphate increases dendritic spine density in adult gerbil hippocampus. *Brain Res* 2007;1182:50–59.

34. Scheltens P, Kamphuis PJ, Verhey FR, et al. Efficacy of a medical food in mild Alzheimer's disease: A randomized controlled trial. *Alzheimers Dement* 2010;6(1):1–10.

35. Scheltens P, Stam CJ, Swinkels SH, et al. Efficacy of Souvenaid in mild Alzheimer's disease: Results from a randomized, controlled trial. *J Alzheimer's Dis* 2012;31(1):225–236.

36. Davenport MH, Hogan DB, Eskes GA, et al. Cerebrovascular reserve: The link between fitness and cognitive function? *Exerc Sport Sci Rev* 2012;40(3):153–158.

37. Erickson KI, Weinstein AM, Lopez OL. Physical activity, brain plasticity, and Alzheimer's disease. *Arch Med Res* 2012;43(8):615–621.

38. Forbes D, Forbes SC, Blake CM, et al. Exercise programs for people with dementia. *Cochrane Database Syst Rev* 2015;2015(4):CD006489.

39. Farina N, Rusted J, Tabet N. The effect of exercise interventions on cognitive outcome in Alzheimer's disease: A systematic review. *Int Psychogeriatr* 2014;26(1):9–18.

40. Zhong K, Cummings J. Healthybrains.org: From registry to randomization. *J Prev Alzheimer's Dis*, 2016;3(3):123–126.

41. Bahar-Fuchs A, Clare L, Woods B. Cognitive training and cognitive rehabilitation for mild to moderate Alzheimer's disease and vascular dementia. *Cochrane Database Syst Rev* 2013;2013(6):CD003260.

42. Buschert V, Bokde AL, Hampel H. Cognitive intervention in Alzheimer disease. *Nat Rev Neurol* 2010;6:508–517.

43. Woods B, Aguirre E, Spector AE, et al. Cognitive stimulation to improve cognitive functioning in people with dementia. *Cochrane Database Syst Rev* 2012;2012(2):CD005562.

44. Huntley JD, Gould RL, Liu K, et al. Do cognitive interventions improve general cognition in dementia? A meta-analysis and meta-regression. *BMJ Open* 2015;5:e005247.

45. Graessel E, Stemmer R, Eichenseer B, et al. Non-pharmacological, multicomponent group therapy in patients with degenerative dementia: A 12-month randomized, controlled trial. *BMC Med* 2011;9:129.

46. Elder GJ, Taylor JP. Transcranial magnetic stimulation and transcranial direct current stimulation: Treatments for cognitive and neuropsychiatric symptoms in the neurodegenerative dementias? *Alzheimers Res Ther* 2014;6(9):74.

FOUR

Cognitive Enhancement in Non-Alzheimer's Dementias

BABAK TOUSI

COGNITIVE ENHANCEMENT IN VASCULAR DEMENTIA

Cognitive impairment in vascular dementia (VaD) results from the disruption of the frontal–subcortical circuits that underlie social behavior, cognitive, and executive cortical functions.[1] Executive dysfunction can be caused by interruption of the dorsolateral prefrontal subcortical circuit, whereas disinhibition, personality change, and emotional lability can be caused by interruption in the orbitofrontal–subcortical loop.[1] The contribution of cholinergic pathways disruption to the clinical presentation of VaD has been the rationale for using cholinesterase inhibitors to treat dementia related to cerebrovascular diseases.[2]

Cholinesterase Inhibitors

Cholinesterase inhibitors, including donepezil, galantamine, and rivastigmine, are considered to be the first-line medicines used for Alzheimer's disease, producing some benefits, but they do not have regulatory approval for treatment of VaD in the United States and most of Europe.[3]

In a double-blind study of galantamine 24 mg/day in patients with VaD or Alzheimer's disease combined with cerebrovascular disease, galantamine showed greater efficacy than placebo on the Alzheimer's Disease Assessment Scale-Cognitive subscale (ADAS-Cog) and the Clinical Interview-Based Impression of Change with Caregiver Input (CIBIC-Plus).[4] Galantamine also showed a therapeutic effect on activities of daily living (ADLs) and behavioral symptoms.[4] During the open-label extension phase of this study, galantamine treatment showed similar sustained benefits in terms of maintenance of or improvement in cognition (ADAS-Cog/11), functional ability (Disability Assessment for Dementia (DAD)), and behavior (Neuropsychiatric Inventory (NPI)) after 12 months.[5]

In a larger study of 788 patients with probable VaD who were randomized to receive galantamine or placebo, the galantamine group showed improvement in cognition in patients with VaD, with greater improvement in ADAS-Cog/11 compared to placebo. However, there was no statistically significant improvement in ADLs with galantamine compared to placebo.[6]

Donepezil has been studied frequently for patients with VaD. The study involving the largest number of patients was a combined analysis using two identical randomized, double-blind, placebo-controlled groups that were studied for a 24-week period in the United States, Europe, and Australia.[7] Patients were randomized to receive donepezil 5 or 10 mg/day after brief titration or placebo. Patients were assessed on cognition and global function. Both donepezil groups showed significant improvements in cognition compared with placebo (ADAS-Cog and Mini-Mental State Examination (MMSE); $p < 0.01$). Significant global function benefits were seen on the CIBIC-Plus in the group receiving donepezil 5 mg/day and on the Clinical Dementia Rating-Sum of Boxes (CDR-SB) in the group receiving 10 mg/day. The authors concluded that donepezil improved cognition, global function, and ability to perform instrumental ADLs in patients with VaD and was well tolerated. This review was sponsored by the manufacturer.[7]

Participants of these two randomized trials were recruited for an open-label, 30-week extension study to determine the long-term tolerability and efficacy of donepezil in patients with VaD.[8] All patients received donepezil 5 mg/day for the first 6 weeks and then 10 mg/day upon clinician approval. Patients treated with donepezil for 54 continuous weeks (double-blind study plus extension study) had ADAS-Cog scores at endpoint that were higher than those at baseline; this included patients who were randomized to donepezil 5 mg/day in the double-blind trial. Patients who initiated donepezil during the open-label extension study exhibited no change in ADAS-Cog scores. The study did not show any significant differences between the groups on function. It was noted that the patients' ability to carry out ADLs generally deteriorated during the course of the study, despite continued donepezil treatment.[8]

Kavirajan and Schneider[3] performed a meta-analysis of available randomized controlled trials (RCTs) of cholinesterase inhibitors and memantine in VaD from 1996 to 2006. Their study included the results of the previously discussed double-blind RCT studies in addition to results of later published trials that lessened the global effects of the 5-mg dose. Eight studies comprising 5183 patients on the study drugs or on placebo met the selection criteria.[4,6,7,9–13] The ADAS-Cog was significantly improved for all drugs, but only 5-mg daily donepezil had an effect on the Clinicians' Global Impression of Change scale (CGIC) (odds ratio, 1:51; 95% confidence interval (CI), 1.11–2.07).[3] There were no behavioral or functional benefits for any of these drugs, except for a –0.95 point difference (95% CI, –1.74 to –0.16) with 10-mg daily donepezil on the Alzheimer's disease Functional Assessment and Change Scale. Kavirajan and Schneider concluded that cholinesterase inhibitors and memantine produce minor benefits in cognitive abilities, as evidenced by testing of patients with mild to moderate VaD, but the clinical significance is uncertain[3] (Table 4.1).

Because previous studies of donepezil in VaD showed inconsistent benefit in global functioning of patients with VaD, the manufacturer sponsored another trial to further evaluate the potential benefits of donepezil in VaD.[14] The design was changed from those of previous large studies; participants were randomized only to donepezil 5 mg or to placebo once daily. A subgroup analysis of hippocampal volume was also performed to determine the extent and frequency of hippocampal atrophy in the VaD population. The researchers achieved their previously reported result: patients treated with donepezil 5 mg/day had significant improvement in cognitive, but they did not show any improvement in global function. Patients with hippocampal atrophy who were treated with donepezil demonstrated stable cognition, but the placebo group showed a decline during the 24-week trial. On the other hand, the cognition of patients without atrophy improved with donepezil, and the placebo group remained relatively stable.[14]

A randomized, double-blind trial of donepezil in patients with subcortical vascular cognitive impairment (cerebral autosomal dominant arteriopathy with subcortical infarcts and leukoencephalopathy (CADASIL)) failed to show any effect on the primary endpoint, which was change from baseline in the score on the Vascular AD Assessment Scale–Cognitive subscale (V-ADAS-Cog) at 18 weeks.[15] Some improvements were noted on a few measures of executive function, such as the Trail Making Test, but the clinical significance was not clear.[15]

TABLE 4.1 Design Characteristics of the Vascular Dementia Trials[a]

Trial	Trial Duration (Weeks)	Treatment	Participants	Outcomes Primary	Outcomes Secondary
Donepezil 319[7]	24	Donepezil 5 mg daily	974 patients with probable or possible NINDS-AIREN VD in USA, Europe, South Africa, and India. MMSE range for inclusion not specified (observed range, 4–30). CT or MRI evidence of VD with central reader of scans	V-ADAS-Cog, CIBIC-Plus	ADAS-Cog, DAD, CDR-SB, MMSE, CLOX 1&2, EXIT25
Donepezil 307[9]	24	Donepezil 5 mg daily and 10 mg daily	603 patients with probable or possible NINDS-AIREN VD in USA, Canada, Europe, and Australia. MMSE 10–26. MRI or CT evidence of VD	ADAS-Cog, CIBIC-Plus	ADFACS, CDR-SB, MMSE
Donepezil 308[13]	24		616 patients with probable or possible NINDS-AIREN VD in USA, Canada, Europe, and Australia. MMSE 10–26. MRI or CT evidence of VD	ADAS-Cog, CIBIC-Plus	ADFACS, CDR-SB, MMSE
GAL-INT-6[4]	24	Galantamine 24 mg daily	592 patients with NINCDS-ADRDA AD with cerebrovascular disease or NINDS-AIREN VD in Europe, Canada, and Israel. MMSE 10–24. MRI or CT evidence of VD	ADAS-Cog, CIBIC-Plus	ADAS-Cog/13, DAD, NPI
GAL-INT-26[6]	26	Flexibly dosed galantamine 16–24 mg daily	788 patients with NINDS-AIREN VD in 21 countries. MMSE 10–26. MRI evidence of VD with central reader of scans	ADAS-Cog, ADCS-ADL	CIBIC-Plus, EXIT-25, NPI

VantagE[10]	24	Rivastigmine flexibly dosed up to 6 mg twice daily	710 patients DSM-IV and probable or possible NINDS-AIREN VD in USA, Canada, Europe, Taiwan, and South Korea. MMSE 10–26. MRI evidence of VD with central reader of scans	V-ADAS-Cog, CIBIC-Plus (ADCS-CGIC)	ADAS-Cog, ADCSADL, MMSE, NPI
MMM300[12]	28	Memantine 20 mg daily	321 patients with probable VD by NINDS-AIREN and MIS ≥5 in France, Belgium, and Switzerland. MMSE 12–20. MRI or CT evidence of VD with central reader	ADAS-Cog, CIBIC-Plus	MMSE, GBS, NOSGER
MMM500[11]	28	Memantine 20 mg daily	579 patients with probable VD by NINDS-AIREN, DSM-III-R, and HIS ≥4 in UK. MMSE 10–22. MRI or CT evidence of VD	ADAS-Cog, CGIC	MMSE, GBS, NOSGER

[a] All trials included were parallel-group, randomized, double-blind, placebo-controlled trials.

ADAS-Cog, Alzheimer's Disease (AD) Assessment Scale, cognitive subscale (possible range, 0–70); ADCS-ADL, AD Cooperative Study Activities of Daily Living Inventory; ADFACS, AD Functional Assessment and Change Scale; CDR-SB, Clinical Dementia Rating–Sum of Boxes score; CIBIC-Plus, Clinicians' Interview-Based Impression of Change with Caregiver's Input (possible range, 1–7); CLOX 1&2, Executive Clock-Drawing Task 1 and 2; CT, computed tomography; DAD, Disability Assessment in Dementia; DSM, Diagnostic and Statistical Manual of Mental Disorders; EXIT25, Executive Interview 25; GBS, Gottfries–Brane–Steen scale; HIS, Hachinski Ischemic Scale; IS, Modified Ischaemic Scale; MMSE, Mini-Mental State Examination; MRI, magnetic resonance imaging; NINCDS-ADRDA, National Institute of Neurological and Communicative Disorders and Stroke–Alzheimer's Disease and Related Disorders Association; NINDS-AIREN, National Institute of Neurological Diseases and Stroke criteria for vascular dementia (VD); NOSGER, Nurses' Observation Scale for Geriatric Patients; NPI, Neuropsychiatric Inventory; V-ADAS-Cog, Vascular ADAS-Cog (i.e., ADAS-Cog plus maze and number cancellation in trial 319, and the maze, number cancellation, digit symbol digit modalities, digits backwards, verbal fluency category tests in VantagE).

Source: Reprinted from The Lancet Neurology, 6(9), 782–92. Kavirajan, H., & Schneider, L. S. (2007). Efficacy and adverse effects of cholinesterase inhibitors and memantine in vascular dementia: A meta-analysis of randomized controlled trials. with permission from Elsevier.

Other Pharmacological Enhancers

Propentofylline is a neuroprotective agent that acts by inhibiting the uptake of adenosine and blocking the enzyme phosphodiesterase. Based on a meta-analysis, there is limited evidence that propentofylline has an impact on cognition, global function, and ADLs in people with VaD.[16]

Evidence from trials with other noncholinergic drugs for cognitive enhancement in VaD has been inconclusive. Drugs such as nicergoline, posatirelin, propentofylline, and pentoxifylline have shown limited benefits in VaD patients.[17]

Physical Exercise

In the Finnish Geriatric Intervention Study to Prevent Cognitive Impairment and Disability (FINGER), a double-blind RCT was designed to assess a multidomain approach to prevent cognitive decline in at-risk elderly people from the general population.[18] These subjects were not necessarily diagnosed with VaD but had a Dementia Risk Score of at least 6 points and cognition at mean level or slightly lower than expected for their age. A total of 1260 participants were assigned to a 2-year multidomain intervention (diet, exercise, cognitive training, and vascular risk monitoring) or a control group (general health advice). The primary outcome was change in cognition as measured through comprehensive neuropsychological test battery z score.[18] Findings from this large, long-term trial suggest that a multidomain intervention may improve or maintain cognitive functioning in at-risk elderly people from the general population.

Currently, there are multiple studies investigating whether physical activity can slow the progression of white matter changes or improve cognition. The PROMoTE study is an RCT of aerobic exercise training in older adults with vascular cognitive impairment.[19] AIBL Active is a single blind RCT in Australia with the goal to determine whether a 24-month physical activity program can delay the progression of white matter changes on magnetic resonance imaging. The participants will be older adults with subjective memory complaints and vascular risk factors.[20] A single-blinded RCT in the Netherlands will be conducted to investigate the effect of an aerobic exercise program on cognition compared with usual care in patients with a transient ischemic attack or minor ischemic stroke within the previous month.[21]

Physical Rehabilitation

A Dutch group compared the effects of combined aerobic and strength training versus aerobic-only training on cognitive and motor function in nursing home residents with dementia during a 9-week trial followed by a consecutive 9 weeks of usual care for all groups. The study did not differentiate types of dementia. The combined group completed two strength training and two walking sessions per week, the aerobic group completed four walking sessions, and the social group only participated in four social visits per week.[22] The combined group gained higher scores compared to the social group for global cognition, visual memory, verbal memory, executive function, walking endurance, leg muscle strength, and balance. Aerobic versus social group scores were higher for executive function.[22] It was noted that subjects reversed to baseline values by the end of 9 weeks of usual care. The authors concluded that a combination of aerobic and strength training is more effective than aerobic-only training in slowing cognitive and motor decline in patients with dementia. This study suggests that improvement in cognitive function seems to be independent of improved motor function.[22]

Cognitive Training and Enhancement

Cognitive rehabilitation has been an evolving concept that primarily originated through work with patients with traumatic brain injury. Cognitive rehabilitation generally refers to an individualized approach to helping people with cognitive impairments, in which those affected and their families work together with an emphasis on improving continuity of everyday functioning.[23] Cognitive training, on the other hand, is guided practice on a set of standard tasks designed to reflect particular cognitive functions, such as memory, attention, or problem-solving (executive function).[23]

Bahar-Fuchs and colleagues[24] reviewed evidence for cognitive training and cognitive rehabilitation in people with mild Alzheimer's disease or VaD. They included 11 RCTs, which provided relevant outcomes for the person with dementia or the caregiver. The authors separated cognitive rehabilitation from cognitive training. The goal of cognitive training was to improve or maintain ability in specific cognitive domains. The goal of cognitive rehabilitation was to enhance the performance and functioning in relation to collaboratively set goals. Their review did not provide evidence to support the efficacy of cognitive training. It was also noted that currently available standardized outcomes may not be able to capture some gains resulting from cognitive training. Only 1 RCT of cognitive rehabilitation done by Clare and colleagues[25] showed promising results. Their intervention targeted patient-derived personal goals. Sessions were supported by components addressing practical aids and strategies, techniques for learning new information, practice in maintaining attention, and techniques for stress reduction. Bahar-Fuchs et al. concluded that further well-designed studies of cognitive training and cognitive rehabilitation are required to provide more definitive evidence.

Cognitive training research has limitations. There is a lack of consistency regarding the content of intervention. Training effects often do not generalize to other functions. There has been variation in the length of intervention, the setting of the trial, and involvement of caregivers. Thus, when there is scarce collaboration of patients and caregivers, cognitive therapy has not always been effective.

Reminiscence Therapy

Reminiscence therapy is one of the most popular interventions in dementia care and is highly rated by care providers. Reminiscence therapy involves the discussion of past activities and experiences with patients in a group, usually using household items, family pictures, music, and old newspapers to stimulate memories. The patients are encouraged to talk about past events. Family caregivers are involved in reminiscence therapy.

Woods and colleagues[26] reviewed the results of four reminiscence therapy studies that had extractable data. After 4–6 weeks of therapy, there was a statistically significant improvement in cognition with reminiscence therapy in comparison with both no treatment and the social contact control group. Caregivers participating in groups with their relatives who had dementia reported significantly lower strain. In view of the limitations of the studies reviewed, such as the limited number and quality of studies and the variation in results between studies, the authors raised the need for more quality research in the field.[26] These studies only identified patients with dementia; no differentiation between types of dementia was made. Despite its popularity, there is no conclusive evidence of the efficacy of reminiscence therapy for dementia.

Cognitive Stimulation Therapy

Cognitive stimulation therapy (CST) is based on prior Cochrane review studies on reality orientation and reminiscence therapy in patients with dementia.[27] Reality orientation was developed in the late 1950s as a response to confusion and disorientation in older hospitalized patients.[28] Cognitive stimulation offers a range of enjoyable activities providing general stimulation for thinking, concentration, and memory usually in a social setting, such as a small group.[28] An earlier Cochrane study showed that reality orientation was associated with cognitive improvement in patients with dementia, but it highlighted the need for large well-designed trials.[29] A single-blind, multicenter trial randomized 115 older people with dementia to the CST group and the control group.[30] The main outcome measures were change in cognitive function and quality of life.[30] At follow-up, the intervention group had significantly improved relative to the control group on the MMSE ($p = 0.044$), the ADAS-Cog ($p = 0.014$), and the Quality of Life–Alzheimer's disease scales ($p = 0.028$). The authors concluded that the results are comparable with those of trials of approved drugs for dementia.

Several authors of the same study performed a meta-analysis of 15 RCTs of CST in dementia in 2012.[28] The studies were conducted in different settings with varying degrees of duration and intensity. The studies had relatively low quality by current standards.[28] The primary analysis was on changes that were evident immediately at the end of the treatment period. A consistent benefit to cognitive function was associated with cognitive stimulation (standardized mean difference, 0.41; 95% CI, 0.25–0.57). This was consistent at 1- and 3-month follow-up visits. However, the authors concluded that trials were of variable quality and suggested that the potential benefits and significance of longer term cognitive stimulation programs should be examined.[28]

The UK Government National Institute of Clinical Excellence's guidance on the management of dementia recommends that patients with mild to moderate dementia of all types should be given the opportunity to participate in a structured group cognitive stimulation program regardless of drug treatments received.[31]

Transcranial Magnetic Stimulation

The discharge of a transient electromagnetic field through the skull, delivered in trains, is the principle of repetitive transcranial magnetic stimulation (rTMS). rTMS can induce lasting modulation of brain activity in the targeted brain region and across brain networks through transcranial induction of electric currents in the brain.[32] rTMS enhances excitability of the motor cortex, which improves procedural learning in normal subjects.[33] rTMS may also have therapeutic and rehabilitative applications because the effects of repeated sessions may persist over time. rTMS has been approved by the US Food and Drug Administration (FDA) for treatment of resistant depression in the United States and Europe.[34] The mechanisms of these changes are not clear, but they seem to be related to synaptic long-term potentiation and long-term depression.[35]

TMS studies have identified a pattern of cortical hyperexcitability probably related to the disruption of the integrity of white matter lesions due to cerebrovascular disease.[36]

In a randomized controlled pilot study of patients with vascular cognitive impairment, one session of high-frequency rTMS applied over the left dorsolateral prefrontal cortex (DLPFC) improved executive performance but had no benefit to any other cognitive functions.[37] Five right-handed patients with post-stroke aphasia received eexcitatory deep transcranial magnetic stimulation over the right homologous Broca's region. The patients underwent a picture-naming task before and immediately after each of three rTMS sessions. The authors concluded that a single session of excitatory deep brain rTMS over the right inferior frontal gyrus significantly improved naming in right-handed chronic post-stroke aphasic patients.[38]

COGNITIVE ENHANCEMENT IN DEMENTIA WITH LEWY BODY DISEASE

Because dementia with Lewy bodies (DLB) and Parkinson's disease dementia (PDD) share many pathological and clinical features, they can be considered two ends of a spectrum of Lewy body disease. There are currently no effective FDA-approved treatments for DLB. Cholinesterase inhibitors have been shown to improve cognition in patients with PDD measured by MMSE[39] or ADAS-Cog.[39,40] However, in a study of the use of rivastigmine in patients with DLB for an 8-week period, there was no statistically significant difference in MMSE between the control and treatment groups, and significant benefit was reported only for behavioral symptoms.[41]

The efficacy of donepezil in patients with DLB was investigated in a 12-week, placebo-controlled, double-blind study in Japan.[42] Patients with probable DLB were randomized to placebo or to 5 or 10 mg of donepezil daily for 12 weeks. The co-primary endpoints were changes in cognition assessed using the MMSE and behavioral and neuropsychiatric symptoms assessed using the NPI. The primary endpoints were not achieved in this trial. However, significant improvement in MMSE score was demonstrated with 10 mg, but not 5 mg, of donepezil. There was no significant difference in NPI scores of the active group compared to the placebo group.[42] The same researchers also published the results of a 36-week, open-label extension phase of the preceding RCT.[43] A total of 110 of 142 DLB patients enrolled in the RCT phase (three arms: placebo, 5 mg, and 10 mg) entered the extension phase. The placebo group initiated active treatment, and the active groups maintained allocated treatment up to 8 weeks into the open-label phase. After that, all patients received 10 mg. The study replicated the initial result from the double-blind phase that donepezil at 10 mg/day improved cognitive function in patients with DLB. In the subgroup of the 5-mg group, further improvement was observed after a dose increase to 10 mg. Both subgroups of placebo and the 5-mg group in the RCT phase showed an improvement of cognition after starting active treatment of 10 mg donepezil daily.[43]

The efficacy and safety of memantine were investigated in patients with DLB.[44] Memantine-treated patients showed greater improvement in total NPI score at week 24 compared to the placebo group. There was noticeable improvement in the treatment arm; there were reductions in delusions and hallucinations; improved sleeping or night-time behavior; and lower instances of appetite or eating disorder. Memantine-treated patients with DLB had significantly greater improvement compared to placebo-treated patients in the Stroop Interference Test-C. Although memantine had mild benefit on the global status of patients with DLB, there were no significant differences between the two treatment groups in most of the cognitive test scores and ADCS ADLs.[44] However, memantine seemed to be beneficial in terms of global clinical status and behavioral symptoms.

In a small Swedish study, early treatment with memantine and a positive clinical response to memantine, measured by CGIC, predicted longer survival in patients with DLB and PDD.[45] This longitudinal prospective study was a continuation of a double-blinded 24-week RCT conducted in 2005–2008. Patients in the memantine group had a better 3-year survival rate compared to patients in the placebo group (log-rank $\chi^2 = 4.02$, $p = 0.045$). Within the active treatment group, the memantine responders, based on CGIC, had higher rates of survival compared to the nonresponders (log-rank $\chi^2 = 6.595$, $p = 0.010$). The authors cautioned that the results only suggest a hypothesis of a possible disease-modifying effect, which needs to be evaluated in larger studies.[45]

A recent systematic review and meta-analysis of trials of cholinesterase inhibitors and memantine in PDD and DLB included 10 trials that met the researchers' criteria.[46] Nine trials measured CGIC scale. Donepezil, rivastigmine, and memantine produced significant efficacy on the global evaluation in the meta-analysis. However, subgroup analysis showed PDD patients benefited from donepezil 10 mg and rivastigmine 12 mg, whereas DLB patients benefited from donepezil 5 and 10 mg based on changes in CGIC score. Cholinesterase inhibitors (donepezil and rivastigmine) improved cognitive function. Memantine showed positive impact on global impression but no benefit on cognitive function. The authors noted a substantial heterogeneity in meta-analyses when PDD and DLB were considered together.[46] This may be due to the fact that these two disorders are different entities despite similarity in clinical presentation and pathology findings.

A pilot randomized trial compared quality of life for patients who had received a diagnosis of dementia (AD, DLB, and VaD) and attended a "Living Well with Dementia" group to a treatment as usual group.[47] The 10-week group intervention trial showed evidence of improvement compared to the control group in the primary outcome, measure of quality of life in Alzheimer's disease, and the secondary outcome, self-esteem. Unexpectedly, there was evidence of a reduction in cognitive functioning in the treatment group compared to the control, which the authors advised to be interpreted cautiously because the results were from a pilot study.[47]

Deep Brain Stimulation

Deep brain stimulation has been previously used in stereotactic and functional neurosurgery for PD patients. Case reports have suggested that electrical stimulation of the cholinergic output of the nucleus basalis of Meynert (NBM) may improve cognitive performances, especially the memory tasks.[48] A trial is underway to assess the effect of bilateral electrical stimulation of the NBM on cognition in patients diagnosed with probable, moderate DLB (NCT01340001 and NCT02263937; https://clinicaltrials.gov).

COGNITIVE ENHANCEMENT IN
FRONTOTEMPORAL DEMENTIA

Frontotemporal dementia (FTD) includes a spectrum of diseases with heterogeneous clinical presentations and different types of underlying neuropathology. FTD can be classified into three clinical syndromes based on the predominant symptoms: behavioral variant frontotemporal dementia (bvFTD), semantic variant primary progressive aphasia (svPPA), and nonfluent variant primary progressive aphasia (nfvPPA).[49]

Currently, there is no disease-specific pharmacological treatment for FTD.[50] Medications for Alzheimer's dementia and other psychiatric disorders have been frequently used as off-label treatments for FTD.

Cholinesterase Inhibitors

In a placebo-controlled study of donepezil involving 24 patients with FTD, with treatment lasting 6 months, 4 patients in the treatment arm had worsening behavior, and the donepezil group had greater worsening on the FTD Inventory. Discontinuation of donepezil improved behavioral symptoms. There were no changes in global cognitive performance or dementia severity.[51]

A 12-month open-label study of rivastigmine with 20 patients did not show any improvement in cognitive measures, including MMSE, although it showed some improvement in NPI score.[52]

Portugal and colleagues[53] performed a systematic review of pharmacological treatment for FTD. They included intervention studies that provided clinical and objective measures published over two decades from 1990 to 2009. They selected 29 studies with a total of 390 participating patients. They noted that all studies had a small number of patients, had short duration of treatment, and used nonuniform measures in evaluating efficacy and tolerability. These trials investigated the role of selective serotonin reuptake inhibitors, trazodone, methyphenidate, cholinesterase inhibitors, stimulants, memantine, moclobemide, antipsychotics, lithium, and mood stabilizers on cognition and behavior in patients with FTD. There were 6 quality A randomized trials, 12 quality B trials, and 11 quality C trials based on "Updated Method Guidelines for Systematic Reviews" by the Cochrane Back Review Group. Considering the quality A study for our purpose, one study randomized 9 patients to be treated with either donepezil 10 mg/day or rivastigmine 12 mg/day immediately after diagnosis for FTD. One group, mainly males with an average younger age, showed improvement in MMSE and clock drawing test with this therapy. Another group, mostly women with an average older age, showed no significant benefit with this treatment.[54] Galantamine was evaluated for 36 patients with bvFTD and PPA in an open-label period of 18 weeks and a randomized, placebo-controlled phase for 8 weeks. Galantamine did not produce any significant differences in behavior or language, but a trend of efficacy was shown in the aphasic subgroup.[55] A study of trazodone showed significant improvement in behavior, with no benefit on cognition.[56] Dextroamphetamine showed significant improvement in apathy and disinhibition in a randomized, double-blind, crossover study of FTD patients with no significant change in cognition.[57] The other two quality A studies investigated paroxetine in small groups of patients. One study reported cognitive improvement in learning and delayed recognition with no significant change in behavior (NPI score),[58] whereas the other study showed improvement in behavior as measured by NPI and the Cornell Scale for Depression in Dementia and worsening cognition measured by the Stroop test and the proverb interpretation task.[59]

Memantine has been used off-label to treat FTD, with open-label studies suggesting some benefit in this group of patients.[60] Two randomized, placebo-controlled clinical trials failed to demonstrate significant benefits on the NPI or CGIC or cognitive measures. The first study tested the efficacy and tolerability of 1-year treatment with memantine (10 mg bid) in bvFTD. The primary endpoint was the CIBIC-Plus, with no significant differences between the memantine group ($n = 23$) and the placebo group ($n = 26$) ($p = 0.4458$). The secondary endpoints included NPI, Frontal Behavioral Inventory, Mattis Dementia Rating Scale (MDRS), MMSE, DAD, and the Zarit Burden Inventory (ZBI). For the secondary endpoints, there were no differences in the evolution of scores between the memantine group and the placebo group (MMSE, $p = 0.63$; MDRS, $p = 0.95$; NPI, $p = 0.25$; ZBI, $p = 0.43$; and DAD, $p = 0.10$).[61]

The second large randomized control study of patients with bvFTD or semantic dementia (SD) also did not show any benefit of memantine treatment on the NPI, CGIC, or cognitive testing (i.e., MMSE, Boston Naming Test (BNT), category fluency, and digital fluency) after 26 weeks of treatment.[62] In fact, memantine treatment was associated with worse performance on tests of naming (BNT) and processing speed (Digit Symbol).[62]

Despite prior open-label studies that initially reported the benefit of memantine in FTD,[60] both of the previously discussed studies provide evidence that memantine is not an effective treatment for FTD.

Stimulants

Rahman and colleagues[63] investigated the effects of a single dose of methylphenidate (40 mg) on a range of different cognitive processes. They studied eight patients with fluent variant FTD (fvFTD) who were randomized into two groups. One group took methylphenidate 40 mg first and then placebo, and the other group took placebo first and then methylphenidate, with the two test sessions for each patient started 90 minutes after administration of the drug or placebo. In both test sessions, the participants were given the same assessment: recognition memory, spatial recognition memory, spatial span, spatial working memory, attentional set shifting, and Tower of London test of spatial planning. The Cambridge Gamble Task was used to assess decision-making cognition.[63] The results showed no effects of methylphenidate on pattern recognition memory, spatial recognition memory, spatial working memory, attentional set shifting, and one-touch Tower of London tasks. However, there was a statistically significant difference in betting behavior, with patients on methylphenidate demonstrating reduced betting ($p = 0.017$), consistently seen across all eight patients. The authors concluded that methylphenidate was effective in "normalizing" the decision-making behavior of patients with fvFTD, although there were no significant effects on other aspects of cognitive function.[63]

Medical Food

The food drug Souvenaid is a compound thought to enhance synaptic function, with some preliminary evidence that it may improve cognitive function in patients with mild Alzheimer's disease. Treatment with Souvenaid (125 ml/day) in subjects with FTD was associated with a significant reduction of behavioral symptoms and an improvement in social cognition skills compared to placebo after 12 weeks.[64] Both effects reverted to baseline 12 weeks after the drug was discontinued. There was no effect on executive functions, and the study enrolled only 26 subjects.[64]

Electrical Stimulation Transcranial Magnetic Stimulation

Noninvasive brain stimulation, TMS, has demonstrated positive effects on depression and possibly cognition, with limited data on the efficacy of this method in neurodegenerative dementias. There are a number of case reports regarding the benefit of TMS in FTD or aphasia. High -frequency repetitive TMS (hf-rTMS) was applied to the left prefrontal cortex in a patient with PPA. Improvement of the patient's performance on verb production following the application of hf-rTMS versus baseline and sham conditions was reported.[65]

In another case, hf-rTMS was delivered over the DLPFC in a right-handed patient with logopenic PPA, and the results were compared to those of a sham stimulation.[66] The subject received two real stimulation cycles and two sham cycles for 5 consecutive days. A temporary but significant improvement in linguistic skills (both oral and written tasks) was noted after active stimulation compared to sham cycle, with no effect in the other cognitive domains tested. The improvement was attributed to enhancing long-term potentiation and synaptic plasticity within the stimulated areas involved in the language network.[66]

CONCLUSION

Identifying effective therapies for neurodegenerative diseases is currently a failure. Patients with Alzheimer's disease may have access to more cognitive enhancers than do patients with DLB or FTD, but even in the case of Alzheimer's disease, the treatments provide minor symptomatic benefit. Trials of cholinesterase inhibitors in patients with VaD are difficult to perform because of heterogeneity of pathology, the location of lesions, and overlap between vascular and neurodegenerative disease pathology.

The available evidence suggests that cholinesterase inhibitors may improve cognitive measures in patients with VaD, but there is no evidence of behavioral or functional benefits. Memantine produces minor benefits in cognitive testing of patients with mild to moderate VaD with uncertain clinical significance.

The role of physical exercise in VaD is not clear, although there seems to be evidence that a multidomain intervention including diet, exercise, cognitive training, and vascular risk monitoring may improve or maintain cognitive functioning in at-risk elderly people. There is some suggestion that physical rehabilitation may improve cognition in dementia, but there are no studies specific to patients with VaD. It is notable that most nonpharmacological interventions used to improve cognition in dementia, such as rehabilitation or cognitive training, do not differentiate types of dementia, and there is inconsistency in measuring scale and the goal for the therapy.

TMS studies suggest possible new approaches, but TMS is in such an early stage that currently conclusions cannot be made.

Despite the relatively high prevalence of DLB, only small numbers of controlled trials have been conducted. Overall, donepezil is well tolerated in patients with DLB, and there is evidence that donepezil at 5- and 10-mg daily doses may improve cognition in patients with DLB. Memantine did not improve cognition but improved global clinical status and behavioral symptoms such as delusions and hallucinations in patients with DLB. However, there is a lack of systematic evidence for the treatment of visual hallucinations in DLB with memantine.

There is an unmet clinical need for additional treatments for DLB, but very few pharmacological clinical trials are underway. Current trials are mostly investigating previously available medications such as cholinesterase inhibitors. Furthermore, large clinical trials are needed to better assess efficacy and safety of cholinesterase inhibitors and memantine on DLB. As new therapeutic modalities are found for Parkinson's disease and Alzheimer's dementia, it is hoped that better designed studies for DLB will be performed.

Currently, there is no strong evidence that cognitive enhancing medications approved for AD (cholinesterase inhibitors and memantine) provide any benefit for patients with FTD, and they actually may worsen behavior in some cases. Trials of other therapeutic modalities suggest a possible minor improvement in a very specific domain of cognition, such as methylphenidate's effect on decision making or TMS on language skills, but these studies have very small samples and the results have not been confirmed by large studies.

During the past decade, hundreds of clinical trials have been conducted for AD, but these attempts to find new treatments have not been successful. This makes the case for FTD even more complicated. None of the pharmacological trials in patients with FTD showed any significant improvement in cognition or function. There is a great heterogeneity among patients with FTD, presenting with different pathology and clinical presentation. That makes designing and performing clinical trials in this group of patients even more challenging. The number of patients randomized in FTD studies is usually small compared to the number of subjects recruited in studies of Alzheimer's dementia.

There is debate regarding what outcome measures for FTD should be considered because there are different predominant features for each subtype of FTD. Clinical trials using standardized diagnostic criteria with well-defined outcome measures specific to FTD symptoms are needed.

REFERENCES

1. Cummings JL. Frontal–subcortical circuits and human behavior. *Arch Neurol* 1993;50(8):873–880.
2. Grantham C, Geerts H. The rationale behind cholinergic drug treatment for dementia related to cerebrovascular disease. *J Neurol Sci* 2002;203-204:131–136.
3. Kavirajan H, Schneider LS. Efficacy and adverse effects of cholinesterase inhibitors and memantine in vascular dementia: A meta-analysis of randomised controlled trials. *Lancet Neurol* 2007;6(9):782–792.
4. Erkinjuntti T, Kurz A, Gauthier S, et al. Efficacy of galantamine in probable vascular dementia and Alzheimer's disease combined with cerebrovascular disease: A randomised trial. *Lancet* 2002;359(9314):1283–1290.
5. Erkinjuntti T, Kurz A, Small GW, et al. An open-label extension trial of galantamine in patients with probable vascular dementia and mixed dementia. *Clin Ther* 2003;25(6):1765–1782.
6. Auchus AP, Brashear HR, Salloway S, et al. Galantamine treatment of vascular dementia: A randomized trial. *Neurology* 2007;69(5):448–458.
7. Roman GC, Wilkinson DG, Doody RS, et al. Donepezil in vascular dementia: Combined analysis of two large-scale clinical trials. *Dement Geriatr Cogn Disord* 2005;20(6):338–344.
8. Wilkinson D, Roman G, Salloway S, et al. The long-term efficacy and tolerability of donepezil in patients with vascular dementia. *Int J Geriatr Psychiatry* 2010;25(3):305–313.
9. Black S, Roman GC, Geldmacher DS, et al. Efficacy and tolerability of donepezil in vascular dementia: Positive results of a 24-week, multicenter, international, randomized, placebo-controlled clinical trial. *Stroke* 2003;34(10):2323–2330.
10. Ballard C, Sauter M, Scheltens P, et al. Efficacy, safety and tolerability of rivastigmine capsules in patients with probable vascular dementia: The VantagE study. *Curr Med Res Opin* 2008;24(9):2561–2574.
11. Wilcock G, Mobius HJ, Stoffler A; MMM 500 group. A double-blind, placebo-controlled multicentre study of memantine in mild to moderate vascular dementia (MMM 500). *Int Clin Psychopharmacol* 2002;17(6):297–305.
12. Orgogozo JM, Rigaud AS, Stoffler A, et al. Efficacy and safety of memantine in patients with mild to moderate vascular dementia: A randomized, placebo-controlled trial (MMM 300). *Stroke* 2002;33(7):1834–1839.
13. Wilkinson D, Doody R, Helme R, et al. Donepezil in vascular dementia: A randomized, placebo-controlled study. *Neurology* 2003;61(4):479–486.
14. Roman GC, Salloway S, Black SE, et al. Randomized, placebo-controlled, clinical trial of donepezil in vascular dementia: Differential effects by hippocampal size. *Stroke* 2010;41(6):1213–1221.
15. Dichgans M, Markus HS, Salloway S, et al. Donepezil in patients with subcortical vascular cognitive impairment: A randomised double-blind trial in CADASIL. *Lancet Neurol* 2008;7(4):310–318.
16. Frampton M, Harvey R, Kirchner V. Propentofylline for dementia. *Cochrane Database Syst Rev* 2003;2003(2):CD002853.
17. Pantoni L. Treatment of vascular dementia: Evidence from trials with non-cholinergic drugs. *J Neurol Sci* 2004;226(1-2):67–70.
18. Ngandu T, Lehtisalo J, Solomon A, et al. A 2 year multidomain intervention of diet, exercise, cognitive training, and vascular risk monitoring versus control to prevent cognitive decline in at-risk elderly people (FINGER): A randomised controlled trial. *Lancet* 2015;385(9984):2255–2263.

19. Liu-Ambrose T, Eng JJ, Boyd LA, et al. Promotion of the mind through exercise (PROMoTE): A proof-of-concept randomized controlled trial of aerobic exercise training in older adults with vascular cognitive impairment. *BMC Neurol* 2010;10:14-2377-10-14.

20. Cyarto EV, Lautenschlager NT, Desmond PM, et al. Protocol for a randomized controlled trial evaluating the effect of physical activity on delaying the progression of white matter changes on MRI in older adults with memory complaints and mild cognitive impairment: The AIBL active trial. *BMC Psychiatry* 2012;12:167.

21. Boss HM, Van Schaik SM, Deijle IA, et al. A randomised controlled trial of aerobic exercise after transient ischaemic attack or minor stroke to prevent cognitive decline: The MoveIT study protocol. *BMJ Open* 2014;4(12):e007065.

22. Bossers WJ, van der Woude LH, Boersma F, et al. A 9-week aerobic and strength training program improves cognitive and motor function in patients with dementia: A randomized, controlled trial. *Am J Geriatr Psychiatry* 2015;23(11):1106–1116.

23. Clare L, Woods RT, Moniz Cook ED, et al. Cognitive rehabilitation and cognitive training for early-stage Alzheimer's disease and vascular dementia. *Cochrane Database Syst Rev* 2003;2003(4):CD003260.

24. Bahar-Fuchs A, Clare L, Woods B. Cognitive training and cognitive rehabilitation for persons with mild to moderate dementia of the Alzheimer's or vascular type: A review. *Alzheimers Res Ther* 2013;5(4):35.

25. Clare L, Linden DE, Woods RT, et al. Goal-oriented cognitive rehabilitation for people with early-stage Alzheimer disease: A single-blind randomized controlled trial of clinical efficacy. *Am J Geriatr Psychiatry* 2010;18(10):928–939.

26. Woods B, Spector A, Jones C, et al. Reminiscence therapy for dementia. *Cochrane Database Syst Rev* 2005;2005(2):CD001120.

27. Knapp M, Thorgrimsen L, Patel A, et al. Cognitive stimulation therapy for people with dementia: Cost-effectiveness analysis. *Br J Psychiatry* 2006;188:574–580.

28. Woods B, Aguirre E, Spector AE, et al. Cognitive stimulation to improve cognitive functioning in people with dementia. *Cochrane Database Syst Rev* 2012;2012(2):CD005562.

29. Spector A, Orrell M, Davies S, et al. Reality orientation for dementia. *Cochrane Database Syst Rev* 2000;2000(2):CD001119.

30. Spector A, Thorgrimsen L, Woods B, et al. Efficacy of an evidence-based cognitive stimulation therapy programme for people with dementia: Randomised controlled trial. *Br J Psychiatry* 2003;183:248–254.

31. National Institute for Health and Care Excellence. *Dementia: Supporting people with dementia and their carers in health and social care* (NICE Clinical Guideline No. 42). November 2006. Retrieved from https://www.nice.org.uk/guidance/cg42

32. Wagner T, Valero-Cabre A, Pascual-Leone A. Noninvasive human brain stimulation. *Annu Rev Biomed Eng* 2007;9:527–565.

33. Pascual-Leone A, Tarazona F, Keenan J, et al. Transcranial magnetic stimulation and neuroplasticity. *Neuropsychologia* 1998;37(2):207–217.

34. Schonfeldt-Lecuona C, Lefaucheur JP, Cardenas-Morales L, et al. The value of neuronavigated rTMS for the treatment of depression. *Neurophysiol Clin* 2010;40(1):37–43.

35. Ziemann U, Hallett M, Cohen LG. Mechanisms of deafferentation-induced plasticity in human motor cortex. *J Neurosci* 1998;18(17):7000–7007.

36. Pennisi G, Ferri R, Cantone M, et al. A review of transcranial magnetic stimulation in vascular dementia. *Dement Geriatr Cogn Disord* 2011;31(1):71–80.

37. Rektorova I, Megova S, Bares M, et al. Cognitive functioning after repetitive transcranial magnetic stimulation in patients with cerebrovascular disease without dementia: A pilot study of seven patients. *J Neurol Sci* 2005;229-230:157–161.

38. Chieffo R, Ferrari F, Battista P, et al. Excitatory deep transcranial magnetic stimulation with H-coil over the right homologous Broca's region improves naming in chronic post-stroke aphasia. *Neurorehabil Neural Repair* 2014;28(3):291–298.

39. Emre M, Aarsland D, Albanese A, et al. Rivastigmine for dementia associated with Parkinson's disease. *N Engl J Med* 2004;351(24):2509–2518.

40. Dubois B, Tolosa E, Katzenschlager R, et al. Donepezil in Parkinson's disease dementia: A randomized, double-blind efficacy and safety study. *Mov Disord* 2012;27(10):1230–1238.

41. McKeith I, Del Ser T, Spano P, et al. Efficacy of rivastigmine in dementia with Lewy bodies: A randomised, double-blind, placebo-controlled international study. *Lancet* 2000;356(9247):2031–2036.

42. Ikeda M, Mori E, Matsuo K, et al. Donepezil for dementia with Lewy bodies: A randomized, placebo-controlled, confirmatory Phase III trial. *Alzheimers Res Ther* 2015;7(1):4.

43. Mori E, Ikeda M, Nagai R, et al. Long-term donepezil use for dementia with Lewy bodies: Results from an open-label extension of Phase III trial. *Alzheimers Res Ther* 2015;7(1):5.

44. Emre M, Tsolaki M, Bonuccelli U, et al. Memantine for patients with Parkinson's disease dementia or dementia with Lewy bodies: A randomised, double-blind, placebo-controlled trial. *Lancet Neurol* 2010;9(10):969–977.

45. Stubendorff K, Larsson V, Ballard C, et al. Treatment effect of memantine on survival in dementia with Lewy bodies and Parkinson's disease with dementia: A prospective study. *BMJ Open* 2014;4(7):e005158.

46. Wang HF, Yu JT, Tang SW, et al. Efficacy and safety of cholinesterase inhibitors and memantine in cognitive impairment in Parkinson's disease, Parkinson's disease dementia, and dementia with Lewy bodies: Systematic review with meta-analysis and trial sequential analysis. *J Neurol Neurosurg Psychiatry* 2015;86(2):135–143.

47. Marshall A, Spreadbury J, Cheston R, et al. A pilot randomised controlled trial to compare changes in quality of life for participants with early diagnosis dementia who attend a "living well with dementia" group compared to waiting-list control. *Aging Ment Health* 2015;19(6):526–535.

48. Freund HJ, Kuhn J, Lenartz D, et al. Cognitive functions in a patient with Parkinson–dementia syndrome undergoing deep brain stimulation. *Arch Neurol* 2009;66(6):781–785.

49. Tsai RM, Boxer AL. Treatment of frontotemporal dementia. *Curr Treat Options Neurol* 2014;16(11):319.

50. Shinagawa S, Nakajima S, Plitman E, et al. Non-pharmacological management for patients with frontotemporal dementia: A systematic review. *J Alzheimers Dis* 2015;45(1):283–293.

51. Mendez MF, Shapira JS, McMurtray A, et al. Preliminary findings: Behavioral worsening on donepezil in patients with frontotemporal dementia. *Am J Geriatr Psychiatry* 2007;15(1):84–87.

52. Moretti R, Torre P, Antonello RM, et al. Rivastigmine in frontotemporal dementia: An open-label study. *Drugs Aging* 2004;21(14):931–937.

53. Portugal MG, Marinho V, Laks J. Pharmacological treatment of frontotemporal lobar degeneration: Systematic review. *Rev Bras Psiquiatr* 2011;33(1):81–90.

54. Lampl Y, Sadeh M, Lorberboym M. Efficacy of acetylcholinesterase inhibitors in frontotemporal dementia. *Ann Pharmacother* 2004;38(11):1967–1968.

55. Kertesz A, Morlog D, Light M, et al. Galantamine in frontotemporal dementia and primary progressive aphasia. *Dement Geriatr Cogn Disord* 2008;25(2):178–185.

56. Lebert F, Stekke W, Hasenbroekx C, et al. Frontotemporal dementia: A randomised, controlled trial with trazodone. *Dement Geriatr Cogn Disord* 2004;17(4):355–359.

57. Huey ED, Garcia C, Wassermann EM, et al. Stimulant treatment of frontotemporal dementia in 8 patients. *J Clin Psychiatry* 2008;69(12):1981–1982.

58. Deakin JB, Rahman S, Nestor PJ, et al. Paroxetine does not improve symptoms and impairs cognition in frontotemporal dementia: A double-blind randomized controlled trial. *Psychopharmacology (Berl)* 2004;172(4):400–408.

59. Moretti R, Torre P, Antonello RM, et al. Frontotemporal dementia: Paroxetine as a possible treatment of behavior symptoms—A randomized, controlled, open 14-month study. *Eur Neurol* 2003;49(1):13–19.

60. Boxer AL, Lipton AM, Womack K, et al. An open-label study of memantine treatment in 3 subtypes of frontotemporal lobar degeneration. *Alzheimer Dis Assoc Disord* 2009;23(3):211–217.

61. Vercelletto M, Boutoleau-Bretonniere C, Volteau C, et al. Memantine in behavioral variant frontotemporal dementia: Negative results. *J Alzheimers Dis* 2011;23(4):749–759.

62. Boxer AL, Knopman DS, Kaufer DI, et al. Memantine in patients with frontotemporal lobar degeneration: A multicentre, randomised, double-blind, placebo-controlled trial. *Lancet Neurol* 2013;12(2):149–156.

63. Rahman S, Robbins TW, Hodges JR, et al. Methylphenidate ("Ritalin") can ameliorate abnormal risk-taking behavior in the frontal variant of frontotemporal dementia. *Neuropsychopharmacology* 2006;31(3):651–658.

64. Pardini M, Serrati C, Guida S, et al. Souvenaid reduces behavioral deficits and improves social cognition skills in frontotemporal dementia: A proof-of-concept study. *Neurodegener Dis* 2015;15(1):58–62.

65. Finocchiaro C, Maimone M, Brighina F, et al. A case study of primary progressive aphasia: Improvement on verbs after rTMS treatment. *Neurocase* 2006;12(6):317–321.

66. Trebbastoni A, Raccah R, de Lena C, et al. Repetitive deep transcranial magnetic stimulation improves verbal fluency and written language in a patient with primary progressive aphasia–logopenic variant (LPPA). *Brain Stimul* 2013;6(4):545–553.

FIVE

Cognitive Interventions in Parkinson's Disease

SARAH BANKS

WHEN FIRST DESCRIBING "THE SHAKING PALSY," JAMES PARKINSON specifically stipulated that his soon-to-be eponymous disease spared the intellect (Parkinson, 2002). However, 50 years later, Charcot observed that cognitive deficits occurred early in the disease and worsened with the tremor. In the 1960s, the contemporaneous development of neuropsychology and groundbreaking treatment of motor symptoms of Parkinson's disease (PD) with levodopa led to greater scrutiny of nonmotor symptoms of PD. The further development of surgical techniques, along with evolving understanding of dementia and Alzheimer's disease (AD), led to increased study of cognition in this group of patients, and in the past few years, there has been widespread agreement on the general patterns of cognitive symptoms seen in PD (Litvan et al., 2011, 2012).

In other neurodegenerative diseases, and in normal aging, cognitive interventions have become highly sought after. These range from tasks and programs developed by scientists to other measures developed in the new "neurogaming genre," with parallel interest from both academic and scientific communities and business. There is evidence that certain lifestyle characteristics promote brain health, but what of cognitive interventions specifically? And how does this apply to the PD population? This chapter addresses these questions with a review of PD and its underlying anatomical disruption, a discussion of the cognitive symptoms often seen in the disease, and a critical review of the few studies that have been completed on cognitive interventions in PD. Finally, the findings to date are integrated, and future directions are suggested to develop empirically validated interventions to help treat cognitive symptoms in PD.

Only one pharmacologic agent—rivastigmine—is approved for treatment of cognitive impairment in PD. In this chapter, I review the non-pharmacologic interventions explored in the treatment of cognitive deficits in PD.

WHAT IS PARKINSON'S DISEASE?

The cardinal triad of symptoms in PD—akinesia/bradykinesia, tremor at rest, and muscular rigidity—results from decreased dopaminergic tone in the motor networks of the basal ganglia. These symptoms are often accompanied by nonmotor symptoms, including mood changes, autonomic dysfunction, sleep dysfunction, and cognitive decline. These changes are thought to be a result of various factors, including the dopamine loss in nonmotor regions of the striatum and more diffuse progressive changes in the basal ganglia, thalamus, and, eventually, the cerebral cortex (Braak et al., 2003). Underlying these changes is a multisystemic synucleinopathy resulting from the vulnerability of certain types of nerve cells to the inclusion body pathology that appears in three forms: Lewy neurites, Lewy bodies, and Lewy plaques. Selective vulnerability of the aforementioned networks to these changes results in a relatively predictable anatomic distribution and spread of pathology and, as a result, expected changes in motor and nonmotor symptoms. The disease starts in the substantia nigra with obliteration of dopaminergic projection neurons in the pars compacta, and it progresses until, at the end stage of the disease, lesions are found in the neocortex. The extent of aggregation in the cortex and other brain regions has been shown to be related with the degree of functional and cognitive change. Although the dopaminergic system is the primary neurotransmitter system to be affected, noradrenergic, serotoninergic, and cholinergic systems are also impacted (Dubois, Ruberg, Javoy-Agid, Ploska, & Agid, 1983; Jellinger, 1991; Scatton, Javoy-Agid, Rouquier, Dubois, & Agid, 1983). For a more in-depth explanation of the circuitry impacted in PD, see the work of Wichmann and Delong (2003a, 2003b, 2006, 2007), and for the pathology, see the work of Braak (Braak et al., 2003; Braak, Rub, & Del Tredici, 2006; Del Tredici & Braak, 2008; Hawkes, Del Tredici, & Braak, 2010).

Substantial overlap exists between AD and PD, with comorbidity evident in approximately one-fourth of PD patients (Irwin et al., 2012). Patients who seem likely to have this comorbidity due to patterns of atrophy on magnetic resonance imaging (MRI) (Weintraub et al., 2012) or possession of an apolipoprotein E epsilon-4 (APOE4) allele are more likely to show early and rapid cognitive decline (Morley et al., 2012). As might be expected given the overlap, there is evidence for a cognitive, behavioral, and activities of daily living benefit of treatment with cholinesterase inhibitors in PD dementia but not in patients with PD and less severe cognitive impairment (Rolinski, Fox, Maidment, & McShane, 2012).

Cognitive dysfunction is ubiquitous, on some level, in PD. As in Alzheimer's research, the level of impairment in PD determines the label that it is given. Although some aspect of pre-dementia cognitive impairment has been noted in PD for many years, it was not until relatively recently that formal criteria for PD–mild cognitive impairment (PD-MCI) have been defined (Box 5.1; Litvan et al., 2012).

The more severe form of cognitive impairment, accompanied by worsening of functional limitations beyond those caused by motor dysfunction, is referred to as PD dementia. PD dementia is defined by a set of core and associated features, including a diagnosis of PD by Queen Square Brain Bank criteria and a dementia syndrome involving cognitive impairment in more than one domain that impairs daily life (Emre et al., 2007). The mean duration of PD prior to development of dementia is 10 years (Aarsland, Andersen, Larsen, Lolk, & Kragh-Sorensen, 2003). PD dementia is a common outcome of PD, with a comprehensive review citing that the point prevalence is approximately 30% and the incidence rate of dementia in PD patients compared to that of age-matched controls is four to six times higher. The same group cites cumulative prevalence as between 48% and 78%, with a follow-up window ranging from 8 to 15 years. Older age and more severe PD symptoms, particularly rigidity, postural instability, and gait disturbance, were all risk factors for dementia (Emre et al., 2007). PD is a type of Lewy body disease. Dementia with Lewy bodies is essentially the same disease, but the cognitive changes predate the motor changes by a year or more in a rather arbitrary cut-off.

WHAT ARE THE COGNITIVE SYMPTOMS USUALLY SEEN IN PARKINSON'S DISEASE?

Although the early cognitive symptoms seen in PD are not entirely predictable, patterns are evident. In one study of 115 newly diagnosed PD patients, executive functioning deficits were highly prevalent in the early stage: Approximately half of the patients showed visuospatial deficits, 45% showed memory deficits, and 20% showed confrontation naming deficits (Muslimovic, Post, Speelman, & Schmand, 2005). Follow-up of the same group 3 years later showed decline mostly in processing speed and attention. Risk factors of decline included later age at disease onset and

BOX 5.1
FORMAL CRITERIA FOR PD-MCI

INCLUSION CRITERIA

- Diagnosis of PD as based on the UK PD Brain Bank Criteria
- Gradual decline, in the context of established PD, in cognitive ability reported by either the patient or the informant *or* observed by the clinician
- Cognitive deficits on either formal neuropsychological testing or a scale of global cognitive abilities
- Cognitive deficits are not sufficient to interfere significantly with functional independence, although subtle difficulties on complex functional tasks may be present.

EXCLUSION CRITERIA

- Diagnosis of PD dementia based on MDS Task Force proposed criteria
- Other primary explanations for cognitive impairment (e.g., delirium, stroke, major depression, metabolic abnormalities, adverse effects of medication, or head trauma)
- Other PD-associated comorbid conditions (e.g., motor impairment or severe anxiety, depression, excessive daytime sleepiness, or psychosis) that, in the opinion of the clinician, significantly influence cognitive testing

SPECIFIC GUIDELINES FOR PD-MCI LEVEL I
AND LEVEL II CATEGORIES

Level I (Abbreviated Assessment)
- Impairment on a scale of global cognitive abilities validated for use in PD *or*
- Impairment on at least two tests, when a limited battery of neuropsychological tests is performed (i.e., the battery includes less than two tests within each of the five cognitive domains, or less than five cognitive domains are assessed)

Level II (Comprehensive Assessment)
- Neuropsychological testing that includes two tests within each of the five cognitive domains (i.e., attention and working memory, executive, language, memory, and visuospatial)
- Impairment on at least two neuropsychological tests, represented by either two impaired tests in one cognitive domain or one impaired test in two different cognitive domains
- Impairment on neuropsychological tests may be demonstrated by
  - Performance approximately 1 or 2 standard deviations below appropriate norms *or*
  - Significant decline demonstrated on serial cognitive testing *or*
  - Significant decline from estimated premorbid levels

SUBTYPE CLASSIFICATION FOR PD-MCI
(OPTIONAL, REQUIRES TWO TESTS FOR EACH OF THE FIVE
COGNITIVE DOMAINS ASSESSED AND IS STRONGLY SUGGESTED
FOR RESEARCH PURPOSES)

- PD-MCI single-domain—abnormalities on two tests within a single cognitive domain (specify the domain), with other domains unimpaired *or*
- PD-MCI multiple-domain—abnormalities on at least one test in two or more cognitive domains (specify the domains)

severity of motor impairment (Muslimovic, Post, Speelman, De Haan, & Schmand, 2009). The profile of worse executive and visuospatial deficits in PD has been shown across numerous studies (Kulisevsky & Pagonabarraga, 2015). However, a range of different symptoms have been reported. This diversity has been used to identify particular test scores that predict negative outcomes. Poor performance on specific tests, such as semantic fluency and copying pentagons, has shown predictive value in determining who will later develop dementia (Williams-Gray et al., 2009).

In order to be motivated for cognitive intervention, and to benefit from it, patients need to have some awareness of their symptoms. Compared with patients on the AD spectrum, patients with PD have more insight into their cognitive dysfunction, although this was the case only for patients who did not have an amnestic MCI profile (Lehrner et al., 2015). This has an important implication for cognitive interventions in PD because it suggests that non-amnestic PD-MCI patients may be more aware of their impairments and thus potentially more motivated and more able to improve their cognition compared to patients with AD-MCI.

Cognitive symptoms have been assessed in relation to medication use in PD. Levodopa use has been shown to provide some benefit on spatial working memory and planning tasks but no difference on attentional set-shifting or visual recognition tasks (Lange et al., 1992). More recent studies have shown a similar distinction (Cools, Stefanova, Barker, Robbins, & Owen, 2002; Lewis, Slabosz, Robbins, Barker, & Owen, 2005).

Overall, cognitive symptoms are very common in PD and should thus be the focus of research into novel neurotherapeutics, including cognitive intervention. In the next section, the impact of cognitive impairment in PD is discussed.

RELEVANCE OF COGNITIVE SYMPTOMS IN PARKINSON'S DISEASE

Some of the important implications of cognitive impairment in PD include reduction in quality of life, increased disability and reliance on others, earlier need for institutionalization, and even earlier mortality. Rahman, Griffin, Quinn, and Jahanshahi (2008) showed that cognitive impairment and depression were the main predictors of quality of life in this disorder. Similarly, another study found worse cognition and more severe depression to be predictive of disability (defined as reduced ability to perform activities of daily living) in PD patients (Weintraub, Moberg, Duda, Katz, & Stern, 2004). It might be hypothesized that any intervention that improves or stabilizes cognition might have an impact on quality of life and functional status.

Impulse control disorders are common in PD. Although it could be argued that these are more of a neuropsychiatric symptom, they warrant mentioning in reviewing cognitive disorders. Impulse control disorders such as compulsive gambling, shopping, eating, and sexual behavior have been described in as many as 14% of patients with PD (Weintraub et al., 2010). In addition, they are sometimes associated with executive dysfunction (Cools, Barker, Sahakian, & Robbins, 2001; Owen et al., 1992), but some studies have found no relationship (Siri et al., 2015). Dopamine replacement therapy is considered a key risk factor in developing impulse control disorders, but its role is likely mediated by other factors, with the catechol-O-methyltransferase genotype having been the most thoroughly researched (Leroi et al., 2013). Treatment with cognitive–behavioral therapy has been shown to produce some improvement in impulse control behaviors in the short term (Okai et al., 2013).

RELEVANCE OF OTHER NONMOTOR SYMPTOMS IN PARKINSON'S DISEASE

Parkinson's disease is a complex disease with several nonmotor symptoms that can have an impact on therapeutic interventions. Neuropsychiatric symptoms are common. Apathy, anxiety, and depression are especially prevalent (Starkstein et al., 1992), and they may each have an impact on cognitive intervention. Hallucinations are also common, but their potential relationship with cognitive interventions is less obvious.

Apathy, in particular, can be a barrier to successful intervention. It is estimated to be present in approximately 10–30% of patients with PD, although the pathophysiology is unclear. Apathy is more common in patients with cognitive dysfunction (Pedersen, Larsen, Alves, & Aarsland, 2009). Treatments with some putative success range from medication to psychotherapy and occupational therapy (Starkstein, 2012). Depression is also common in PD and may be related to cognition, particularly memory loss (Norman, Troster, Fields, & Brooks, 2002). Cognitive–behavioral interventions have been studied in PD and have shown to result in some reduction in both anxiety and depression, although concomitant change in cognition was not studied (Yang, Sajatovic, & Walter, 2012). Hallucinations are very common in PD, affecting approximately 25% of patients, and may be related to breakdown in the visuoperceptual networks (Goldman et al., 2014). They are more common in patients with cognitive loss (Fenelon, Mahieux, Huon, & Ziegler, 2000), but it is unclear if this would have an impact on cognitive intervention. According to one study, hallucinations rarely affect quality of life unless the patient is not aware that they are not "real," which is rare (Goetz, Leurgans, Pappert, Raman, & Stemer, 2001).

Neuropsychiatric symptoms could have an important impact on the potential for cognitive interventions to be successful in PD. Their presence and severity should be taken into account when assessing the efficacy of such interventions. To date, there is insufficient evidence to make any conclusive statement about their role in predicting success of interventions.

A NOTE ON NOMENCLATURE

Several terms are used for cognitive interventions, including brain training, cognitive training, cognitive rehabilitation, and cognitive stimulation. In this chapter, *cognitive intervention* is used as an umbrella term. *Cognitive training* has been defined as drilled and practiced tasks designed to exercise specific cognitive skills, whereas *cognitive rehabilitation* is more of a comprehensive approach incorporating cognitive training within a larger, individualized rehabilitation program (Clare & Woods, 2004).

COGNITIVE INTERVENTIONS

The design of cognitive interventions in any disease builds on the concepts of neuroplasticity and cognitive reserve. *Neuroplasticity* is the change in brain form and function with development, usually in response to experience. In several studies, it has been shown to continue into adulthood (Maguire et al., 2000; Rosenzweig & Bennett, 1972). *Cognitive reserve* is the concept that some brains have more resilience to injury or damage due to being better at coping with or compensating for pathology (Stern, 2002). The classic finding is that people with more education appear to demonstrate less clinical decline with AD compared to those with less education and a similar pathological burden. Combining these concepts, it can be concluded that the brain should be, to some degree, manipulable in response to experience and that a brain with more cognitive strength should be less vulnerable to the outward manifestations of neurodegeneration. This premise has led to a recent growth of interest in cognitive interventions in normal aging and diseases and disorders such as AD, traumatic brain injury, and, to a lesser extent, PD. One important criticism of cognitive intervention is that it often does not generalize beyond the particular skill or skills on which it focuses, and there is no concomitant "functional" improvement, such as an improvement in activities of daily living or quality of life.

A recent review of the limited literature on this topic concluded that the data so far point to the potential for improvement at least in executive functioning (Hindle, Petrelli, Clare, & Kalbe, 2013). Here, the literature is reviewed based on the domains that each study focused on for remediation. The studies are summarized in Table 5.1.

TABLE 5.1 Summary of Studies of Cognitive Intervention in PD

First Author	Year	N (Groups)	Study Design	Findings	Domains Targeted
Mohlman	2011	16 PD, nondemented, mean MMSE 28. No controls	Four sessions of standardized attentional training with homework over a month. Assessed fatigue, effort, process, enjoyment	Improvement on 4 tests of executive functioning Feasibility of cognitive intervention	Executive functioning
Disbrow	2012	14 Impaired PD 16 unimpaired PD 21 healthy control	Non-randomized, 10 day at home, computer based training	More improvement in impaired group, especially on sequence initiation and completion, and this generated to a related pencil-and-paper task	Attention (Reaction time) Executive (sequencing and switching)
Sammer	2006	26 PD inpatients specifically for rehabilitation (in Germany) split into groups of 13. Presence or severity of cognitive impairment not reported.	Controlled trial, working memory task requiring executive function, control with no targeted cognitive intervention. Control group had "standard rehabilitation", the other had additional "executive function treatment" consisting of 10 30 minute sessions.	Improvement in both groups on executive function, greater in intervention group especially on a "rule shift" tasks	Executive functioning

Paris	2011	33 PD (MMSE>23) Random allocation Experimental group (n=18) vs. control group (n=15). Approximately half of patients in each group had MCI.	Blinded randomized control trial, 45 minute training 2 times a week for 4 weeks targeting several domains. Active control of speech therapy	Improvement in attention, information processing speed, memory, visuospatial and visuoconstructive ability and executive functioning. MCI status did not predict success. No improvement in mood or QOL were seen	multiple cognitive domains
Sinforiani	2004	20 PD, mean MMSE=25, none had "severe cognitive impairment compatible with dementia". No control group or control condition.	Intervention using software aimed at stimulating cognition. Outcome measures were phonemic fluency, story memory and nonverbal reasoning. These were administered at the end of training and 6 months later. 12 sessions were administered (twice a week for 6 weeks).	Patients improved on all three cognitive outcome measures and there was no difference between the post-training results and those 6 months later.	Executive functioning (attention, abstract reasoning) Visuospatial abilities
Naismith	2013	50 PD (15 = waitlist control) 62% of the sample had MCI (36% amnestic)	Single-blinded wait-list controlled design: 1 hr psychoeducation and cognitive training evaluations, twice weekly over 7 weeks. Computerized training was individualized and depended on individuals strengths and weaknesses.	Improvement on memory (Logical Memory) after cognitive training, no change in other cognitive domains. Data not analyzed by MCI status	Primary outcome memory; secondary outcomes other cognition./knowledge of psychoeducation topics

(continued)

TABLE 5.1 Continued

First Author	Year	N (Groups)	Study Design	Findings	Domains Targeted
Reuter	2012	240 PD-MCI patients, random allocation to cognitive training, cognitive training + transfer or mixed training	4-week inpatient training, then 6 weeks at home. Training was tailored to the patient's individual needs and inpatient training was delivered in individual 60-minute lessons occurring 4 times a week. At home training was completed via paper and pencil and a computer training session, three times a week for 45 minutes. Cognition was assessed before the training, at discharge and six months later.	Combination training group showed most improvements on cognitive measures, although all groups improved. Caregivers of patients in all group reported improvement in ADLs, although this was highest in the combined group and lowest in the cognitive training only group.	Primary: ADAS-Cog Secondary: SCOPA-Cog
Nombela	2011	10 PD (5 of whom went into a "trained" group; 10 healthy controls	Non-randomized, fMRI Stroop, one Soduku game per day for 6 months, control group no Soduku	Positive effects in all domains because activation patterns in PD post-intervention similar to controls; behavioral results showed improvement in reaction time	Executive function (Stroop fMRI task)

Executive Functions

Executive functions are perhaps an obvious target in this population, in which executive deficits are abundant. As such, most studies that are specific in their target, target this domain. In one of the earliest cognitive remediation studies, Sinforiani, Banchieri, Zucchella, Pacchetti, and Sandrini (2004) assessed a 6-week-long computer-based intervention program aimed at executive functioning and visuospatial abilities. There was no control group, but the authors reported improvement on three neuropsychological measures—one assessing memory, a phonemic fluency test, and a nonverbal reasoning test—which were unchanged 6 months later. Two years later, Sammer, Reuter, Hullmann, Kaps, and Vaitl (2006) compared standard inpatient rehabilitation in 13 patients to a similar rehabilitation with an added executive function training program in another 13 patients. There was no description of the baseline level of impairment overall, just on the specific scores assessed. The executive training group improved on the executive tasks, whereas the nontargeted training group had no significant improvement. No functional outcome measure was reported. The design of the intervention did not incorporate the same tasks used in the evaluation. This was an encouraging early look at executive intervention in PD.

In a study utilizing pre- and post-intervention functional magnetic resonance imaging (fMRI), Nombela and colleagues (2011) trained five PD patients in Sudoku during a 6-month-long intervention. They compared the these patients' results on a Stroop task while undergoing fMRI with those of 5 untrained patients and 10 controls. They found that following the intervention there were improvements in reaction time in the trained patient group and also an alteration in the activation patterns, such that trained patients' brain activation was more similar to that of controls following the training. Although small, this study is an important indicator of how fMRI might be utilized to demonstrate shifts in functional neuroanatomy in response to training.

Multiple Cognitive Domains

Other studies have assessed multiple domains in addition to executive functioning. Mohlman, Chazin, and Georgescu (2011) used a standardized training of "attention process" designed and implemented in traumatic brain injury during four 90-minute sessions, with additional homework sessions. Tasks were specifically selected to target those aspects of attention that the authors' believed were most impacted by PD: sustained, selective, alternating, and divided. Positive feedback was provided. They studied 16 noninstitutionalized patients with a diagnosis of PD without dementia. They also used "feasibility measures" (discussed later) to assess the patients' experience of, and level of engagement with, the intervention. The homework was not completed consistently by participants. Improvement was reported on four neuropsychological measures of executive functioning (Digits Backward, Stroop Color–Word Trial, Trailmaking Test Part B, and Controlled Oral Word Association Test). However, without a control group, there was no way to determine if this represented practice effects or specific executive functional improvement. Although mood was measured in this study, the results relative to the success of the intervention were not reported. There was no report of measure of functional ability or quality of life.

In a single-blinded, wait-list-control study, Naismith, Mowszowski, Diamond, and Lewis (2013) used both psychoeducation and a computerized cognitive training program, twice a week for 7 weeks, in an all-PD sample of 50 patients. The primary outcome domain was memory, although the computer-based training was tailor-made to the individual patients, depending on their own pretesting neuropsychological profiles. They found some improvements in memory in the intervention group compared to wait-list controls. In contrast, there were no improvements on various attentional and executive measures, including mental flexibility, verbal fluency, and psychomotor speed. Although a substantial proportion of the group had MCI, Naismith et al. did not report results of their analyses stratified by MCI group. The authors acknowledged the limitation of a lack of randomization and long-term follow-up to assess maintenance of improvements.

Paris and colleagues (2011) studied 33 patients with PD who all had MMSE scores of 23 or greater. The patients were randomly allocated into either an experimental or a control group. Half of the participants in each group met criteria for MCI. The training consisted of 4 weeks of 45 minutes of combined computerized and pencil-and-paper exercises, compared with speech therapy in the control group. It was found that the experimental groups improved on several domains, including attention, memory, visuospatial skills, and executive functions, although no improvements were noted in quality of life or ability to complete activities of daily living. Paris et al. also stratified the patients by MCI status, finding that on tests of visuospatial skill and executive function, those with MCI had more improvement compared to those without MCI. Despite the small sample size and lack of long-term follow-up, this study shows the promise of cognitive intervention in PD.

In the largest study to date, Reuter, Mehnert, Sammer, Oechsner, and Engelhardt (2012) randomized 240 PD-MCI patients into three intervention groups: cognitive training only; cognitive training and transfer training; and a combined group receiving cognitive training, transfer training, and psychomotor and endurance training. This study is also the most prolonged, with a 4-week inpatient rehabilitation program initially and then 6 months of at-home training. The authors employed cognitive batteries used frequently in clinical trials, the Alzheimer's Disease Assessment Scale–Cognitive subscale (ADAS-Cog) and the Scales for Outcomes of Parkinson's Disease–Cognition (SCOPA-Cog), to assess cognition. They found improvements in all groups, but the greatest changes were seen in patients with combined training. These patients also showed the most benefit in caregiver-assessed activities of daily living functioning 6 months after the end of the trial. There was no group without the additional training, so it cannot be determined if the cognitive training itself was actually beneficial beyond the standard-of-care rehabilitation training. However, this study is promising, and it demonstrates a role for combining physical therapy with cognitive interventions.

Summary of the Evidence

The literature on cognitive intervention in PD, summarized here, is brief. Although we do not know of any studies with negative findings, which may not have been published, the initial available data are encouraging. There is initial evidence of changes across multiple domains, which are enduring and appear to also be associated with underlying changes in network activity. No one has yet reported a change in functional status or mood. Some suggest particular improvement in those who are impaired. The one study that assessed feasibility suggests that the intervention used was not overly burdensome. Larger scale studies and studies with specifically identified PD-MCI groups would be useful. Similarly, the use of well-defined, publically available interventions would improve the practical utility of the research. Finally, using imaging to learn more about how the brain changes in response to these activities might be useful because it could lead to further understanding of underlying mechanisms.

WHAT ELSE CAN WE LEARN FROM COGNITIVE INTERVENTIONS IN NON-PARKINSON'S DISEASE POPULATIONS?

The work done so far on cognitive interventions in the PD population has only scratched the surface. In comparison to similar work in the normal aging or memory-disordered populations, there is a great disparity in the number of studies completed. However, given the relative maturity in the field of cognitive intervention in non-PD patients, future studies aimed at PD can build on prior research.

In traumatic injury, for example, cognitive interventions are divided into "restorative" techniques, those that are aimed at repairing and retraining lost abilities, and "compensatory" techniques, which are built around adapting intact cognitive domains to fulfill the tasks normally completed by the impaired domain. Compensatory techniques could rely heavily on executive abilities and could be used as a model for retraining the brain to mediate lost abilities.

In AD, cognitive interventions have shown mixed results, with a review that assessed only randomized controlled trials revealing the absence of improvement in most cognitive domains assessed but some improvement on screening measures (Alves et al., 2013). MCI is often considered a precursor, or at least a risk factor, for AD. A review synthesizing results from cognitive intervention studies of amnestic MCI revealed a high level of variability in quality and characteristics of studies. Naturally, in AD and MCI, studies usually emphasize memory, which is the primary domain impaired in AD. The results were somewhat promising, but the lack of large, well-powered studies with standardized interventions was identified as a limitation in interpreting this literature (Jean, Bergeron, Thivierge, & Simard, 2010). Another review, which incorporated meta-analysis and pooled memory training data across trials, specifically indicated that there were no improvements above and beyond control conditions for either healthy people or those with MCI (Martin, Clare, Altgassen, Cameron, & Zehnder, 2011). Other reviews of healthy individuals have shown very small effect sizes for cognition in general improving with training, although they are slightly larger if they are measured specifically within the domain that is the focus of training (Papp, Walsh, & Snyder, 2009). Overall, the results for memory training specifically are not overly promising either in the MCI-AD spectrum or in healthy aging.

Others have examined nonmemory domains, such as executive functions. In perhaps the most encouraging study to date—given its size, the thoroughness of the scientific approach, and its 10-year follow-up window—the Advanced Cognitive Training for Independent and Vital Elderly (ACTIVE) study has shown enduring effects of intervention on processing speed and executive functioning (reasoning) in healthy older adults, in addition to improvement in subjectively reported activities of daily living. Memory improvements did not last, however (Rebok et al., 2014). Other studies have also pointed to executive functions as being particularly compatible with positive response to training. For example, one study used a computer game involving strategizing and planning (Rise of Nations) and found impressive post-training improvement on executive control, working memory, visual short-term memory and reasoning, as well as task switching. No improvement was seen in a series of visuospatial tests or reaction time (Basak, Boot, Voss, & Kramer, 2008).

Other positive results in studies of older adults have been obtained using specially designed computer games that have had a positive impact on executive functioning—for example, the NeuroRacer game, which has shown sustainable and generalizable improvements in this domain (Anguera et al., 2013). These kinds of improvements could be particularly pertinent for the PD population, in which executive dysfunction is the most prevalent form of cognitive impairment.

There is a gap in the current understanding of cognitive interventions in PD with regard to how they might affect patients' lives beyond cognition. Although it might seem obvious that the "success" of cognitive interventions should be in improved cognition or stabilized cognitive decline, other factors might play an equal or more important role, such as improving perceived quality of life or mood. In non-PD populations, others have focused on noncognitive characteristics such as level of motivation, perceived support, and positive feedback—all important but often neglected features of the training model—which may well be independent predictors of success (Choi & Twamley, 2013). Although often overlooked, level of engagement is important. Mohlman and colleagues added four "feasibility dimensions" to their trial of cognitive remediation—fatigue, effort, progress, and enjoyment—which were each predictors of success in their program (Mohlman et al., 2011).

There is also other research on PD and other disorders that has examined non-cognitive interventions, such as physical treatments. Although this topic is beyond the scope of this chapter, it is important to note that studies of physical interventions to improve cognition have positive results in non-PD conditions (Hotting & Roder, 2013), and results are also encouraging in animal models of PD as well as human patients with PD (Petzinger et al., 2013). Other potential avenues of noncognitive targets for neuroplasticity that could have a cognitive impact include olfactory training, which has shown within-modality success in PD patients (Haehner et al., 2013), although it has yet to be investigated whether this had a positive impact on cognition.

CONCLUSION

Interventions for cognitive dysfunction in PD are an area of continued research interest with translational potential. Cognitive dysfunction in PD has a clear impact on quality of life and independence; hence, there is a need to identify treatments that will reliably improve this important nonmotor symptom. Executive dysfunction appears to be the primary target, both due to its prevalence in PD and due to encouraging data indicating that cognitive interventions can provide real and enduring change in this domain. Noncognitive aspects of PD, including motor but also common nonmotor symptoms such as apathy and depression, should be taken into account in studies, as should awareness of cognitive decline and motivation for change. Although neuroimaging has been incorporated into a few cognitive intervention studies to date, the potential to include MRI and positron emission tomography technology in the future is important for understanding mechanisms of change that may, in turn, inform improvements on future interventions. Finally, cognitive interventions should be studied in isolation but also in combination with other promising interventions such as physical activity and pharmacologic interventions. It is hoped that in the coming years, treatment for cognitive dysfunction in PD will be similarly successful and life changing as treatment for the motor aspects, but there is still a long way to go.

REFERENCES

Aarsland, D., Andersen, K., Larsen, J. P., Lolk, A., & Kragh-Sorensen, P. (2003). Prevalence and characteristics of dementia in Parkinson disease: An 8-year prospective study. *Archives of Neurology*, *60*(3), 387–392.

Alves, J., Magalhaes, R., Thomas, R. E., Goncalves, O. F., Petrosyan, A., & Sampaio, A. (2013). Is there evidence for cognitive intervention in Alzheimer disease? A systematic review of efficacy, feasibility, and cost-effectiveness. *Alzheimer Disease and Associated Disorders*, *27*(3), 195–203. doi:10.1097/WAD.0b013e31827bda55

Anguera, J. A., Boccanfuso, J., Rintoul, J. L., Al-Hashimi, O., Faraji, F., Janowich, J., . . . Gazzaley, A. (2013). Video game training enhances cognitive control in older adults. *Nature*, *501*(7465), 97–101. doi:10.1038/nature12486

Basak, C., Boot, W. R., Voss, M. W., & Kramer, A. F. (2008). Can training in a real-time strategy video game attenuate cognitive decline in older adults? *Psychology and Aging*, *23*(4), 765–777. doi:10.1037/a0013494

Braak, H., Del Tredici, K., Rub, U., de Vos, R. A., Jansen Steur, E. N., & Braak, E. (2003). Staging of brain pathology related to sporadic Parkinson's disease. *Neurobiology of Aging*, *24*(2), 197–211.

Braak, H., Rub, U., & Del Tredici, K. (2006). Cognitive decline correlates with neuropathological stage in Parkinson's disease. *Journal of the Neurological Sciences*, *248*(1-2), 255–258. doi:10.1016/j.jns.2006.05.011

Choi, J., & Twamley, E. W. (2013). Cognitive rehabilitation therapies for Alzheimer's disease: A review of methods to improve treatment engagement and self-efficacy. *Neuropsychology Review*, *23*(1), 48–62. doi:10.1007/s11065-013-9227-4

Clare, L., & Woods, R. T. (2004). Cognitive training and cognitive rehabilitation for people with early stage Alzheimer's disease. *Neuropsychological Rehabilitation*, *14*, 385–401.

Cools, R., Barker, R. A., Sahakian, B. J., & Robbins, T. W. (2001). Enhanced or impaired cognitive function in Parkinson's disease as a function of dopaminergic medication and task demands. *Cerebral Cortex*, *11*(12), 1136–1143.

Cools, R., Stefanova, E., Barker, R. A., Robbins, T. W., & Owen, A. M. (2002). Dopaminergic modulation of high-level cognition in Parkinson's disease: The role of the prefrontal cortex revealed by PET. *Brain*, *125*(Pt. 3), 584–594.

Del Tredici, K., & Braak, H. (2008). A not entirely benign procedure: Progression of Parkinson's disease. *Acta Neuropathologica*, *115*(4), 379–384. doi:10.1007/s00401-008-0355-5

Dubois, B., Ruberg, M., Javoy-Agid, F., Ploska, A., & Agid, Y. (1983). A subcortico-cortical cholinergic system is affected in Parkinson's disease. *Brain Research*, *288*(1-2), 213–218.

Emre, M., Aarsland, D., Brown, R., Burn, D. J., Duyckaerts, C., Mizuno, Y., . . . Dubois, B. (2007). Clinical diagnostic criteria for dementia associated with Parkinson's disease. *Movement Disorders*, *22*(12), 1689–1707; quiz 1837. doi:10.1002/mds.21507

Fenelon, G., Mahieux, F., Huon, R., & Ziegler, M. (2000). Hallucinations in Parkinson's disease: Prevalence, phenomenology and risk factors. *Brain*, *123*(Pt. 4), 733–745.

Goetz, C. G., Leurgans, S., Pappert, E. J., Raman, R., & Stemer, A. B. (2001). Prospective longitudinal assessment of hallucinations in Parkinson's disease. *Neurology*, *57*(11), 2078–2082.

Goldman, J. G., Stebbins, G. T., Dinh, V., Bernard, B., Merkitch, D., deToledo-Morrell, L., & Goetz, C. G. (2014). Visuoperceptive region atrophy independent of cognitive status in patients with Parkinson's disease with hallucinations. *Brain*, *137*(Pt. 3), 849–859. doi:10.1093/brain/awt360

Haehner, A., Tosch, C., Wolz, M., Klingelhoefer, L., Fauser, M., Storch, A., . . . Hummel, T. (2013). Olfactory training in patients with Parkinson's disease. *PLoS One*, *8*(4), e61680. doi:10.1371/journal.pone.0061680

Hawkes, C. H., Del Tredici, K., & Braak, H. (2010). A timeline for Parkinson's disease. *Parkinsonism & Related Disorders*, *16*(2), 79–84. doi:10.1016/j.parkreldis.2009.08.007

Hindle, J. V., Petrelli, A., Clare, L., & Kalbe, E. (2013). Nonpharmacological enhancement of cognitive function in Parkinson's disease: A systematic review. *Movement Disorders*, *28*(8), 1034–1049. doi:10.1002/mds.25377

Hotting, K., & Roder, B. (2013). Beneficial effects of physical exercise on neuroplasticity and cognition. *Neuroscience and Biobehavioral Reviews*, *37*(9 Pt. B), 2243–2257. doi:10.1016/j.neubiorev.2013.04.005

Irwin, D. J., White, M. T., Toledo, J. B., Xie, S. X., Robinson, J. L., Van Deerlin, V., . . . Trojanowski, J. Q. (2012). Neuropathologic substrates of Parkinson disease dementia. *Annals of Neurology*, *72*(4), 587–598. doi:10.1002/ana.23659

Jean, L., Bergeron, M. E., Thivierge, S., & Simard, M. (2010). Cognitive intervention programs for individuals with mild cognitive impairment: Systematic review of the literature. *American Journal of Geriatric Psychiatry*, *18*(4), 281–296. doi:10.1097/JGP.0b013e3181c37ce9

Jellinger, K. A. (1991). Pathology of Parkinson's disease: Changes other than the nigrostriatal pathway. *Molecular and Chemical Neuropathology*, *14*(3), 153–197.

Kulisevsky, J., & Pagonabarraga, J. (2015). Neurocognitive screening and assessment in parkinsonism. In A. I. Troster (Ed.), *Clinical neuropsychology and cognitive neurology of Parkinson's disease and other movement disorders*. New York, NY: Oxford University Press.

Lange, K. W., Robbins, T. W., Marsden, C. D., James, M., Owen, A. M., & Paul, G. M. (1992). L-Dopa withdrawal in Parkinson's disease selectively impairs cognitive performance in tests sensitive to frontal lobe dysfunction. *Psychopharmacology (Berlin)*, *107*(2-3), 394–404.

Lehrner, J., Kogler, S., Lamm, C., Moser, D., Klug, S., Pusswald, G., . . . Auff, E. (2015). Awareness of memory deficits in subjective cognitive decline, mild cognitive impairment, Alzheimer's disease and Parkinson's disease. *International Psychogeriatrics*, *27*(3), 357–366. doi:10.1017/S1041610214002245

Leroi, I., Barraclough, M., McKie, S., Hinvest, N., Evans, J., Elliott, R., & McDonald, K. (2013). Dopaminergic influences on executive function and impulsive behaviour in impulse control disorders in Parkinson's disease. *Journal of Neuropsychology*, *7*(2), 306–325. doi:10.1111/jnp.12026

Lewis, S. J., Slabosz, A., Robbins, T. W., Barker, R. A., & Owen, A. M. (2005). Dopaminergic basis for deficits in working memory but not attentional set-shifting in Parkinson's disease. *Neuropsychologia*, *43*(6), 823–832. doi:10.1016/j.neuropsychologia.2004.10.001

Litvan, I., Aarsland, D., Adler, C. H., Goldman, J. G., Kulisevsky, J., Mollenhauer, B., . . . Weintraub, D. (2011). MDS Task Force on mild cognitive impairment in Parkinson's disease: Critical review of PD-MCI. *Movement Disorders*, *26*(10), 1814–1824. doi:10.1002/mds.23823

Litvan, I., Goldman, J. G., Troster, A. I., Schmand, B. A., Weintraub, D., Petersen, R. C., . . . Emre, M. (2012). Diagnostic criteria for mild cognitive impairment in Parkinson's disease: Movement Disorder Society Task Force guidelines. *Movement Disorders*, *27*(3), 349–356. doi:10.1002/mds.24893

Maguire, E. A., Gadian, D. G., Johnsrude, I. S., Good, C. D., Ashburner, J., Frackowiak, R. S., & Frith, C. D. (2000). Navigation-related structural change in the hippocampi of taxi drivers. *Proceedings of the National Academy of Sciences of the USA*, *97*(8), 4398–4403. doi:10.1073/pnas.070039597

Martin, M., Clare, L., Altgassen, A. M., Cameron, M. H., & Zehnder, F. (2011). Cognition-based interventions for healthy older people and people with mild cognitive impairment. *Cochrane Database of Systematic Reviews, 2011*(1), CD006220. doi:10.1002/14651858.CD006220.pub2

Mohlman, J., Chazin, D., & Georgescu, B. (2011). Feasibility and acceptance of a nonpharmacological cognitive remediation intervention for patients with Parkinson disease. *Journal of Geriatric Psychiatry and Neurology, 24*(2), 91–97. doi:10.1177/0891988711402350

Morley, J. F., Xie, S. X., Hurtig, H. I., Stern, M. B., Colcher, A., Horn, S., . . . Siderowf, A. (2012). Genetic influences on cognitive decline in Parkinson's disease. *Movement Disorders, 27*(4), 512–518. doi:10.1002/mds.24946

Muslimovic, D., Post, B., Speelman, J. D., De Haan, R. J., & Schmand, B. (2009). Cognitive decline in Parkinson's disease: A prospective longitudinal study. *Journal of the International Neuropsychological Society, 15*(3), 426–437. doi:10.1017/S1355617709090614

Muslimovic, D., Post, B., Speelman, J. D., & Schmand, B. (2005). Cognitive profile of patients with newly diagnosed Parkinson disease. *Neurology, 65*(8), 1239–1245. doi:10.1212/01.wnl.0000180516.69442.95

Naismith, S. L., Mowszowski, L., Diamond, K., & Lewis, S. J. (2013). Improving memory in Parkinson's disease: A healthy brain ageing cognitive training program. *Movement Disorders, 28*(8), 1097–1103. doi:10.1002/mds.25457

Nombela, C., Bustillo, P. J., Castell, P. F., Sanchez, L., Medina, V., & Herrero, M. T. (2011). Cognitive rehabilitation in Parkinson's disease: Evidence from neuroimaging. *Frontiers in Neurology, 2*, 82. doi:10.3389/fneur.2011.00082

Norman, S., Troster, A. I., Fields, J. A., & Brooks, R. (2002). Effects of depression and Parkinson's disease on cognitive functioning. *Journal of Neuropsychiatry and Clinical Neurosciences, 14*(1), 31–36.

Okai, D., Askey-Jones, S., Samuel, M., O'Sullivan, S. S., Chaudhuri, K. R., Martin, A., . . . David, A. S. (2013). Trial of CBT for impulse control behaviors affecting Parkinson patients and their caregivers. *Neurology, 80*(9), 792–799. doi:10.1212/WNL.0b013e3182840678

Owen, A. M., James, M., Leigh, P. N., Summers, B. A., Marsden, C. D., Quinn, N. P., . . . Robbins, T. W. (1992). Fronto-striatal cognitive deficits at different stages of Parkinson's disease. *Brain, 115*(Pt. 6), 1727–1751.

Papp, K. V., Walsh, S. J., & Snyder, P. J. (2009). Immediate and delayed effects of cognitive interventions in healthy elderly: A review of current literature and future directions. *Alzheimer's & Dementia, 5*(1), 50–60. doi:10.1016/j.jalz.2008.10.008

Paris, A. P., Saleta, H. G., Crespo Maraver, M., Silvestre, E., Freixa, M. G., Torrellas, C. P., Pont, S. A., Nada, M. F., Garcia, S. A., Perea Bartolome, M. V., Fernandez, V. L., & Rusinol, A. B. (2011). Blind randomized controlled study of the efficacy of cognitive training in Parkinson's disease. *Movement Disorders, 26*(7), 1251–1258; doi:10.1002/mds.23688

Parkinson, J. (2002). An essay on the shaking palsy: 1817. *Journal of Neuropsychiatry and Clinical Neurosciences, 14*(2), 223–236; discussion 222.

Pedersen, K. F., Larsen, J. P., Alves, G., & Aarsland, D. (2009). Prevalence and clinical correlates of apathy in Parkinson's disease: A community-based study. *Parkinsonism & Related Disorders, 15*(4), 295–299. doi:10.1016/j.parkreldis.2008.07.006

Petzinger, G. M., Fisher, B. E., McEwen, S., Beeler, J. A., Walsh, J. P., & Jakowec, M. W. (2013). Exercise-enhanced neuroplasticity targeting motor and cognitive circuitry in Parkinson's disease. *Lancet Neurology, 12*(7), 716–726. doi:10.1016/S1474-4422(13)70123-6

Rahman, S., Griffin, H. J., Quinn, N. P., & Jahanshahi, M. (2008). Quality of life in Parkinson's disease: The relative importance of the symptoms. *Movement Disorders, 23*(10), 1428–1434. doi:10.1002/mds.21667

Rebok, G. W., Ball, K., Guey, L. T., Jones, R. N., Kim, H. Y., King, J. W., . . . Willis, S. L.; ACTIVE Study Group. (2014). Ten-year effects of the advanced cognitive training for independent and vital elderly cognitive training trial on cognition and everyday functioning in older adults. *Journal of the American Geriatrics Society, 62*(1), 16–24. doi:10.1111/jgs.12607

Reuter, I., Mehnert, S., Sammer, G., Oechsner, M., & Engelhardt, M. (2012). Efficacy of a multimodal cognitive rehabilitation including psychomotor and endurance training in Parkinson's disease. *Journal of Aging Research, 2012*, 235765. doi:10.1155/2012/235765

Rolinski, M., Fox, C., Maidment, I., & McShane, R. (2012). Cholinesterase inhibitors for dementia with Lewy bodies, Parkinson's disease dementia and cognitive impairment in Parkinson's disease. *Cochrane Database of Systematic Reviews, 2012*(3), CD006504. doi:10.1002/14651858. CD006504.pub2

Rosenzweig, M. R., & Bennett, E. L. (1972). Cerebral changes in rats exposed individually to an enriched environment. *Journal of Comparative and Physiological and Psychology, 80*(2), 304–313.

Sammer, G., Reuter, I., Hullmann, K., Kaps, M., & Vaitl, D. (2006). Training of executive functions in Parkinson's disease. *Journal of the Neurological Sciences, 248*(1-2), 115–119. doi:10.1016/j.jns.2006.05.028

Scatton, B., Javoy-Agid, F., Rouquier, L., Dubois, B., & Agid, Y. (1983). Reduction of cortical dopamine, noradrenaline, serotonin and their metabolites in Parkinson's disease. *Brain Research, 275*(2), 321–328.

Sinforiani, E., Banchieri, L., Zucchella, C., Pacchetti, C., & Sandrini, G. (2004). Cognitive rehabilitation in Parkinson's disease. *Archives of Gerontology and Geriatrics Supplement* (9), 387–391. doi:10.1016/j.archger.2004.04.049

Siri, C., Cilia, R., Reali, E., Pozzi, B., Cereda, E., Colombo, A., . . . Pezzoli, G. (2015). Long-term cognitive follow-up of Parkinson's disease patients with impulse control disorders. *Movement Disorders, 30*(5), 696–704. doi:10.1002/mds.26160

Starkstein, S. E. (2012). Apathy in Parkinson's disease: Diagnostic and etiological dilemmas. *Movement Disorders, 27*(2), 174–178. doi:10.1002/mds.24061

Starkstein, S. E., Mayberg, H. S., Preziosi, T. J., Andrezejewski, P., Leiguarda, R., & Robinson, R. G. (1992). Reliability, validity, and clinical correlates of apathy in Parkinson's disease. *Journal of Neuropsychiatry and Clinical Neurosciences, 4*(2), 134–139.

Stern, Y. (2002). What is cognitive reserve? Theory and research application of the reserve concept. *Journal of the International Neuropsychological Society, 8*(3), 448–460.

Weintraub, D., Dietz, N., Duda, J. E., Wolk, D. A., Doshi, J., Xie, S. X., . . . Siderowf, A. (2012). Alzheimer's disease pattern of brain atrophy predicts cognitive decline in Parkinson's disease. *Brain, 135*(Pt. 1), 170–180. doi:10.1093/brain/awr277

Weintraub, D., Koester, J., Potenza, M. N., Siderowf, A. D., Stacy, M., Voon, V., . . . Lang, A. E. (2010). Impulse control disorders in Parkinson disease: A cross-sectional study of 3090 patients. *Archives of Neurology, 67*(5), 589–595. doi:10.1001/archneurol.2010.65

Weintraub, D., Moberg, P. J., Duda, J. E., Katz, I. R., & Stern, M. B. (2004). Effect of psychiatric and other nonmotor symptoms on disability in Parkinson's disease. *Journal of the American Geriatrics Society, 52*(5), 784–788. doi:10.1111/j.1532-5415.2004.52219.x

Wichmann, T., & DeLong, M. R. (2003a). Functional neuroanatomy of the basal ganglia in Parkinson's disease. *Advances in Neurology, 91*, 9–18.

Wichmann, T., & DeLong, M. R. (2003b). Pathophysiology of Parkinson's disease: The MPTP primate model of the human disorder. *Annals of the New York Academy of Science, 991*, 199–213.

Wichmann, T., & DeLong, M. R. (2006). Basal ganglia discharge abnormalities in Parkinson's disease. *Journal of Neural Transmission Supplement* (70), 21–25.

Wichmann, T., & Delong, M. R. (2007). Anatomy and physiology of the basal ganglia: Relevance to Parkinson's disease and related disorders. *Handbook of Clinical Neurology, 83*, 1–18. doi:10.1016/S0072-9752(07)83001-6

Williams-Gray, C. H., Evans, J. R., Goris, A., Foltynie, T., Ban, M., Robbins, T. W., . . . Barker, R. A. (2009). The distinct cognitive syndromes of Parkinson's disease: 5 year follow-up of the CamPaIGN cohort. *Brain, 132*(Pt. 11), 2958–2969. doi:10.1093/brain/awp245

Yang, S., Sajatovic, M., & Walter, B. L. (2012). Psychosocial interventions for depression and anxiety in Parkinson's disease. *Journal of Geriatric Psychiatry and Neurology, 25*(2), 113–121. doi:10.1177/0891988712445096

SIX

Cognitive Enhancement in Traumatic Brain Injury

TESSA HART

TRAUMATIC BRAIN INJURY (TBI) IS A MAJOR PUBLIC HEALTH CONCERN. In the US alone, an estimated 275,000 people annually sustain TBI serious enough to warrant hospitalization.[1] Of these, as many as 124,000 per year may be left with permanent disability.[2] According to the Centers for Disease Control and Prevention (CDC), approximately 5.3 million Americans are living with disability due to TBI, at a high cost to health care and social support systems.[3]

Although physical impairments in the form of hypertonia, hemiparesis, incoordination, or ataxia may occur after moderate to severe TBI, cognitive dysfunction is nearly ubiquitous and accounts for more of the disruption in social, community, and vocational functioning.[3,4] Because many survivors are young adults just entering their most productive years, the "silent epidemic" of TBI has stimulated many attempts to remediate the characteristic cognitive impairments. This chapter provides a selective review of pharmacologic, behavioral, and other methods used to enhance cognitive functioning in TBI. The focus is on moderate to severe TBI because persons with severe injury are overwhelmingly more likely to be left with persistent cognitive impairment compared to those with mild TBI (concussion).[5] In addition, the focus is on adult TBI. Less attention has been devoted to cognitive rehabilitation in pediatric

TBI, partly because it is assumed that such services for children will be delivered through special education rather than health care delivery systems.[6]

THE COGNITIVE SEQUELAE OF
TRAUMATIC BRAIN INJURY

The CDC defines TBI as an injury to the brain caused by external mechanical forces that disrupts normal function.[7] In the United States, falls now exceed motor vehicle collisions as the primary cause of TBI, with other injuries resulting from assault, sports mishaps, and falling objects. Blast-induced TBI has received a great deal of study since the conflicts in the Middle East revealed the potential importance of this mechanism to persisting disability.[8] Although moderate/severe TBI can happen at any age, the distribution is roughly bimodal with a peak in late adolescence and early adulthood and a smaller peak among the elderly. At the older ages, however, the gender ratio is 2:1 to 3:1 male.[9]

The pathophysiology of TBI is complex, accounting in part for wide variation in symptoms and outcomes from person to person.[10] Mechanical forces, both direct contact and ensuing inertial forces within the brain matter, lead to structural changes as well as cytotoxic processes that perpetuate cellular damage following the initial insult.[11] Secondary injury also occurs from hypoxia and hemorrhage. The chief pathology that leads to permanent cognitive impairment is diffuse axonal injury (DAI) resulting from rotational forces that cause shearing and stretching of axons and blood vessels. The resulting disconnections within networks that subserve arousal and wakefulness cause immediate loss or alteration of consciousness.[3] Return of consciousness is gradual and typically merges into a period of confusion and disorientation during which ongoing events are not consolidated into long-term memory store (post-traumatic amnesia (PTA)). The duration of PTA is considered the most reliable index of the extent of diffuse brain damage,[12] which may or may not be visible on clinical neuroimaging. In the most severe TBI, the person does not emerge from PTA but, rather, is permanently amnestic and disoriented. Most regain day-to-day memory, but with some degree of impairment in learning and recalling new information and events; biographical and long-term memories are generally spared. Thus, deficits in *memory*, especially "short-term memory," are a chief complaint of survivors of TBI even many years post injury.[13]

The resolution of consciousness, for those not left in persistent vegetative or minimally conscious states, is also typically followed by residual impairments in *attention*. Attention is a multifaceted construct that includes basic arousal and alertness, the ability to focus on specific stimuli to the exclusion of others (selective attention), and the ability to maintain focus over time (vigilance). Resistance to environmental distraction and multitasking (divided attention) are also included. Careful research on attention following TBI suggests that the most common persistent impairments involve the strategic control over attention rather than automatic processes such as orienting to external stimuli.[14] Speed of information processing is also affected and is exacerbated by increased complexity or demand.[3] Although survivors of TBI do complain of attention problems (being distractible and losing one's train of thought), some attention problems lead to problems with everyday memory and may be reported as such.

The third major area of cognition affected by TBI is *executive function*, sometimes referred to as *cognitive control*. These terms are inconsistently defined, but they refer to the interrelated cognitive operations needed to support goal-directed behavior that is internally directed and persistent but flexible in response to changes in the social and physical environment.[4] Recognizing problems that need to be solved, setting goals, generating and executing plans of action, and monitoring their outcomes are among the uniquely human abilities included in most conceptualizations of executive function. Thus, the "dysexecutive syndrome" describes a person whose behavior appears disorganized, aimless or unmotivated, or inappropriate to the situation.[15] There may be an inability to appreciate one's limitations—that is, impaired self-awareness.[16] Executive functions are also considered to regulate other cognitive and emotional functions; thus, emotional lability, apathy, and mood disturbances are common following TBI.[17] In addition, some failures in memory and attention may be due more to a failure in strategic control than to dysfunction in the basic neural systems supporting those functions. In particular, prospective memory—that is, remembering to remember future events such as appointments—may be affected more by the integrity of executive function than that of basic memory systems.[18]

Problems with executive function, which relies heavily on tertiary prefrontal cortex and its connections, are prevalent in TBI not only because of network disconnections caused by DAI but also due to the predilection of prefrontal and anterior temporal cortex to focal lesions (bruising and contusions) following application of external force that causes the brain to slide over the bony ridges supporting its ventral surface.[15,19]

Although it is obvious that the "big three" areas of cognitive dysfunction in TBI—attention, memory, and executive function—are interrelated, they are often approached separately in treatment, and they are addressed separately in later sections of this chapter. Cognitive deficits in other domains, such as language or visual–spatial perception, may occur after TBI due to focal injuries in more posterior regions of the brain, such as contusions, hemorrhages, or cell death due to vasospasm. It is beyond the scope of this chapter to review treatment approaches for all such impairments. In general, treatment approaches for language and visual–spatial impairments would be similar in TBI as in stroke.

MODELS OF COGNITIVE ENHANCEMENT IN TRAUMATIC BRAIN INJURY

TBI rehabilitation, like other subspecialties of the field, lacks theoretical models with which to guide the majority of treatments.[20] Rehabilitation has tended to be pragmatic rather than theory driven, and the multidisciplinary nature of the field has also inhibited the development of unifying theories. One overarching model distinguishes *restorative* from *compensatory* approaches. This dates at least to the seminal paper by Oliver Zangwill, published in 1947, on methods for "re-education" of persons with brain injury.[21] Restorative approaches are meant to reinstate a damaged function to the pre-injury condition, usually through repetitive practice, by analogy to muscle exercise. Pharmacologic treatments may also be considered restorative, in that they are usually intended to replenish the depleted neurotransmitters involved in cognitive functions. In contrast, compensatory approaches are designed to circumvent the damaged functions, using "work-arounds" so that cognitively demanding tasks may still be accomplished, albeit differently than pre-injury.

Several types of compensatory approaches may be identified. *Internal strategies* may include mnemonic devices such as visualization methods for associating names to faces. "Metacognitive" strategies are those that can be applied to multiple situations, such as an algorithm of general steps to follow when solving everyday problems. *External strategies* are limited only by the imagination. Common strategies include using a checklist to organize a multistep activity or to ensure that tasks are completed, using the alarm function on a cell phone to initiate a desired activity on time, and using a pill dispenser to track whether medications have been taken. Note that in contrast to restorative approaches, the underlying cognitive deficit is not assumed to change. In general, clinicians plan treatments around restorative approaches early after TBI and switch to compensatory strategy training after the phase of rapid spontaneous recovery has ended and it is more apparent what deficits will need to be compensated. This approach may result in better acceptance of compensatory strategies by the patient, who may reject them while he or she is still improving.[22]

Although some find it worthwhile in clinical practice, the restorative/compensatory distinction has not been very useful in stimulating cognitive rehabilitation research. This may be because in many cases, the distinction between restoration and compensation is more apparent than real. For example, if a person learns a problem-solving sequence and applies it successfully in everyday life, is that an example of a restored problem-solving function or a compensatory mechanism that is taking over for a lost natural ability? Similarly, if a person is accustomed to using a planner to organize daily activities, is using a planner after TBI "restorative" for him or her but "compensatory" for someone who has never used one before?

Compensatory approaches may be further subdivided into those taught to the affected person, as in the previous examples, versus those based on *environmental modifications*. For example, the physical environment might be simplified by labeling cabinets with their contents or removing unnecessary clutter so that items are easier to find. The social environment might be modified by asking that only one person speak to the patient at any given time to help compensate for attention problems. Caregiver training may be thought of as another type of environmental modification. As a general rule, environmental modifications are emphasized to the degree that the injured person is less able to learn or apply internal or external strategies. However, in many instances, a wide variety of strategies will be applied. For example, vocational rehabilitation for people with TBI may include modifications to simplify work tasks or to limit the number of people with whom the patient must interact (environmental changes), coupled with strategies used by the patient such as task lists, alarms to keep track of time, and so on.

Very few other conceptual frameworks have influenced research or practice in cognitive enhancement following TBI. One that bears mention is the concept of *contextualized* cognitive rehabilitation[23] as contrasted with treatment of cognitive functions in relative isolation, also known as the modular approach. An assumption of the latter model is that when the cognitive skill is strengthened, the person's performance will then improve on a range of real-world activities that require that skill. This assumption tends to apply more to restorative approaches, although compensatory techniques may also be applied outside of a realistic context. For example, a patient may be taught to practice taking notes to support recall during a television show, based on the assumption that the ability to take notes will transfer to a classroom lecture situation.

In the contextualized cognitive rehabilitation model, cognitive functions are conceptualized not as isolated modules but, rather, as interactive with one another, with other aspects of function (e.g., emotions), and with the social and physical environments. The primary focus is not on improving function but, rather, on helping the person to attain or regain meaningful activities and societal roles. Cognitive limitations are addressed with restorative or compensatory techniques as appropriate, but they are primarily managed with *natural supports* that allow successful participation to take place. These supports may include creative modification of the job or other social role and coaching, strategy development, or other assistance from people on-site. Support people may include a mixture of professionals and "everyday people" such as supervisors, teachers, friends/family, and coworkers. As the person with cognitive limitations develops new habits in personally meaningful activities, independence may improve and the supports may be faded over time. However, generalization of cognitive skills from one situation to another is neither assumed nor required.

For some, an advantage of the contextualized approach is that it avoids labeling the person with brain injury as "defective" or "needing to be fixed," as assumed in a primarily medical model of rehabilitation. Instead, the community is the focus of change, with the goal of supporting the universal human need to participate and contribute to the full extent of one's abilities. A similar framework has been offered by Malec,[24] who argues for a social rather than medical perspective on TBI rehabilitation beyond the early stage of acute medical need. In a social framework, the "system" in which the patient resides is the target for change, and the outcomes are determined not by professional evaluations that determine the problems of the injured person but, rather, by their importance to the patient and

TABLE 6.1 Modular/Medical and Contextual/Social Models of Cognitive Rehabilitation for Traumatic Brain Injury

	Modular/Medical	Contextual/Social
Target of treatment	Cognitive deficits (impaired attention, memory, etc.)	Social and/or physical environment in which the patient will use cognitive functions
Locus of change	Within the person	System or community surrounding the person in a given context
Therapeutic modalities	Therapy exercises geared toward changing cognitive functions, or compensatory strategy training if restorative approach fails	Supports and accommodations; incorporation and training of everyday people to serve as supports; compensatory strategy training
Timing of treatment	Early after injury, to maximize extent of natural recovery	Any time after injury, with adjustments for changes in the person/environment over time
Setting of treatment	Clinic, with expected generalization to real world	Real-world contexts individualized to each person
Desired outcome	The person improves and can then reintegrate into society.	The environment/community changes to include the person.

family. Table 6.1 summarizes the main contrasts between the contextualized/social model and the more traditional medical model as applied to cognitive rehabilitation. Unfortunately, in practice, contextualized or social approaches to rehabilitation are quite labor-intensive and, lacking the economy of scale of clinic-based treatments, are less likely than traditional modular treatments to be funded or maintained by third-party payers.

In summary, only a few theoretical models have guided the development of cognitive rehabilitation treatments for TBI. Neuroscientists concerned with rehabilitation have commented that theories explaining cognitive function in the uninjured brain have contributed relatively little to theories about how to repair those functions.[20] It is likely that models of *change* (e.g., learning theories) will be more fruitful for advances at the conceptual level.[25]

COGNITIVE ENHANCEMENT IN EARLY STAGES OF TRAUMATIC BRAIN INJURY RECOVERY

For decades, TBI researchers have sought a "magic bullet"—an early physiologic treatment that could reverse the damage or prevent the cascade leading to cell death in the hours, days, and weeks after injury. Promising preclinical and Phase II studies have led to failure after failure in Phase III trials, probably due to the variability of neuropathophysiology in this population.[26] Most neuroprotection trials have focused not on cognitive outcome but on global outcome using broad categories such as those captured by the Glasgow Outcome Scale,[27] which ranges from "death" to "good outcome." A notable exception was the Citicoline Brain Injury Treatment (COBRIT) trial, in which citicoline or placebo was administered for 90 days, starting within 24 hours of moderate/severe TBI.[28] This trial was unusual for its inclusion of an extensive cognitive test battery administered at 30, 90, and 180 days in addition to the global outcome measures that are standard for such trials. The reasoning was that administration of citicoline, an acetylcholine precursor, in the early stages of TBI might preserve memory or other cognitive functions even if global outcome measures were insensitive to the treatment. Unfortunately, citicoline did not improve outcome at all, and there was even a suggestion of worse cognitive outcome in the patients with less severe TBI. The search for neuroprotective agents continues, but currently there is no compound with an evidence base for emergent administration in this population. The consensus in the field is that success may depend on improved characterization of subgoups of TBI[10] and/or use of combination therapies.[29] However, improved preclinical studies and widespread adoption of more sensitive outcome measures may also be required.[30]

Studying the efficacy of cognitive enhancement in the subacute phase of TBI (up to 3–6 months post injury) is challenging because most survivors of TBI show rapid gains in cognition during this time, making it difficult to estimate the effects of superimposed treatment.[31,32] However, Willmott and Ponsford[33] showed that methylphenidate improved cognitive processing speed in people with moderate/severe TBI treated on an inpatient unit, at a mean of 2 months post injury. As discussed later, improved processing speed is a chief effect of methylphenidate for those with chronic TBI as well.[34] In people with very severe TBI and persistent disorders of consciousness (i.e., those in vegetative or minimally conscious state at 4–16 weeks post TBI), an international clinical trial showed that administration of amantadine hydrochloride for 4 weeks accelerated improvements in responsiveness to the environment.[35] Hence, this agent should be considered the first-line treatment for patients with persistent disorders of consciousness in the subacute phase of TBI.

As noted previously, recovery of consciousness is typically followed by a phase of altered consciousness, often resembling delirium, which is known as PTA. During this period, patients are amnestic from day-to-day and may be restless and agitated. Although there are no known treatments to accelerate recovery from this phase, there are practices that should be incorporated into patient care to prevent worsening or reinjury. Patients should be allowed to "roam" in a safe environment, and restraint should be avoided as much as possible. Frequent reorientation to circumstances should be provided; this serves to reduce anxiety but does not actually reduce the duration of PTA. Overstimulation should be avoided and physically, rather than cognitively, oriented therapies emphasized. There is evidence that patients in this phase can learn procedures and routines even though they are amnestic for daily events.[36,37] Most important, neuroleptic medications should be avoided because they inhibit recovery overall and can actually prolong PTA.[38,39]

COGNITIVE ENHANCEMENT IN CHRONIC TRAUMATIC BRAIN INJURY

Although "spontaneous" recovery may continue for years after TBI, it occurs at a slower pace after approximately 6 months. The majority of attempts to enhance cognition in this population have been conducted in this chronic phase, with the ultimate aim of improving psychosocial and community functioning. The following sections describe both pharmacologic and behavioral methods (e.g., strategy training) that have been tested for attention, memory, and executive function.

Enhancement of Attention in Traumatic Brain Injury

Pharmacologic Treatments for Attention

A variety of noradrenergic agonists have been studied for their effects on attention in chronic TBI. The best evidence is available for methylphenidate, which improves sustained attention and information processing speed[38,40,41] without lowering the seizure threshold.[29] Dopaminergic agents such as amantadine have also been examined; although global arousal may improve as noted, there is limited evidence for enhancement of more complex attention functions.[41] The cholinergic agonist donepezil has also been noted to improve attention in persons with TBI.[42]

Behavioral Treatments for Attention

One of the best-validated approaches to TBI-related attention deficits is attention process training (APT), a manualized treatment that includes repeated practice on computerized task modules addressing a hierarchy of exercises requiring attention skills that are hypothesized to be successively more difficult: sustained, selective, alternating, and divided.[43–45] The developers of APT emphasize that these tasks should be conducted with therapist guidance and that a major component is the identification, training, and evaluation of strategies to manage attention difficulties. Thus, APT may be considered a compensatory, rather than restorative, treatment even though it features repetitive practice on attention-demanding tasks. Controlled studies of a 10-week course of APT suggest that its effects may extend to "real-world" measures whose content is relatively dissimilar from the training materials.[46] APT has been incorporated into multicomponent rehabilitation programs that use attention training as a "base" on which to build more sophisticated reasoning and self-regulation abilities. Note, however, that independent practice on computerized "brain-training"-type attention tasks is not recommended for TBI due to lack of evidence of efficacy.[41]

Another training approach, called time pressure management (TPM), has also been found efficacious for TBI-related attention deficits. In TPM, patients learn strategies to compensate for slowed information processing in real-world activities. These strategies include becoming more self-aware of vulnerability to time pressure, planning ahead to prevent pressure, and creating emergency plans to deal with "information overload." TPM led to superior gains compared to a generic "concentration training" condition in which patients performed tasks while receiving instructions such as "try not to get distracted."[47] TPM appears to generalize well to a range of outcome measures.[41,48]

Taken in aggregate, this research has led to the conclusion that strategic training of attention should be considered a practice standard for persons with TBI in the chronic phase.[46] A systematic review and meta-analysis resulted in an overlapping but different conclusion—that training of attention in the context of real-world activities showed greater efficacy than more isolated modular training.[49] That is, studies focusing on functional skills training with gradually increasing demands on attention showed more efficacy than those focusing on decontextualized attention tasks.

Other behavioral strategies attempted for remediation of attention have met with less success in rigorous testing. Mindfulness meditation does not appear efficacious for this purpose and is not recommended despite its high face validity for improving attention.[41] Dual-task training on activities that need to be performed together (e.g., walking and talking) usually results in improved performance on the specific tasks addressed, but without carryover to other situations requiring divided attention.[41,50]

Enhancement of Memory in Traumatic Brain Injury

Pharmacologic Treatments for Memory

In view of the prominent role of cholinergic systems in anterograde memory, acetylcholine agonists have been the primary agents tested. Donepezil is the most promising of these, associated with substantial improvements in both attention and memory; physostigmine and lecithin have shown less promise.[38,42,51]

Behavioral Treatments for Memory

Purely restorative approaches to memory retraining, such as drilling on list-learning tasks or playing "Concentration," show no general effects on memory unless the material is used to develop or practice compensatory techniques.[52,53] Internal strategies, such as the use of visual imagery to enhance verbal recall, generating mnemonics, or learning to search one's memory more systematically, are most effective for those with relatively mild memory impairment and some preservation of executive functions.[40,52,54] Group-based treatment focused on internal strategy development may be valuable for those with mild to moderate disorders.[55,56]

Perhaps more than for any other cognitive impairment associated with TBI, the evidence is very strong that limitations in memory can be compensated with the use of external aids, even for those with severe deficits.[40,48,57] External aids may be paper based, such as planner books or pocket note cards, or electronic devices such as smartphones. These commonplace devices have high face validity, are familiar to many people, and may require less new learning compared to other strategies.

However, people with TBI frequently have difficulty with the executive demands of using external memory aids, particularly the skills involved in knowing when to use the aid, how to use it effectively in different situations, and using recorded information prospectively. Although clinicians may assume that patients will use a prescribed external aid appropriately on their own, research has shown that intensive, systematic training and practice are needed to use aids such as memory notebooks effectively.[58] A recent randomized controlled trial compared trial-and-error-based instruction with *systematic instruction* for people with TBI learning to use the calendar function on an electronic aid.[59] Systematic instruction is a "package" of training methods that includes direct instruction, modeling, supervised practice with immediate corrective feedback, and gradual withdrawal of support. Performance errors are minimized while a new skill is being acquired, practice is distributed (rather than massed), and training is conducted in a variety of environments to promote generalization. In the trial that compared systematic and trial-and-error-based instruction, both conditions resulted in learning, but systematic instruction resulted in better performance at 30-day follow-up and better generalization across environments. A review of evidence for instructional methods used in cognitive rehabilitation found general support for systematic instruction but emphasized that this approach needs to be modified for specific learning targets and patient characteristics.[60]

In addition to training factors, the success of an external aid depends on an individual's awareness of memory deficits and acceptance of the need to use external strategies, both of which may need to be addressed before any system is introduced. It is important to ask for details as to what strategies have been used by the person both before and after disability and how well those strategies have worked, as well as explore attitudes toward external aids. Younger, better educated people who used memory devices before TBI are likely to use them after injury as well.[61] Compensatory memory strategies should be developed collaboratively with the user and practiced in the context of what the person is doing in everyday life in order to be sustained. With severe memory deficits, it is ideal to involve caregivers in the training so that support will be ongoing.[52]

One of the best-studied electronic memory aids is the NeuroPage, a small portable pager that alerts the person with brief text messages to do specific tasks (e.g., take medications, feed the dog, and leave for the bus stop) at preset times. Times and tasks may be programmed into a centralized computer system by caregivers or therapists in addition to, or instead of, the person with TBI. Wilson and colleagues[62] showed in a large, randomized crossover trial that the NeuroPage enabled people with brain injury to keep appointments and complete other prospective assignments more independently. The effects were so robust that in Britain, the NeuroPage service became part of the national health benefit. A 10-year follow-up examining trends in usage reported that the vast majority of messages were used to help patients remember to take medications at the correct times; other frequently used messages pertained to meal preparation and general time management (e.g., "plan your weekend").

A theoretically motivated training method, *errorless learning* (EL), may help patients with severe memory disorders not only to learn how to use compensatory strategies more effectively but also to learn new information of personal importance such as name–face associations and novel routes.[63] EL provides maximal cues and support during the learning process, with gradual fading as mastery is achieved, ideally without error. Although it is seldom possible to prevent all errors during learning, EL minimizes the error interference that can occur when the explicit memory system is impaired—that is, when there is significant impairment of episodic recall. EL has been used to help people with brain injury to learn the routines involved in effective use of memory notebooks[64] and, more recently, in the use of smartphones as a multipurpose compensatory memory aid.[65] Most impressively, a follow-up conducted 12–19 months after the completion of EL and systematic instruction training in smartphone use showed that 9 of 10 trained individuals maintained accurate use of the phones, with concomitant maintenance of gains in the ability to participate in desired home and community activities.[66]

The challenges of using EL in the clinical setting are to prevent errors while still allowing for active engagement in the task and to know when to fade cueing even though an error may occur. Findings from EL research have implications for typical clinical practice. For example, a procedure commonly used by clinicians and family members with memory-impaired patients—"quizzing" them on orientation items and other information in declarative memory—may actually be detrimental because of the probability that errors will be reinforced.[52] Clinicians must also keep in mind that EL is best used to teach tasks or information that is constrained to only one "right answer" (e.g., transfers and other consistent sequences, names and addresses, and routes) and that training, however successful in leading to persistent improvement, will not generalize to other material.

Enhancement of Executive Function in Traumatic Brain Injury

Pharmacologic Treatments for Executive Function

The cognitive operations involved in executive function are subserved by many different neurotransmitter systems. Depending on the specific aspect of executive function one wishes to change (e.g., disinhibition or apathy), psychoactive medications may be tried on a case-by-case basis; however, no guidelines for specific medications are available.[29,42] One controlled study demonstrated that bromocriptine, a dopamine agonist, improved specific cognitive operations associated with executive function on laboratory tasks in a TBI sample,[67] but this finding was not replicated or followed with additional trials.

Behavioral Treatments for Executive Function

Considering the complexity and scope of the cognitive processes within executive function, it is difficult to summarize the range of treatments that have been studied to try to help people with TBI regain mastery over goal-directed behavior. There is no evidence to date for a purely restorative approach to remediating executive function. For example, providing patients with reasoning puzzles or computer games that appear to "exercise" cognitive control operations does not enhance executive function in everyday life.[68] In contrast, one type of compensatory training appears to be quite effective, according to several systematic reviews of this literature.[48,69,70] This approach involves teaching the affected person a "metacognitive" strategy to apply in problem situations. The intervention consists of training and practice in a step-by-step process for such components as (1) identifying a situation in which action needs to be taken, (2) generating possible courses of action, (3) weighing the advantages and disadvantages of each possibility and deciding on one, (4) planning the specific actions that fit with the decision, (5) executing those actions, (6) checking the results against the original intention, and (7) adjusting the plan as needed. There are several variations on this theme, including an extensively studied treatment called goal management training (GMT),[71] in which the patient learns the steps involved in defining tasks, breaking them into steps, and checking one's performance. GMT has been adapted and combined with problem-solving training and/or attention training in several randomized controlled trials. In one, the GMT-based treatment led to more involvement in work and leisure activities, as well as better ability to set and plan real-life goals, compared to computer-based attention and executive function exercises.[72] In another study, GMT plus attention training led to greater improvements in mental flexibility and other cognitive functions compared to an education control condition.[73] Moreover, participants exposed to the goals training condition exhibited differences on functional magnetic resonance imaging: enhanced processing in extrastriate cortex, interpreted as "tuning" of attention toward goal-relevant visual stimuli.[74] In a similar vein, Rath and colleagues[75] compared a 2- or 3-hour per week, 24-week program of group problem-solving treatment to a more conventional group therapy focused on coping and support for people with chronic TBI and social/vocational dysfunction. The problem-solving group experienced more improvement in both self-perceived problem-solving skill and ratings of that skill provided by outside observers during simulated problem situations, and gains were maintained at 6-month follow-up.[75] These investigators emphasize that change in self-efficacy regarding one's belief that one can solve problems is as important as, or more so, than changing the actual skill set used in problem-solving.[76]

Although results of these metacognitive strategy training approaches are generally reported as positive, rigorous testing has been conducted primarily in persons with relatively milder levels of cognitive impairment. Thus, it is not clear whether there is a minimal level of remaining executive function that is necessary for patients to implement these methods after treatment is concluded. Nonetheless, a meta-analysis of studies using step-by-step metacognitive strategy instruction concluded that there was sufficient evidence to recommend such training for persons with TBI when everyday problem-solving was the goal of treatment.[69]

An interesting variation on the idea of training people with executive dysfunction to set specific goals, or solve specific problems, is the use of "content-free cueing." This involves the use of quasi-randomly timed altering tones to remind patients to stop, re-evaluate what they are doing, and compare it to what they had intended to do. It has been hypothesized that such content-free cues may help to counteract the so-called "goal neglect"[77] seen in some patients with TBI, who can remember their intentions but fail to carry them out due to inadequate self-monitoring. Indeed, the construct of goal neglect was influential in the development of GMT as a remediation strategy. Several studies have shown that such alerting tones do enable better performance on complex tasks and real-life planned activities among people with executive dysfunction.[78,79]

In somewhat more complex treatment approaches, problem-solving or goal management training may be blended with other components in a group-based format. For example, the Short-Term Executive Plus (STEP) program included APT, emotional regulation training, and training in the use of external memory aids in addition to problem-solving focused on real-world situations. Treatment was administered 3 half-days per week for 12 weeks. In a randomized wait-list control group, STEP resulted in enhanced problem-solving and decreased executive dysfunction (both based on self-report).[80] Even more time-intensive programs may be termed "holistic" or "neuropsychological" rehabilitation programs and often include vocational interventions, psychotherapy, and training in compensatory memory strategies as well as executive function treatments. Cicerone and colleagues[81] performed a randomized trial of such a program (15 hours per week for 16 weeks) compared to a more standard outpatient program offering treatments in individual rehabilitation disciplines. The holistic program resulted in more gains in community function and perceived quality of life; improvements were maintained at 6-month follow-up.

Another promising approach to the rehabilitation of executive function is the *gist reasoning* training developed by Chapman and Mudar.[82] In this group-based treatment, patients are systematically taught to extract relevant points from complex information. In a controlled study of persons with chronic TBI, this training resulted in positive changes in community activity as well as gains in reasoning through materials similar to those used in training.[83]

Even if the person with executive dysfunction learns a routine for problem-solving or a new way to extract the gist of important information, the same question arises as for memory compensation: How will he or she know when to use these strategies? Recognition of everyday problem situations may be compromised after TBI, partly due to impaired self-awareness of deficit.[84] Ownsworth and colleagues[85] designed a 16-week group treatment that targeted a broad range of executive skills, including problem-solving and self-awareness. The authors reported that one effect of this treatment was to improve so-called *emergent* and *anticipatory* awareness.[86] Emergent self-awareness refers to recognizing situations in which one's limitations are causing problems; anticipatory awareness allows one to pre-plan preventive or compensatory strategies for situations that are likely to be problematic. A review and discussion of self-awareness interventions by Fleming and Ownsworth[87] highlighted the importance of selecting key tasks and environments, providing clear feedback and structured learning experiences, including peer feedback via group therapy, and carefully considering the emotional consequences of improving self-awareness. Self-awareness training can best be accomplished by using direct feedback, in any modality, in the context of functionally relevant activity and a trusting relationship.[70] Video feedback has been reported to be effective in several studies, including a well-controlled investigation comparing video + verbal feedback, verbal feedback, or experiential feedback (i.e., practice) on performance of a repeated cooking task. The combination of video and verbal feedback resulted in fewer errors over the repeated trials compared to the other two conditions.[88]

For severe cases of inappropriate behavior of which the patient seems to be unaware, several controlled single-case studies have shown benefit of self-monitoring training, in which patients are taught systematically to monitor specific aspects of their behavior in comparison with the observations of other people. Interestingly, self-monitoring training has led to reduction in undesirable behaviors, even when there is no instruction to reduce the behavior nor reinforcement for doing so.[89,90] This strategy might work best with individuals who realize at an intellectual level that certain behaviors are not appropriate but lack the ability to monitor or inhibit the behavior as it is occurring.

The severity of executive deficits may also help determine whether compensatory interventions should be targeted to the affected person (e.g., strategy training) or to modifying the environment. Such modifications may include use of highly repetitive schedules and routines to keep people "on task." In addition, residential and day-treatment facilities for severely affected people may use operant techniques to change stimulus control over behavior.[91] Analyzing and changing the antecedent conditions that appear to trigger dysexecutive behavior is thought to produce better outcomes for severe TBI than manipulating consequences of behavior via reward or punishment. Simplified forms of motivational interviewing and other nonaversive methods may be fruitfully combined with traditional operant conditioning techniques.[92]

EMERGING METHODS OF COGNITIVE ENHANCEMENT IN TRAUMATIC BRAIN INJURY

Despite the promise of the interventions described, very few treatments for cognition in TBI have strong enough evidence of efficacy to support practice guidelines. This is especially true for pharmacologic treatments, which to date have not met with as much success, nor been explored in as many careful trials, compared to the interventions based on behavior change. With few practice guidelines or standards to follow, researchers continue to explore alternative treatments that may prove to ameliorate the cognitive sequelae of TBI. For example, a few studies have examined the role of physical exercise in enhancing cognition after TBI, based largely on the known benefits in other populations. An uncontrolled trial reported that individuals with TBI improved on several neuropsychological measures after engaging in a 12-week program of vigorous physical exercise. Although the lack of a control group precludes definitive causal interpretation, it was notable that the degree of cognitive change was strongly related to the degree of cardiovascular fitness attained. Also, measures of sleep quality and mood remained unchanged, suggesting that the effect was specific to cognition.[93]

Noninvasive neuromodulation techniques have also been explored in TBI rehabilitation. In a double-blind crossover study with nine patients with TBI and residual attention deficits, Kang and colleagues[94] applied a single session of transcranial direct current stimulation (tDCS) versus sham treatment to the left dorsolateral frontal cortex. Modest improvement in reaction time was associated with tDCS, although the conditions did not differ on other objective or subjective indices of attention. Moreover, a sham-controlled study found that tDCS applied to the left dorsolateral prefrontal cortex of TBI patients with disorders of consciousness was associated with significant, transient improvement in responsiveness.[95]

A recent review[96] outlined the rationale and parameters for use of tDCS, transcranial magnetic stimulation, and other neuromodulation methods in TBI. It is very likely that the next decade will see further trials of these methods to enhance cognition in this population.

RESOURCES FOR FURTHER STUDY

Since 2000, a task force within the American Congress of Rehabilitation Medicine (ACRM) Brain Injury Interdisciplinary Special Interest Group has published a series of systematic reviews on nonpharmacologic cognitive rehabilitation in TBI and stroke, with updates every 5 or 6 years.[46,48,97] As of this writing, a fourth update is in preparation with expected publication in 2017 or 2018 in *Archives of Physical Medicine and Rehabilitation*. Members of this group have also published a *Cognitive Rehabilitation Manual*,[98] which purports to translate the systematic reviews into procedures for everyday practice and which has been the focus of clinician training sessions throughout the United States and internationally.

Web resources include PsycBITE (http://www.psycbite.com), which was developed by a group of prominent TBI rehabilitation researchers in Australia and comprises a searchable database of thousands of articles on cognitive rehabilitation for acquired brain injury, as well as ratings of their methodologic rigor. Also, Evidence-Based Review of Moderate to Severe Acquired Brain Injury (http://www.abiebr.com), a project based in Canada, produced its first summary in 2005 and has issued periodic updates of the evidence base thereafter.

CONCLUSION

Cognitive enhancement for TBI continues to grow as a clinical specialty and a focus for research. There remains a need to specify what treatments are most effective for what kinds of patients and problems and also a need to specify treatments in greater detail to facilitate comparisons across studies.[99] Nonetheless, there is increasing evidence that cognitive rehabilitation is effective for this population. The most recent of the ACRM task force reviews reported that 370 interventions had been reviewed altogether, across many domains of cognition; in every study in which cognitive rehabilitation was compared to no active treatment, the cognitive rehabilitation was superior. In studies in which the comparison was to usual care, cognitive rehabilitation was superior in 94%.[48] Both the accelerating pace of research on this topic and the continued attempts to secure funding for evidence-based cognitive remediation appear to be justified.

REFERENCES

1. Faul M, Xu L, Wald MM, et al. *Traumatic brain injury in the United States: Emergency department visits, hospitalizations and deaths, 2002–2006*. Atlanta, GA: Centers for Disease Control and Prevention, National Center for Injury Prevention and Control; 2010.

2. Zaloshnja E, Miller T, Langlois JA, et al. Prevalence of long-term disability from traumatic brain injury in the civilian population of the United States, 2005. *J Head Trauma Rehabil* 2008;23(6):394–400.

3. Whyte J, Ponsford J, Watanabe T, et al. Traumatic brain injury. In Frontera WR (Ed.), *Delisa's physical medicine and rehabilitation: Principles and practice* (5th ed.). Philadelphia, PA: Lippincott Williams & Wilkins; 2010:575–623.

4. Chen AJW, D'Esposito M. Traumatic brain injury: From bench to bedside to society. *Neuron* 2010;66(1):11–14.

5. Schretlen DJ, Shapiro AM. A quantitative review of the effects of traumatic brain injury on cognitive functioning. *Int Rev Psychiatry* 2003;15(4):341–349.

6. Laatsch L, Harrington D, Hotz G, et al. An evidence-based review of cognitive and behavioral rehabilitation treatment studies in children with acquired brain injury. *J Head Trauma Rehabil* 2007;22(4):248–256.

7. Centers for Disease Control and Prevention. *Traumatic brain injury & concussion*. Retrieved from https://www.cdc.gov/TraumaticBrainInjury. Accessed June 1, 2015.

8. MacDonald CL, Johnson AM, Cooper D, et al. Detection of blast-related traumatic brain injury in US military personnel. *N Engl J Med* 2011;364(22):2091–2100.

9. Langlois JA, Rutland-Brown W, Wald MM. The epidemiology and impact of traumatic brain injury: A brief overview. *J Head Trauma Rehabil* 2006;21(5):375–378.

10. Saatman KE, Duhaime A-C, Bullock R, et al. Classification of traumatic brain injury for targeted therapies. *J Neurotrauma* 2008;25(7):719–738.

11. Arciniegas DB. Cholinergic dysfunction and cognitive impairment after traumatic brain injury: Part 2. Evidence from basic and clinical investigations. *J Head Trauma Rehabil* 2011;26(4):319–323.

12. Povlishock JT, Katz DI. Update of neuropathology and neurological recovery after traumatic brain injury. *J Head Trauma Rehabil* 2005;20(1):76–94.

13. Jacobs HE. The Los Angeles Head Injury Survey: Procedures and preliminary findings. *Arch Phys Med Rehabil* 1988;69:425–431.

14. Whyte J, Ponsford J, Snow P. Attentional function after traumatic brain injury: What's impaired, what's preserved and why? In *International Perspectives in Traumatic Brain Injury: Fifth International Association for the Study of Traumatic Brain Injury*. Melbourne, Australia: Australian Academic Press; 1998:154–159.

15. Stuss DT. Traumatic brain injury: Relation to executive dysfunction and the frontal lobes. *Curr Opin Neurol* 2011;24(6):584–589.

16. Hart T, Sherer M, Whyte J, et al. Awareness of behavioral, cognitive and physical deficits in acute traumatic brain injury. *Arch Phys Med Rehabil* 2004;85:1450–1456.

17. Bryant RA, O'Donnell ML, Creamer M, et al. The psychiatric sequelae of traumatic injury. *Am J Psychiatry* 2010;167(3):312–320.

18. McFarland C, Glisky E. Implementation intentions and imagery: Individual and combined effects on prospective memory among young adults. *Mem Cognit* 2012;40(1):62–69.

19. Cicerone KD, Levin H, Malec JF, et al. Cognitive rehabilitation interventions for executive function: Moving from bench to bedside in patients with traumatic brain injury. *J Cogn Neurosci* 2006;18:1212–1222.

20. Whyte J. A grand unified theory of rehabilitation (we wish!). The 57th John Stanley Coulter Memorial Lecture. *Arch Phys Med Rehabil* 2008;89(2):203–209.

21. Boake C, Wilson BA. Stages in the history of neuropsychological rehabilitation. In *Neuropsychological rehabilitation: Theory and practice*. Lisse, the Netherlands: Swets & Zeitlinger; 2003:11–22.

22. Wilson BA. Compensating for cognitive deficits following brain injury. *Neuropsychol Rev* 2000;10(4):233–243.

23. Ylvisaker M, Hanks R, Johnson-Greene D. Perspectives on rehabilitation of individuals with cognitive impairment after brain injury: Rationale for reconsideration of theoretical paradigms. *J Head Trauma Rehabil* 2002;17(3):191–209.

24. Malec JF. Ethical and evidence-based practice in brain injury rehabilitation. *Neuropsychol Rehabil* 2009;19(6):790–806.

25. Hart T, Ehde DM. Defining the treatment targets and active ingredients of rehabilitation: Implications for rehabilitation psychology. *Rehabil Psychol* 2015;60(2):126.

26. Doppenberg EM, Choi SC, Bullock R. Clinical trials in traumatic brain injury: Lessons for the future. *J Neurosurg Anesthesiol* 2004;16(1):87–94.

27. Jennett B, Bond MR. Assessment of outcome after severe brain damage: A practical scale. *Lancet* 1975;305(7905):480–484.

28. Zafonte RD, Bagiella E, Ansel BM, et al. Effect of citicoline on functional and cognitive status among patients with traumatic brain injury: Citicoline Brain Injury Treatment Trial (COBRIT). *JAMA* 2012;308(19):1993–2000.

29. Chew E, Zafonte RD. Pharmacological management of neurobehavioral disorders following traumatic brain injury—A state-of-the-art review. *J Rehabil Res Dev* 2009;46(6):851–879.

30. Stein DG. Embracing failure: What the Phase III progesterone studies can teach about TBI clinical trials. *Brain Injury* 2015;29(11):1259–1272.

31. Novack TA, Caldwell SG, Duke LW, et al. Focused versus unstructured intervention for attention deficits after traumatic brain injury. *J Head Trauma Rehabil* 1996;11(3):52–60.

32. Wheaton P, Mathias JL, Vink R. Impact of early pharmacological treatment on cognitive and behavioral outcome after traumatic brain injury in adults: A meta-analysis. *J Clin Psychopharmacol* 2009;29(5):468–477.

33. Willmott C, Ponsford J. Efficacy of methylphenidate in the rehabilitation of attention following traumatic brain injury: A randomised, crossover, double blind, placebo controlled inpatient trial. *J Neurol Neurosurg Psychiatry* 2009;80(5):552–557.

34. Whyte J, Hart T, Vaccaro M, et al. The effects of methylphenidate on attention deficits after traumatic brain injury: A multi-dimensional randomized controlled trial. *Am J Phys Med Rehabil* 2004;83(6):401–420.

35. Giacino JT, Whyte J, Bagiella E, et al. Placebo-controlled trial of amantadine for severe traumatic brain injury. *N Engl J Med* 2012;366(9):819–826.

36. Ewert J, Levin HS, Watson MG, et al. Procedural memory during posttraumatic amnesia in survivors of severe closed head injury: Implications for rehabilitation. *Arch Neurol* 1989;46(8):911–916.

37. Ptak R, Gurbrod K, Schnider A. Association learning in the acute confusional state. *J Neurol Neurosurg Psychiatry* 1998;65:390–392.

38. Warden DL, Gordon B, McAllister TW, et al. Guidelines for the pharmacologic treatment of neurobehavioral sequelae of traumatic brain injury. *J Neurotrauma* 2006;23(10):1468–1501.

39. Ponsford J, Janzen S, McIntyre A, et al. INCOG recommendations for management of cognition following traumatic brain injury: Part I. Posttraumatic amnesia/delirium. *J Head Trauma Rehabil* 2014;29(4):307–320.

40. Rees L, Marshall S, Hartridge C, et al.; Erabi Group. Cognitive interventions post acquired brain injury. *Brain Injury* 2007;21(2):161–200.

41. Ponsford J, Bayley M, Wiseman-Hakes C, et al. INCOG recommendations for management of cognition following traumatic brain injury: Part II. Attention and information processing speed. *J Head Trauma Rehabil* 2014;29(4):321–337.

42. Arciniegas DB, Silver JM. Pharmacotherapy of cognitive impairments. In *Brain injury medicine: Principles and practice* (2nd ed.). New York, NY: Demos Medical; 2013:1215–1226.

43. Sohlberg MM, Johnson L, Paule L, et al. *Attention process training II: A program to address attentional deficits for persons with mild cognitive dysfunction.* Puyallup, WA: Association for the Neuropsychological Research and Development; 1993.

44. Sohlberg MM, Mateer CA. Effectiveness of an attention-training program. *J Clin Exp Neuropsychol* 1987;9:117–130.

45. Sohlberg MM, McLaughlin KA, Pavese A, et al. Evaluation of attention process training and brain injury education in persons with acquired brain injury. *J Clin Exp Neuropsychol* 2000;22:656–676.

46. Cicerone KD, Dahlberg C, Malec JF, et al. Evidence-based cognitive rehabilitation: Updated review of the literature from 1998 through 2002. *Arch Phys Med Rehabil* 2005;86:1681–1692.

47. Fasotti L, Kovacs F, Eling PATM, et al. Time pressure management as a compensatory strategy training after closed head injury. *Neuropsychol Rehabil* 2000;10(1):47–65.

48. Cicerone KD, Langenbahn DM, Braden C, et al. Evidence-based cognitive rehabilitation: Updated review of the literature from 2003 through 2008. *Arch Phys Med Rehabil* 2011;92(4):519–530.

49. Park NW, Ingles JL. Effectiveness of attention rehabilitation after an acquired brain injury: A meta-analysis. *Neuropsychology* 2001;15(2):199–210.

50. Manly T, Murphy FC. Rehabilitation of executive function and social cognition impairments after brain injury. *Curr Opin Neurol* 2012;25(6):656–661.

51. Wheaton P, Mathias JL, Vink R. Impact of pharmacological treatments on cognitive and behavioral outcome in the post-acute stages of adult traumatic brain injury: A meta-analysis. *J Clin Psychopharmacol* 2011;31(6):745–757.

52. Velikonja D, Tate R, Ponsford J, et al. INCOG recommendations for management of cognition following traumatic brain injury: Part V. Memory. *J Head Trauma Rehabil* 2014;29(4):369–386.

53. Glisky EL, Halligan PW, Wade DT. Can memory impairment be effectively treated? In *The effectiveness of rehabilitation for cognitive deficits*. New York, NY: Oxford University Press; 2005:135–142.

54. Kaschel R, Della Sala S, Cantagallo A, et al. Imagery mnemonics for the rehabilitation of memory: A randomised group controlled trial. *Neuropsychol Rehabil* 2002;12(2):127–153.

55. O'Neil-Pirozzi TM, Strangman GE, Goldstein R, et al. A controlled treatment study of internal memory strategies (I-MEMS) following traumatic brain injury. *J Head Trauma Rehabil* 2010;25(1):43–51.

56. Thickpenny-Davis KL, Barker-Collo SL. Evaluation of a structured group format memory rehabilitation program for adults following brain injury. *J Head Trauma Rehabil* 2007;22(5):303–313.

57. Wilson BA. *Memory rehabilitation*. New York, NY: Guilford; 2009.

58. Schmitter-Edgecombe M, Fahy JF, Whelan JP, et al. Memory remediation after severe closed head injury: Notebook training versus supportive therapy. *J Consult Clin Psychol* 1995;63(3):484–489.

59. Powell LE, Glang A, Ettel D, et al. Systematic instruction for individuals with acquired brain injury: Results of a randomised controlled trial. *Neuropsychol Rehabil* 2012;22(1):85–112.

60. Ehlhardt LA, Sohlberg MM, Kennedy M, et al. Evidence-based practice guidelines for instructing individuals with neurogenic memory impairments: What have we learned in the past 20 years? *Neuropsychol Rehabil* 2008;18(3):300–342.

61. Evans J, Wilson B, Needham P, et al. Who makes good use of memory aids? Results of a survey of people with acquired brain injury. *J Int Neuropsychol Soc* 2003;9(6):925–935.

62. Wilson BA, Emslie HC, Quirk K, et al. Reducing everyday memory and planning problems by means of a paging system: A randomised control crossover study. *J Neurol Neurosurg Psychiatry* 2001;70(4):477–482.

63. Kessels RPC, de Haan EHF. Implicit learning in memory rehabilitation: A meta-analysis on errorless learning and vanishing cues methods. *J Clin Exp Neuropsychol* 2003;25(6):805–814.

64. Squires EJ, Hunkin NM, Parkin AJ. Memory notebook training in a case of severe amnesia: Generalising from paired associate learning to real life. *Neuropsychol Rehabil* 1996;6(1):55–65.

65. Svoboda E, Richards B, Leach L, et al. PDA and smartphone use by individuals with moderate-to-severe memory impairment: Application of a theory-driven training programme. *Neuropsychol Rehabil* 2012;22(3):408–427.

66. Svoboda E, Richards B, Yao C, et al. Long-term maintenance of smartphone and PDA use in individuals with moderate to severe memory impairment. *Neuropsychol Rehabil* 2015;25(3):353–373.

67. McDowell S, Whyte J, D'Esposito M. Differential effect of a dopaminergic agonist on prefrontal function in traumatic brain injury patients. *Brain* 1998;121:1155–1164.

68. D'Esposito M, Gazzaley A. Neurorehabilitation of executive function. In *Neural rehabilitation and repair*. Cambridge, UK: Cambridge University Press; 2006:475–487.

69. Kennedy MR, Coelho C, Turkstra L, et al. Intervention for executive functions after traumatic brain injury: A systematic review, meta-analysis and clinical recommendations. *Neuropsychol Rehabil* 2008;18(3):257–299.

70. Tate R, Kennedy M, Ponsford J, et al. INCOG recommendations for management of cognition following traumatic brain injury: Part III. Executive function and self-awareness. *J Head Trauma Rehabil* 2014;29(4):338–352.

71. Levine B, Robertson IH, Clare L, et al. Rehabilitation of executive functioning: An experimental–clinical validation of Goal Management Training. *J Int Neuropsychol Soc* 2000;6:299–312.

72. Spikman JM, Boelen DH, Lamberts KF, et al. Effects of a multifaceted treatment program for executive dysfunction after acquired brain injury on indications of executive functioning in daily life. *J Int Neuropsychol Soc* 2010;16(01):118–129.

73. Novakovic-Agopian T, Chen AJ, Rome S, et al. Rehabilitation of executive functioning with training in attention regulation applied to individually defined goals: a pilot study bridging theory, assessment, and treatment. *J Head Trauma Rehabil* 2011;26(5):325–338.

74. Chen AJW, Novakovic-Agopian T, Nycum TJ, et al. Training of goal-directed attention regulation enhances control over neural processing for individuals with brain injury. *Brain* 2011;134(5):1541–1554.

75. Rath JF, Simon D, Langenbahn DM, et al. Group treatment of problem-solving deficits in outpatients with traumatic brain injury: A randomised outcome study. *Neuropsychol Rehabil* 2003;13(4):461–488.

76. Rath JF, Hradil AL, Litke DR, et al. Clinical applications of problem-solving research in neuropsychological rehabilitation: Addressing the subjective experience of cognitive deficits in outpatients with acquired brain injury. *Rehabil Psychol* 2011;56(4):320.

77. Duncan J, Johnson R, Swales M, et al. Frontal lobe deficits after head injury: Unity and diversity of function. *Cogn Neuropsychol* 1997;14(5):713–741.

78. Fish J, Evans JJ, Nimmo M, et al. Rehabilitation of executive dysfunction following brain injury: "Content-free" cueing improves everyday prospective memory performance. *Neuropsychologia* 2007;45(6):1318–1330.

79. Manly T, Heutink J, Davison B, et al. An electric knot in the handkerchief: "Content free cueing" and the maintenance of attentive control. *Neuropsychol Rehabil* 2004;14(1/2):89–116.

80. Cantor J, Ashman T, Dams-O'Connor K, et al. Evaluation of the Short-Term Executive Plus intervention for executive dysfunction after traumatic brain injury: A randomized controlled trial with minimization. *Arch Phys Med Rehabil* 2014;95(1):1–9.

81. Cicerone KD, Mott T, Azulay J, et al. A randomized controlled trial of holistic neuropsychologic rehabilitation after traumatic brain injury. *Arch Phys Med Rehabil* 2008;89:2239–2249.

82. Chapman SB, Mudar RA. Enhancement of cognitive and neural functions through complex reasoning training: Evidence from normal and clinical populations. *Front Syst Neurosci* 2014;8.

83. Vas AK, Chapman SB, Cook LG, et al. Higher-order reasoning training years after traumatic brain injury in adults. *J Head Trauma Rehabil* 2011;26(3):224–239.

84. Hart T, Whyte J, Kim J, et al. Executive function and self-awareness of "real-world" behavior and attention deficits following traumatic brain injury. *J Head Trauma Rehabil* 2005;20(4):333–347.

85. Ownsworth T, McFarland K, Young RM. Self-awareness and psychosocial functioning following acquired brain injury: An evaluation of a group support programme. *Neuropsychol Rehabil* 2000;10:465–484.

86. Crosson B, Barco PP, Velozo CA, et al. Awareness and compensation in post-acute head injury rehabilitation. *J Head Trauma Rehabil* 1989;4(3):46–54.

87. Fleming JM, Ownsworth T. A review of awareness interventions in brain injury rehabilitation. *Neuropsychol Rehabil* 2006;16(4):474–500.

88. Schmidt J, Fleming J, Ownsworth T, et al. Video feedback on functional task performance improves self-awareness after traumatic brain injury: A randomized controlled trial. *Neurorehabil Neural Repair* 2013;27(4):316–324.

89. Dayus B, van den Broek M. Treatment of stable delusional confabulations using self-monitoring training. *Neuropsychol Rehabil* 2000;10(4):415–427.

90. Knight C, Rutterford NA, Aldermam N, et al. Is accurate self-monitoring necessary for people with acquired neurological problems to benefit from the use of differential reinforcement methods? *Brain Injury* 2002;16(1):75–87.

91. Worthington A, Halligan PW, Wade DT. Rehabilitation of executive deficits: Effective treatment of related disabilities. In *The effectiveness of rehabilitation for cognitive deficits*. New York, NY: Oxford University Press; 2005:257–267.

92. Giles GM, Manchester D. Two approaches to behavior disorder after traumatic brain injury. *J Head Trauma Rehabil* 2006;21(2):168–178.

93. Chin LM, Keyser RE, Dsurney J, et al. Improved cognitive performance following aerobic exercise training in people with traumatic brain injury. *Arch Phys Med Rehabil* 2015;96(4):754–759.

94. Kang E, Kim D, Paik N. Transcranial direct current stimulation of the left prefrontal cortex improves attention in patients with traumatic brain injury: A pilot study. *J Rehabil Med* 2012;44:346–350.

95. Thibaut A, Bruno M-A, Ledoux D, et al. tDCS in patients with disorders of consciousness: Sham-controlled randomized double-blind study. *Neurology* 2014;82(13):1112–1118.

96. Demirtas-Tatlidede A, Vahabzadeg-Hagh AM, Bernabeu M, et al. Noninvasive brain stimulation in traumatic brain injury. *J Head Trauma Rehabil* 2012;27:274–292.

97. Cicerone KD, Dahlberg C, Kalmar K, et al. Evidence-based cognitive rehabilitation: Recommendations for clinical practice. *Arch Phys Med Rehabil* 2000;81:1596–1615.

98. Haskins EC, Cicerone KD, Trexler LE. *Cognitive rehabilitation manual: Translating evidence-based recommendations into practice*. Reston, VA: ACRM Publishing; 2012.

99. Institute of Medicine. *Cognitive rehabilitation therapy for traumatic brain injury: Evaluating the evidence*. Washington, DC: National Academies Press; 2011.

SEVEN

Cognitive Enhancement in Epilepsy

BETH A. LEEMAN-MARKOWSKI

AND KIMFORD J. MEADOR

COGNITIVE DEFICITS ARE COMMON IN THE SETTING OF EPILEPSY, affecting patients who are newly diagnosed as well as those with chronic seizures.[1-5] Approximately 50–75% of patients with newly diagnosed, untreated seizures demonstrate cognitive dysfunction.[3,5] Deficits may affect multiple domains, including attention, executive function, visuospatial skills, language, and memory.[3] Cognitive dysfunction in epilepsy is often multifactorial and may relate to the underlying etiology or epilepsy syndrome, comorbid psychiatric disease, interictal epileptiform discharges (IEDs), effects of seizures, antiepileptic drugs (AEDs), and surgical interventions.[6-13] Few clinical trials, however, have examined cognitive enhancement in epilepsy patients. More commonly, studies have assessed prevention of impairment. This chapter examines the possible underlying mechanisms of cognitive deficits in epilepsy, methods for prevention of dysfunction, issues in trial design, data regarding cognitive enhancement, and agents currently under study.

MOLECULAR BASIS OF COGNITIVE DYSFUNCTION IN EPILEPSY

The cellular mechanisms underlying memory formation are based on long-term potentiation (LTP), the alteration of synaptic structure and activity resulting from high-frequency input. The mechanisms of LTP and the neuronal circuits involved, however, overlap to a large extent with the process of epileptogenesis.[14] One difference is that LTP can be very selective in the synapses affected, whereas the effects of epileptogenic kindling are more diffuse. Like epileptogenic kindling, LTP is most readily produced in the hippocampus, requires exquisitely timed high-frequency neuronal activity across pre- and postsynaptic neurons, depends on protein synthesis, and results in structural changes. Normal gamma synchronization between the hippocampus and parahippocampus, for example, induces LTP in the CA3 region of the hippocampus. The CA3 cells modulated by the gamma oscillations may signal stimulus features to be encoded.[15] It follows that epileptic activity causing abnormal CA3 excitation or interruption of gamma oscillations in this region could disrupt the process of LTP. LTP is indeed markedly reduced in hippocampal tissue from epilepsy patients with hippocampal-onset seizures and mesial temporal sclerosis[16] Hence, it may be expected that a longer duration of epilepsy or more frequent epileptiform discharges may lead to greater disruption of LTP and predispose patients to memory or other cognitive deficits.

RISK FACTORS AND PREVENTION

Interictal Epileptiform Discharges

Interictal epileptiform discharges are intermittent spikes or sharp waves evident on the electroencephalograms (EEGs) of many epilepsy patients. IEDs are abnormal, but they do not evolve into seizures. They are considered to be markers of epilepsy but are not typically treated with medications. Prior studies have found an association between disruptions of cognitive task performance and the presence of either focal or generalized IEDs. The IED-related disruptions are termed "transient cognitive impairment," although the true duration of IED effects is unknown.

Data revealed poorer intelligence test performance associated with the presence of IEDs.[17–19] Studies also demonstrated longer reaction times, greater numbers of nonresponses, and increased error rates related to abnormal discharges during tests of motor speed and target detection,[8,20–26] continuous visual–motor performance,[27] and driving.[28] Wilkus and Dodril[29] suggested that memory processes may be particularly sensitive to the effects of IEDs. In an animal model, hippocampal spikes resulted in longer spatial memory task completion times, more long-term spatial memory errors, and impaired object recognition compared to controls without epileptiform activity.[30] In humans, IEDs impaired verbal and nonverbal short-term[10] and long-term[31] memory and correlated with accelerated rates of long-term forgetting.[31] Hippocampal interictal discharges have been shown to impair memory when occurring during the retrieval period, as opposed to encoding, in both animals and humans.[32,33]

Whether reduction of IEDs improves cognitive performance remains unknown. The answer will depend on (1) the ability of medications to suppress discharges, (2) the cognitive effects of discharge suppression, and (3) a lack of adverse cognitive effects of the treatment used. Anticonvulsants are typically used to raise the seizure threshold, not inhibit IEDs. Data suggest, however, that some anticonvulsants have IED-reducing effects, including lamotrigine,[34] levetiracetam,[35,36] and topiramate.[37] Preliminary studies also suggest that IED suppression is associated with improvements in behavior[34] and memory,[35] as well as better performance across a broad battery of neuropsychological tests.[38]

Effects of Seizures

The duration of epilepsy, age of onset, seizure frequency, and other seizure-related factors may also affect cognition. Theodore et al.[39] found that a longer duration of epilepsy corresponded to more severe hippocampal sclerosis, suggesting that chronic seizures lead to progressive sclerosis and corresponding cognitive decline in temporal lobe epilepsy (TLE). Consistent with this finding, a longer duration of the seizure disorder in patients with refractory TLE was associated with greater cognitive impairment, as patients with epilepsy of greater than 30 years' duration had lower IQ scores than patients with less than 15 years or 15–30 years of ongoing seizures.[40] Earlier age of onset, at younger than age 5 years, also resulted in lower IQ and measures of attention and executive function,[41] which may indicate that seizures occurring during critical periods of development are more likely to disrupt structural and functional maturation. In children, secondary generalized seizures may pose more risk than simple or complex partial seizures, leading to impairment on a test of spatial memory and overall lower scores across multiple domains.[41] At the time of diagnosis, children with generalized seizures, particularly those with absence seizures, were found to have more impaired cognitive test performance compared to children with partial seizures.[42]

In localization-related epilepsy, the location of seizure-onset plays an important role. Patients with frontal lobe seizures, for example, may have impaired motor coordination and response inhibition.[43] Memory impairment is particularly common with TLE, with material-specific deficits reflecting the site of seizure onset. Patients with dominant hemisphere TLE are at risk for verbal memory loss, whereas those with nondominant hemisphere TLE may have nonverbal memory dysfunction.[12,44] The specific etiology is also significant, in that patients with hippocampal sclerosis may have more diffuse impairments compared to patients with TLE from other causes.[15] As a general rule, idiopathic generalized epilepsy syndromes carry a better cognitive prognosis than epilepsy due to focal lesions, hereditary metabolic syndromes, or neurodegenerative disorders. The generalized epileptic encephalopathies of childhood are classically associated with cognitive regression or delay, including Ohtahara, West, Lennox–Gastaut, and Landau–Kleffner syndromes. Although these disorders involve diffuse cerebral abnormalities, specific deficits may reflect areas in which there is a greater burden of epileptiform or ictal discharges. Landau–Kleffner syndrome is a prime example of an epileptic encephalopathy with a specific language deficit, as patients typically present with verbal auditory agnosia and language regression. Children with continuous spikes and waves during slow-wave sleep syndrome may also exhibit prominent language dysfunction when discharges frequently involve temporal regions, and they may exhibit behavioral abnormalities when discharges largely affect frontal cortex.[46]

Better cognitive outcomes may be attained if epileptiform discharges and seizures can be controlled. Although the goal may be seizure freedom, approximately 30% of adults have medically refractory epilepsy, despite best efforts at treatment. In addition, as discussed in the following sections, anticonvulsant medications, surgical resections, and device implantations may have their own cognition-impairing effects.

Antiepileptic Drugs

The risk of cognitive dysfunction due to AEDs is greater with rapid titration rates, higher dosage and blood levels, and polypharmacy. Time for habituation, individual susceptibility, and type of anticonvulsant must also be considered. In general, the older AEDs, including phenobarbital, benzodiazepines, carbamazepine, phenytoin, and valproate, cause greater deficits compared to the majority of new-generation medications (Figure 7.1). The older drugs have been shown to cause objective deficits in response inhibition, verbal fluency, attention, psychomotor speed, P3 potentials, and verbal recall, as well as subjective confusion and memory loss.[47–50] Phenobarbital can cause greater impairment than other older agents, with poorer performance on tests of psychomotor speed, response inhibition, and attention compared

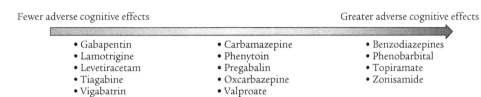

Fewer adverse cognitive effects   Greater adverse cognitive effects

- Gabapentin
- Lamotrigine
- Levetiracetam
- Tiagabine
- Vigabatrin

- Carbamazepine
- Phenytoin
- Pregabalin
- Oxcarbazepine
- Valproate

- Benzodiazepines
- Phenobarbital
- Topiramate
- Zonisamide

FIGURE 7.1 *Relative risk of cognitive side effects with anticonvulsants.*

to carbamazepine, valproate, and phenytoin.[47,49] Benzodiazepines may also produce particularly significant impairments in reaction time, sensory discrimination, vigilance, short-term memory, and divided attention compared to placebo.[50]

Data regarding the new generation of AEDs are mixed, with decrements in performance on isolated tasks and improvement or no effects on other measures. Results also vary across studies. Overall, the newer AEDs are believed to cause fewer cognitive side effects compared to older drugs. Topiramate and zonisamide, however, have cognitive effects that are comparable to, or perhaps worse than, those of the older AEDs. These agents have consistently demonstrated an association with dysfunction across multiple domains, with language deficits being most common. Up to nearly 50% of patients taking zonisamide report mild cognitive complaints,[51] with deficits documented in verbal intelligence,[52] verbal learning and delayed verbal and nonverbal memory,[51,53] and verbal fluency.[51] Effects of zonisamide appear to be dose-related and may resolve with dosage reduction.[51–53]

Adverse effects of topiramate have been documented by testing of IQ, verbal comprehension, verbal and nonverbal memory, verbal and nonverbal fluency, response inhibition, working memory, attention, processing and psychomotor speed, visuospatial skills, naming, and problem-solving.[52,54–59] Up to 50% of patients report anomia or other expressive difficulties with topiramate,[56–58] which may be of sufficient severity to impact daily life.[60] Thompson et al.[60] found that the most significant difficulties occurred with verbal IQ, verbal fluency, and verbal learning. Effects are typically reversible upon drug discontinuation.[52,58,60]

Levetiracetam is unique among the AEDs in that it is generally considered to be "nootropic" or cognition enhancing. After 6 months of treatment, subjective improvement was reported in 58% of patients and objective improvement was noted in 23–29% of patients on measures of executive function, memory, fluency, comprehension, and visuospatial skills. These positive effects may be due to reduction of seizures or interictal discharges because levetiracetam does not produce substantial positive or negative effects in healthy adults,[61] outside of possible improvement in attention span.[62] In patients, positive effects were related to greater baseline function, later-onset seizures, fewer concurrent AEDs, and better seizure control.[63] In newly diagnosed epilepsy patients, levetiracetam monotherapy was associated with improved verbal and visual attention, psychomotor speed, mental flexibility, executive function, verbal fluency, and word generation after approximately 1 year of treatment.[64] Cieslielski et al.[65] noted a trend for improved visual short-term memory and subjective increases in alertness after 2 weeks of treatment with adjunctive levetiractam. However, longer term studies are needed.

Surgical Interventions

Surgical resection of the region of seizure onset may be performed in selected patients with medically refractory epilepsy. Anterior temporal lobectomy (ATL) is the most common surgical procedure performed and may result in freedom from seizures that impair awareness in approximately 60% of patients.[66] In a minority of cases, cognition improves postoperatively, likely due to the removal of nociferous tissue. Stroup et al.[67] noted that 3% of dominant and 7% of nondominant ATL patients had postoperative improvement of verbal memory. Other data suggest improvement in up to 25% of patients.[68–70]

More often, however, surgical resection risks postoperative cognitive dysfunction due to removal of eloquent tissue or damage to connecting fibers. Patients may suffer from postoperative word-finding difficulties[71] and memory dysfunction,[67,72–76] particularly in the setting of dominant-hemisphere resections. Verbal memory decline occurs in an estimated 20% and 40–60% of patients undergoing nondominant and dominant ATL, respectively.[67,75] The resulting deficits are severe in 21% of patients, with performance declining greater than 60% from baseline.[72] Memory deficits are considered disabling in 1–4% of cases.[76]

A focus of preoperative evaluations is to assess the risk of postsurgical cognitive decline in an attempt to avoid deficits and appropriately counsel patients. A number of factors may be considered:

- Preoperative EEG: Bilateral abnormalities on EEG may indicate greater risk of postoperative deficits because removal of the epileptogenic region will leave behind abnormally functioning contralateral tissue.[77]
- Structural magnetic resonance imaging (MRI): Removal of a normal-appearing hippocampus on MRI poses a risk for postoperative learning and memory deficits[78] because it suggests that functional tissue has been resected. Abnormal MRI findings other than unilateral mesial temporal sclerosis also pose some risk because remaining tissue may have less functional reserve.[67] MRI findings are one of the most predictive factors for postsurgical cognitive outcome.[67]

- Neuropsychological testing: Neuropsychological testing is administered routinely pre- and post-epilepsy surgery to evaluate cognitive performance across a variety of measures (Table 7.1). It is expected that deficits will reflect the impairment of functions normally supported by the site of seizure onset (i.e., verbal memory deficits in the setting of dominant temporal lobe seizures). When preoperative testing is normal, there is greater risk for postoperative deficits because properly functioning tissue will be removed.[67,79] Atypical patterns (i.e., impaired spatial memory but intact verbal memory with dominant temporal lobe seizures) are particularly concerning because functional tissue may be removed and nonfunctional tissue may remain.

- Wada testing: Wada testing may be performed preoperatively to assess memory function and lateralization of language. The test involves administration of cognitive testing during selective anesthetization of the anterior circulation of each hemisphere in turn to simulate the outcome of surgery. The anesthesia deafferents the hippocampus and renders cortical language areas nonfunctional for a brief period of time. Injecting the surgical side indicates what tasks can be performed in the absence of that tissue (functional reserve). Injecting the

TABLE 7.1 Neuropsychological Testing[a]

Cognitive Domains Commonly Tested	Recommended Measures
Verbal memory	Rey Auditory Verbal Learning Test
	California Verbal Learning Test-2
	Selective Reminding Test
Spatial memory[b]	Wechsler Memory Scale Visual Reproduction
	Rey–Osterrieth Complex Figure Test
	Brief Visuospatial Memory Test–Revised
	Nonverbal Selective Reminding Test
Naming	Boston Naming Test
Verbal and performance IQ	Wechsler Adult Intelligence Test–Fourth Edition
	Wechsler Abbreviated Scale of Intelligence
Frontal/executive function	Wisconsin Card Sorting
	Trails A and B
	Digit Span
Behavior	No specific tests recommended; Minnesota Multiphasic Personality Inventory and Personality Assessment Inventory commonly used

[a]*Domains assessed and recommended tests per the National Institute of Neurological Disorders and Stroke (NINDS) Common Data Elements.*[188]

[b]*No test was recommended; however, the scales listed were noted by NINDS as measures to consider.*

nonsurgical side demonstrates what functions the to-be-resected tissue performs (functional adequacy). If testing suggests that the contralateral hemisphere cannot support memory functions, resection would pose a great risk of postoperative amnesia.[67,80]

- Functional imaging: Because Wada testing requires angiography for the injection of anesthesia, there is a desire to develop less invasive methods for the assessment of lateralization of function and risks of epilepsy surgery. Limited data have demonstrated the ability of functional MRI (fMRI) to predict postoperative naming ability.[81] Other noninvasive approaches for language and memory lateralization, such as magnetoencephalography, positron emission tomography, transcranial magnetic stimulation, single-photon emission computed tomography, functional transcranial Doppler monitoring, and near infrared spectroscopy, have been investigated.[82,83] In general, neuroimaging methods are less constrained by timing and have the advantages of being able to provide information regarding localization; being easily repeatable; and investigating functions outside of language and memory, such as vision, attention, or motor skills. They share the disadvantage, however, of showing activity in brain regions that may not be essential for task performance, making interpretation of findings challenging. Currently, the clinical utility of fMRI and other imaging modalities is limited, and Wada testing remains in common use.

- Cortical mapping: In patients undergoing intracranial seizure monitoring prior to resection, cortical function may be mapped through direct electrical stimulation of implanted electrodes. Electrical current is gradually increased until it disrupts the function of the underlying tissue. With concurrent cognitive testing, the regions subserving various tasks can be determined. Surgery may then be tailored to avoid resection of eloquent cortex.[84]

In some cases of temporal lobe epilepsy, more restricted resections are performed with the goal of minimizing potential cognitive deficits. Leaving the lateral temporal cortex intact (selective amygdalohippocampectomy (SAH)) may result in better cognitive outcomes,[85] although data are conflicting.[86] Even with limited resections, however, the disruption of connecting fibers and neighboring tissue may still lead to cognitive deficits.[87,88]

Less commonly, the technique of multiple subpial transections (MST) is used in an attempt to spare cognitive function. This approach has been used for decades in the neocortex, typically to treat seizures involving the motor cortex. More recently, MST has been applied to the hippocampus (multiple hippocampal transections (MHT)), particularly in patients with mesial temporal lobe seizures without mesial temporal sclerosis, who are at high risk for postoperative memory loss. The procedure does not remove tissue but, rather, disrupts epileptic networks by transecting the pyramidal layer of the hippocampus while leaving fibers subserving memory intact. In selected cases, the procedure may be combined with MST of the neocortex and resection of the amygdala and/or temporal tip. Shimizu et al.[89] noted no changes in IQ or spatial memory in patients with either left- or right-sided MHT. Of the eight patients with left MHT, one patient had transiently worsened verbal memory, which resolved within 6 months. The remaining patients had no postoperative verbal memory decline. Uda et al.[90] reported that no adverse effects of MHT on verbal or nonverbal memory were noted at 6 months to 1 year postsurgery, with right-sided procedures leading to improvements in verbal memory and left-sided procedures resulting in no significant changes. Similarly, Patil and Andrews[91] found no decrement in verbal memory in nine subjects tested 3–6 months after MHT. Verbal memory improved in seven patients and was unchanged in the others. Nonverbal memory improved in four, slightly deteriorated in two, and was unchanged in the remaining three patients. One patient exhibited transient word-finding difficulty. The effect of hippocampal transections on other cognitive functions (e.g., naming and attention) is unknown.

Minimally invasive techniques, such as radiofrequency amygdalohippocampectomy, were first performed in the 1970s, with minimal success. Advances in imaging technology and surgical approaches have led investigators to re-evaluate these methods. Recent data concerning radiofrequency amygdalohippocampectomy suggest seizure outcomes comparable to those of open surgeries, with improvements in measures of memory, attention, and IQ at 2 years postsurgery.[92] Surgical lesions may also be restricted by new minimally invasive techniques such as gamma knife surgery and laser ablation.

Gamma knife radiosurgery focuses gamma radiation to create lesions restricted to the amygdala, anterior hippocampus, and parahippocampal gyrus, with limited data suggesting a lower rate of postsurgical verbal memory deficits than sustained with standard anterior temporal lobectomy. At 1 and 2 years post-treatment, 25% of patients with dominant radiosurgeries and 7% of patients with nondominant radiosurgeries showed verbal memory impairment. Significant improvements were evident in 16% of patients with dominant radiosurgeries and 7% of patients with nondominant radiosurgeries.[93] Régis et al.[94] found that no declines in visual or verbal memory were evident 2 years after treatment, with 20% experiencing improvements.

Stereotactic laser ablation involves MRI-guided insertion of a laser fiber into the region of seizure onset, which uses heat to cause tissue destruction. Drane et al.[95] demonstrated that laser amygdalohippocampotomy (SLAH), by preserving white matter pathways and neocortex, minimizes face and object naming and facial recognition deficits compared to open resection (standard ATL, tailored ATL, or SAH). None of the SLAH patients in this series experienced any performance declines on these tasks. In contrast, 21 of 22 subjects with open resections of the dominant hemisphere sustained naming deficits, and 11 of 17 nondominant open surgeries led to facial recognition deficits. Preliminary data from this center also suggest beneficial effects of SLAH on memory.[88]

Stimulation Therapies for Epilepsy

A number of implantable devices are now available for the treatment of refractory epilepsy, including vagal nerve stimulators (VNS), responsive neurostimulation (RNS), and deep brain stimulation (DBS). No tissue is resected in such procedures, potentially leading to better cognitive outcomes.

VNS consists of a programmable pulse generator positioned in the chest, with stimulation applied to the left vagus nerve. Epilepsy patients generally experience no overall adverse effects of VNS on cognition, although the positive effects demonstrated in animal models have not been confirmed.[96,97] In children, an initial positive effect of high-level stimulation on IQ was evident, although it was not sustained after a longer term open follow-up period.[97]

In RNS, intracranial electrodes are implanted directly into the seizure-onset zone. The apparatus detects when a seizure occurs and delivers electrical stimulation to abort the event. The pivotal clinical trial involving 191 subjects demonstrated improvements in verbal functioning, visuospatial ability, and memory when tested at 1 and 2 years post-RNS implantation.[98] Recent studies evaluated the effects of stimulation location. Patients receiving hippocampal or extrahippocampal RNS demonstrated no declines in naming or verbal memory when evaluated at 1 and 2 years post-implantation.[99] Exploratory analyses suggested robust naming improvement in neocortical RNS, particularly in the setting of frontal-onset epilepsy, and a smaller beneficial effect on verbal memory in subjects with medial temporal and temporal lobe RNS.[99]

DBS may also have a role in the management of refractory epilepsy, although it is not currently approved by the US Food and Drug Administration. The thalamus has recently been investigated as a potential target, with anterior thalamic DBS approved for adjunctive treatment of partial-onset epilepsy in Canada, Europe, and elsewhere. In a double-blind randomized trial of bilateral DBS of the anterior nuclei of the thalamus for epilepsy (SANTE), no cognitive effects of stimulation were demonstrated at 2-year follow-up.[100] Although subjects receiving active stimulation reported subjective memory impairments more frequently, all complaints ultimately resolved.

Oh et al.[101] studied patients at a mean of 16 months after DBS implantation in the anterior nucleus of the thalamus, and they found improvements in verbal fluency and verbal delayed recall, with no changes on tests of IQ, psychomotor speed, attention, or executive function.

The previously discussed devices result in significant reduction of seizure frequency; however, they do not offer the same likelihood of seizure freedom as resection. Such procedures are typically reserved for patients with refractory seizures who are not candidates for, or do not desire, epilepsy surgery. Hence, a lower likelihood of cognitive deficits must be balanced against the likelihood of seizure freedom for each patient.

Psychosocial Factors

Patients with epilepsy have poorer overall health-related quality of life, more activity limitations, greater social isolation, increased unemployment rates, and lower educational attainment and income than those without seizures.[102–106] Limited school, work, and social engagement may be due in part to continued seizures, effects of AEDs, social stigma, fear of having seizures in public, and comorbid psychiatric disorders.[106,107] Epilepsy patients have a greater incidence of anxiety and depression, with suicide rates 10 times higher than that of the general population.[104] These psychosocial factors may, in turn, further impair cognition with respect to attention and other frontal-executive functions.

Data indicate that using certain coping strategies and maintaining a positive attitude can diminish the negative psychosocial consequences of epilepsy.[107–109] Specific coping mechanisms, such as learned resourcefulness, global problem-solving strategies, and self-efficacy, have been associated with lower levels of depression and anxiety, better subjective health, increased self-esteem, decreased feelings of stigma, and a lessened negative impact of epilepsy.[107] In this regard, cognitive behavioral therapy, self-help and support groups, and educational programs may be helpful.[108] However, the impact of psychosocial interventions on cognition is unknown.

COGNITIVE ENHANCEMENT

Issues in Trial Design

A limited number of studies have investigated cognitive enhancement in patients with epilepsy, perhaps due in part to the difficulties of trial design. As with all studies of cognitive enhancement, administration of test batteries must be standardized across study sites, trials must control for practice effects, and effects of rehearsal should be considered. Intrasubject variability in performance, ceiling effects, and floor effects may obscure improvements. Appropriate control groups are necessary, matched for characteristics such as IQ and age.[110] In addition, the time course of drug effects is unknown, and long-term trials may not be feasible due to cost or subject withdrawal from participation over time.

Other issues may be more specific to the study of an epilepsy patient sample. In many epilepsy-related trials, subject groups are heterogeneous, with multiple seizure types, localizations, etiologies, and concurrent medications. Consequently, drug effects in a specific subset may be difficult to detect, and prohibitively large groups may be required to assess all subgroups and control variables.

The effects of seizure localization must also be considered. Patients with left TLE often have verbal memory loss, for example, whereas patients with right TLE have variable visuospatial deficits.[44] Trials of cognition enhancing agents must use appropriate subject groups and outcome measures. Study designs employing a broad battery of tests may determine whether drug effects are specific to a certain domain or reflect a generalized cognition enhancing effect. It may be particularly difficult to document cognitive improvement in patients with nondominant TLE, however, because visuospatial functions are less strongly lateralized.[111,112] Currently, there are no cognitive tests that have been shown to specifically assess right temporal function.

The outcome measures must also be carefully designed because baseline memory impairment in patients with epilepsy may not be identified using routine measures of 30- to 40-minute delayed recall. Eliciting memory deficits may require delayed testing at hours to weeks to detect accelerated long-term forgetting.[110]

In addition, patients with epilepsy often require multiple anticonvulsants, each with potential cognitive effects. Dosing of the nonstudy drugs should remain unchanged during a trial to avoid confounding due to anticonvulsant side effects or improved seizure control. Maintaining an unchanged anticonvulsant regimen for a prolonged period, however, may not be feasible in patients with breakthrough seizures. In the setting of polypharmacy, it may also be challenging to determine whether an effect is due to the study drug or synergy between agents. In addition, many anticonvulsants have P-450 enzyme-inducing (e.g., phenytoin, phenobarbital, primidone, and carbamazepine) or -inhibiting (i.e., valproic acid) properties,[113] and interactions with cognition enhancing agents should be considered.

Cognitive Rehabilitation

Cognitive rehabilitation is not a unitary approach. Many different rehabilitative techniques have been employed, with varying success.[114] Rehabilitation programs often achieve only partial compensation, with less efficacy in left TLE patients, who are likely the most in need of treatment for verbal memory deficits.

Methods for improving memory function include use of external aids (e.g., calendars and alarms) and internal strategies (e.g., semantic associations and mental imagery). Jones[115] examined the use of mental imagery for the recall of verbal material and showed that post left temporal lobectomy patients can have partial compensation and patients post right temporal lobectomy can make gains similar to those of healthy controls. Bresson et al.[116] demonstrated benefits of deep processing, use of cues, and self-generated elaboration when assessing verbal memory in patients with TLE. Similarly, Schefft et al.[117] showed that using a self-generated encoding strategy was beneficial in subjects with temporal and frontal lobe epilepsy when combined with cues for verbal recall or recognition. Following SAH or temporal lesionectomy, Helmstaedter et al.[118] demonstrated limited effects of a holistic rehabilitation approach that involved metacognitive neuropsychological group therapy, occupational therapy, sociotherapy, individual counseling, and computer-based cognitive exercises, with medical care, physical therapy, and sports therapy utilized as needed. The authors found no benefits with respect to figural memory or verbal delayed recall. Although verbal learning and recognition improved in patients post right temporal lobectomy, no effect was seen for patients with left temporal resections. Finally, Koorenhof et al.[119] encouraged the use of external and internal strategies (e.g., mental imagery, elaboration, and computer-based training), with rehabilitation administered pre- or postoperatively in patients with left TLE. They demonstrated improved verbal learning and recall, as well as improved subjective memory ratings, regardless of the timing of rehabilitation relative to surgery. Greater gains in verbal learning were evident with use of the computer-based program and reduction in depressive symptoms, with benefits similar to those of healthy controls.

Strategies for rehabilitation of attentional impairments have included direct training and compensatory methods. Engelberts et al.[120] studied direct retraining of divided attention using computerized tasks, compensation methods (e.g., external aids, daily routines, and reducing task complexity), and a non-intervention control in patients with localization-related epilepsy treated with carbamazepine monotherapy. Both active interventions resulted in improvements on objective and subjective measures involving attention compared to the control group, particularly in patients with breakthrough seizures. The benefits, however, did not extend to a test of divided attention and response inhibition not directly related to the training program. In postoperative patients, however, Helmstaedter et al.[118] showed that attention improved post-temporal lobectomy regardless of rehabilitation.

The cognitive rehabilitation literature is limited by short-term follow-up, small sample sizes, a lack of data regarding generalization of techniques to daily life, and a paucity of controlled studies with objective outcome measures. In addition, much of the rehabilitation work focuses on psychiatric disease rather than cognition. Although few data are available to support its efficacy, cognitive rehabilitation may be useful for the treatment of epilepsy-related cognitive impairment in selected patients. In designing a rehabilitation program, a holistic rehabilitation approach may be more useful than selective interventions to treat memory and attention deficits.[114] The goals of rehabilitation should be individualized, small, concrete, and reflect the patient's interests (i.e., returning to work).

Future Treatments

Acetylcholinesterase Inhibitors

Animal models have demonstrated that hippocampal cholinergic transmission is diminished in epilepsy, similar to Alzheimer's disease, suggesting that acetylcholinesterase inhibitors used for the treatment of Alzheimer's disease might improve memory function in the setting of epilepsy.[121] In mouse models of epilepsy, pentylenetetrazole (PTZ) has been used to induce kindling and corresponding memory deficits. Coadministration of an acetylcholinesterase inhibitor (tacrine) prevented the seizure-associated memory loss as assessed by tests of active avoidance and spatial memory.[121,122] Similar benefits were attained with donepezil, with improved performance on social discrimination, acoustic fear conditioning, water maze, and passive avoidance tasks after PTZ kindling in mice.[123]

Human trials, however, have demonstrated inconsistent results and questionable benefits. Whereas a pilot study found improved verbal short-term memory after 3 months of open-label treatment with donepezil,[124] a randomized, double-blind, placebo-controlled crossover trial showed no effect of donepezil on verbal delayed recall.[125] Galantamine also failed to demonstrate effects on verbal and nonverbal memory in patients with epilepsy.[126]

Acetylcholinesterase inhibitors may pose a risk of seizure exacerbation in this population, potentially limiting their use. Fisher et al.[124] reported a significant increase in the frequency of generalized tonic–clonic seizures during donepezil treatment. Cholinergic agents have been shown to cause seizures and facilitate kindling in animal models as well.[121,122,127] Given isolated reports of seizures associated with donepezil use, the manufacturer issued an advisory note warning of a possible relationship, although data have been insufficient to establish causality. Although an increase in seizures was not noted by Hamberger et al.,[125] seizure exacerbation remains a concern regarding the use of this drug in patients with epilepsy.

Stimulants

The effectiveness of stimulant medications, such as methylphenidate, for the treatment of attention deficit hyperactivity disorder (ADHD) might suggest a role for these agents in the treatment of epilepsy-related cognitive dysfunction. The greatest concern regarding this class of drugs is the potential for seizure exacerbation, as reported in isolated cases.[128] The prescribing information for methylphenidate warns of a lowered seizure threshold, particularly in patients with a history of seizures or EEG abnormalities, and recommends discontinuation of the drug in the setting of seizures. An increased risk of seizures, however, has not been clearly demonstrated in the limited number of studies conducted to date.[129–131] No alteration in seizure frequency or occurrence of new-onset seizures with use of methylphenidate, for example, was noted by McBride et al.[132] in their case series of 23 children with ADHD and epilepsy and/or epileptiform discharges on EEG. Hemmer et al.[133] suggested that a pretreatment EEG may help to assess risk. In children without a history of epilepsy, seizures occurred with stimulant treatment in 1 of 175 patients with a normal EEG but 3 of 30 children with epileptiform abnormalities, all 4 of whom had been taking methylphenidate prior to or at the time of the seizure.

Multiple studies in children with epilepsy and ADHD have demonstrated improved attention and impulsivity with use of the drug.[134] In an open-label study of osmotic-controlled release oral delivery system (OROS) methylphenidate in children with well-controlled epilepsy and ADHD, Yoo et al.[135] reported improved attention, hyperactivity, impulsivity, and quality of life, with 2 of 25 children having breakthrough seizures with treatment. a study by Gucuyener et al.,[136] children with ADHD and active seizures and/or EEG abnormalities took open-label methylphenidate. The drug was effective for symptoms of ADHD without an overall change in seizure frequency, although in an individual subject analysis, 5 of 57 patients with active seizures had an increase in frequency. Efficacy for ADHD symptoms without worsening seizure control in pediatric epilepsy patients was also noted by Finck et al.[137] In a small sample of adults with epilepsy and ADHD, the drug was similarly effective, with no changes in seizure frequency or severity.[138]

Methylphenidate is the only stimulant for which there are prospective, double-blind, placebo-controlled data on subjects with epilepsy. Feldman et al.[139] found improvements in measures of hyperactivity and attention without breakthrough seizures in 10 children with well-controlled epilepsy and ADD with or without hyperactivity. Gross-Tsur et al.[140] found similar results, with no overall changes in seizure frequency. Those who were seizure-free had no breakthrough seizures, and of 5 children with active epilepsy, 3 had an increase in seizure frequency and 2 demonstrated no change or a reduction in frequency.

One study to date has assessed the open-label use of methylphenidate in adults without ADHD, who had cognitive deficits related to focal-onset epilepsy and the use of multiple AEDs.[141] Attention, memory, spatial processing, information processing speed, overall measures of cognition, fatigue, and quality of life were improved post-treatment, with one of eight patients having increased seizure frequency.

When changes in AEDs or improved seizure control are not indicated, methylphenidate may be a reasonable option for treatment of cognitive impairments in patients with well-controlled seizures. However, further research is needed with larger samples and patients with more frequent seizures, varying seizure types, and long-term use.

None of the other stimulants have controlled data in the setting of epilepsy. No systematic investigations of the effects of amphetamines on cognition in patients with epilepsy have been reported to date, with open-label use in one published study of children with ADHD and epilepsy suggesting symptomatic benefit only in a small percentage of cases.[142] No prospective, controlled trials have been published regarding the use of other ADHD treatments, such as atomoxetine, clonidine, or guanfacine, for the treatment of cognitive deficits in the setting of epilepsy.

Although not chemically related to the classic stimulants, modafinil has stimulating effects that have been studied in a small number of trials. A case report suggested benefits of modafinil for the treatment of cognitive deficits due to anticonvulsant use in a patient with epilepsy.[143] Artsy et al.[144] assessed the safety of modafinil in the setting of epilepsy in a retrospective chart review. The authors identified 4 patients with new-onset seizures in the setting of modafinil use, and 6 out of 205 patients with a diagnosis of epilepsy who were receiving modafinil had a concern for seizure exacerbation. No effect of dosage was evident. Rodent models have suggested an anti-epileptic effect of the drug.[145,146] Although some authors are encouraged by these results,[147] others are more cautious regarding the use of modafinil due to non-seizure-related side effects (i.e., Stevens–Johnson syndrome).[129]

N-Methyl-D-Aspartate Receptor Antagonists

It is believed that excitotoxicity, mediated by glutamate acting on N-methyl-D-aspartate (NMDA) receptors in the hippocampus, causes hippocampal sclerosis. This process leads to further seizures and memory dysfunction. Alteration of this excitotoxic pathway by NMDA antagonists would offer a novel approach to the treatment of memory loss.

An NMDA antagonist, memantine, is prescribed in humans for treatment of moderate to severe Alzheimer's disease,[148–150] with significant cognitive improvements as measured by the Severe Impairment Battery. NMDA antagonists have also shown promising results with respect to learning and memory in animal models of epilepsy. In rats, MK-801 injection prior to seizure induction with perforant path electrical stimulation reduced seizure frequency and intensity, and it mitigated impairments in the Morris water maze spatial memory test.[151] *N*-[1-(2-thienyl)cyclohexyl] piperidine (TCP), also acting by NMDA receptor blockade, improved active avoidance and spatial memory test performance in the setting of soman-induced seizures in guinea pigs.[152] Memantine administered to PTZ-kindled rats led to improved spatial learning and memory task performance, in contrast to task impairment evident when memantine alone was administered, suggesting benefit only in the setting of excitotoxicity.[153]

It is unknown, however, if NMDA antagonists would be of benefit in humans with memory dysfunction and seizures. An ongoing study (Leeman-Markowski et al., unpublished data) is testing the hypothesis that treatment with memantine would improve memory test performance in patients with localization-related epilepsy. If beneficial, this would provide a much-needed treatment option with a favorable safety profile. The manufacturer reported a seizure incidence of 0.2% with memantine use in clinical trials, which is lower than that of placebo,[154] although not studied specifically in patients with seizure disorders. Although seizures secondary to memantine have been noted in isolated case reports,[155] there is generally less concern about seizure induction than with the cholinergic medications.

Vinpocetine (Herbal Supplement)

Vinpocetine is a synthetic ethyl ester of apovincamine, a vinca alkaloid derived from the lesser periwinkle (*Vinca minor*). Vinpocetine inhibits Ca^{2+}/calmodulin-dependent phosphodiesterase (PDE) type 1,[156] which prevents the breakdown of cAMP to 5′-AMP, maintaining activation of cyclic AMP response element binding protein (CREB) and protein kinases implicated in memory formation and synaptic plasticity. Vinpocetine's action as a PDE type 1 inhibitor may underlie its ability to facilitate LTP,[157] enhance the structural dynamics of dendritic spines,[158] improve memory retrieval,[159] reverse scopolamine- and hypoxia-induced learning deficits,[150,160] and restore LTP impaired by medial septal lesions[161] in animal models. In addition, neuroprotective effects of vinpocetine have been demonstrated in animal models of ischemia[162–164] and glutamate- and NMDA-related toxicity.[165]

A limited number of human trials suggest positive cognitive effects of vinpocetine as well. Randomized, double-blind crossover studies demonstrated enhanced short-term memory after 2-day trials of vinpocetine in young healthy human volunteers.[166–168] Vinpocetine may also be beneficial in the setting of dementia, although evidence is insufficient to recommend clinical use. A Cochrane review examined double-blind, placebo-controlled randomized trials of vinpocetine in subjects with cognitive impairment due to vascular disease, Alzheimer's disease, mixed (vascular and Alzheimer's disease), and other dementias.[169] The review included three investigations[170–172] showing a statistically significant improvement on the Clinical Global Index after treatment with vinpocetine compared to placebo.

One published study to date has evaluated the use of vinpocetine in subjects with epilepsy-related cognitive impairment.[173] In this trial, vinpocetine was shown to improve attention and memory in patients with cognitive deficits due to epilepsy or dementia, with greater benefit in epilepsy patients. The study was limited, however, by the unblinded design, the absence of placebo control, and lack of control for practice effects because the healthy control group only had baseline testing. An ongoing randomized, double-blind, single-dose, placebo-controlled crossover study in subjects with localization-related epilepsy and healthy controls, followed by an open-label extension in epilepsy patients, is assessing the effects of vinpocetine on memory, attention, executive function, and psychomotor speed (K. J. Meador et al., unpublished data).

The putative anticonvulsant effects of vinpocetine make this agent an attractive candidate for cognitive enhancement in epilepsy. Vinpocetine blocks voltage-gated sodium channels,[174] and compared to carbamazepine, phenytoin, valproate, oxcarbazepine, lamotrigine, and topiramate, vinpocetine is far more potent and effective in inhibiting both sodium and calcium channel-mediated release of glutamate.[175] In animal models, vinpocetine prevented PTZ-induced seizures at lower concentrations than those of carbamazepine, phenytoin, and valproic acid,[176] and it prevented seizures induced by 4-aminopyridine at concentrations lower than that of carbamazepine.[176–179] Although no significant changes in seizure frequency were noted in the study by Ogunrin,[173] two small clinical trials found that vinpocetine reduced seizures in children and adults with epilepsy.[180,181]

Brain Stimulation for Cognitive Enhancement

Trials have evaluated the potential cognitive enhancing effects of DBS in patients with TLE, with variable results. Low-frequency stimulation of the fornix during intracranial monitoring led to improved Mini-Mental Status Exam (MMSE) scores, primarily due to better delayed verbal recall.[182] Possible practice effects, however, may complicate data interpretation. Stimulation of the entorhinal cortex delivered during a spatial learning task resulted in better subsequent recall,[183] whereas hippocampal stimulation had variable effects across subjects. Although direct hippocampal stimulation is generally believed to impair memory formation, Fell et al.[184] demonstrated that low-amplitude synchronous stimulation of rhinal cortex and hippocampal tissue led to a trend for improved verbal recall. In their investigation of continuous, long-term, unilateral amygdalo-hippocampal DBS, Boëx et al.[185] demonstrated reversible memory impairment in two of five patients, but only with higher stimulation settings. Vonck et al.[186] found no neuropsychological effects of either long-term unilateral amygdalo-hippocampal or bilateral hippocampal stimulation. Clearly, effects of DBS will depend on location, stimulation parameters, and underlying structural abnormalities, among other factors.[187] Brain stimulation techniques for improvement of cognitive function remain an active area of investigation.

CONCLUSION

Cognitive deficits often occur in the setting of epilepsy and can negatively impact social, work, and school activities. Cognitive dysfunction in epilepsy is multifactorial. While continued seizures and IEDs may cause impairment, treatments for epilepsy may also lead to cognitive deficits. Cognitive rehabilitation remains the standard treatment modality, but strategies for compensation do not address the underlying mechanisms, and benefits are limited. Much of the time, the goal is prevention of deficits by controlling seizures, minimizing anticonvulsant drug loads, selecting medications with fewer cognitive risks, completing detailed presurgical cognitive evaluations to guide surgical recommendations, and using less invasive or less extensive surgical approaches. A number of therapies for cognitive enhancement, however, are currently under investigation, including stimulant medications, acetylcholinesterase inhibitors, NMDA receptor antagonists, vinpocetine, and deep brain stimulation, with some encouraging results. Cognitive enhancement in epilepsy is an area of great clinical importance and a topic of active research. Effective treatments may have a significant impact on quality of life, employability, or need for assistance with activities of daily living in patients with epilepsy.

DISCLOSURES

Dr. Leeman-Markowski received research funding from University of California, Berkeley (UCB), the Epifellows Foundation, and the American Academy of Neurology.

Dr. Meador received research funding from the National Institutes of Health, the Patient-Centered Outcomes Research Institute, the Epilepsy Foundation, and UCB. The Epilepsy Study Consortium pays Dr. Meador's university for his research consultant time related to Eisai, GW Pharmaceuticals, NeuroPace, Novartis, Supernus, Upsher Smith Laboratories, UCB, and Vivus Pharmaceuticals. He has received travel support from UCB.

REFERENCES

1. Aikiä M, Salmenperä T, Partanen K, et al. Verbal memory in newly diagnosed patients and patients with chronic left temporal lobe epilepsy. *Epilepsy Behav* 2001;2(1):20–27.
2. Pulliainen V, Kuikka P, Jokelainen M. Motor and cognitive functions in newly diagnosed adult seizure patients before antiepileptic medication. *Acta Neurol Scand* 2000;101(2):73–78.
3. Taylor J, Kolamunnage-Dona R, Marson AG, et al. Patients with epilepsy: Cognitively compromised before the start of antiepileptic drug treatment? *Epilepsia* 2010;51(1):48–56.
4. Jokeit H, Ebner A. Effects of chronic epilepsy on intellectual functions. *Prog Brain Res* 2002;135:455–463.
5. Witt J-A, Helmstaedter C. Should cognition be screened in new-onset epilepsies? A study in 247 untreated patients. *J Neurol* 2012;259(8):1727–1731.
6. Lennox WG. Brain injury, drugs, and environment as causes of mental decay in epilepsy. *Am J Psychiatry* 1942;99(2):174–180.
7. Lesser RP, Lüders H, Wyllie E, et al. Mental deterioration in epilepsy. *Epilepsia* 1986;27(Suppl 2):S105–S123.
8. Tromp SC, Weber JW, Aldenkamp AP, et al. Relative influence of epileptic seizures and of epilepsy syndrome on cognitive function. *J Child Neurol* 2003;18(6):407–412.
9. Aldenkamp A, Arends J. The relative influence of epileptic EEG discharges, short nonconvulsive seizures, and type of epilepsy on cognitive function. *Epilepsia* 2004;45(1):54–63.
10. Aarts JH, Binnie CD, Smit AM, et al. Selective cognitive impairment during focal and generalized epileptiform EEG activity. *Brain* 1984;10(Pt 1):293–308.
11. Motamedi G, Meador K. Epilepsy and cognition. *Epilepsy Behav* 2003;4(Suppl 2):S25–S38.
12. Meador KJ. Cognitive outcomes and predictive factors in epilepsy. *Neurology* 2002;58(8 Suppl 5):S21–S26.
13. Leeman BA, Meador KJ. Cognitive effects of epilepsy therapies. In St. Louis E, Ficker DM, O'Brien TJ (Eds.), *Epilepsy and the interictal state: Comorbidities and quality of life*. Oxford, UK: Wiley-Blackwell; 2015:74–87.
14. Meador KJ. The basic science of memory as it applies to epilepsy. *Epilepsia* 2007;48(Suppl 9):23–25.
15. Axmacher N, Mormann F, Fernández G, et al. Memory formation by neuronal synchronization. *Brain Res Rev* 2006;52(1):170–182.
16. Beck H, Goussakov IV, Lie A, et al. Synaptic plasticity in the human dentate gyrus. *J Neurosci* 2000;20(18):7080–7086.
17. Hovey HB, Kooi KA. Transient disturbances of thought processes and epilepsy. *AMA Arch Neurol Psychiatry* 1955;74(3):287–291.
18. Dodrill CB, Wilkus RJ. Relationships between intelligence and electroencephalographic epileptiform activity in adult epileptics. *Neurology* 1976;26(6 Pt 1):525–531.
19. Kooi KA, Hovey HB. Alterations in mental function and paroxysmal cerebral activity. *AMA Arch Neurol Psychiatry* 1957;78(3):264–271.
20. Browne TR, Penry JK, Proter RJ, et al. Responsiveness before, during, and after spike-wave paroxysms. *Neurology* 1974;24(7):659–665.
21. Selldén U. Psychotechnical performance related to paroxysmal discharges in EEG. *Clin Electroencephal* 1971; 2(1):18–27.
22. Schwab RS. Reaction time in petit mal epilepsy. *Res Publ Assoc Res Nerv Ment Dis* 1947:339–341.
23. Shewmon DA, Erwin RJ. The effect of focal interictal spikes on perception and reaction time: I. General considerations. *Electroencephalogr Clin Neurophysiol* 1988;69(4):319–337.
24. Shewmon DA, Erwin RJ. The effect of focal interictal spikes on perception and reaction time: II. Neuroanatomic specificity. *Electroencephalogr Clin Neurophysiol* 1988;69(4):338–352.
25. Tizard B, Margerison JH. The relationship between generalized paroxysmal E.E.G. discharges and various test situations in two epileptic patients. *J Neurol Neurosurg Psychiatry* 1963;26:308–313.

26. Tizard B, Margerison JH. Psychological functions during wave-spike discharge. *Br J Soc Clin Psychol* 1963;3:6–15.

27. Goode, DJ, Penry, JK, Dreifuss, FE. Effects of paroxysmal spike-wave and continuous visual motor performance. *Epilepsia* 1970;11:241–254.

28. Kasteleijn-Nolst Trenité DG, Riemersma JB, Binnie CD, et al. The influence of subclinical epileptiform EEG discharges on driving behaviour. *Electroencephalogr Clin Neurophysiol* 1987;67(2):167–170.

29. Wilkus RJ, Dodrill CB. Neuropsychological correlates of the electroencephalogram in epileptics: I. Topographic distribution and average rate of epileptiform activity. *Epilepsia* 1976;17:89–100.

30. Shatskikh TN, Raghavendra M, Zhao Q, et al. Electrical induction of spikes in the hippocampus impairs recognition capacity and spatial memory in rats. *Epilepsy Behav* 2006;9:549–556.

31. Mameniskiene R, Jatuzis D, Kaubrys G, et al. The decay of memory between delayed and long-term recall in patients with temporal lobe epilepsy. *Epilepsy Behav* 2006;8(1):278–288.

32. Kleen JK, Scott RC, Holmes GL, et al. Hippocampal interictal spikes disrupt cognition in rats. *Ann Neurol* 2010;67:250–257.

33. Kleen JK, Scott RC, Holmes GL, et al. Hippocampal interictal epileptiform activity disrupts cognition in humans. *Neurology* 2013;81:18–24.

34. Pressler RM, Robinson RO, Wilson GA, et al. Treatment of interictal epileptiform discharges can improve behavior in children with behavioral problems and epilepsy. *J Pediatr* 2005;146(1):112–117.

35. Mintz M, Legoff D, Scornaienchi J, et al. The underrecognized epilepsy spectrum: The effects of levetiracetam on neuropsychological functioning in relation to subclinical spike production. *J Child Neurol* 2009;24(7):807–815.

36. Gallagher MJ, Eisenman LN, Brown KM, et al. Levetiracetam reduces spike-wave density and duration during continuous EEG monitoring in patients with idiopathic generalized epilepsy. *Epilepsia* 2004;45(1):90–91.

37. Placidi F, Tombini M, Romigi A, et al. Topiramate: Effect on EEG interictal abnormalities and background activity in patients affected by focal epilepsy. *Epilepsy Res* 2004;58(1):43–52.

38. Leeman BA, Moo LR, Leveroni CL, et al. Cognitive effects of treatment of focal interictal discharges with levetiracetam. *Epilepsia* 2008;49(Suppl 7):136–177. [Abstract]

39. Theodore WH, Bhatia S, Hatta J, et al. Hippocampal atrophy, epilepsy duration, and febrile seizures in patients with partial seizures. *Neurology* 1999;52:132–136.

40. Jokeit H, Ebner A. Long term effects of refractory temporal lobe epilepsy on cognitive abilities: A cross sectional study. *J Neurol Neurosurg Psychiatry* 1999;67(1):44–50.

41. O'Leary DS, Lovell MR, Sackellares JC, et al. Effects of age of onset of partial and generalized seizures on neuropsychological performance in children. *J Nerv Ment Dis* 1983;171(10):624–629.

42. Mandelbaum DE, Burack GD. The effect of seizure type and medication on cognitive and behavioral functioning in children with idiopathic epilepsy. *Dev Med Child Neurol* 1997;39(11):731–735.

43. Helmstaedter C, Kemper B, Elger CE. Neuropsychological aspects of frontal lobe epilepsy. *Neuropsychologia* 1996;34(5):399–406.

44. Barr WB. Examining the right temporal lobe's role in nonverbal memory. *Brain Cogn* 1997;35(1):26–41.

45. York MK, Rettig GM, Grossman RG, et al. Seizure control and cognitive outcome after temporal lobectomy: A comparison of classic Ammon's horn sclerosis, atypical mesial temporal sclerosis, and tumoral pathologies. *Epilepsia* 2003;44(3):387–398.

46. Van Rijckevorsel K. Cognitive problems related to epilepsy syndromes, especially malignant epilepsies. *Seizure* 2006;15(4):227–234.

47. Meador KJ, Loring DW, Huh K, et al. Comparative cognitive effects of anticonvulsants. *Neurology* 1990;40(3 Pt 1):391–394.

48. Meador KJ, Loring DW, Allen ME, et al. Comparative cognitive effects of carbamazepine and phenytoin in healthy adults. *Neurology* 1991;41(10):1537–1540.

49. Meador KJ, Loring DW, Moore EE, et al. Comparative cognitive effects of phenobarbital, phenytoin, and valproate in healthy adults. *Neurology* 1995;45(8):1494–1499.

50. Hindmarch I, Trick L, Ridout F. A double-blind, placebo- and positive-internal-controlled (alprazolam) investigation of the cognitive and psychomotor profile of pregabalin in healthy volunteers. *Psychopharmacology (Berl)* 2005;183(2):133–143.

51. Park S-P, Hwang Y-H, Lee H-W, et al. Long-term cognitive and mood effects of zonisamide monotherapy in epilepsy patients. *Epilepsy Behav* 2008;12(1):102–108.

52. Ojemann LM, Ojemann GA, Dodrill CB, et al. Language disturbances as side effects of topiramate and zonisamide therapy. *Epilepsy Behav* 2001;2(6):579–584.

53. Berent S, Sackellares JC, Giordani B, et al. Zonisamide (CI-912) and cognition: Results from preliminary study. *Epilepsia* 1987;28(1):61–67.

54. Martin R, Kuzniecky R, Ho S, et al. Cognitive effects of topiramate, gabapentin, and lamotrigine in healthy young adults. *Neurology* 1999;52(2):321–327.

55. Meador KJ, Loring DW, Vahle VJ, et al. Cognitive and behavioral effects of lamotrigine and topiramate in healthy volunteers. *Neurology* 2005;64(12):2108–2114.

56. Reife R, Pledger G, Wu SC. Topiramate as add-on therapy: Pooled analysis of randomized controlled trials in adults. *Epilepsia* 2000;41(Suppl 1):S66–S71.

57. Meador KJ, Loring DW, Hulihan JF, et al. Differential cognitive and behavioral effects of topiramate and valproate. *Neurology* 2003;60(9):1483–1488.

58. Lee S, Sziklas V, Andermann F, et al. The effects of adjunctive topiramate on cognitive function in patients with epilepsy. *Epilepsia* 2003;44(3):339–347.

59. Burton LA, Harden C. Effect of topiramate on attention. *Epilepsy Res* 1997;27(1):29–32.

60. Thompson PJ, Baxendale SA, Duncan JS, et al. Effects of topiramate on cognitive function. *J Neurol Neurosurg Psychiatry* 2000;69(5):636–641.

61. Meador KJ, Gevins A, Loring DW, et al. Neuropsychological and neurophysiologic effects of carbamazepine and levetiracetam. *Neurology* 2007;69(22):2076–2084.

62. Mecarelli O, Vicenzini E, Pulitano P, et al. Clinical, cognitive, and neurophysiologic correlates of short-term treatment with carbamazepine, oxcarbazepine, and levetiracetam in healthy volunteers. *Ann Pharmacother* 2004;38(11):1816–1822.

63. Helmstaedter C, Witt J-A. The effects of levetiracetam on cognition: A non-interventional surveillance study. *Epilepsy Behav* 2008;13(4):642–649.

64. Koo DL, Hwang KJ, Kim D, et al. Effects of levetiracetam monotherapy on the cognitive function of epilepsy patients. *Eur Neurol* 2013;70(1-2):88–94.

65. Ciesielski A-S, Samson S, Steinhoff BJ. Neuropsychological and psychiatric impact of add-on titration of pregabalin versus levetiracetam: A comparative short-term study. *Epilepsy Behav* 2006;9(3):424–431.

66. Wiebe S, Blume WT, Girvin JP, et al. Effectiveness and efficiency of surgery for temporal lobe epilepsy study group: A randomized, controlled trial of surgery for temporal-lobe epilepsy. *N Engl J Med* 2001;345(5):311–318.

67. Stroup E, Langfitt J, Berg M, et al. Predicting verbal memory decline following anterior temporal lobectomy (ATL). *Neurology* 2003;60(8):1266–1273.

68. Leijten FSS, Alpherts WCJ, Van Huffelen AC, et al. The effects on cognitive performance of tailored resection in surgery for nonlesional mesiotemporal lobe epilepsy. *Epilepsia* 2005;46(3):431–439.

69. Cukiert A, Buratini JA, Machado E, et al. Seizure-related outcome after corticoamygdalohippocampectomy in patients with refractory temporal lobe epilepsy and mesial temporal sclerosis evaluated by magnetic resonance imaging alone. *Neurosurg Focus* 2002;13(4):ecp2.

70. Sanyal SK, Chandra PS, Gupta S, et al. Memory and intelligence outcome following surgery for intractable temporal lobe epilepsy: Relationship to seizure outcome and evaluation using a customized neuropsychological battery. *Epilepsy Behav* 2005;6(2):147–155.

71. Langfitt JT, Rausch R. Word-finding deficits persist after left anterotemporal lobectomy. *Arch Neurol* 1996;53(1):72–76.

72. Ivnik RJ, Sharbrough FW, Laws ER. Anterior temporal lobectomy for the control of partial complex seizures: Information for counseling patients. *Mayo Clin Proc* 1988;63(8):783–793.

73. Rausch R, Kraemer S, Pietras CJ, et al. Early and late cognitive changes following temporal lobe surgery for epilepsy. *Neurology* 2003;60(6):951–959.

74. Téllez-Zenteno JF, Dhar R, Hernandez-Ronquillo L, et al. Long-term outcomes in epilepsy surgery: Antiepileptic drugs, mortality, cognitive and psychosocial aspects. *Brain* 2007;130(Pt 2):334–345.

75. Paglioli E, Palmini A, Paglioli E, et al. Survival analysis of the surgical outcome of temporal lobe epilepsy due to hippocampal sclerosis. *Epilepsia* 2004;45(11):1383–1391.

76. Spencer SS. Long-term outcome after epilepsy surgery. *Epilepsia* 1996;37(9):807–813.

77. Tuunainen A, Nousiainen U, Hurskainen H, et al. Preoperative EEG predicts memory and selective cognitive functions after temporal lobe surgery. *J Neurol Neurosurg Psychiatry* 1995; 58(6):674–680.

78. Trenerry MR, Jack CR, Ivnik RJ, et al. MRI hippocampal volumes and memory function before and after temporal lobectomy. *Neurology* 1993;43(9):1800–1805.

79. Hermann BP, Seidenberg M, Haltiner A, et al. Relationship of age at onset, chronologic age, and adequacy of preoperative performance to verbal memory change after anterior temporal lobectomy. *Epilepsia* 1995;36(2):137–145.

80. Jokeit H, Ebner A, Holthausen H, et al. Individual prediction of change in delayed recall of prose passages after left-sided anterior temporal lobectomy. *Neurology* 1997;49(2):481–487.

81. Sabsevitz DS, Swanson SJ, Hammeke TA, et al. Use of preoperative functional neuroimaging to predict language deficits from epilepsy surgery. *Neurology* 2003;60(11):1788–1792.

82. Pelletier I, Sauerwein HC, Lepore F, et al. Non-invasive alternatives to the Wada test in the presurgical evaluation of language and memory functions in epilepsy patients. *Epileptic Disord* 2007;9(2):111–126.

83. Papanicolaou AC, Rezaie R, Narayana S, et al. Is it time to replace the Wada test and put awake craniotomy to sleep? *Epilepsia* 2014;55(5):629–632.

84. Shimizu H, Suzuki I, Ishijima B, et al. Modifications of temporal lobectomy according to the extent of epileptic foci and speech-related areas. *Surg Neurol* 1990;34(4):229–234.

85. Morino M, Uda T, Naito K, et al. Comparison of neuropsychological outcomes after selective amygdalohippocampectomy versus anterior temporal lobectomy. *Epilepsy Behav* 2006;9(1):95–100.

86. Wolf RL, Ivnik RJ, Hirschorn KA, et al. Neurocognitive efficiency following left temporal lobectomy: Standard versus limited resection. *J Neurosurg* 1993;79(1):76–83.

87. Lutz MT, Clusmann H, Elger CE, et al. Neuropsychological outcome after selective amygdalo-hippocampectomy with transsylvian versus transcortical approach: A randomized prospective clinical trial of surgery for temporal lobe epilepsy. *Epilepsia* 2004;45(7):809–816.

88. Gross RE, Mahmoudi B, Riley JP. Less is more: Novel less-invasive surgical techniques for mesial temporal lobe epilepsy that minimize cognitive impairment. *Curr Opin Neurol* 2015;28(2):182–191.

89. Shimizu H, Kawai K, Sunaga S, et al. Hippocampal transection for treatment of left temporal lobe epilepsy with preservation of verbal memory. *J Clin Neurosci* 2006;13(3):322–328.

90. Uda T, Morino M, Ito H, et al. Transsylvian hippocampal transection for mesial temporal lobe epilepsy: Surgical indications, procedure, and postoperative seizure and memory outcomes. *J Neurosurg* 2013;119(5):1098–1104.

91. Patil AA, Andrews R. Long term follow-up after multiple hippocampal transection (MHT). *Seizure* 2013;22(9):731–734.

92. Malikova H, Kramska L, Vojtech Z, et al. Stereotactic radiofrequency amygdalohippocampectomy: Two years of good neuropsychological outcomes. *Epilepsy Res* 2013;106(3):423–432.

93. Barbaro NM, Quigg M, Broshek DK, et al. A multicenter, prospective pilot study of gamma knife radiosurgery for mesial temporal lobe epilepsy: Seizure response, adverse events, and verbal memory. *Ann Neurol* 2009;65(2):167–175.

94. Régis J, Rey M, Bartolomei F, et al. Gamma knife surgery in mesial temporal lobe epilepsy: A prospective multicenter study. *Epilepsia* 2004;45(5):504–515.

95. Drane DL, Loring DW, Voets NL, et al. Better object recognition and naming outcome with MRI-guided stereotactic laser amygdalohippocampotomy for temporal lobe epilepsy. *Epilepsia* 2015;56(1):101–113.

96. Boon P, Moors I, De Herdt V, et al. Vagus nerve stimulation and cognition. *Seizure* 2006;15(4):259–263.

97. Klinkenberg S, van den Bosch CNCJ, Majoie HJM, et al. Behavioural and cognitive effects during vagus nerve stimulation in children with intractable epilepsy—A randomized controlled trial. *Eur J Paediatr Neurol* 2013;17(1):82–90.

98. Morrell MJ; RNS System in Epilepsy Study Group. Responsive cortical stimulation for the treatment of medically intractable partial epilepsy. *Neurology* 2011;77(13):1295–1304.

99. Loring DW, Kapur R, Meador K, et al. Long-term memory and language outcomes with responsive cortical stimulation do not differ by stimulation localization. Platform Presentation, American Epilepsy Society, Seattle, WA, December 8, 2014.

100. Fisher R, Salanova V, Witt T, et al. Electrical stimulation of the anterior nucleus of thalamus for treatment of refractory epilepsy. *Epilepsia* 2010;51(5):899–908.

101. Oh Y-S, Kim HJ, Lee KJ, et al. Cognitive improvement after long-term electrical stimulation of bilateral anterior thalamic nucleus in refractory epilepsy patients. *Seizure* 2012;21(3):183–187.

102. Centers for Disease Control and Prevention. Prevalence of epilepsy and health-related quality of life and disability among adults with epilepsy—South Carolina, 2003 and 2004. *MMWR Morb Mortal Wkly Rep* 2005;54(42):1080–1082.

103. Kobau R, DiIorio CA, Price PH, et al. Prevalence of epilepsy and health status of adults with epilepsy in Georgia and Tennessee: Behavioral Risk Factor Surveillance System, 2002. *Epilepsy Behav* 2004;5(3):358–366.

104. Strine TW, Kobau R, Chapman DP, et al. Psychological distress, comorbidities, and health behaviors among US adults with seizures: Results from the 2002 National Health Interview Survey. *Epilepsia* 2005;46(7):1133–1139.

105. Sillanpää M, Jalava M, Kaleva O, et al. Long-term prognosis of seizures with onset in childhood. *N Engl J Med* 1998;338(24):1715–1722.

106. McCagh J, Fisk JE, Baker GA. Epilepsy, psychosocial and cognitive functioning. *Epilepsy Res* 2009;86(1):1–14.

107. Livneh H, Wilson LM, Duchesneau A, et al. Psychosocial adaptation to epilepsy: The role of coping strategies. *Epilepsy Behav* 2001;2(6):533–544.

108. May TW, Pfäfflin M. The efficacy of an educational treatment program for patients with epilepsy (MOSES): Results of a controlled, randomized study. *Epilepsia* 2002;43(5):539–549.

109. DiIorio C, Shafer PO, Letz R, et al. Project EASE: A study to test a psychosocial model of epilepsy medication management. *Epilepsy Behav* 2004;5(6):926–936.

110. Elliott G, Isaac CL, Muhlert N. Measuring forgetting: A critical review of accelerated long-term forgetting studies. *Cortex* 2014;54:16–32.

111. Lee TMC, Yip JTH, Jones-Gotman M. Memory deficits after resection from left or right anterior temporal lobe in humans: A meta-analytic review. *Epilepsia* 2002;43(3):283–291.

112. Glikmann-Johnston Y, Saling MM, Chen J, et al. Structural and functional correlates of unilateral mesial temporal lobe spatial memory impairment. *Brain* 2008;131(Pt 11):3006–3018.

113. Tanaka E. Clinically significant pharmacokinetic drug interactions between antiepileptic drugs. *J Clin Pharm Ther* 1999;24(2):87–92.

114. Farina E, Raglio A, Giovagnoli AR. Cognitive rehabilitation in epilepsy: An evidence-based review. *Epilepsy Res* 2015;109C:210–218.

115. Jones MK. Imagery as a mnemonic aid after left temporal lobectomy: Contrast between material-specific and generalized memory disorders. *Neuropsychologia* 1974;12(1):21–30.

116. Bresson C, Lespinet-Najib V, Rougier A, et al. Verbal memory compensation: Application to left and right temporal lobe epileptic patients. *Brain Lang* 2007;102(1):13–21.

117. Schefft BK, Dulay MF, Fargo JD, et al. The use of self-generation procedures facilitates verbal memory in individuals with seizure disorders. *Epilepsy Behav* 2008;13(1):162–168.

118. Helmstaedter C, Loer B, Wohlfahrt R, et al. The effects of cognitive rehabilitation on memory outcome after temporal lobe epilepsy surgery. *Epilepsy Behav* 2008;12(3):402–409.

119. Koorenhof L, Baxendale S, Smith N, et al. Memory rehabilitation and brain training for surgical temporal lobe epilepsy patients: A preliminary report. *Seizure* 2012;21(3):178–182.

120. Engelberts NHJ, Klein M, Ade HJ, et al. The effectiveness of cognitive rehabilitation for attention deficits in focal seizures: A randomized controlled study. *Epilepsia* 2002;43(6):587–595.

121. Mishra A, Goel RK. Adjuvant anticholinesterase therapy for the management of epilepsy-induced memory deficit: A critical pre-clinical study. *Basic Clin Pharmacol Toxicol* 2014;115(6):512–517.

122. Getova DP, Dimitrova DS. Effects of the anticholinesterase drug tacrine on the development of PTZ kindling and on learning and memory processes in mice. *Folia Med (Plovdiv)* 2000;42(4):5–9.

123. Jia F, Kato M, Dai H, et al. Effects of histamine H(3) antagonists and donepezil on learning and mnemonic deficits induced by pentylenetetrazol kindling in weanling mice. *Neuropharmacology* 2006;50(4):404–411.

124. Fisher RS, Bortz JJ, Blum DE, et al. A pilot study of donepezil for memory problems in epilepsy. *Epilepsy Behav* 2001;2(4):330–334.

125. Hamberger MJ, Palmese CA, Scarmeas N, et al. A randomized, double-blind, placebo-controlled trial of donepezil to improve memory in epilepsy. *Epilepsia* 2007;48(7):1283–1291.

126. Griffith HR, Martin R, Andrews S, et al. The safety and tolerability of galantamine in patients with epilepsy and memory difficulties. *Epilepsy Behav* 2008;13(2):376–380.

127. Turski L, Ikonomidou C, Turski WA, et al. Review: Cholinergic mechanisms and epileptogenesis. The seizures induced by pilocarpine: A novel experimental model of intractable epilepsy. *Synapse* 1989;3(2):154–171.

128. Chamberlain RW. Letter: Convulsions and Ritalin? *Pediatrics* 1974;54(5):658–659.

129. Torres AR, Whitney J, Gonzalez-Heydrich J. Attention-deficit/hyperactivity disorder in pediatric patients with epilepsy: Review of pharmacological treatment. *Epilepsy Behav* 2008;12(2):217–233.

130. Baptista-Neto L, Dodds A, Rao S, et al. An expert opinion on methylphenidate treatment for attention deficit hyperactivity disorder in pediatric patients with epilepsy. *Expert Opin Investig Drugs* 2008;17(1):77–84.

131. Koneski JA, Casella EB. Attention deficit and hyperactivity disorder in people with epilepsy: Diagnosis and implications to the treatment. *Arq Neuropsiquiatr* 2010;68(1):107–114.

132. McBride MC, Wang DD, Torres CF. Methylphenidate in therapeutic doses does not lower seizure threshold. *Ann Neurol* 1986;20:428.

133. Hemmer SA, Pasternak JF, Zecker SG, et al. Stimulant therapy and seizure risk in children with ADHD. *Pediatr Neurol* 2001;24(2):99–102.

134. Semrud-Clikeman M, Wical B. Components of attention in children with complex partial seizures with and without ADHD. *Epilepsia* 1999;40(2):211–215.

135. Yoo HK, Park S, Wang H-R, et al. Effect of methylphenidate on the quality of life in children with epilepsy and attention deficit hyperactivity disorder: An open-label study using an osmotic-controlled release oral delivery system. *Epileptic Disord* 2009;11(4):301–308.

136. Gucuyener K, Erdemoglu AK, Senol S, et al. Use of methylphenidate for attention-deficit hyperactivity disorder in patients with epilepsy or electroencephalographic abnormalities. *J Child Neurol* 2003;18(2):109–112.

137. Finck S, Metz-Lutz MN, Becache E, et al. Attention-deficit hyperactivity disorder in epileptic children: A new indication for methylphenidate? *Ann Neurol* 1995;38:520. [Abstract]

138. Van der Feltz-Cornelis CM, Aldenkamp AP. Effectiveness and safety of methylphenidate in adult attention deficit hyperactivity disorder in patients with epilepsy: An open treatment trial. *Epilepsy Behav* 2006;8(3):659–662.

139. Feldman H, Crumrine P, Handen BL, et al. Methylphenidate in children with seizures and attention-deficit disorder. *Am J Dis Child* 1989;143(9):1081–1086.
140. Gross-Tsur V, Manor O, van der Meere J, et al. Epilepsy and attention deficit hyperactivity disorder: Is methylphenidate safe and effective? *J Pediatr* 1997;130(4):670–674.
141. Moore JL, McAuley JW, Long L, et al. An evaluation of the effects of methylphenidate on outcomes in adult epilepsy patients. *Epilepsy Behav* 2002;3(1):92–95.
142. Ounsted C. The hyperkinetic syndrome in epileptic children. *Lancet* 1955;269(6885):303–311.
143. Smith BW. Modafinil for treatment of cognitive side effects of antiepileptic drugs in a patient with seizures and stroke. *Epilepsy Behav* 2003;4(3):352–353.
144. Artsy E, McCarthy DC, Hurwitz S, et al. Use of modafinil in patients with epilepsy. *Epilepsy Behav* 2012;23(4):405–408.
145. Chatterjie N, Stables JP, Wang H, et al. Anti-narcoleptic agent modafinil and its sulfone: A novel facile synthesis and potential anti-epileptic activity. *Neurochem Res* 2004;29(8):1481–1486.
146. Chen CR, Qu WM, Qiu MH, et al. Modafinil exerts a dose-dependent antiepileptic effect mediated by adrenergic alpha1 and histaminergic H1 receptors in mice. *Neuropharmacology* 2007;53(4):534–541.
147. Garcia VA, Matos G, Tufik S, et al. Demystifying the effect of modafinil in epilepsy. *Epilepsy Behav* 2012;24(2):287.
148. Tariot PN, Farlow MR, Grossberg GT, et al. Memantine treatment in patients with moderate to severe Alzheimer disease already receiving donepezil: A randomized controlled trial. *JAMA* 2004;291(3):317–324.
149. Reisberg B, Doody R, Stöffler A, et al. Memantine in moderate-to-severe Alzheimer's disease. *N Engl J Med* 2003;348(14):1333–1341.
150. Reisberg B, Doody R, Stöffler A, et al. A 24-week open-label extension study of memantine in moderate to severe Alzheimer disease. *Arch Neurol* 2006;63(1):49–54.
151. Kelsey JE, Sanderson KL, Frye CA. Perforant path stimulation in rats produces seizures, loss of hippocampal neurons, and a deficit in spatial mapping which are reduced by prior MK-801. *Behav Brain Res* 2000;107(1-2):59–69.
152. De Groot DM, Bierman EP, Bruijnzeel PL, et al. Beneficial effects of TCP on soman intoxication in guinea pigs: Seizures, brain damage and learning behaviour. *J Appl Toxicol* 2001;21(Suppl 1):S57–S65.
153. Jia L-J, Wang W-P, Li Z-P, et al. Memantine attenuates the impairment of spatial learning and memory of pentylenetetrazol-kindled rats. *Neurol Sci* 2011;32(4):609–613.
154. Memantine [package insert]. St. Louis, MO: Forest Laboratories; 2013.
155. Peltz G, Pacific DM, Noviasky JA, et al. Seizures associated with memantine use. *Am J Health Syst Pharm* 2005;62(4):420–421.
156. Beavo JA. Cyclic nucleotide phosphodiesterases: Functional implications of multiple isoforms. *Physiol Rev* 1995;75(4):725–748.
157. Molnár P, Gaál L. Effect of different subtypes of cognition enhancers on long-term potentiation in the rat dentate gyrus in vivo. *Eur J Pharmacol* 1992;215(1):17–22.
158. Lendvai B, Zelles T, Rozsa B, et al. A vinca alkaloid enhances morphological dynamics of dendritic spines of neocortical layer 2/3 pyramidal cells. *Brain Res Bull* 2003;59(4):257–260.
159. DeNoble VJ. Vinpocetine enhances retrieval of a step-through passive avoidance response in rats. *Pharmacol Biochem Behav* 1987;26(1):183–186.
160. DeNoble VJ, Repetti SJ, Gelpke LW, et al. Vinpocetine: Nootropic effects on scopolamine-induced and hypoxia-induced retrieval deficits of a step-through passive avoidance response in rats. *Pharmacol Biochem Behav* 1986;24(4):1123–1128.
161. Molnár P, Gaál L, Horváth C. The impairment of long-term potentiation in rats with medial septal lesion and its restoration by cognition enhancers. *Neurobiology (Bp)* 1994;2(3):255–266.
162. Rischke R, Krieglstein J. Protective effect of vinpocetine against brain damage caused by ischemia. *Jpn J Pharmacol* 1991;56(3):349–356.

163. Romanova GA, Voronina TA, Dugina YL, et al. Neuroprotective activity of proproten in rats with experimental local photothrombosis of the prefrontal cortex. *Bull Exp Biol Med* 2005;139(4):404–407.

164. Sauer D, Rischke R, Beck T, et al. Vinpocetine prevents ischemic cell damage in rat hippocampus. *Life Sci* 1988;43(21):1733–1739.

165. Miyamoto M, Murphy TH, Schnaar RL, et al. Antioxidants protect against glutamate-induced cytotoxicity in a neuronal cell line. *J Pharmacol Exp Ther* 1989;250(3):1132–1140.

166. Subhan Z, Hindmarch I. Psychopharmacological effects of vinpocetine in normal healthy volunteers. *Eur J Clin Pharmacol* 1985;28(5):567–571.

167. Bhatti JZ, Hindmarch I. Vinpocetine effects on cognitive impairments produced by flunitrazepam. *Int Clin Psychopharmacol* 1987;2(4):325–331.

168. Coleston DM, Hindmarch I. Possible memory-enhancing properties of vinpocetine. *Drug Dev Res* 1988;14(3-4):191–193.

169. Szatmari SZ, Whitehouse PJ. Vinpocetine for cognitive impairment and dementia. *Cochrane Database Syst Rev* 2003;2003(1):CD003119.

170. Blaha L, Erzigkeit H, Adamczyk A, et al. Clinical evidence of the effectiveness of vinpocetine in the treatment of organic psychosyndrome. *Hum Psychopharmacol Clin Exp* 1989;4(2):103–111.

171. Fenzl E, Apecechea M, Schaltenbrand R, et al. Long-term study concerning tolerance and efficacy of vinpocetine in elderly patients suffering from a mild to moderate organic psychosyndrome. In Bes A, Cahn J, Cahn R, et al. (Eds.), *Senile dementias: Early detection*. London: John Libby Eurotext; 1986:580–585.

172. Hindmarch I, Fuchs HH, Erzigkeit H. Efficacy and tolerance of vinpocetine in ambulant patients suffering from mild to moderate organic psychosyndromes. *Int Clin Psychopharmacol* 1991;6(1):31–43.

173. Ogunrin A. Effect of vinpocetine (Cognitol) on cognitive performances of a Nigerian population. *Ann Med Health Sci Res* 2014;4(4):654–661.

174. Molnár P, Erdö SL. Vinpocetine is as potent as phenytoin to block voltage-gated Na⁺ channels in rat cortical neurons. *Eur J Pharmacol* 1995;273(3):303–306.

175. Sitges M, Chiu LM, Guarneros A, et al. Effects of carbamazepine, phenytoin, lamotrigine, oxcarbazepine, topiramate and vinpocetine on Na⁺ channel-mediated release of [³H]glutamate in hippocampal nerve endings. *Neuropharmacology* 2007;52(2):598–605.

176. Nekrassov V, Sitges M. Additive effects of antiepileptic drugs and pentylenetetrazole on hearing. *Neurosci Lett* 2006;406(3):276–280.

177. Nekrassov V, Sitges M. Vinpocetine inhibits the epileptic cortical activity and auditory alterations induced by pentylenetetrazole in the guinea pig in vivo. *Epilepsy Res* 2004;60(1):63–71.

178. Nekrassov V, Sitges M. Comparison of acute, chronic and post-treatment effects of carbamazepine and vinpocetine on hearing loss and seizures induced by 4-aminopyridine. *Clin Neurophysiol* 2008;119(11):2608–2614.

179. Sitges M, Nekrassov V. Vinpocetine prevents 4-aminopyridine-induced changes in the EEG, the auditory brainstem responses and hearing. *Clin Neurophysiol* 2004;115(12):2711–2717.

180. Dutov AA, Tolpyshev BA, Petrov AP, et al. [Use of cavinton in epilepsy]. *Zh Nevropatol Psikhiatr Im S S Korsakova* 1986;86(6):850–855.

181. Dutov AA, Gal'tvanitsa GA, Volkova VA, et al. [Cavinton in the prevention of the convulsive syndrome in children after birth injury]. *Zh Nevropatol Psikhiatr Im S S Korsakova* 1991;91(8):21–22.

182. Koubeissi MZ, Kahriman E, Syed TU, et al. Low-frequency electrical stimulation of a fiber tract in temporal lobe epilepsy. *Ann Neurol* 2013;74(2):223–231.

183. Suthana N, Haneef Z, Stern J, et al. Memory enhancement and deep-brain stimulation of the entorhinal area. *N Engl J Med* 2012;366(6):502–510.

184. Fell J, Staresina BP, Do Lam AT, et al. Memory modulation by weak synchronous deep brain stimulation: A pilot study. *Brain Stimul* 2013;6(3):270-273.

185. Boëx C, Seeck M, Vulliémoz S, et al. Chronic deep brain stimulation in mesial temporal lobe epilepsy. *Seizure* 2011;20(6):485–490.
186. Vonck K, Sprengers M, Carrette E, et al. A decade of experience with deep brain stimulation for patients with refractory medial temporal lobe epilepsy. *Int J Neural Syst* 2013;23(1):1250034.
187. Suthana N, Fried I. Deep brain stimulation for enhancement of learning and memory. *Neuroimage* 2014;85(Pt 3):996–1002.
188. National Institute of Neurological Disorders and Stroke. *NINDS common data elements* [online]. Retrieved from https://www.commondataelements.ninds.nih.gov/#page=Default; 2010; Accessed August 24, 2014.

EIGHT

Cognitive Enhancement at the Mild Cognitive Impairment Stage of Alzheimer's Disease

ZARA MELIKYAN, HEATHER ROMERO, AND KATHLEEN A. WELSH-BOHMER

INTRODUCTION

Alzheimer's disease (AD) is by far the most common cause of dementia in aging and among the most feared health conditions in adults older than age 65 years (MetLife Foundation, 2011). Finding an effective treatment has been an urgent health priority. A number of promising compounds have been identified that show good target engagement in the brain. Despite this success, no effective treatment has been found to reverse or slow the progression of AD (Cummings, Morstorf, & Zhong, 2014). Part of the difficulty is believed to be due to the timing of therapies in the mild to moderate stages of dementia, a point too late in the pathogenesis (Feldman et al., 2014). Therapeutic interventions are being initiated earlier in the disease course, enabled by advances in biomarkers, making it possible to reliably identify individuals in the early stages of disease. The rationale of this strategy is to take advantage of the still healthy neuronal systems to optimize function, slow cognitive decline, and facilitate adaptive compensation in deficient brain networks.

This chapter provides an overview and critique of the evidence supporting the enhancement of cognitive function at the early symptomatic stage of AD, so-called mild cognitive impairment due to AD (MCI-AD). It reviews the clinical diagnosis of MCI-AD, underscoring the differences between this condition and healthy brain aging and highlighting the importance of fluid and imaging biomarkers in ensuring reliable diagnosis and providing targets for therapeutic modification. Next, it discusses techniques to enhance cognition in MCI, with an emphasis on nonpharmacological interventional approaches. It concludes with a discussion of future challenges and opportunities in the treatment of MCI-AD.

DIAGNOSIS OF ALZHEIMER'S DISEASE AND MILD COGNITIVE IMPAIRMENT

Alzheimer's disease is now well recognized as a chronic illness that evolves over the course of decades, involving inexorable worsening in cognition and function that parallels the neuropathological progression across brain systems (Ballard et al., 2011; Jack et al., 2010; Katzman, 2008). In recent years, three sets of diagnostic criteria have been proposed that parse the disease into fundamentally three identifiable stages (Vos et al., 2015). The diagnostic criteria from the International Working Group (IWG) were introduced first and include specificity in the clinical features and require biomarkers (Dubois et al., 2007). Later, the National Institute on Aging–Alzheimer's Association (NIA-AA) criteria were issued, an approach that uses biomarker data in support of the clinical criteria (Albert et al., 2011). The criteria in the fifth edition of the *Diagnostic and Statistical Manual of Mental Disorders* (DSM-5) begin with a clinical diagnosis of mild or major neurocognitive disorder, based on the presence or absence of functional impairment. Clinical assignment of causation is then determined based on disease-specific supporting evidence including genetics. Although biomarkers are recognized in the DSM-5 criteria as likely valuable, they are not included in the criteria and are cited as "not yet fully validated" (American Psychiatric Association, 2013).

Despite the differences in the three criteria, each nosology separates out different levels of cognitive disorder along the continuum of disease. The first stage in the expression of the brain disease is a clinically silent phase in which the neuropathology is beginning to accrue but there are no evident symptoms (Sperling et al., 2011). This is followed by a prodromal stage, often referred to as the MCI-AD stage, in which symptoms begin to emerge but the ability to function independently remains largely intact (Albert et al., 2011). Later, functional impairments become evident, at which point a diagnosis of AD dementia, major neurocognitive disorder, or fully expressed AD can be made (American Psychiatric Association, 2013; Dubois et al., 2007; McKhann et al., 2011). To appreciate more fully the differences across the various criteria, Table 8.1 contrasts each approach for the diagnosis of early symptomatic AD—that is, MCI-AD, prodromal AD, and mild neurocognitive disorder due to AD—according to the NIA-AA, IWG, and DSM-5 criteria, respectively.

The neurocognitive features across the continuum of symptomatic AD are now well recognized, described, and included with varying degrees of specificity within each diagnostic approach (Vos et al., 2015). From the earliest stages in its clinical expression, AD presents with a profound impairment in recent episodic memory, characterized by a rapid forgetting of new information. Subtle at first, the memory disorder becomes increasingly extreme, and the patient may not be able to remember events occurring just minutes before. As the disease progresses, other impairments in cognition become apparent, including problems in higher order executive functions, language expression, motor praxis, and visuospatial abilities (Welsh, Butters, Hughes, Mohs, & Heyman, 1991, 1992). Note that although cognitively healthy older adults can also demonstrate increased forgetfulness with advancing age, the memory problem in normative aging is fundamentally quite different from that in AD. In normal aging, memory problems emerge from difficulties in encoding and retrieving recent information. As a consequence, these memory weaknesses will be mild, not disabling, and largely mitigated through reminders or recognition prompts.

In contrast to cognitively healthy aging, the amnestic syndrome of AD benefits very little from recognition prompting or other retrieval supports. This is because the memory problem of AD involves impaired consolidation of recently experienced events into long-term storage. In this setting, reminders will have little impact because the information to be recalled is no longer accessible. This does not mean that AD patients cannot benefit from compensatory strategies. Early in the illness, particularly during the MCI stage, compensatory strategies can be employed that build on the patient's retained cognitive capacities to bolster memory. Language-based skills, procedural learning, and aspects of problem-solving are retained early in the condition. Hence, the development of regular habits and routines minimizes the problem of losing objects. Use of auxiliary aids (e.g., calendars) and other devices (e.g., calculators, pill boxes, and electronic reminders) can be employed to support function and maintain independence. Eventually, however, as the disease continues to progress, this capacity to compensate becomes more difficult, impairments in meeting daily demands emerge, and the patient can no longer function independently.

Distinguishing between the early symptoms of AD and the more benign effects of healthy cognitive aging can be challenging, particularly in the earliest stages of symptomatic MCI-AD. Detailed neuropsychological assessment can help disentangle

TABLE 8.1 Diagnostic Criteria for the Mild Predementia Stage of Alzheimer's Disease

	Criteria	
International Working Group Prodromal AD (Dubois et al., 2007)	National Institute on Aging–Alzheimer's Association Mild Cognitive Impairment (Albert et al., 2011)	DSM-5 Mild Neurocognitive Disorder (American Psychiatric Association, 2013)
Presence of early and significant episodic memory impairment (alone or with other cognitive-behavioral problems) and, includes both <ul><li>a gradual and progressive course from family or patient report over >6 months; and</li><li>objective evidence of impaired memory on memory tests such as cued recall or encoding tests.</li></ul>	Cognitive concern reflecting a change in cognition from usual baseline reported by the individual, a knowledgeable informant (e.g., a family member), or the clinician's own observation. This can be based on historical information from the subject and/or informant, or it includes actual observed evidence of decline.	Evidence of modest cognitive decline from previous level of performance in one or more cognitive domains based on either an informant report or objective evidence such as neuropsychological testing. Capacity to perform everyday activities (instrumental activities of daily living) is maintained, although greater effort or compensatory strategies may be needed.
In vivo evidence of AD pathology from <ul><li>CSF tau/Aβ levels studies;</li><li>amyloid PET imaging; or</li><li>AD autosomal dominant genetic mutations.</li></ul>	Objective evidence of impairment in one or more cognitive domains, typically episodic memory early in the course. This can be established by formal or bedside testing of multiple domains.	Not occurring exclusively in the context of delirium. Not explained by another mental disorder, such as major depression or schizophrenia.
No sudden onset or early occurrence of gait disturbance, seizures, or major or minor prevalent behavior changes.	Preservation of function in abilities to carry out instrumental activities of daily living, although greater effort, time, and/or compensatory strategies needed.	The disorder is not better explained by cerebrovascular disease, another neurodegenerative disorder, or another medical explanation.
No focal neurological signs, no early extrapyramidal signs, and no early hallucinations or cognitive fluctuations.	Etiology is consistent with AD pathophysiological process with evidence of longitudinal decline when possible and history of AD genetic factors when relevant.	Probable AD as cause of the mild neurocognitive disorder is supported if there is a genetic mutation from family history or genetic testing.

TABLE 8.1 Continued

Criteria		
No other medical condition that is severe enough to account for the presentation.	Vascular, traumatic, and other medical causes responsible for cognitive decline are excluded.	Mild neurocognitive disorder due to possible AD is diagnosed in the absence of a causative gene, and all three of following are met: • Clear evidence of decline in learning/memory and one other domain based on history or serial neuropsychological testing. • Slow and indolent decline in cognition without extended plateaus. • No evidence of mixed etiology.

AD, Alzheimer's disease; CSF, cerebrospinal fluid; PET, positron emission tomography.

the two conditions (Romero, Hayes, & Welsh-Bohmer, 2010; Twamley, Ropacki, & Bondi, 2006). Impaired delayed recall of new information with little improvement following cuing provides evidence of the AD memory disorder. Deficits across other domains are also commonly observed when an individual's cognitive test performance is compared to normative values that are derived from individuals with a similar age and education background. Areas of impairment occur typically in (1) higher executive functions placing demands on multitasking and flexible behavior; (2) language expression, with problems on confrontation naming and semantic fluency; and (3) visuospatial judgment, leading to problems in spatial planning, navigation, and motor praxis (Backman, Jones, Berger, Laukka, & Small, 2005). Typically, the aspects of cognition that are well preserved early in the disease and indistinguishable from normal aging are attentional function, vision perception, and language comprehension (Chen et al., 2001).

Any ambiguity in the clinical diagnosis can be further resolved with repeated testing separated by 12–18 months. Test–retest improvement is common on episodic memory assessment in normal aging, whereas this effect is absent or muted in MCI-AD (Salthouse, 2010). Consequently, a pattern of no improvement or decline on repeated examination signals the likelihood of a neurodegenerative process that can be explored further with a detailed clinically history.

In cases of mild cognitive disorders, in which the diagnosis is still in question, the inclusion of cerebrospinal fluid (CSF) and brain imaging biomarkers for AD may allow further clarity (see Table 8.1; Johnson et al., 2013). In CSF, biomarkers of interest include the two major proteins abnormally processed in AD: amyloid and tau. Levels of the amyloid beta peptide (Aβ), total tau concentrations, and measures of abnormally phosphorylated tau in the CSF can be contrasted to normative values to allow clinical inferences of disease. Neuroimaging permits a direct assessment of abnormal processing of the same key proteins with regional specificity. Brain amyloid aggregation and high levels of phosphorylated tau can be detected and measured using highly specific radioactive tracers and positron emission tomography (PET). Although the methods are not fully validated for clinical use in asymptomatic individuals, the use of imaging and fluid biomarkers in research has proven highly valuable, both as an enrichment tool to identify individuals likely in the very earliest stages of AD and as surrogate markers of disease, capable of monitoring target engagement during the silent stage of the disease. Biomarker testing will no doubt become more commonly ordered as effective therapeutic compounds to treat AD become available and as the tests become reimbursed by third-party insurance payers (Johnson et al., 2013). This, no doubt, will drive personalized medicine in which the requisites for prescribing a drug to prevent AD may require demonstration that the patient has biomarker-affirmed disease before starting a medicine aimed at reducing AD pathology.

ADVANCES IN INTERVENTIONAL APPROACHES

Therapeutic Trials in MCI and Alzheimer's Disease

A goal in diagnosing AD early in its pathogenesis is to begin treating patients before the disease has become entrenched, allowing a greater potential for therapeutic success. Clinical trials in AD have focused on a number of different disease targets and have examined the efficacy of investigational agents, dietary supplements, behavioral–lifestyle approaches, and cognitive interventions. Before the introduction of biomarkers to identify early disease, these trials were largely conducted in clinically affected people with mild to moderate AD dementia (Birks & Harvey, 2006). This work met with some success and also provided the methodological foundation and important safety data crucial to the current generation of clinical trials now aimed at earlier staged disease.

The five available US Food and Drug Administration (FDA)-approved medications for the treatment of AD (Table 8.2) were issued in the early 1990s through

2003 and are not disease modifying but, rather, target neurotransmitter systems implicated in episodic memory and hippocampal memory systems (Karakaya, Fusser, Schroder, & Pantel, 2013). Three of these compounds are cholinesterase inhibitors (ChEIs) and are typically prescribed early in the dementia process. An additional compound is an *N*-methyl-ᴅ-aspartate (NMDA) receptor antagonist. Approved more recently in 2003, this latter compound is commonly used as an add-on medication at the moderate stages of dementia in combination with a ChEI. The fifth compound is a combination pill that encapsulates a ChEI and NMDA antagonist. It has been available since 2014, simplifying medication management and enhancing compliance. All these compounds provide limited symptomatic benefit for some patients (Doody et al., 2009; Feldman et al., 2007; Petersen et al., 2005; Salloway et al., 2004; Winblad et al., 2008). Unfortunately, they do not alter the underlying pathological trajectory. A systematic review of the three

TABLE 8.2 FDA-Approved Compounds for Alzheimer's Disease and Difference on ADAS-Cog Scores at 24 Weeks of Treatment

Compound (Dose)	Year of FDA Approval	Indication	Mechanism of Action	Difference on ADAS-Cog[a]
Donepezil (5 mg)	1996	All stages of AD	Cholinesterase inhibitor	−1.95 (CI: −2.60, −1.29)
Donepezil (10 mg)				−2.48 (CI: −3.23, −1.73)
Galantamine (24 mg)	2000	Mild to moderate stages of AD	Cholinesterase inhibitor	−3.03 (CI: −3.66, −2.41)
Galantamine (32 mg)				−3.20 (CI: −4.36, −2.04)
Rivistigamine (12 mg)	2001	Mild to moderate stages of AD	Cholinesterase inhibitor	−2.01 (CI: −2.69, −1.32)
Memantine (20 mg)	2003	Moderate to severe AD dementia	NMDA receptor antagonist	−1.29 (CI: −2.30, −0.28)
Donepezil and memantine combination (Namzaric)	2014	Moderate to severe AD dementia	Cholinesterase inhibitor and NMDA receptor antagonist	n/a

[a]*Negative numbers favor improvement on a 70-point scale.*

AD, Alzheimer's disease; ADAS-Cog, Alzheimer's Disease Assessment Scale–Cognition; CI, confidence interval; n/a, not applicable; NMDA, N-methyl-ᴅ-aspartate.

Source: Schneider et al. (2014).

ChEIs (donepezil, rivastigmine, and galantamine) in randomized controlled trials among persons with abnormal memory function and/or those who met the MCI diagnostic criteria concluded that use of ChEIs was not associated with any delay in the onset of AD or dementia (Raschetti, Albanese, Vanacore, & Maggini, 2007). Consequently, any improvements in cognition are not sustained, and inevitably the disease progresses (Kaduszkiewicz, Zimmermann, Beck-Bornholdt, & van den Bussche, 2005; Pelosi, McNulty, & Jackson, 2006).

More current therapeutic attempts have focused primarily on reducing Aβ accumulation (Hyman, 2011; Sperling et al., 2011). However, these trials have failed to show a drug–placebo difference in the primary outcomes, despite encouraging evidence of target engagement and amyloid reduction (Cummings et al., 2014). Whereas this lack of efficacy may suggest that the amyloid hypothesis for disease pathogenesis is wrong, other explanations focus on methodological issues, including the inappropriate targeting of disease initiation events (i.e., amyloid deposition accumulation) in patients who are at the end stage of disease (Vellas et al., 2012). Consequently, at least for these anti-Aβ therapies, it may be more effective if treatment was begun early in the disease pathogenesis before significant neuronal injury has accrued (Aisen, Vellas, & Hampel, 2013). Support for this general idea derives from the Aβ immunotherapy trials Expedition 1 and Expedition 2 (Doody et al., 2009). A pre-planned analysis of disease subgroups revealed positive treatment effects at the mild stage of disease. As such, primary and secondary prevention trials are now underway with some of the same amyloid-lowering agents in patients who are at risk of AD or are in the early symptomatic stages.

Clinical Trials to Prevent or Delay Symptom Onset in Alzheimer's Disease

A number of new lines of investigation are now aiming at the preclinical AD stage of disease and target key pathophysiological mechanisms informed by an improved understanding of mechanistic pathways involved at each stage of disease (Bredesen & John, 2013; Sperling et al., 2011). Four prominent multisite trials to delay the onset of MCI-AD were announced in 2011 and started enrollment in 2013 (Reiman et al., 2016). In contrast to prior clinical trial efforts, the four announced trials involve partnerships of academic scientists, industry, and, in some instances, public funds from the National Institutes of Health (NIH). The studies leverage expertise across a number of disciplines to evaluate relatively quickly a number of promising therapeutic compounds, designed to prevent or delay symptomatic AD and simultaneously test the predictive and therapeutic value of a number of AD biomarker endpoints.

The first of the studies, the Anti-Amyloid Treatment in Asymptomatic Alzheimer's or A4 study, is being conducted through the Alzheimer's Disease Cooperative Study group (see https://clinicaltrials.gov, study No. NCT02008357). For this study, subjects aged 65–85 years are randomized to treatment after being screened using amyloid PET scans for the presence of elevated fibrillar amyloid in brain. Those who have evidence of elevated amyloid are invited to participate in the 3-year, placebo-controlled trial of solanezumab, a humanized monoclonal antibody directed against the Aβ peptide and the same compound that was tested in the Expedition 1 and Expedition 2 studies of mild to moderate AD, in which signals of therapeutic benefit were noted in the mild cases of AD (Liu-Seifert et al., 2015).

The Alzheimer's Prevention Initiative (API) Autosomal Dominant AD (ADAD) and Apolipoprotein E4 (APOE4) trials are focused on cognitively unimpaired persons who, based on their genetic background and age, are at particularly high risk for progression to the clinical onset of AD (see https://clinicaltrials.gov, study No. NCT01998841). The API ADAD trial examines efficacy of crenezumab, an experimental antibody targeting Aβ peptide, in approximately 300 people from an extraordinarily large extended family in Colombia, who share a rare genetic mutation that typically triggers AD symptoms at approximately age 45 years. The API APOE4 trial randomizes individuals who are homozygous for the APOE4 risk allele to promising therapeutics. Both API trials are examining Aβ-lowering drugs based on a rationale that AD genetic risk conditions are tightly correlated to high amyloid accumulation in the brain, a fundamental initiating step in the disease. Outcomes in both studies include a novel, empirically derived measure of cognitive performance as well as a variety of embedded AD biomarkers to determine whether treatments affect putative AD biomarkers and whether these effects ultimately predict clinical benefit.

The Dominantly Inherited Alzheimer's Network Trials Unit (DIAN-TU) Biomarker and Adaptive Prevention trials are two studies that are built off of an international, multicenter observational study, DIAN, which has been enrolling more than 400 participants from families with known causative mutations for AD (see https://clinicaltrials.gov, study No. NCT00869817). The DIAN-TU biomarker trial randomizes subjects to either gantenerumab (an antibody targeting aggregated Aβ), solanezumab (an antibody targeting soluble Aβ), or placebo and examines effects on a comprehensive set of AD biomarkers, including amyloid deposition in the brain, CSF Aβ and tau, magnetic resonance imaging brain atrophy, and other functional imaging measures using fluorodeoxyglucose PET imaging and new tau imaging methods. The study intends to also test future drugs as they become available in asymptomatic to mildly symptomatic AD mutation carriers. The DIAN-TU Adaptive Prevention Trial (APT) parallels the biomarker study and leverages the existing infrastructure of the DIAN-TU biomarker trial to perform a registration enabling trial of prevention of cognitive decline. The goal of DIAN-TU APT is to determine whether drugs with proven safety and biomarker efficacy can slow or prevent cognitive and clinical impairment of AD.

The TOMMORROW trial is a unique global trial that does not have NIH public funding but does involve academic researchers and industry partners and is entirely supported via Takeda and Zinfandel Pharmaceuticals (see https://clinicaltrials.gov, study No. NCT01931566). It is a Phase III, double-blind, randomized, placebo-controlled clinical trial involving more than 59 sites globally with two goals: (1) to qualify a genetic biomarker risk assignment algorithm (BRAA) for assigning 5-year risk for developing MCI-AD based on genotype at APOE and another AD risk allele (TOMM40) in relation to age and (2) to evaluate the efficacy of low-dose pioglitazone as a treatment to delay the onset of MCI-AD in cognitively normal, high-risk individuals, as identified by the BRAA. Unlike the other prevention trials, the goal of this study is to delay the onset of MCI due to AD, as determined clinically. The investigation is also testing a novel therapeutic agent that is believed to exert its effects primarily through a mitochondrial mechanism while also having broader effects on AD pathogenesis, including amyloid accumulation.

Nonpharmacological Intervention in Preclinical Alzheimer's Disease and MCI Due to Alzheimer's Disease

In parallel to the drug development efforts, much attention has been directed toward disease prevention through behavioral approaches targeting lifestyle change and other nonpharmacological approaches. The rationale is based on a considerable literature from epidemiological studies throughout the world suggesting that greater than 60% of the risk for AD is related to modifiable risk factors often acquired in midlife (Norton, Matthews, Barnes, Yaffe, & Brayne, 2014). In particular, cardiovascular disease and cerebrovascular disease are modifiable risk factors that can increase the incidence of MCI and AD and accelerate the progression of cognitive decline in MCI and AD. Cardiovascular risk factors (e.g., arterial hypertension, obesity, hypercholesterolemia, atrial fibrillation, smoking, type 2 diabetes, and metabolic syndrome) and cerebrovascular disease (e.g., stroke), especially when combined with AD risk factors, have adverse effects on cognitive functioning for both normal elderly and those with MCI (Middleton & Yaffe, 2009). Also, the likelihood of clinical dementia increases up to twofold in the presence of concurrent cerebrovascular pathology (Schneider, Wilson, Bienias, Evans, & Bennett, 2004).

Because the cardiovascular risk conditions associated with AD are treatable, either through medications or through lifestyle changes, reducing these factors in cognitively healthy adults and patients with memory problems appears to be both a logical and a promising strategy for optimizing brain health and potentially slowing or preventing AD altogether. Evidence to support this assertion derives from the population health literature and has not always been consistent. Studies examining population health trends suggest that reducing the relative prevalence of the seven key negative risk factors (diabetes, hypertension, obesity, physical inactivity, low education, depression, and smoking) by 10–20% during the next three decades could reduce the global prevalence of AD by more than 15% by 2050 (Smith & Yaffe, 2014). Studies examining the treatment of vascular risk factors in relation to disease trends suggest that this approach can be successful, but it may depend on when these treatments are started during the life span and in relation to AD onset (Safouris et al., 2015). Statin use has been linked to lower risk of AD (Rockwood et al., 2002). However, anti-diabetic or antihypertensive medications have not revealed steadily positive association with AD prevention (Forette et al., 2002; Huang et al., 2014; Launer et al., 2011; Prince, Bird, Blizard, & Mann, 1996), and treatment of vascular risk factors in individuals with already diagnosed dementia has demonstrated little success (Fillit, Nash, Rundek, & Zuckerman, 2008).

Approaches to modify lifestyle factors contributing to vascular disease and dementia have focused on physical exercise, heart-smart dietary habits, and cognitive engagement through either mental and social activity or cognitive training interventions. Other nonpharmacological approaches include the use of new technology such as computerized brain training programs or actual neuronal alterations through transcranial magnetic stimulation. Each of these nonpharmacological strategies is designed to enhance brain plasticity either through sustainable lifestyle changes or by directly changing key neural circuits through noninvasive means (Petersen et al., 2014). Each of these approaches shows promise in MCI populations, and all are reviewed in the following sections.

Physical Exercise

There is increasing evidence that aerobic exercise may be protective against cognitive deterioration among individuals with cognitive impairment and dementia (Heyn, Abreu, & Ottenbacher, 2004). The mechanisms for this effect are not clear. However, the benefits of aerobic physical exercises are mainly on vascular health, including (1) improved cerebral circulation and perfusion, (2) lowered blood pressure and lipid levels, (3) prophylaxis of metabolic syndrome, (4) improved endothelial function, (5) increased brain plasticity and brain volume, (6) enhanced vascular reserve, (7) a positive effect on inflammatory markers and enhancement of brain-derived neurotrophic factor, and (8) neurogenesis (Ohman, Savikko, Strandberg, & Pitkala, 2014). Multimodal physical exercise has demonstrated positive effects on reducing pro-inflammatory cytokines levels (tumor necrosis factor-α and interleukin-6) and increasing peripheral concentration of brain-derived neurotrophic factor, as well as some improvement in cognitive functioning in MCI (Nascimento et al., 2014). Furthermore, physical exercise also helps to normalize cortisol levels and circadian rhythms in amnestic MCI (aMCI) patients (Tortosa-Martinez et al., 2015).

Clinical trials in cases of significant cognitive disorder suggest that aerobic exercise may be protective against further cognitive deterioration (Heyn et al., 2004). A systematic review evaluating the effects of aerobic exercise on cognitive performance in patients with dementia found moderate improvements in several cognitive domains (McDonnell, Smith, & Mackintosh, 2011). Epidemiological studies demonstrate decreased risk of developing dementia later in life for those practicing aerobic exercises at least twice a week, although outcomes may be more beneficial for reducing risk of vascular dementia compared to dementia of the Alzheimer's type (Larson et al., 2006; Ravaglia et al., 2008).

There is increasing evidence that the benefits of exercise found in dementia populations also occur earlier in the disease process. Large randomized controlled trials are needed to determine the effects of aerobic exercise on improving cognitive performance in MCI patients. Review of recent randomized controlled trials indicates that systematic aerobic physical exercise (three or four times per week for 1.5 up to 6 months) improves cognition and overall functioning in individuals with MCI. Positive effects were found on measures of global cognition (based on the Mini-Mental State Exam, the Alzheimer's Disease Assessment Scale–Cognition, and Clinical Dementia Rating Sum of Boxes scores), executive function (as measured by verbal fluency tests administered together with the Clock Drawing Test, Trail Making Test A and B, Symbol Digit Substitution, or task switching tests), attention (measured by Stroop Color–Word Test and the digit span test), verbal immediate and delayed recall, as well as performance in activities of daily living (Hu et al., 2014). In addition, observational clinical studies demonstrate a lower rate to AD progression in individuals with MCI systematically involved in physical leisure activities (Grande et al., 2014).

Several studies are currently underway examining the effects of structured physical activity on disease progression; overall cognitive functioning; and cognitive domains most affected by AD pathology, such as processing speed and verbal memory in MCI populations (Sink et al., 2014). A limited number of studies are examining whether the combination of physical activity with other nonpharmacological approaches (e.g., diet) can afford even greater benefits among individuals with MCI. For example, the ENLIGHTEN study is examining whether exercise and the Dietary Approaches to Stop Hypertension (DASH) diet can delay the progression of cognitive impairment among individuals with MCI.

Benefits of Diet

The evidence supporting a role of diet in AD risk derives from a number of large epidemiological studies suggesting that adherence to a heart-smart diet lowers the risk of AD in adults older than age 65 years and leads to improved cognitive health outcomes (Wengreen et al., 2013). Daily intake of fruits and vegetables and weekly intake of fish were associated with a 30–40% decrease in the risk of AD in a 4-year follow-up. At least some of the benefits were restricted to non-APOE4 carriers (Barberger-Gateau et al., 2007; Dai, Borenstein, Wu, Jackson, & Larson, 2006; Nurk et al., 2007; van Gelder, Tijhuis, Kalmijn, & Kromhout, 2007). Attention to diet components suggests that foods rich in antioxidants may affect disease progression. Antioxidants either in supplements or through dietary sources have been associated with a reduced risk of AD as well as better memory performance in the elderly (Perrig, Perrig, & Stahelin, 1997; Wengreen et al., 2013; Zandi et al., 2005).

   Common diets examined in clinical trials are the DASH diet and the Mediterranean diet. The DASH diet is characterized by high consumption of fruits, vegetables, legumes, seeds, meat, fish, poultry, and low-fat dairy and by low consumption of sweets, saturated fat, and sodium. The Mediterranean-style diet is characterized by consumption of extra virgin olive oil, grains, legumes, vegetables, fruit, nuts, fish, and modest intake of wine or alcohol (Tangney, 2014). Both diets have been shown to be protective against AD risk factors such as hypertension, cardiovascular disease, and diabetes. However, the Mediterranean-style diet, rich in omega-3 fatty acids, is considered more beneficial in protecting from AD pathology.

   In cognitively impaired populations, there have also been trials of dietary components, such as omega-3 fatty acids (usually in fish consumptions) or vitamin nutraceutical supplements. One study conducted in patients with mild to moderate AD suggested some limited benefit of antioxidant vitamins, reporting that the combined use of selegeline and vitamin E had a modest effect on the rate of cognitive decline measured during the 2-year trial period (Sano et al., 1997). Similarly, in one study, gingko biloba had a modest effect in patients with mild AD observed during a 1-year trial (Le Bars et al., 2002); however, there was no effect in another large study of individuals with MCI (DeKosky et al., 2008).

Although research has focused on AD populations, there is evidence that diet can protect against cognitive decline in elderly and MCI populations as well. Among individuals with MCI, higher dietary consumption of antioxidants is associated with some improvements in executive functions and constructional praxis (Rita Cardoso et al., 2016). Superior performance in a range of cognitive domains for omega-3 fatty acid consumers from fish and other food was demonstrated in a 5-year follow-up study, although the effects were dose dependent. Benefits of a fish diet are likely mediated by omega-3 fatty acids, especially docosahexaenoic acid (DHA), which is found in oils such as canola oil, flaxseed oil, and walnut oil. Other epidemiological studies of adults aged 55 years old or older have also demonstrated a reduced rate of cognitive decline in 1- and 2-year follow-up for tea intake, especially evident for black (fermented) and oolong (semifermented) regular tea consumers. The benefits were dose dependent and appear specifically related to tea consumption because no benefits have been convincingly demonstrated for coffee intake (Ng, Feng, Niti, Kua, & Yap, 2008).

Cognitive Engagement

Converging lines of evidence from population-based studies (Stern et al., 1995), community cohort studies (Hall et al., 2009), and clinical trials (Rebok, Carlson, & Langbaum, 2007) suggest that engaging in cognitively stimulating activities throughout the life span is important for maintaining optimal cognitive health, delaying the onset of cognitive decline related to AD, and reducing overall dementia risk. Epidemiological studies have shown an inverse association between educational and occupational attainment and later dementia risk, suggesting that these experiences create a "cognitive reserve" that may buffer against the clinical manifestations of AD (Stern, Albert, Tang, & Tsai, 1999). Further evidence suggests that the incidence of AD and other dementias is reduced in individuals who as a group continue to maintain high levels of cognitive stimulation through engaging social and leisure activities (Wilson et al., 2002). This observation suggests that programs that enhance cognitive stimulation into late life may provide a promising prevention tool, leading to better health outcomes at the individual level and potentially reducing the overall public health burden of dementia at a societal level (Mowszowski, Batchelor, & Naismith, 2010).

Clinical trials of cognitive interventions show overall positive benefits in healthy adults and in patients with cognitive disorders, including early AD (Rebok et al., 2014). The evidence is very strong in healthy older adults that cognitive interventions can lead to improvements in performance on tests of memory and executive function domains (Rebok et al., 2007; Smith et al., 2009). The Advanced Cognitive Training for Independent and Vital Elderly (ACTIVE) study was the first large-scale, randomized trial to explore whether cognitive training could have an impact on cognitive function in community-dwelling older adults. Early reports from the study indicated that the cognitive training led to improvements in short-term cognitive abilities and everyday function 5 years later (Willis et al., 2006). Follow-up assessments of the cohort demonstrated that the effects persisted 10 years after the training and generalized beyond the trained domain, leading to improvements in daily function for the active training arms compared to the control group (Rebok et al., 2014).

The effectiveness of cognitive training in patients with diagnosed MCI or early stage AD is more mixed in terms of whether the interventions are effective and sustainable over time (Maci et al., 2012). Some studies note an immediate benefit for different areas of cognition, including executive function, working memory, delayed recall, and global cognition, even after accounting for confounding variables such as baseline score and educational status, whereas others show no benefit (Barnes et al., 2009; Buschert et al., 2011; Carretti, Borella, Fostinelli, & Zavagnin, 2013; Moro et al., 2012; Olchik, Farina, Steibel, Teixeira, & Yassuda, 2013; Rapp, Brenes, & Marsh, 2002; Troyer, Murphy, Anderson, Moscovitch, & Craik, 2008; Tsolaki et al., 2011).

It is likely that within the MCI stage of AD, cognitive interventions alone will be more variable in their effectiveness. Supporting this suggestion, the Finish Geriatric Study to Prevent Cognitive Impairment and Disability (FINGER) found encouraging results among elderly in the general population at high risk for developing dementia who used multidomain approaches including diet, exercise, cognitive training, and vascular risk monitoring (Ngandu et al., 2015). Although this study was not conducted in MCI patients, the notion of combined approaches across the AD continuum, from silent to fully expressed disease, is encouraged given the complexity of the disease (Bredesen & John, 2013). Emerging evidence indicates that a combination of pharmacological and cognitive interventions is one of the promising approaches in clinically symptomatic disease (Rozzini et al., 2007).

Computerized Cognitive Training

A popular and promising cognitive intervention strategy is the use of computer- and Internet-based training approaches. Built around the same goals as conventional cognitive training methods to strengthen cognitive function and buffer against decline with aging, computerized cognitive training has become a growing industry, with numerous companies entering the market claiming to be "brain training" programs (Max Planck Institute for Human Development and Stanford Center on Longevity, 2014). It is estimated that these companies generated $2–$8 billion in revenue through 2015. Although many make promises of improving cognition, memory, and attention, and in some instances have made claims of helping to protect against AD and other cognitive disorders, few of these claims are supported by scientific evidence such as randomized placebo-controlled clinical trials. Despite these criticisms, a number of systematic reviews within the past few years have suggested that Internet- and computer-based brain training approaches may have some merit with regard to both healthy aging and MCI (Gross et al., 2012; Zhuang et al., 2013). A meta-analysis showed that the effect sizes from computer training were as large as, and in some instances larger than, those of cognitive training done using more conventional, in-person methods involving mnemonic strategies (Martin, Clare, Altgassen, Cameron, & Zehnder, 2011). Furthermore, the results suggest that techniques that are aimed at multiple cognitive domain targets and have built-in opportunities for practice and periodic booster training are important for success (Gross et al., 2012).

It is clear that as more individuals in the Baby Boomer generation age and as the risk for dementia continues to grow in the population, the demand for effective, broadly available prevention therapies that are also affordable will become increasingly urgent. Computer brain training is an attractive option should these products prove to live up to their claims. The ubiquitous availability of computers, smartphones, and wearable devices across all demographics suggests that the methods would be available to a broad demographic. Improvements in the technology allowing subjects to track their performance gains in real time and to potentially engage with others collaboratively may offer subjects many of the benefits of in-person cognitive training at minimal cost and inconvenience.

Transcranial Magnetic Stimulation and Transcranial Direct Current Stimulation

Other alternative treatment options that are under clinical investigation include the application of noninvasive brain stimulation methods. Transcranial magnetic stimulation (TMS) modulates cortical plasticity by a brief electrical current that is delivered through a coiled wire placed on the scalp, resulting in a time-varying magnetic field across the scull, which induces an electric field and subsequently alters neuronal activity. Using a weak electric current delivered through two scalp electrodes, transcranial direct current stimulation (tDCS) is another method designed to strategically modulate cortical excitability in brain circuits important for memory processing—typically the dorsolateral prefrontal cortex (DLPFC), temporal and temporoparietal regions, or a combination of these regions.

To date, there are a few studies of the effects of TMS and tDCS on cognitive functioning in MCI. Most of these studies have small sample sizes and are very heterogeneous methodologically; therefore, they may suggest only preliminary inferences. One comprehensive literature review reported some temporary improvements following TMS and tDCS in AD. Although more TMS and tDCS studies have been conducted on AD patients, there is reason to believe that the technique will be more beneficial in MCI patients because less severely impaired individuals have tended to benefit more from the treatment (Cotelli, Manenti, Cappa, Zanetti, & Miniussi, 2008).

Indeed, a limited number of studies have shown modest benefits of TMS in MCI samples (Drumond Marra et al., 2015). Improvements in nonverbal recognition in patients with MCI were seen in one study following repetitive TMS inhibition of the right DLPFC (Turriziani et al., 2012). In another study, semantic word retrieval improved in MCI following decreased bilateral prefrontal activation (using anodal tDCS) (Meinzer et al., 2015). Improvement of memory for face–name association in aMCI was seen following application of daily high-frequency repetitive TMS to the left parietal area (Cotelli et al., 2008). In addition, a single case report demonstrated improvements in the patient's associative memory after TMS (Cotelli et al., 2012). It remains to be seen how useful TMS will be as a treatment option. However, some work suggests that combining TMS with other treatment approaches, such as cognitive training, will be optimally beneficial in MCI (Bentwich et al., 2011; Rabey et al., 2013).

CONCLUSION

If there is one lesson from more than 30 years of research on treatments for AD, it is that this disease is a highly complex, chronic disease evolving over decades in the brain and involving not only multiple pathological mechanisms but also a broad network of interconnected brain systems. It would be foolhardy to believe that the optimal therapeutic approach in this context would be confined to a single method or monotherapy. Alzheimer's disease, like other chronic diseases, will likely require a combination of compounds that are applied strategically either alone or in combinations at different points during the illness. With regard to other chronic diseases, it may be the case that a cocktail of chemicals provides optimal treatment at different phases of disease. In the case of AD, it may be that each constituent exerts only modest effects in isolation, but in combination they provide a synergistic effect (Bredesen & John, 2013). In addition, it is likely that the most effective therapies will not be limited to pharmacological interventions; optimal approaches will involve both pharmacological and nonpharmacological components. One of the challenges to identifying the most effective approaches is to determine the optimal combinations for clinical use and how to personalize these therapies to each patient. Current continuing work with multimodal therapeutic approaches should inform their application in routine clinical practice.

Developing effective compounds to address the public health urgency will also require some streamlining of the current system for drug development and approval. This process includes harmonization of clinical methods across trials, when possible, to facilitate cross-comparisons. Ideally, an expedited sharing of clinical trial data across drug company sponsors will also speed discovery and allow a clearer understanding of disease pathogenesis while also allowing more direct comparisons of factors contributing to efficacy. Clinical trial data are becoming more readily available through federally developed data-sharing efforts such as the National Institute on Drug Abuse's NIDA Data Share website for completed clinical trials (https://datashare.nida.nih.gov). However, the ability to access data earlier in the drug approval process is essential if effective therapeutics are to be developed quickly for AD. Merging data sets earlier in the approval process without having an impact on regulatory approval will have its own set of challenges, but ultimately this harmonized approach could allow for more powerful data sets to inform basic questions of disease mechanisms and targets for interventions across different populations and classes of compounds. The Collaboration for Alzheimer's Prevention (CAP) is a group of major AD prevention trials addressing some of these complex issues in order to determine new ways to work together in support of common goals so as to help stakeholders advance AD prevention research expeditiously with rigor, care, and maximal impact (Reiman et al., 2016).

REFERENCES

Aisen, P. S., Vellas, B., & Hampel, H. (2013). Moving towards early clinical trials for amyloid-targeted therapy in Alzheimer's disease. *Nature Reviews Drug Discovery, 12*(4), 324. doi:10.1038/nrd3842-c1

Albert, M. S., DeKosky, S. T., Dickson, D., Dubois, B., Feldman, H. H., Fox, N. C., . . . Phelps, C. H. (2011). The diagnosis of mild cognitive impairment due to Alzheimer's disease: Recommendations from the National Institute on Aging–Alzheimer's Association workgroups on diagnostic guidelines for Alzheimer's disease. *Alzheimer's & Dementia, 7*(3), 270–279. doi:10.1016/j.jalz.2011.03.008

American Psychiatric Association. (2013). *Diagnostic and statistical manual of mental disorders* (5th ed.). Arlington, VA: American Psychiatric Association.

Backman, L., Jones, S., Berger, A. K., Laukka, E. J., & Small, B. J. (2005). Cognitive impairment in preclinical Alzheimer's disease: A meta-analysis. *Neuropsychology, 19*(4), 520–531. doi:2005-08223-013

Ballard, C., Gauthier, S., Corbett, A., Brayne, C., Aarsland, D., & Jones, E. (2011). Alzheimer's disease. *Lancet*, *377*(9770), 1019–1031. doi:10.1016/S0140-6736(10)61349-9

Barberger-Gateau, P., Raffaitin, C., Letenneur, L., Berr, C., Tzourio, C., Dartigues, J. F., & Alperovitch, A. (2007). Dietary patterns and risk of dementia: The three-city cohort study. *Neurology*, *69*(20), 1921–1930. doi:69/20/1921

Barnes, D. E., Yaffe, K., Belfor, N., Jagust, W. J., DeCarli, C., Reed, B. R., & Kramer, J. H. (2009). Computer-based cognitive training for mild cognitive impairment: Results from a pilot randomized, controlled trial. *Alzheimer Disease and Associated Disorders*, *23*(3), 205–210. doi:10.1097/WAD.0b013e31819c6137

Bentwich, J., Dobronevsky, E., Aichenbaum, S., Shorer, R., Peretz, R., Khaigrekht, M., . . . Rabey, J. M. (2011). Beneficial effect of repetitive transcranial magnetic stimulation combined with cognitive training for the treatment of Alzheimer's disease: A proof of concept study. *Journal of Neural Transmission*, *118*(3), 463–471. doi:10.1007/s00702-010-0578-1

Birks, J., & Harvey, R. J. (2006). Donepezil for dementia due to Alzheimer's disease. *Cochrane Database of Systematic Reviews*, *2006*(1), CD001190. doi:10.1002/14651858.CD001190.pub2

Blumenthal, J. A., Smith, P. J., Welsh-Bohmer, K., Babyak, M. A., Browndyke, J., Lin, P. H., . . . Sherwood, A. (2013). Can lifestyle modification improve neurocognition? Rationale and design of the ENLIGHTEN clinical trial. *Contemporary Clinical Trials*, *34*(1), 60–69. doi:10.1016/j.cct.2012.09.004

Bredesen, D. E., & John, V. (2013). Next generation therapeutics for Alzheimer's disease. *EMBO Molecular Medicine*, *5*(6), 795–798. doi:10.1002/emmm.201202307

Buschert, V. C., Friese, U., Teipel, S. J., Schneider, P., Merensky, W., Rujescu, D., & Buerger, K. (2011). Effects of a newly developed cognitive intervention in amnestic mild cognitive impairment and mild Alzheimer's disease: A pilot study. *Journal of Alzheimer's Disease*, *25*(4), 679–694. doi:10.3233/JAD-2011-100999

Carretti, B., Borella, E., Fostinelli, S., & Zavagnin, M. (2013). Benefits of training working memory in amnestic mild cognitive impairment: Specific and transfer effects. *International Psychogeriatrics*, *25*(4), 617–626. doi:10.1017/S1041610212002177

Chen, P., Ratcliff, G., Belle, S. H., Cauley, J. A., DeKosky, S. T., & Ganguli, M. (2001). Patterns of cognitive decline in presymptomatic Alzheimer disease: A prospective community study. *Archives of General Psychiatry*, *58*(9), 853–858. doi:yoa20218

Cotelli, M., Calabria, M., Manenti, R., Rosini, S., Maioli, C., Zanetti, O., & Miniussi, C. (2012). Brain stimulation improves associative memory in an individual with amnestic mild cognitive impairment. *Neurocase*, *18*(3), 217–223. doi:10.1080/13554794.2011.588176

Cotelli, M., Manenti, R., Cappa, S. F., Zanetti, O., & Miniussi, C. (2008). Transcranial magnetic stimulation improves naming in Alzheimer disease patients at different stages of cognitive decline. *European Journal of Neurology*, *15*(12), 1286–1292. doi:10.1111/j.1468-1331.2008.02202.x

Cummings, J. L., Morstorf, T., & Zhong, K. (2014). Alzheimer's disease drug-development pipeline: Few candidates, frequent failures. *Alzheimer's Research & Therapy*, *6*(4), 37. doi:10.1186/alzrt269

Dai, Q., Borenstein, A. R., Wu, Y., Jackson, J. C., & Larson, E. B. (2006). Fruit and vegetable juices and Alzheimer's disease: The kame project. *American Journal of Medicine*, *119*(9), 751–759. doi:S0002-9343(06)00677-2

DeKosky, S. T., Williamson, J. D., Fitzpatrick, A. L., Kronmal, R. A., Ives, D. G., Saxton, J. A., . . . Furberg, C. D.; Ginkgo Evaluation of Memory (GEM) Study Investigators. (2008). Ginkgo biloba for prevention of dementia: A randomized controlled trial. *JAMA*, *300*(19), 2253–2262. doi:10.1001/jama.2008.683

Doody, R. S., Ferris, S. H., Salloway, S., Sun, Y., Goldman, R., Watkins, W. E., . . . Murthy, A. K. (2009). Donepezil treatment of patients with MCI: A 48-week randomized, placebo-controlled trial. *Neurology*, *72*(18), 1555–1561. doi:10.1212/01.wnl.0000344650.95823.03

Drumond Marra, H. L., Myczkowski, M. L., Maia Memoria, C., Arnaut, D., Leite Ribeiro, P., Sardinha Mansur, C. G., . . . Marcolin, M. A. (2015). Transcranial magnetic stimulation to address mild cognitive impairment in the elderly: A randomized controlled study. *Behavioural Neurology*, *2015*, 287843. doi:10.1155/2015/287843

Dubois, B., Feldman, H. H., Jacova, C., Dekosky, S. T., Barberger-Gateau, P., Cummings, J., . . . Scheltens, P. (2007). Research criteria for the diagnosis of Alzheimer's disease: Revising the NINCDS-ADRDA criteria. *Lancet Neurology*, *6*(8), 734–746. doi:S1474-4422(07)70178-3

Feldman, H. H., Ferris, S., Winblad, B., Sfikas, N., Mancione, L., He, Y., . . . Lane, R. (2007). Effect of rivastigmine on delay to diagnosis of Alzheimer's disease from mild cognitive impairment: The InDDEx study. *Lancet Neurology*, *6*(6), 501–512. doi:S1474-4422(07)70109-6

Feldman, H. H., Haas, M., Gandy, S., Schoepp, D. D., Cross, A. J., . . . Mayeux, R.; One Mind for Research and the New York Academy of Sciences. (2014). Alzheimer's disease research and development: A call for a new research roadmap. *Annals of the New York Academy of Sciences*, *1313*, 1–16. doi:10.1111/nyas.12424

Fillit, H., Nash, D. T., Rundek, T., & Zuckerman, A. (2008). Cardiovascular risk factors and dementia. *American Journal of Geriatric Pharmacotherapy*, *6*(2), 100–118. doi:10.1016/j.amjopharm.2008.06.004

Forette, F., Seux, M. L., Staessen, J. A., Thijs, L., Babarskiene, M. R., Babeanu, S., . . . Birkenhäger, W. H.; Systolic Hypertension in Europe Investigators. (2002). The prevention of dementia with antihypertensive treatment: New evidence from the systolic hypertension in Europe (Syst-Eur) study. *Archives of Internal Medicine*, *162*(18), 2046–2052. doi:ioi10730

Grande, G., Vanacore, N., Maggiore, L., Cucumo, V., Ghiretti, R., Galimberti, D., . . . Clerici, F. (2014). Physical activity reduces the risk of dementia in mild cognitive impairment subjects: A cohort study. *Journal of Alzheimer's Disease*, *39*(4), 833–839. doi:10.3233/JAD-131808

Gross, A. L., Parisi, J. M., Spira, A. P., Kueider, A. M., Ko, J. Y., Saczynski, J. S., . . . Rebok, G. W. (2012). Memory training interventions for older adults: A meta-analysis. *Aging & Mental Health*, *16*(6), 722–734. doi:10.1080/13607863.2012.667783

Hall, C. B., Lipton, R. B., Sliwinski, M., Katz, M. J., Derby, C. A., & Verghese, J. (2009). Cognitive activities delay onset of memory decline in persons who develop dementia. *Neurology*, *73*(5), 356–361. doi:10.1212/WNL.0b013e3181b04ae3

Heyn, P., Abreu, B. C., & Ottenbacher, K. J. (2004). The effects of exercise training on elderly persons with cognitive impairment and dementia: A meta-analysis. *Archives of Physical Medicine and Rehabilitation*, *85*(10), 1694–1704. doi:S0003999304003971

Hu, J. P., Guo, Y. H., Wang, F., Zhao, X. P., Zhang, Q. H., & Song, Q. H. (2014). Exercise improves cognitive function in aging patients. *International Journal of Clinical and Experimental Medicine*, *7*(10), 3144–3149.

Huang, C. C., Chung, C. M., Leu, H. B., Lin, L. Y., Chiu, C. C., Hsu, C. Y., . . . Chan, W. L. (2014). Diabetes mellitus and the risk of Alzheimer's disease: A nationwide population-based study. *PLoS One*, *9*(1), e87095. doi:10.1371/journal.pone.0087095

Hyman, B. T. (2011). Amyloid-dependent and amyloid-independent stages of Alzheimer disease. *Archives of Neurology*, *68*(8), 1062–1064. doi:10.1001/archneurol.2011.70

Jack, C. R., Knopman, D. S., Jagust, W. J., Shaw, L. M., Aisen, P. S., Weiner, M. W., . . . Trojanowski, J. Q. (2010). Hypothetical model of dynamic biomarkers of the Alzheimer's pathological cascade. *Lancet Neurology*, *9*(1), 119–128.

Johnson, K. A., Minoshima, S., Bohnen, N. I., Donohoe, K. J., Foster, N. L., . . . Herscovitch, P.; Amyloid Imaging Task Force of the Alzheimer's Association and Society for Nuclear Medicine and Molecular Imaging. (2013). Update on appropriate use criteria for amyloid PET imaging: Dementia experts, mild cognitive impairment, and education. amyloid imaging task force of the Alzheimer's Association and Society for Nuclear Medicine and Molecular Imaging. *Alzheimer's & Dementia*, *9*(4), e106–e109. doi:10.1016/j.jalz.2013.06.001

Kaduszkiewicz, H., Zimmermann, T., Beck-Bornholdt, H. P., & van den Bussche, H. (2005). Cholinesterase inhibitors for patients with Alzheimer's disease: Systematic review of randomised clinical trials. *BMJ*, *331*(7512), 321–327. doi:331/7512/321

Karakaya, T., Fusser, F., Schroder, J., & Pantel, J. (2013). Pharmacological treatment of mild cognitive impairment as a prodromal syndrome of Alzheimer's disease. *Current Neuropharmacology*, *11*(1), 102–108. doi:10.2174/1570159138049994879

Katzman, R. (2008). The prevalence and malignancy of Alzheimer disease: A major killer. *Alzheimer's & Dementia, 4*(6), 378–380. doi:10.1016/j.jalz.2008.10.003

Larson, E. B., Wang, L., Bowen, J. D., McCormick, W. C., Teri, L., Crane, P., & Kukull, W. (2006). Exercise is associated with reduced risk for incident dementia among persons 65 years of age and older. *Annals of Internal Medicine, 144*(2), 73–81. doi:144/2/73

Launer, L. J., Miller, M. E., Williamson, J. D., Lazar, R. M., Gerstein, H. C., Murray, A. M., . . . Bryan, R. N.; ACCORD MIND Investigators. (2011). Effects of intensive glucose lowering on brain structure and function in people with type 2 diabetes (ACCORD MIND): A randomised open-label substudy. *Lancet Neurology, 10*(11), 969–977. doi:10.1016/S1474-4422(11)70188-0

Le Bars, P. L., Velasco, F. M., Ferguson, J. M., Dessain, E. C., Kieser, M., & Hoerr, R. (2002). Influence of the severity of cognitive impairment on the effect of the ginkgo biloba extract EGb 761 in Alzheimer's disease. *Neuropsychobiology, 45*(1), 19–26. doi:nps45019

Liu-Seifert, H., Siemers, E., Holdridge, K. C., Andersen, S. W., Lipkovich, I., Carlson, C., . . . Aisen, P. (2015). Delayed-start analysis: Mild Alzheimer's disease patients in solanezumab trials, 3.5 years. *Alzheimer's & Dementia, 1*(2), 111–121. doi:10.1016/j.trci.2015.06.006

Maci, T., Pira, F. L., Quattrocchi, G., Nuovo, S. D., Perciavalle, V., & Zappia, M. (2012). Physical and cognitive stimulation in Alzheimer disease: The GAIA project—A pilot study. *American Journal of Alzheimer's Disease and Other Dementias, 27*(2), 107–113. doi:10.1177/1533317512440493

Martin, M., Clare, L., Altgassen, A. M., Cameron, M. H., & Zehnder, F. (2011). Cognition-based interventions for healthy older people and people with mild cognitive impairment. *Cochrane Database of Systematic Reviews, 2011*(1), CD006220. doi:10.1002/14651858.CD006220.pub2

Max Planck Institute for Human Development and Stanford Center on Longevity. (2014). *A consensus on the brain training industry from the scientific community.* Retrieved from http://longevity3.stanford.edu.proxy.library.nd.edu/blog/2014/10/15/the-consensus-on-the-brain-training-industry-from-the-scientific-community. Accessed March 20, 2016.

McDonnell, M. N., Smith, A. E., & Mackintosh, S. F. (2011). Aerobic exercise to improve cognitive function in adults with neurological disorders: A systematic review. *Archives of Physical Medicine and Rehabilitation, 92*(7), 1044–1052. doi:10.1016/j.apmr.2011.01.021

McKhann, G. M., Knopman, D. S., Chertkow, H., Hyman, B. T., Jack, C. R., Jr., Kawas, C. H., . . . Phelps, C. H. (2011). The diagnosis of dementia due to Alzheimer's disease: Recommendations from the National Institute on Aging–Alzheimer's Association workgroups on diagnostic guidelines for Alzheimer's disease. *Alzheimer's & Dementia, 7*(3), 263–269. doi:10.1016/j.jalz.2011.03.005

Meinzer, M., Lindenberg, R., Phan, M. T., Ulm, L., Volk, C., & Floel, A. (2015). Transcranial direct current stimulation in mild cognitive impairment: Behavioral effects and neural mechanisms. *Alzheimer's & Dementia, 11*(9), 1032–1040. doi:10.1016/j.jalz.2014.07.159

MetLife Foundation. (2011). *What America thinks: MetLife foundation Alzheimer's survey.* Retrieved from https://www.metlife.com/assets/cao/foundation/alzheimers-2011.pdf

Middleton, L. E., & Yaffe, K. (2009). Promising strategies for the prevention of dementia. *Archives of Neurology, 66*(10), 1210–1215. doi:10.1001/archneurol.2009.201

Moro, V., Condoleo, M. T., Sala, F., Pernigo, S., Moretto, G., & Gambina, G. (2012). Cognitive stimulation in a-MCI: An experimental study. *American Journal of Alzheimer's Disease and Other Dementias, 27*(2), 121–130. doi:10.1177/1533317512441386

Mowszowski, L., Batchelor, J., & Naismith, S. L. (2010). Early intervention for cognitive decline: Can cognitive training be used as a selective prevention technique? *International Psychogeriatrics, 22*(4), 537–548. doi:10.1017/S1041610209991748

Nascimento, C. M., Pereira, J. R., de Andrade, L. P., Garuffi, M., Talib, L. L., Forlenza, O. V., . . . Stella, F. (2014). Physical exercise in MCI elderly promotes reduction of pro-inflammatory cytokines and improvements on cognition and BDNF peripheral levels. *Current Alzheimer Research, 11*(8), 799–805. doi:CAR-62250

Ng, T. P., Feng, L., Niti, M., Kua, E. H., & Yap, K. B. (2008). Tea consumption and cognitive impairment and decline in older Chinese adults. *American Journal of Clinical Nutrition, 88*(1), 224–231. doi:88/1/224

Ngandu, T., Lehtisalo, J., Solomon, A., Levalahti, E., Ahtiluoto, S., Antikainen, R., . . . Kivipelto, M. (2015). A 2 year multidomain intervention of diet, exercise, cognitive training, and vascular risk monitoring versus control to prevent cognitive decline in at-risk elderly people (FINGER): A randomised controlled trial. *Lancet*, *385*(9984), 2255–2263. doi:10.1016/S0140-6736(15)60461-5

Norton, S., Matthews, F. E., Barnes, D. E., Yaffe, K., & Brayne, C. (2014). Potential for primary prevention of Alzheimer's disease: An analysis of population-based data. *Lancet Neurology*, *13*(8), 788–794. doi:10.1016/S1474-4422(14)70136-X

Nurk, E., Drevon, C. A., Refsum, H., Solvoll, K., Vollset, S. E., Nygard, O., . . . Smith, A. D. (2007). Cognitive performance among the elderly and dietary fish intake: The Hordaland Health Study. *American Journal of Clinical Nutrition*, *86*(5), 1470–1478. doi:86/5/1470

Ohman, H., Savikko, N., Strandberg, T. E., & Pitkala, K. H. (2014). Effect of physical exercise on cognitive performance in older adults with mild cognitive impairment or dementia: A systematic review. *Dementia and Geriatric Cognitive Disorders*, *38*(5-6), 347–365. doi:10.1159/000365388

Olchik, M. R., Farina, J., Steibel, N., Teixeira, A. R., & Yassuda, M. S. (2013). Memory training (MT) in mild cognitive impairment (MCI) generates change in cognitive performance. *Archives of Gerontology and Geriatrics*, *56*(3), 442–447. doi:10.1016/j.archger.2012.11.007

Pelosi, A. J., McNulty, S. V., & Jackson, G. A. (2006). Role of cholinesterase inhibitors in dementia care needs rethinking. *BMJ*, *333*(7566), 491–493. doi:333/7566/491

Perrig, W. J., Perrig, P., & Stahelin, H. B. (1997). The relation between antioxidants and memory performance in the old and very old. *Journal of the American Geriatrics Society*, *45*(6), 718–724.

Petersen, R. C., Caracciolo, B., Brayne, C., Gauthier, S., Jelic, V., & Fratiglioni, L. (2014). Mild cognitive impairment: A concept in evolution. *Journal of Internal Medicine*, *275*(3), 214–228. doi:10.1111/joim.12190

Petersen, R. C., Thomas, R. G., Grundman, M., Bennett, D., Doody, R., Ferris, S., . . . Thal, L. J.; Alzheimer's Disease Cooperative Study Group. (2005). Vitamin E and donepezil for the treatment of mild cognitive impairment. *New England Journal of Medicine*, *352*(23), 2379–2388. doi:NEJMoa050151

Prince, M. J., Bird, A. S., Blizard, R. A., & Mann, A. H. (1996). Is the cognitive function of older patients affected by antihypertensive treatment? Results from 54 months of the Medical Research Council's trial of hypertension in older adults. *BMJ*, *312*(7034), 801–805.

Rabey, J. M., Dobronevsky, E., Aichenbaum, S., Gonen, O., Marton, R. G., & Khaigrekht, M. (2013). Repetitive transcranial magnetic stimulation combined with cognitive training is a safe and effective modality for the treatment of Alzheimer's disease: A randomized, double-blind study. *Journal of Neural Transmission*, *120*(5), 813–819. doi:10.1007/s00702-012-0902-z

Rapp, S., Brenes, G., & Marsh, A. P. (2002). Memory enhancement training for older adults with mild cognitive impairment: A preliminary study. *Aging & Mental Health*, *6*(1), 5–11. doi:10.1080/13607860120101077

Raschetti, R., Albanese, E., Vanacore, N., & Maggini, M. (2007). Cholinesterase inhibitors in mild cognitive impairment: A systematic review of randomized trials. *PLoS Medicine*, *4*(11), e338. doi:07-PLME-RA-0189

Ravaglia, G., Forti, P., Lucicesare, A., Pisacane, N., Rietti, E., Bianchin, M., & Dalmonte, E. (2008). Physical activity and dementia risk in the elderly: Findings from a prospective Italian study. *Neurology*, *70*(19 Pt. 2), 1786–1794. doi:01.wnl.0000296276.50595.86

Rebok, G. W., Ball, K., Guey, L. T., Jones, R. N., Kim, H. Y., King, J. W., . . . Willis, S. L.; ACTIVE Study Group. (2014). Ten-year effects of the advanced cognitive training for independent and vital elderly cognitive training trial on cognition and everyday functioning in older adults. *Journal of the American Geriatrics Society*, *62*(1), 16–24. doi:10.1111/jgs.12607

Rebok, G. W., Carlson, M. C., & Langbaum, J. B. (2007). Training and maintaining memory abilities in healthy older adults: Traditional and novel approaches. *Journals of Gerontology. Series B, Psychological Sciences and Social Sciences*, *62*(Spec. No. 1), 53–61. doi:62/suppl_Special_Issue_1/53

Reiman, E. M., Langbaum, J. B., Tariot, P. N., Lopera, F., Bateman, R. J., Morris, J. C., . . . Weninger, S. (2016). CAP-advancing the evaluation of preclinical Alzheimer disease treatments. *Nature Reviews Neurology, 12*(1), 56–61. doi:10.1038/nrneurol.2015.177

Rita Cardoso, B., Apolinario, D., da Silva Bandeira, V., Busse, A. L., Magaldi, R. M., Jacob-Filho, W., & Cozzolino, S. M. (2016). Effects of Brazil nut consumption on selenium status and cognitive performance in older adults with mild cognitive impairment: A randomized controlled pilot trial. *European Journal of Nutrition, 55*(1), 107–116. doi:10.1007/s00394-014-0829-2

Rockwood, K., Kirkland, S., Hogan, D. B., MacKnight, C., Merry, H., Verreault, R., . . . McDowell, I. (2002). Use of lipid-lowering agents, indication bias, and the risk of dementia in community-dwelling elderly people. *Archives of Neurology, 59*(2), 223–227. doi:noc10195

Romero, H. R., Hayes, S., & Welsh-Bohmer, K. A. (2010). Cognitive domains affected by conditions of aging and the role of neuropsychological testing. In M. Abou-Saleh, C. Katona, & A. Kumar (Eds.), *Principles and practices of geriatric psychiatry* (3rd ed., pp. 389–396). Hoboken, NJ: Wiley-Blackwell.

Rozzini, L., Costardi, D., Chilovi, B. V., Franzoni, S., Trabucchi, M., & Padovani, A. (2007). Efficacy of cognitive rehabilitation in patients with mild cognitive impairment treated with cholinesterase inhibitors. *International Journal of Geriatric Psychiatry, 22*(4), 356–360. doi:10.1002/gps.1681

Safouris, A., Psaltopoulou, T., Sergentanis, T. N., Boutati, E., Kapaki, E., & Tsivgoulis, G. (2015). Vascular risk factors and Alzheimer's disease pathogenesis: Are conventional pharmacological approaches protective for cognitive decline progression? *CNS & Neurological Disorders Drug Targets, 14*(2), 257–269. doi:CNSNDDT-EPUB-65268

Salloway, S., Ferris, S., Kluger, A., Goldman, R., Griesing, T., Kumar, D., & Richardson, S.; Donepezil 401 Study Group. (2004). Efficacy of donepezil in mild cognitive impairment: A randomized placebo-controlled trial. *Neurology, 63*(4), 651–657. doi:63/4/651

Salthouse, T. A. (2010). Influence of age on practice effects in longitudinal neurocognitive change. *Neuropsychology, 24*(5), 563–572. doi:10.1037/a0019026

Sano, M., Ernesto, C., Thomas, R. G., Klauber, M. R., Schafer, K., Grundman, M., . . . Thal, L. J. (1997). A controlled trial of selegiline, alpha-tocopherol, or both as treatment for Alzheimer's disease: The Alzheimer's Disease Cooperative Study. *New England Journal of Medicine, 336*(17), 1216–1222. doi:10.1056/NEJM199704243361704

Schneider, J. A., Wilson, R. S., Bienias, J. L., Evans, D. A., & Bennett, D. A. (2004). Cerebral infarctions and the likelihood of dementia from Alzheimer disease pathology. *Neurology, 62*(7), 1148–1155.

Schneider, L. S., Mangialasche, F., Andreasen, N., Feldman, H., Giacobini, E., Jones, R., . . . Kivipelto, M. (2014). Clinical trials and late-stage drug development for Alzheimer's disease: An appraisal from 1984 to 2014. *Journal of Internal Medicine, 275*(3), 251–283. doi:10.1111/joim.12191

Sink, K. M., Espeland, M. A., Rushing, J., Castro, C. M., Church, T. S., Cohen, R., . . . Williamson, J. D.; LIFE Investigators. (2014). The LIFE cognition study: Design and baseline characteristics. *Clinical Interventions in Aging, 9*, 1425–1436. doi:10.2147/CIA.S65381

Smith, A. D., & Yaffe, K. (2014). Dementia (including Alzheimer's disease) can be prevented: Statement supported by international experts. *Journal of Alzheimer's Disease, 38*(4), 699–703. doi:10.3233/JAD-132372

Smith, G. E., Housen, P., Yaffe, K., Ruff, R., Kennison, R. F., Mahncke, H. W., & Zelinski, E. M. (2009). A cognitive training program based on principles of brain plasticity: Results from the Improvement in Memory with Plasticity-Based Adaptive Cognitive Training (IMPACT) study. *Journal of the American Geriatrics Society, 57*(4), 594–603. doi:10.1111/j.1532-5415.2008.02167.x

Sperling, R. A., Aisen, P. S., Beckett, L. A., Bennett, D. A., Craft, S., Fagan, A. M., . . . Phelps, C. H. (2011). Toward defining the preclinical stages of Alzheimer's disease: Recommendations from the National Institute on Aging–Alzheimer's Association workgroups on diagnostic guidelines for Alzheimer's disease. *Alzheimer's & Dementia, 7*(3), 280–292. doi:10.1016/j.jalz.2011.03.003

Stern, Y., Albert, S., Tang, M. X., & Tsai, W. Y. (1999). Rate of memory decline in AD is related to education and occupation: Cognitive reserve? *Neurology, 53*(9), 1942–1947.

Stern, Y., Alexander, G. E., Prohovnik, I., Stricks, L., Link, B., Lennon, M. C., & Mayeux, R. (1995). Relationship between lifetime occupation and parietal flow: Implications for a reserve against Alzheimer's disease pathology. *Neurology, 45*(1), 55–60.

Tangney, C. C. (2014). DASH and Mediterranean-type dietary patterns to maintain cognitive health. *Current Nutrition Reports, 3*(1), 51–61. doi:10.1007/s13668-013-0070-2

Tortosa-Martinez, J., Clow, A., Caus-Pertegaz, N., Gonzalez-Caballero, G., Abellan-Miralles, I., & Saenz, M. J. (2015). Exercise increases the dynamics of diurnal cortisol secretion and executive function in people with amnestic mild cognitive impairment. *Journal of Aging and Physical Activity, 23*(4), 550–558. doi:10.1123/japa.2014-0006

Troyer, A. K., Murphy, K. J., Anderson, N. D., Moscovitch, M., & Craik, F. I. (2008). Changing everyday memory behaviour in amnestic mild cognitive impairment: A randomized controlled trial. *Neuropsychological Rehabilitation, 18*(1), 65–88. doi:783032173

Tsolaki, M., Kounti, F., Agogiatou, C., Poptsi, E., Bakoglidou, E., Zafeiropoulou, M., . . . Vasiloglou, M. (2011). Effectiveness of nonpharmacological approaches in patients with mild cognitive impairment. *Neurodegenerative Diseases, 8*(3), 138–145. doi:10.1159/000320575

Turriziani, P., Smirni, D., Zappala, G., Mangano, G. R., Oliveri, M., & Cipolotti, L. (2012). Enhancing memory performance with rTMS in healthy subjects and individuals with mild cognitive impairment: The role of the right dorsolateral prefrontal cortex. *Frontiers in Human Neuroscience, 6*, 62. doi:10.3389/fnhum.2012.00062

Twamley, E. W., Ropacki, S. A., & Bondi, M. W. (2006). Neuropsychological and neuroimaging changes in preclinical Alzheimer's disease. *Journal of the International Neuropsychological Society, 12*(5), 707–735. doi:S1355617706060863

van Gelder, B. M., Tijhuis, M., Kalmijn, S., & Kromhout, D. (2007). Fish consumption, n-3 fatty acids, and subsequent 5-y cognitive decline in elderly men: The Zutphen Elderly Study. *American Journal of Clinical Nutrition, 85*(4), 1142–1147. doi:85/4/1142

Vellas, B., Hampel, H., Rouge-Bugat, M. E., Grundman, M., Andrieu, S., Abu-Shakra, S., . . . Aisen, P.; Task Force Participants. (2012). Alzheimer's disease therapeutic trials: EU/US task force report on recruitment, retention, and methodology. *Journal of Nutrition, Health & Aging, 16*(4), 339–345.

Vos, S. J., Verhey, F., Frolich, L., Kornhuber, J., Wiltfang, J., Maier, W., . . . Visser, P. J. (2015). Prevalence and prognosis of Alzheimer's disease at the mild cognitive impairment stage. *Brain, 138*(Pt. 5), 1327–1338. doi:10.1093/brain/awv029

Welsh, K., Butters, N., Hughes, J., Mohs, R., & Heyman, A. (1991). Detection of abnormal memory decline in mild cases of Alzheimer's disease using CERAD neuropsychological measures. *Archives of Neurology, 48*(3), 278–281.

Welsh, K. A., Butters, N., Hughes, J. P., Mohs, R. C., & Heyman, A. (1992). Detection and staging of dementia in Alzheimer's disease: Use of the neuropsychological measures developed for the Consortium to Establish a Registry for Alzheimer's Disease. *Archives of Neurology, 49*(5), 448–452.

Wengreen, H., Munger, R. G., Cutler, A., Quach, A., Bowles, A., Corcoran, C., . . . Welsh-Bohmer, K. A. (2013). Prospective study of dietary approaches to stop hypertension- and Mediterranean-style dietary patterns and age-related cognitive change: The Cache County Study on Memory, Health and Aging. *American Journal of Clinical Nutrition, 98*(5), 1263–1271. doi:10.3945/ajcn.112.051276

Willis, S. L., Tennstedt, S. L., Marsiske, M., Ball, K., Elias, J., Koepke, K. M., . . . Wright, E.; ACTIVE Study Group. (2006). Long-term effects of cognitive training on everyday functional outcomes in older adults. *JAMA, 296*(23), 2805–2814. doi:296/23/2805

Wilson, R. S., Mendes De Leon, C. F., Barnes, L. L., Schneider, J. A., Bienias, J. L., Evans, D. A., & Bennett, D. A. (2002). Participation in cognitively stimulating activities and risk of incident Alzheimer disease. *JAMA, 287*(6), 742–748. doi:joc11682

Winblad, B., Gauthier, S., Scinto, L., Feldman, H., Wilcock, G. K., Truyen, L., . . . Nye, J. S.; GAL-INT-11/18 Study Group. (2008). Safety and efficacy of galantamine in subjects with mild cognitive impairment. *Neurology*, *70*(22), 2024–2035. doi:10.1212/01.wnl.0000303815.69777.26

Zandi, P. P., Sparks, D. L., Khachaturian, A. S., Tschanz, J., Norton, M., Steinberg, M., . . . Breitner, J. C.; Cache County Study Investigators. (2005). Do statins reduce risk of incident dementia and Alzheimer disease? The Cache County Study. *Archives of General Psychiatry*, *62*(2), 217–224. doi:62/2/217

Zhuang, J. P., Fang, R., Feng, X., Xu, X. H., Liu, L. H., Bai, Q. K., . . . Chen, S. D. (2013). The impact of human–computer interaction-based comprehensive training on the cognitive functions of cognitive impairment elderly individuals in a nursing home. *Journal of Alzheimer's Disease*, *36*(2), 245–251. doi:10.3233/JAD-130158

NINE

Cognitive Enhancement in Schizophrenia

JAMES GILLEEN

INTRODUCTION

Cognitive deficits are common in schizophrenia and are associated with significant impairments in functional, social, and employment outcomes. Cognitive impairments are, accordingly, also widely researched, and we have a good understanding of the profile of cognitive deficits observed in the disorder. Despite this understanding, there are currently no approved compounds to treat the cognitive impairments in schizophrenia.

The lack of effective treatments for cognitive impairment is a testimony to the interaction of multiple factors—the complexity of the disease, our somewhat limited understanding of the neurobiology of cognition, our understanding of available pharmacological compounds, and the challenges of drug development and of conducting clinical trials.

This chapter provides a selective rather than exhaustive review of the current status of approaches that have been developed to improve cognition in schizophrenia, including pharmacological as well as cognitive training and cognitive remediation techniques. It also explores the various study design issues and challenges that contribute to the difficulties in discovering reliable and efficacious means of ameliorating the cognitive deficits in schizophrenia.

Schizophrenia is characterized by a constellation of heterogeneous symptoms, which predominantly include hallucinations and delusions, as well as motivational and social deficits and cognitive impairments. Together, the positive, negative, and cognitive deficits form a triptych of potential pharmacological targets. Although positive symptoms have historically been the target for drug development, in recent years, attention has turned to cognitive and negative symptoms—with the aim being to treat these to improve the lives of people with schizophrenia.

COGNITIVE FUNCTIONING IN SCHIZOPHRENIA

Cognitive deficits are widely spread across patients with schizophrenia and are critical to patients' functional outcomes (Green, 1996; Green, Kern, & Heaton, 2004; Milev, Ho, Arndt, & Andreasen, 2005), real-world adaptive skills (Bowie et al., 2010), employment status and capacity for activities of daily living (D. I. Velligan et al., 1997), and ultimately quality of life (Green, 1996; Green et al., 2004). Longitudinal studies have demonstrated the importance of cognitive functioning as a strong predictor of functional outcome (Green et al., 2004), employment outcome (McGurk, Mueser, & Pascaris, 2005), compliance and relapse (Burton, 2005; Keefe, Bilder, et al., 2007; Keefe, Sweeney, et al., 2007), and psychosocial outcomes (Prouteau et al., 2005). The degree of deficit across these aspects of life further impacts the tertiary financial burden to society (Patel et al., 2006) and interpersonal burden to family (Hjarthag, Helldin, Karilampi, & Norlander, 2010). Cognition is weakly to moderately associated with severity of the clinical symptoms of schizophrenia. Similarly, change in cognition is associated with change in symptom severity (Davidson et al., 2009; Keefe, Bilder, et al., 2007), and it remains plausible that treatment of cognitive deficits may improve or prevent worsening of clinical symptoms.

The Cognitive Phenotype

Patients with schizophrenia present with a wide range of cognitive impairments across multiple domains (Figure 9.1). Cognitive deficits in schizophrenia have been demonstrated in all key cognitive faculties: memory, executive function, working memory, attention, and processing speed. Importantly, in some patients, they are evident before symptom onset, and in the overwhelming majority, they persist after symptoms have been treated (Heinrichs, 2005). Nevertheless, cognitive deficits do not constitute any diagnostic criteria for the disorder.

Meta-analyses have demonstrated that there is a generalized cognitive impairment in schizophrenia. Dickinson, Ramsey, and Gold (2007) analyzed data from

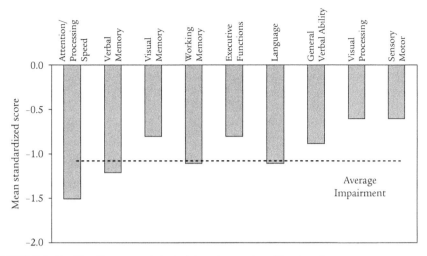

FIGURE 9.1 *Profile of neuropsychological impairment in schizophrenia.* SOURCE: ADAPTED FROM REICHENBERG AND HARVEY (2007).

37 cognitive measures in 1,961 patients and 1,444 comparison subjects across 37 studies. Results showed a generalized mean effect in patients with schizophrenia, with an effect size of 0.98. The greatest deficit was in the Digit Symbol Coding Test (a complex cognitive measure involving attention, processing speed, memory, and executive functions), on which patients score more than 1.5 standard deviations below healthy controls. Although there is a considerable heterogeneity between patients in the cognitive domains that are impaired and in the severity of impairment in individual measures, the overwhelming majority of schizophrenia patients have a cognitive impairment that is judged to be of clinical significance (Reichenberg et al., 2009).

Developmental Origins of the Cognitive Impairment

Cognitive impairments in schizophrenia are identifiable before the onset of the disease, and they have been shown to originate in childhood (Fuller et al., 2002; Reichenberg et al., 2005, 2010). These cognitive deficits have been shown to remain largely stable after disease is first diagnosed (Heaton et al., 2001) and are persistent throughout the life course (Friedman et al., 2001).

By the time the first episode happens, cognitive deficits are already widespread. A meta-analysis of 43 studies of more than 2,200 patients and 2,700 matched control participants demonstrated medium to large impairments across 10 neurocognitive domains (mean effect sizes ranged from ~0.64 to ~1.20), with greatest deficits in processing speed and verbal memory (Mesholam-Gately, Giuliano, Goff, Faraone, & Seidman, 2009). Deficits were largely of a similar magnitude to those seen in chronic patients with established illness, but they were greater than those seen in the premorbid period, suggesting that deterioration occurs between the prodrome and first episode (Mesholam-Gately et al., 2009).

These deficits cannot be explained by medication alone because cognitive deficits are also apparent in patients off antipsychotics. A meta-analysis that used data from 23 studies involving 1,106 drug-naive patients and 1,385 controls showed that patients performed significantly worse on all measures compared to the healthy group, and deficits were of a medium to large effect size (Fatouros-Bergman, Cervenka, Flyckt, Edman, & Farde, 2014). Verbal memory, processing speed, and working memory were the three domains most impaired, broadly consistent with findings from the medicated population outlined.

CAUTIONARY NOTES AND REPORTING OF EFFECTS FROM HEALTHY STUDIES

Overall, there are many avenues of research aiming to discover reliable pharmacological and nonpharmacological means of enhancing cognition. It should be kept in mind that the US Food and Drug Administration (FDA) does not require an explanation of the *mechanism* by which cognitive enhancement may occur. This is likely the explanation for the plethora of speculative studies in this field in which there is limited a priori rationale for the choice of drug with respect to the putative mechanism by which it may improve cognitive impairments.

There also appears to be a limited correspondence between improvements observed in cognition due to a compound when given to healthy individuals and when given to schizophrenia patients. For example, pro-cognitive results observed with modafinil in healthy individuals (Gilleen et al., 2014) did not translate into positive findings in patients with schizophrenia (Michalopoulou et al., 2015), despite careful methodological control to ensure similarity of methods and increased sample size. This could be due to the specific neurobiology of schizophrenia or to the failure to spot true effects due to design issues such as low numbers and statistical power (discussed later). It could also be because "normalizing" impaired cognition (as is the goal for patients with schizophrenia) is not the same as enhancing cognition above normal levels (as is the goal in studies with healthy individuals).

It should also be kept in mind that cognitive deficits may also be, at least in part, or in certain cognitive domains, secondary to, or exacerbated, by antipsychotic medication. Antipsychotic medications affect symptoms by predominantly acting to reduce dopamine transmission, but these compounds also act more widely on other neurotransmitter systems (Sumiyoshi, 2008). Furthermore, although the full neural and cognitive repertoire of dopamine is not fully characterized, it is known that dopamine plays a role in learning, working memory, movement, salience attribution, and attention. Thus, antipsychotics, which reduce dopamine transmission, have a negative impact on attention, reaction time, and speed of processing in healthy individuals (Saeedi, Remington, & Christensen, 2006; Vernaleken et al., 2006), and they prevent practice effects on the Digit Symbol Substitution Test (Veselinovic et al., 2013). In addition, low D2-receptor binding is associated with poorer cognition (Cervenka, Backman, Cselenyi, Halldin, & Farde, 2008; Cropley, Fujita, Innis, & Nathan, 2006; Takahashi et al., 2007).

In summary, the findings from the extensive literature demonstrate that cognitive impairments are apparent at all stages of illness. Cognitive deficits precede illness, increase in magnitude over its development, and are largely independent of the trajectory of the psychotic symptoms. Next, the most common pharmacological and nonpharmacological approaches used to try to improve cognition are discussed.

NONPHARMACOLOGICAL INTERVENTIONS

Cognitive Remediation

As indicated later in this chapter, antipsychotics alone do not sufficiently improve cognitive and functional performance measures. Demonstrating capacity to improve cognitive performance in schizophrenia by nonpharmacological means would be ideal because this would eliminate the need for long-term medication as well as any concerns about drug sensitivity effects or side effects from drug–drug interactions. Nonpharmacological intervention may also be more cost-effective if a limited number of sessions could produce long-lasting effects. First, the evidence for cognitive remediation training to elevate cognitive functioning in schizophrenia is discussed.

Cognitive remediation training (CRT) has been defined as "behavioral training based intervention that aims to improve cognitive processes (attention, memory, executive function, social cognition or metacognition) with the goal of durability and generalization" (Wykes, Huddy, Cellard, McGurk, & Czobor, 2011). CRT usually involves a series of sessions, ranging from a few to more than 40, in which a patient is administered behavioral and and/or cognitive training, which is often computerized and may also be supported by a therapist. The goal of these training sessions is to improve performance on a range of tests or games spanning many domains of cognitive functioning. There are many so-called "brain training" software suits, which were originally designed for the consumer market but have been adopted for efficacy trials in patients with schizophrenia.

Within CRT trial designs, a range of parameters of CRT can be manipulated, and this is reflected in the large heterogeneity in published studies: number of sessions, duration and frequency of sessions, supported or nonsupported (by a psychologist) learning, as well as differences in the specific cognitive domains targeted. In addition, the means by which the tests are expected to produce improvements also vary. Some CRT interventions use the "drill and practice" (repeat exposure only) approach, which may involve an inbuilt mechanism to "drive" learning by challenging the patient (i.e., making the task slightly more difficult as the patient improves) or by discussing and encouraging adoption of strategies to improve performance. An alternative approach is to supplement practice with strategy used to increase generalization to real-world problems (Cella, Reeder, & Wykes, 2015).

Wykes et al. (2011) conducted a meta-analysis of 40 CRT trials in schizophrenia including 2,104 participants. The average length of CRT treatment was 16 weeks, with 32 hours of CRT using either drill and practice or drill and practice plus strategy. CRT showed a significant effect on global cognition (effect size = 0.45). Also, significant effects were apparent in most, but not all, domains of cognition. Effects on global cognition at follow-up visits remained significant (effect size = 0.43), indicating they were durable. Interestingly, the higher order domains of social cognition and executive function showed the most improvement (effect size = 0.65 and 0.57, respectively).

The strongest effects have been seen in studies that adopted a rehabilitation strategy in addition to CRT. However, training in this manner improves test scores by teaching a different approach to the task per se (e.g., rehearsal techniques), which is not the same as improving the intrinsic underlying (and therefore the targeted) cognitive ability (Shipstead, Redick, & Engle, 2012).

Interventions are more effective in younger patients, possibly due to greater potential for neuroplasticity (Wykes et al., 2009). However, there is considerable study heterogeneity with respect to sample size and study quality, and CRT studies often suffer from small sample sizes and lack of methodological rigor (Wykes et al., 2011).

Murthy et al. (2012) conducted a study that involved six sites and 55 patients with schizophrenia who completed hour-long sessions on Brainfit (PositScience) every workday for 40 days. Brainfit aims to improve cognition using a bottom-up model—drill and practice with a "challenge" component, whereby low-level attentional function (auditory and visual perception and discrimination) is driven by training over many sessions. This is done by using staircase training algorithms that are pitched at a level at which participants get items correct but also incorrect on more difficult items—thus elevating demands and improvements over time.

A study by Vinogradov et al. (2009) demonstrated positive effects on cognition using these approaches, and improvements were associated with normalization of decreased brain-derived neurotrophic factor levels. Despite the intensity and duration of the intervention, and the use of staircase algorithms, brain training did not improve performance on untrained tasks compared to baseline (Murthy et al., 2012).

Such results demonstrate a critical point (discussed in detail later): Even training patients on the same task over a considerable number of sessions may fail to reap any rewards, let alone lead to improvements in untrained tasks. These results also illustrate the importance of the underlying training principle being relied on for cognitive improvement. The study by Murthy et al. (2012) aimed, and failed, to improve performance via bottom-up attentional mechanisms, which contrasts with structured CRT sessions in which top-down processes (e.g., strategy development) are putatively engaged and which evidence suggests are more successful (Wykes et al., 2011).

There may also be specific windows during illness progression at which cognitive interventions can be successful. Revell, Neill, Harte, Khan, and Drake (2015) examined whether CRT is effective when delivered in the early phase of illness. Their meta-analysis of 11 studies using CRT in the first-episode schizophrenia showed that although CRT had significant effects on verbal learning and memory domains (effect size = 0.23), neither global cognitive functioning nor the other cognitive domains that were studied showed improvement. In three studies with a 6-month follow-up, no cognitive outcome was significantly better in the CRT group compared to the control group. The authors suggested that the lower baseline functioning in chronic patients may allow more scope for improvement.

Evidence suggests that cognitive remediation is most effective at improving functional outcomes when delivered in combination with supported employment (Bell, Zito, Greig, & Wexler, 2008) or other rehabilitative interventions (Cella et al., 2015). McGurk et al. (2005) showed that patients given supported employment and cognitive remediation demonstrated significantly greater neurocognitive and employment outcomes compared to patients receiving supported employment only.

The mechanisms by which cognitive remediation can improve cognition are unclear. It has been suggested that neuroplasticity may be central, and indeed cognitive remediation has been shown to improve prefrontal activation (Cella et al., 2015; Wexler, Anderson, Fulbright, & Gore, 2000; Wykes et al., 2002) and white matter anisotropy (Penades et al., 2013) and to reduce gray matter loss over time (Eack et al., 2010).

Neurostimulation

If the effects of cognitive remediation are indeed reliant on neuroplastic processes, then it is possible that techniques that directly modulate neural processes will be able to mimic these effects and may thus be an alternative, even a "shortcut," to multiple and effortful cognitive remediation sessions. The role of neuroplastic effects can be investigated with transcranial magnetic stimulation (TMS) and transcranial direct current stimulation (tDCS) (Antal, Nitsche, & Paulus, 2006). Application of neurostimulation techniques has demonstrated working memory improvements in healthy people (Andrews, Hoy, Enticott, Daskalakis, & Fitzgerald, 2011), but these techniques have not been used extensively to treat cognitive deficits in schizophrenia. Although positive effects across a range of cognitive domains have been found in small samples (reviewed by Minzenberg & Carter, 2012), a recent review (Hasan, Strube, Palm, & Wobrock, 2016) concluded that most studies fail to find a positive effect, but there is an indication that visual, verbal, and working memory, as well as source monitoring, may be improved by repetitive TMS. For example, in one study, patients receiving 4 weeks of 20-Hz stimulation to the dorsolateral prefrontal cortex (DLPFC) showed increased 3-back performance compared to sham (Barr et al., 2013). Several other studies reported evidence of cognitive enhancement via TMS in treatment refractory patients (Demirtas-Tatlidede et al., 2010; Levkovitz, Rabany, Harel, & Zangen, 2011). A range of methodological differences between studies, poor study design, and small numbers are limiting a consensus about the efficacy of TMS for cognitive deficits in schizophrenia (Hasan et al., 2016).

An alternative neurostimulation technique, tDCS, has also shown some efficacy. Hoy, Arnold, Emonson, Daskalakis, and Fitzgerald (2014) administered a single 20-minute session of anodal tDCS to the DLPFC and found a significant improvement in working memory functioning at the higher strength stimulation only (2 mA). Other studies, however, did not find significant improvements (Vercammen et al., 2011). Further work in this field is required to determine the optimal set of parameters to elicit cognitive gains.

PHARMACOLOGICAL INTERVENTIONS

Antipsychotics

Because patients are invariably already taking antipsychotic medication, it would of course be preferable if some antipsychotics, given as treatment-as-usual, were able to induce positive change in cognitive functioning without the need for additional medications. The predominant action of all antipsychotics occurs via blockade of striatal D2 receptors, although considerable differences in action of antipsychotics on other neurotransmitter systems are apparent, particularly between typical and atypical medications (Sumiyoshi, 2008).

It has been proposed that atypical medications may be beneficial to cognition compared to typicals (Keefe, Silva, Perkins, & Lieberman, 1999; Meltzer & McGurk, 1999), and that this may be due to, in part, the differential affinity of these compounds to 5-HT_{2A} (Tyson, Roberts, & Mortimer, 2004). There is considerable evidence that increased levels of serotonin can result in impairments in cognitive functioning (Canli & Lesch, 2007; Cowen & Sherwood, 2013; Schmitt, Wingen, Ramaekers, Evers, & Riedel, 2006), and it has been proposed that this may be due to 5-HT_{2A} receptors exerting a secondary effect on prefrontal dopamine.

However, the Clinical Antipsychotic Trials for Intervention Effectiveness (CATIE; see Lieberman et al., 2005) dispelled some of these assumptions. CATIE, which was primarily conducted to compare clinical outcomes associated with five common antipsychotic medications in 817 patients, also measured cognition at baseline and at 2, 6, and 18 months. All treatment groups showed improvements in cognition, but there were no differences in the degree of change associated with the different compounds. Improvements were only small (0.25 standard deviations at most), and they occurred mostly in the first few months of treatment.

Previous reports of the superiority of atypical antipsychotics have been criticized for drawing conclusions from studies with various design problems. As explained by Keefe, Sweeney, et al. (2007), these studies are often characterized by low numbers of participants; short durations; no comparator drug; industry sponsorhip; or failure to account for symptom change, extrapyramidal side effects, or anticholinergic treatment. Thus, there remain substantial controversies relating to findings that antipsychotic medication has a positive impact on cognition. Furthermore, clozapine, the most atypical of antipsychotics, was once considered favorable to cognitive functioning compared to other antipsychotic treatments but is no longer considered to be so (Harvey et al., 2008). The current consensus is that the effects of antipsychotic medications on cognition in schizophrenia, if present, are only minimal (Tandon, Nasrallah, & Keshavan, 2010; Young & Geyer, 2015).

Cognitive Enhancers

An obvious advantage of pharmacology compared to CRT is the fact that fewer resources are needed to support the intervention. CRT requires frequent, supported cognitive remediation sessions, whereas prescription of a drug, although potentially financially costly, does not place demands on clinicians' time. An additional advantage is that pharmacological enhancement may allow to avoid the difficulties that positive as well as negative symptoms pose for engagement with the content and structure of a CRT session.

A large number of compounds have been investigated, and plausible biological pathways targeted, in an attempt to treat the cognitive impairments in schizophrenia. Clinical trials can be classified into two main categories: those attempting to repurpose existing drugs by testing their efficacy on cognitive targets in schizophrenia, and those developing new therapeutics aimed at schizophrenia. This section presents a selective review of the literature focusing on compounds that modulate dopamine, serotonin, γ-aminobutyric acid (GABA), glutamate, histamine, and cholinergic targets. It is important to keep in mind that studies differ considerably in design, duration, dose, and sample size. In addition, each compound is unlikely to have neurobiological specificity and, as such, is likely to affect multiple neurotransmitters and therefore multiple cognitive systems.

Modafinil

Modafinil, a wake-promoting compound prescribed for sleep disorders and narcolepsy, has been widely researched for its cognitive enhancing potential. The compound acts non-specifically on a range of neurotransmitter systems, including catecholamines, serotonin, glutamate, orexin, and histamine systems. If modafinil could be used to enhance cognition, it would confer potential clinical advantage compared to other compounds, such as amphetamine, because it has a low side effect profile, including a low risk of exacerbating psychotic symptoms (however, see Narendran, Young, Valenti, Nickolova, & Pristach, 2002), and little potential for abuse.

In patients with schizophrenia, Turner et al. (2004) showed that 200 mg of modafinil improved verbal memory and set-shifting, but not visual memory, spatial planning, or stop-signal performance. In the first-episode patients, 200 mg modafinil improved verbal and spatial working memory but had no effects on sustained attention, set-shifting, learning, or fluency measures (Scoriels, Barnett, Soma, Sahakian, & Jones, 2012). Changes have also been demonstrated in PFC activation with functional magnetic resonance imaging (Hunter, Ganesan, Wilkinson, & Spence, 2006) and in anterior cingulate activity during a working-memory task (Spence, Green, Wilkinson, & Hunter, 2005).

There is evidence that modafinil may only facilitate cognitive enhancement for more difficult levels of cognitive function (Bayley et al., submitted; Muller, Steffenhagen, Regenthal, & Bublak, 2004). For example, Bayley et al. found significant (off-drug) improvements following combination modafinil and cognitive training, but only for more difficult tasks. They also demonstrated that 2 weeks of modafinil and cognitive training results in changes in brain activity during working memory tasks that are consistent with improved neural efficiency and potential for task-relevant engagement. Recently, the potential of 200 mg daily modafinil to enhance the effects of cognitive training in schizophrenia was investigated, after seeing positive effects in a healthy control trial (Gilleen et al., 2014; Michalopoulou et al., 2015). However, no positive effects were demonstrated in any cognitive outcome.

Differences are also apparent in findings from drug studies with a single dose and those with adjunct medication given over a period of months. In contrast to the study previously discussed, several studies have shown no effects for adjunct modafinil alone given over time (Freudenreich et al., 2009; Pierre, Peloian, Wirshing, Wirshing, & Marder, 2007; Sevy et al., 2005).

Armodafinil, the long-lasting isomer of modafinil, has shown no cognitive benefits when given as an adjunct for 4 weeks (Kane et al., 2010) or 6 weeks (Bobo, Woodward, Sim, Jayathilake, & Meltzer, 2011) compared to placebo. Although not widely reported, there is evidence that modafinil can lead to exacerbated psychotic symptoms and increased blood pressure (Gilleen et al., 2014; Minzenberg & Carter, 2008), which calls into question any potential long-term use of this compound.

Amphetamine

The action of amphetamine is predominantly via inhibition of the dopamine transporter. Cognitive enhancing effects of amphetamine have been frequently reported. A meta-analysis concluded that when used at low doses in healthy adults, amphetamine produces modest improvements in memory, working memory, and attention (Ilieva, Hook, & Farah, 2015).

Barch and Carter (2005) reported that a single dose of 0.25 mg/kg D-amphetamine improved working memory, inhibitory control, and language production (amount of speech and formal thought disorder) in a group of 10 patients with schizophrenia, although the improvements in working memory may reflect a capacity for amphetamine to improve prefrontal signal-to-noise ratio during working memory. Prior studies showed improved set-shifting performance in schizophrenia (Daniel et al., 1991; Goldberg, Bigelow, Weinberger, Daniel, & Kleinman, 1991), which was associated with amphetamine-induced increases in DLPFC activation (Daniel et al., 1991). A double-blind, placebo-controlled crossover study of 32 patients with schizophrenia showed improvement on measures of executive function and visual attention and vigilance, and it showed modest improvements on a measure of speed of processing. However, no effects on MATRICS Consensus Cognitive Battery (MCCB) scores were apparent from 20 mg amphetamine in a single-dose crossover study in a larger sample of 60 healthy people (Chou, Talledo, Lamb, Thompson, & Swerdlow, 2013). Interestingly, a secondary analysis showed that whereas amphetamine enhanced performance in those with low placebo performance, it impaired performance in those with high placebo performance. Such contrasting effects may be due to genetic variation, specifically differential levels of dopamine regulation by catechol O-methyltransferase val[158]met polymorphisms (Mattay et al., 2003).

Although amphetamine does demonstrate a potential to improve cognition, given the capacity of amphetamine to induce psychotic-like symptoms in healthy people, its use in schizophrenia, particularly as a long-term (repeat-dose) medication to maintain cognitive improvements, remains inadvisable.

Cholinergic Targets

The cholinergic system is involved in a range of cognitive processes known to be impaired in schizophrenia, including memory, attention, processing speed, and sensory gating. In the CATIE trial, adjunct anticholinergic medication was associated with greater cognitive impairment (Keefe, Sweeney, et al., 2007). The nicotinic cholinergic system is involved in various domains of cognition, including attention and memory. Stimulation of the α_7 nicotinic receptors increases cholinergic transmission and results in these receptors interacting with all other major neurotransmitters in the brain (Wonnacott, Barik, Dickinson, & Jones, 2006). Nicotine has been demonstrated to improve cognitive functioning in schizophrenia (for a summary, see Hahn et al., 2013). Adler, Hoffer, Wiser, and Freedman (1993) reported that nicotine (smoking) produced a "normalization" of P50 auditory gating (effect size = 0.8). Harris et al. (2004) reported that the effects of nicotine on cognition were limited to attention. The impact of nicotine on cognitive performance may be dependent on smoking status. For example, nicotine reversed abstinence-induced deficits in spatial working memory and attention (Sacco et al., 2005). It has been suggested that in healthy nonsmokers, nicotine actually impairs cognitive performance (Newhouse, Potter, & Singh, 2004) and that nicotine administration improves performance for those with lower baseline cognitive functioning but impairs performance for those with higher baseline cognitive function (Niemegeers et al., 2014), similar to reported effects of amphetamine.

Adler et al. (1993) also reported that nicotine effects were only present in schizophrenic patients who smoked, whereas Harris et al. (2004) reported that nicotine administration enhanced cognitive performance in nonsmokers but impaired cognitive performance in the nicotine abstinent smokers. Quisenaerts et al. (2014) found no effects of nicotine on measures of visual memory, working memory, processing speed, psychomotor speed, or social cognitive functioning, although the sample size was small.

DMXB-A, a partial α_7 nicotinic agonist, improved Repeatable Battery for the Assessment of Neuropsychological Status (RBANS) total scale score compared to placebo, especially in the lower DMXB-A dose (Olincy et al., 2006), albeit with a small sample size. A very large study of three doses of AZD3480 ($N = 440$), a selective agonist of alpha $\alpha_4\beta_2$ nicotinic receptors, given for 12 weeks found no effects on cognition compared to placebo (D. Velligan et al., 2012). Lieberman et al. (2013) reported that TC-5619, another α_7 partial agonist, improved executive functioning as measured by the Cogstate Maze Learning task.

Aside from agonizing ACh receptors, acetylcholinesterase, an enzyme responsible for metabolizing acetylcholine in the synaptic cleft, inhibits levels of acetylcholine at cholinergic receptors (both muscarinic and nicotinic). Zhu et al. (2014) administered daily 5 mg donepezil (an anticholinesterase inhibitor) to 31 nonsmoking patients with schizophrenia and compared performance at 12 weeks to that of 30 patients administered placebo. The group receiving donepezil showed moderate (effect size = ~0.5) improvement in working memory, speed of processing, visual learning, and memory. A 12-week adjunct study using 5 or 10 mg donepezil (Friedman et al., 2002) failed to show positive effects. Similarly, Sharma, Reed, Aasen, and Kumari (2006) reported no improvements in participants given rivastigmine for 24 weeks. Also, Kumari, Aasen, ffytche, Williams, and Sharma (2006) reported only minor improvements in *n*-back accuracy after 12 weeks.

In a large trial conducted by Keefe et al. (2008) that included 121 patients randomized to receive donepezil (5 mg for 6 weeks followed by 10 mg for 6 weeks) and 124 patients randomized to receive a placebo for the same duration, donepezil failed to improve cognitive measures relative to placebo, although this could have been due to a large placebo/practice effect in the control group. Ultimately, the evidence for the use of donzepil in schizophrenia is disappointing (for review, see Thakurathi, Vincenzi, & Henderson, 2013).

Galantamine is a cholinesterase inhibitor with additional nicotinic agonist effects. In a small trial involving patients with schizophrenia, participants given galantamine demonstrated significant improvement in RBANS total score and particularly in the attention and delayed memory subscale score (effect size = 1.0) (Schubert, Young, & Hicks, 2006). A larger trial comparing 42 patients given galantamine for 12 weeks to 44 patients on placebo found no improvements in global cognition, working memory, or motor speed, although improvements on measures of processing speed and verbal memory were apparent (R. W. Buchanan et al., 2008). A follow-up study in which galantamine was administered for 6 weeks did not find evidence for cognitive enhancement compared with placebo on a range of cognitive and social tasks (D. Kelly, 2015), although sample size was small in this study. Several other adjunct studies failed to find any significant effects on a range of measures (Dyer et al., 2008; S. W. Lee, Lee, Lee, & Kim, 2007; Lindenmayer & Khan, 2011).

Encenicline, a selective α_7 nicotinic ACh receptor agonist, showed some efficacy for composite cognitive (Cogstate test battery) and functional (Schizophrenia Cognition Rating Scale) (Keefe, Poe, Walker, Kang, & Harvey, 2006) outcomes in a Phase II trial in which approximately 300 schizophrenia patients were given placebo or low- or high-dose encenicline for 12 weeks (Keefe et al., 2015). However, in 2016, it was reported that a subsequent 26-week Phase III trial involving approximately 1,500 patients with schizophrenia failed to show improvements in primary cognitive outcomes (MATRICS). It was noted that both Phase II and Phase III studies observed that placebo group improvement was unexpectedly high.

Glutamate Targets

Ketamine and MK801 models of schizophrenia indicate a role of glutamate in schizophrenia. NMDA functioning is thought to impact cognition through its effects on synaptic plasticity, memory, and cognition (Coyle, 1996; Goff & Coyle, 2001; McDonald & Johnston, 1990), most likely via modulation of long-term potentiation and long-term depression (Bear & Malenka, 1994; Nicoll & Malenka, 1999).

The glutamate system has multiple points of entry, and glutamate transmission can be enhanced by direct agonists (D-serine and glycine), by partial agonism (D-cycloserine), or by inhibition of the transporter. R. W. Buchanan et al. (2007) conducted a 16-week double-blind, double-dummy, parallel group, randomized clinical trial of adjunctive glycine, D-cycloserine, or placebo that included 157 schizophrenia patients. They found no significant differences in cognition between glycine and placebo or D-cycloserine and placebo subjects. A further trial that included 195 patients gave a low dose of 2 g/day adjunct D-serine for 16 weeks and found no differences compared to placebo (Weiser et al., 2012). Glycine transporter inhibitors (GlyTi), which play a pivotal role in maintaining the concentration of glycine, attenuate the psychomimetic effects of ketamine in healthy individuals (D'Souza et al., 2012). The GlyTi sarcosine has been shown to improve cognition in patients with schizophrenia; for example, after 6 weeks of 2 g/day, subjects in one study showed improvements in cognition when assessed by the Positive and Negative Syndrome Scale (PANSS; clinician-rated) (Tsai, Lane, Yang, Chong, & Lange, 2004). These improvements were not seen in a separate study with clozapine patients (Lane et al., 2006). These results do not currently support the hypothesis that glutamate targets are an effective therapeutic option for treating cognitive impairments in schizophrenia.

Oxytocin

Oxytocin is a nonapeptide that has a role in social bonding across mammalian species including humans, and so there has been a focus on targeting *social* cognition with this compound. Oxytocin has been shown to improve social cognitive processes (Feifel, Macdonald, Cobb, & Minassian, 2012), identification of false beliefs (Pedersen et al., 2011), and emotion recognition and high-order social cognition (Averbeck, Bobin, Evans, & Shergill, 2012). Davis et al. (2013), for example, found that schizophrenia patients significantly improved on detection of sarcasm, deception, and empathy, and Guastella et al. (2015) found improvements in appreciation of indirect hints and recognition of social faux pas. Gibson et al. (2014) conducted a 6-week double-blind, placebo-controlled trial of adjunct oxytocin compared to placebo. Oxytocin improved fear recognition and perspective taking but no other outcomes. Adjunct oxytocin administered for 6 weeks did not show superiority to placebo in a randomized trial measuring a range of cognitive and social tasks (M. R. Lee et al., 2013).

The potential for oxytocin to improve cognition has also been investigated longitudinally by combining its administration with social or cognitive social training (Cacciotti-Saija et al., 2015; Davis et al., 2013). Davis et al. gave patients either oxytocin or placebo before 30 minutes of social training that included training in facial affect recognition, social perception, and empathy for 12 sessions. Oxytocin enhanced empathy but not social or facial affect outcomes relative to placebo. However, Cacciotti-Saija et al., who conducted a similar study on early psychosis, gave patients oxytocin nasal spray twice daily for 6 weeks combined with social cognitive training that was defined as training on four social–cognitive domains: emotion recognition, understanding intentions of others, correction of cognitive biases, and skill integration. Oxytocin-facilitated training did not, however, demonstrate enhancement of social skills relative to placebo.

It is worth noting that there is no clearly identified mechanism by which oxytocin may directly improve cognition. It is furthermore plausible that oxytocin may reduce performance anxiety during administration of cognitive and social measures such that apparent cognitive improvements are actually only indirectly achieved.

GABA

Because GABA is the main inhibitory neurotransmitter in the brain, inhibition of its activity should theoretically promote excitatory activity neural systems (for a broad discussion, see Wallace, Ballard, Pouzet, Riedel, & Wettstein, 2011). A $GABA_A$ α_2/α_3 partial agonist was used in a 4-week double-blind trial with 3 and 8 mg versus placebo (R. W. Buchanan et al., 2011). No effects on MCCB composite score were observed, and the placebo group actually performed significantly better on visual memory and reasoning/problem-solving tests compared to participants assigned to either dose level. However, Lewis et al. (2008) reported improved performance on the *n*-back, AX Continuous Performance Test, delayed memory, and Preparing to Overcome Prepotency tests, but not on composite scores. A small study using a single-dose design reported that flumazenil, a $GABA_A$ receptor antagonist, showed efficacy in improving working memory, whereas lorazepam, a GABA agonist, impaired working memory.

Serotonin

Serotonin depletion with tryptophan causes cognitive deficits, including perseveration (Clarke, Dalley, Crofts, Robbins, & Roberts, 2004), whereas stimulation of $5\text{-}HT_{1A}$ and blockade of $5\text{-}HT_{2A}$ are suggested to improve cognitive functioning (Meltzer & Massey, 2011; Terry, Buccafusco, & Wilson, 2008), a reflection of their opposing effects on cortical neuron excitability (Roth, Hanizavareh, & Blum, 2004).

The role of serotonin in cognition is not well understood. There is a controversy regarding whether agonism or antagonism of the 5-HT system is pro-cognitive, with studies showing cognitive enhancing effects for both. It has been suggested that this may reflect differential effects of 5-HT receptor subunit systems on cognition (M. L. Wallace, Frank, & Kraemer, 2013). $5\text{-}HT_{2A}$ antagonism may prove effective for schizophrenia due to a close association between NMDA and $5\text{-}HT_{2A}$ receptors (T. L. Wallace et al., 2011), whereby NMDA receptor function may be normalized (Terry et al., 2008).

Aripiprazole, clozapine, olanzapine, perospirone, quetiapine risperidone, and ziprasidone are atypical antipsychotic drugs that are either direct or indirect $5\text{-}HT_{2A}$ antagonists, and they have been shown to improve cognitive function in patients with schizophrenia (Meltzer & Sumiyoshi, 2008). The pro-cognitive effects of amisulpride may be via $5\text{-}HT_7$ because it does not act on any other 5-HT receptor (Meltzer & Massey, 2011). However, risperidone is a $5\text{-}HT_{1A}$ antagonist, so it appears that antagonism also improves cognition (Roth et al., 2004).

Buspirone (30 mg/day), a $5\text{-}HT_{1A}$ partial agonist, has been shown to improve digit symbol substitution test performance but not performance on other cognitive measures (Sumiyoshi et al., 2007). Adjunct tandospirone, another serotonin-$5\text{-}HT_{1A}$ partial agonist, has been shown to improve executive function and verbal learning and memory (Sumiyoshi et al., 2001). Tandospirone may enhance cognition by increasing cortical dopamine via the $5\text{-}HT_{1A}$ mechanism, but it has wide effects on multiple other neurotransmitters (Meltzer & Massey, 2011).

Norepinephrine

The noradrenergic system is particularly important in attention, and a focus has been on compounds that upregulate transmission at α_2 adrenergic receptors. Atomoxetine, a selective norepinephrine reuptake inhibitor that elevates norepinephrine and has cascading effects that enhance other neurotransmitter systems such as dopamine, shows efficacy in treating attentional deficits in attention deficit hyperactivity disorder (Michelson et al., 2001). In schizophrenia, there were no effects of atomoxetine on standard cognitive testing, but there were greater increases in working memory-related neural activation (Friedman et al., 2008). Kelly et al. (2009) also found no effects on a range of cognitive tests following an 8-week trial of 80 mg/day. Guanfacine, a noradrenergic α_2 receptor agonist, failed to show effects on cognition compared with placebo after 4 weeks; however, post-hoc analysis observed specific effects on measures of working memory and attention in participants treated with atypical antipsychotics (Friedman et al., 2001).

COMBINING COGNITIVE TRAINING/COGNITIVE REMEDIATION AND PHARMACOLOGY

The previous sections provided an overview of the current status of pharmacological and cognitive remediation approaches. Relatively recently, there have been attempts to combine these approaches.

Cognitive exercise might be necessary to realize the benefits of cognitive enhancers (Keefe et al., 2011), in much the same way that physical exercise is required to profit from steroid administration. In essence, combining pharmacological and nonpharmacological methods may improve functioning beyond that achieved by either approach alone (Swerdlow, 2012).

A combined approach has indeed shown additive effects in several experimental paradigms in patient groups: L-DOPA improves motor rehabilitation after stroke (Scheidtmann, Fries, Muller, & Koenig, 2001); amphetamine enhances language learning in patients with post-stroke aphasia (Walker-Batson et al., 2001); and both of these compounds, when combined with repeated testing, elevate the performance of healthy volunteers on an artificial language learning task relative to that of healthy volunteers given placebo and repeated testing (Breitenstein et al., 2004; Knecht et al., 2004). D-Cycloserine, a partial agonist at the glycine site of the NMDA receptor, has also been shown to enhance the effects of cognitive behavioral therapy for delusions in schizophrenia (Gottlieb et al., 2011).

Combining pharmacological compounds with task exposure or training, relative to combining with placebo, may therefore be a plausible approach to demonstrate efficacy of pharmacological compounds to enhance cognition. D'Souza et al. (2013) combined D-serine with CRT on the basis that NMDA agonism may enhance neuroplasticity. However, D-serine did not enhance CRT gains—although no effects of D-serine alone or CRT alone were observed either. Sample sizes were small, and there were strong gains in the control arms (see sections on placebo and practice effects). Gilleen et al. (2014) demonstrated improvements in implicit learning in healthy individuals when modafinil was given before daily cognitive training over 10 days (compared to placebo), but these effects were not apparent in a subsequent study of schizophrenia (Michalopoulou et al., 2015), either due to no real effects, insufficient sample size and/or large between-patient and between-session variability in this group—a common occurrence in trials using repeated administration of tasks.

Combining a drug with repeated exposure to tasks to improve cognition also highlights the importance of drug choice. Whereas in traditional studies drug choice would be best dictated by the potential for the drug to directly improve the cognitive domain being targeted (e.g., to affect attention or working memory capacity), improving performance over time may instead be best achieved by a drug that enhances learning or plasticity because these would be expected to improve the brain's capacity to show cognitive adaptation. This, in turn, may facilitate brain changes that help achieve task improvements. Thus, the drug may not, by itself, necessarily directly improve cognition.

DESIGN AND METHODOLOGY CONSIDERATIONS FOR TRIALS TO ENHANCE COGNITION IN SCHIZOPHRENIA

In any trial that aims to show efficacy of a cognitive enhancer, evidence for cognitive enhancement depends on three factors: true treatment effect, placebo effect, and practice effect (Keefe et al., 2008). This section discusses methodological and design issues that may reduce the potential to find positive effects of a cognitive enhancer, and describes important factors that should be considered in order to facilitate the success of trials.

Placebo Effects

Placebo effects are well documented in drug development more generally, and these are equally a concern in the development of cognitive enhancers. Large improvements in a control group minimize the potential to show real drug effects—as noted with various compounds including the relatively recent failure of encenecline. The positive response in control groups may, for example, arise due to expectancy or monetary incentives for study participation. However, it is important to note that only 3 of the 40 CRT trials analyzed by Wykes et al. (2011) paid patients, suggesting that this factor does not contribute to effects in this type of intervention at least.

In addition, there is a real concern about the impact of "professional patients." These are patients who are less unwell; who are taking part, or have taken part, in multiple clinical trials; and who may produce gains in performance—either consciously to try to "please" the researchers or inadvertently because of previous experience with the assessment procedures. One risk of this is the potential for apparent elevation of placebo effects and, simultaneously, obfuscation of real drug effects. Another factor that may contribute to the magnitude of the placebo effect is the inclusion of patients who were required to be clinically stable upon inclusion and to remain clinically stable throughout the study (Keefe et al., 2008). Practice effects may be artificially high for these patients compared to a clinically more representative sample.

There are also issues with the constitution of control interventions. The development of new treatments for cognition is hindered by the lack of current treatments; that is, there are no positive control compounds to which the efficacy of new compounds can be compared (Floresco, Geyer, Gold, & Grace, 2005). Similar issues arise in CRT protocols: Should a control group receive no intervention, active comparators such as video games, or training games designed to improve "control" cognitive domains? Each option is justifiable but would in turn likely reduce the potential for gains to be found in the active group.

Finally, subjective effects are also likely to be critical particularly, for example, in a crossover design. Drugs that change physiological arousal are implicitly unblinded, and this may create a two-hit effect—a combination of a compound's real effects coupled with effects congruent with expectations of "taking the real drug." It is critical that a central aim of the manufacture of the placebo should be to match the drug for taste and scent, not just color and size of tablet—this is particularly taxing for liquid formulations.

Practice Effects and Measuring Change

A cognitive test battery must demonstrate the following characteristics for sufficient utility when assessing the impact of a cognitive enhancer: good reliability and validity, sensitivity to the deficits apparent in the clinical population as well as to drug effects, minimal practice effects, and a difficulty level (lack of floor and ceiling effects) appropriate for the population being targeted.

For schizophrenia, the MCCB (Nuechterlein et al., 2008) was developed with these goals in mind. The MCCB is reported to have good reliability and validity and appropriate difficulty levels for schizophrenia patients, although practice effects are reported in the test manual for some tests following repeated administration. Critically, the MCCB's sensitivity to drug effects has not been well established. Nevertheless, these issues are not specific to the MCCB, and other available assessment batteries have limitations as well (e.g., Cogstate and RBANS).

Legitimate concerns arise about test psychometrics when tests from different batteries, which claim to measure the same domain of cognition, show the presence and/or the absence of significant effects on performance (Keefe et al., 2015). This is critical because the choice of which test battery to use may result in discrepancies in identification of drug effects and in turn whether a drug proceeds to the next phase of development and testing (for an example of battery outcome differences, see Keefe et al., 2015).

Study Design

Study design in this field remains a challenge. Consistent with clinical trial guidelines, the majority of studies use traditional placebo-controlled, randomized, double-blind designs. With adjunct medication trials, a placebo should be given rather than treatment as usual. Of course, the inclusion of a placebo group is essential to isolate positive drug effects from placebo and practice effects.

Studies using a combination therapy approach may require a greater number of trial "arms." However, because costs and resources severely limit sample size, this places constraints on the number of participants per condition and may lead to studies being underpowered. Table 9.1 illustrates the number of cells (conditions) required for a study examining the combination effects of a drug combined with cognitive training in the simple case of a single "dose" for either the drug or cognitive training. It can be argued that not all cells are necessary to demonstrate efficacy. In measuring the efficacy of modafinil to enhance cognitive training gains, Gilleen et al. (2014) contrasted only two cells (see Table 9.1). This was justified by the research question, which was whether modafinil enhances cognitive training gains. Thus, a placebo plus cognitive training is a baseline by which to compare modafinil plus cognitive training. D'Souza et al. (2013), examining D-serine plus cognitive training, used four cells (see Table 9.1). This approach limits the sample size but allows separation of drug and cognitive training effects.

TABLE 9.1 Possible Conditions in a Randomized Control Trial Examining the Effects of a Combination of a Drug and Cognitive Training

	Drug	Placebo Drug	No Drug
CT	Combined[a]	CT accounting for placebo effects of IMP[a]	CT alone
Placebo CT	Drug with "inactive" (control) CT[b]	"Active baseline" (placebo–placebo)[b]	Inactive (control) CT alone
No CT	Drug alone[c]	Placebo alone[c]	Absolute baseline[c]

[a]*Cells used in Gilleen et al. (2014).*
[b]*Cells used in D'Souza et al. (2013).*
[c]*Cells required to fully contrast placebo and drug effects.*
CT, cognitive training; IMP, investigational medicinal product.

Practice Effects

Discerning real effects from positive effects in repeated cognitive testing remains an important issue. Two review papers concluded that practice effects occur for many neuropsychological tests used in clinical trials in chronic schizophrenia (T. Buchanan et al., 2010; Goldberg, Keefe, Goldman, Robinson, & Harvey, 2010). Pietrzak, Snyder, and Maruff (2010) showed the impact of practice effects on the potential to reveal true cognitive enhancement effects. In their study, a version of a repeatable maze-learning task was used. A condition using the same maze showed practice effects with repeated administrations, whereas a condition using alternate mazes produced constant performance. When adjunct amphetamine was given to participants, drug effects were present only in the alternate test version (when practice effects were absent), suggesting practice effects in the constant version obfuscated the drug effects. More generally, repeated testing runs a further risk that participants may develop different strategies to complete the task over the multiple administrations. Thus, in effect, participants will do different cognitive tasks.

Inclusion of a placebo group may address some of the issues related to practice effects. It is expected that members of both groups (drug and placebo), on average, will demonstrate the same gains through practice alone, such that differential gains in the active group should be due to the compound. However, as discussed previously, many studies report high placebo effects, which is concerning because the placebo effects may obfuscate real drug effects. Furthermore, practice effects in a placebo group may push real drug effects (if present) toward ceiling, making it more difficult for real effects to be seen. This is a further reason to ensure that baseline functioning on a primary outcome is included as a randomization factor.

A related study design that may address this concern involves inclusion of an initial shorter phase for all participants during which everyone takes placebo. Test scores after this phase can be compared to baseline, and placebo responders can then be removed. This also has the added benefit of saturating practice effects. After this phase, randomization to drug or placebo can begin with a greater potential for true drug effects to be observed. A drawback to this design is the large initial sample size required to be left with a sufficient number of eligible participants.

A common procedure in clinical trials is to include a familiarization technique for cognitive outcome measures in which an initial repeat testing of cognitive measures is conducted (two or three sessions) to saturate practice effects. It is only after this is done that drug/placebo are given. This approach is recommended to mitigate practice effects obfuscating true treatment effects on a task. Specifically, this approach can help reduce the effect of differential learning *rates* among participants, limit the risk of an interaction between the investigational compound and individual learning rates, and remove gains associated with differences in participants' understanding and accommodating the nature of what to do during the task per se—cognitive performance may improve just from understanding the task and/or becoming accustomed to the interface and "gist" of the test.

However, this technique has some limitations. It requires multiple forms of the test with similar psychometric characteristics, including level of difficulty, to be available. The MCCB battery, for example, has five forms for some tests, and some, albeit minor, differences in mean test performance scores across test formats do exist. A large number of repeated assessments, even on different days, of the same test can result in fatigue or "study ennui." Last, the number of formats is limited, which is a significant issue for longer trials with more than four or five testing points.

Patient Selection

In general, schizophrenia patients recruited to clinical trials are greatly constrained in terms of permitted inclusion and exclusion criteria. Patients with a history of drug or alcohol addiction, with medical conditions of a variety of types, who are heavier than a certain weight, with excessive positive or negative or total symptom scores, and with a range of other factors have often been excluded from clinical trials. The obvious sequelae to this is that reducing patient heterogeneity runs the risk that findings will not generalize to the broader patient population.

Clinical trials are associated with high dropout rates, particularly with cognitive training (due to long schedules of repetitive sessions) and adjunct studies, because some last 6–12 months. Only patients already very motivated to engage with the research project will remain in the study, and these patients may be less ill, perhaps having lower positive and negative symptoms or higher motivation levels than "average" patients. Furthermore, this results in a group that has less room in which to improve cognitively, risking again the potential to demonstrate true positive effects.

Last, patients with good or very poor cognition are also sometimes excluded. Very impaired patients may have learning disabilities or nondiagnosed neurological problems, whereas those with good functioning have little room for improvement.

Sample Size and Power

Keefe et al. (2013) analyzed trials of cognitive enhancers for schizophrenia listed on https://clinicaltrials.gov and reported that the large majority of studies were underpowered to detect moderate effect sizes—an issue exacerbated by low reliability coefficients of cognitive outcome measures (Figure 9.2). The lower the test–retest reliability, the greater the number of patients required to show drug effects. Furthermore, the duration of interventions was also too short, lasting 8–12 weeks on average rather than the 6 months recommended by guidelines.

Administration, Scoring, Coding, and Other Measurement Errors

Thorough training and certification, as well as intermittent retraining, are required for large multisite trials, although subtle differences in administration methods

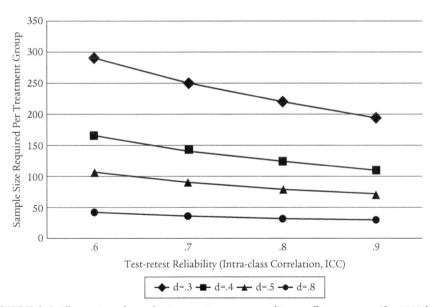

FIGURE 9.2 *Illustration of sample size requirements to achieve sufficient power (ß = .80) based on estimated effect size (Cohen's* d*) and test–retest reliability (intraclass correlation (ICC)).* SOURCE: REPRINTED FROM KEEFE ET AL. (2011).

and characteristics may still affect cognitive test scores. The CATIE trial, which made use of 57 sites for patient recruitment and analyses, found that approximately 13% of the variance in neurocognitive composite score at baseline was due to differences across sites. This may have serious implications for clinical trials (Keefe, Bilder, et al., 2006). D'Souza et al. (2013) also found site effects in a trial of D-serine and CRT that used sites in the United States and India. Patients may also have prior exposure to neuropsychological test batteries from taking part in other clinical trials or observational studies, and whether or not the tests are remembered, which may be problematic (Keefe, Bilder, et al., 2006) because it would alter practice effects, learning rates, and estimation of baseline functioning for these patients. The counterpoint is that within-subject designs should be immune to this problem because each participant has his or her own original cognitive performance as his or her baseline. However, as discussed previously, repeat administration and improvements toward ceiling make drug effects less likely to produce observable improvement in test scores.

Baseline Functioning

There is evidence in the literature that the magnitude of cognitive effects is related to baseline functioning of study participants. For example, in trials using modafinil, several studies reported effects only in those with low baseline functioning (Finke et al., 2010; Hunter et al., 2006; Kalechstein, De La Garza, & Newton, 2010; Randall, Shneerson, & File, 2005). Spence et al. (2005) further reported that pro-cognitive effects in their study of modafinil were seen only in patients treated with typical, but not atypical, antipsychotics. Thus, baseline parameters and the related room for cognitive improvement may be important factors in potential gains.

Wykes et al. (2011) also reported that patients with higher baseline functioning (and fewer symptoms) showed greater improvements following CRT. Thus, selection of patients with specifically high or low cognitive functioning gives rise to the potential to miss real drug effects or to demonstrate drug effects that would not occur in a more representative sample. This points to a need to balance participants according to cognitive function at baseline so that groups are balanced for these effects.

Motivation and Indirect Effects

There is considerable within-subject (between-session) variability in cognitive performance in trials involving patients with schizophrenia. In addition, intra-day variation in cognitive function is considerable. Test administration should be done at the same time of the day to mitigate the effects of circadian rhythms, sleepiness, and even the effects of consumption of food, caffeine, and so on that may bias the effect of the investigational compound. Motivation as well as clinical variability, fatigue, mood, and the presence and fluctuation of clinical symptoms undoubtedly play a role in cognitive test performance. Ideally, daily measures of each of these factors should be taken and included as covariates in the analysis of trial data.

Transfer

In trials that aim to improve cognitive performance via cognitive training (repeated administration), improvement on trained tasks is of limited interest if this improvement is not accompanied by improvement in performance on *untrained* tasks. Improvement in trained tasks indicates that there may be potential for cognitive training to facilitate improvement in real-life functioning. Distal effects (to tasks that are as dissimilar as possible to the trained task) are therefore more of interest than proximal effects, and this is the purpose of the FDA's requirement to demonstrate changes in functional outcomes. For example, showing that gains "transfer" from a task involving working memory of letters to one involving working memory of numbers is of limited value per se, whereas improvement in a measure of fluid intelligence is of considerable interest.

Dahlin, Neely, Larsson, Backman, and Nyberg (2008) demonstrated transfer effects from one working memory task to another (proximal transfer) and found evidence that common reliance of brain activity in specific regions may constitute the critical foundation for transfer effects. Clearly, the greater the "cognitive distance" between training and transfer tasks, the less likely transfer will occur. Shipstead et al. (2012) showed that major increases can be lost if even minor changes are made to task parameters. Effects do appear to be stronger in distal transfer with greater duration and intensity of training (Alloway, Bibile, & Lau, 2013; Schmiedek, Lovden, & Lindenberger, 2010). With respect to working memory, a meta-analysis suggested that training produces short-term gains, but overall there is no convincing evidence that working memory training generalizes to other skills in healthy individuals (Melby-Lervag & Hulme, 2013); however, one study reported improvement in fluid IQ following repeated working memory training (Jaeggi, Buschkuehl, Jonides, & Perrig, 2008).

Owen et al. (2010) investigated cognitive gains and transfer effects in a large study involving approximately 11,400 healthy participants who engaged via a BBC website. Participants completed an average of 24.5 sessions during 6 weeks, and tasks were designed to challenge performance. Performance on trained tasks improved, but transfer effects were largely absent, even in tasks that were closely related. The authors reported that "the increase in the number of digits that could be remembered following training on tests designed, at least in part, to improve memory, was three-hundredths of a digit." In healthy participants at least, transfer effects may be elusive, and currently there is little evidence of transfer effects in schizophrenia.

The Question of Premorbid Functioning

Finally, as discussed previously, the cognitive impairments in schizophrenia are apparent at all stages of illness and are moderate to severe in the overwhelming majority of patients. For a substantial group, however, the cognitive deficits precede illness and increase in magnitude over development.

This pattern may constrain the potential for cognitive enhancers to improve cognition. Recovering a level of impairment, for which an individual patient only very recently and suddenly declined, is a different prospect than generating cognitive improvement in a patient who has been at a low cognitive level since childhood. Understanding the factors that determine decline, perhaps by understanding the rate of decline, could inform development of treatment strategies. A sudden cognitive decline may have different causes from those of a slow progressing decline and, accordingly, perhaps require a different means of intervention.

CONCLUSION

This chapter provided an overview of the current status of cognitive enhancement in schizophrenia. It discussed multiple pharmacological as well as psychological interventions and approaches that have been developed and tested. It also presented and discussed methodology and study design issues that likely affect trials of cognitive enhancement in schizophrenia. The current evidence-based is mixed, and findings should be interpreted with caution because studies are too frequently underpowered.

Investigators should consider the neurobiology and neuropsychology of the disorder, the neurobiology of cognition, and the pharmacology of the compound when choosing compounds and/or psychological interventions and when designing studies. Attention to study design, duration, choice of cognitive battery, choice of participants, administration training, quality control, and consideration of learning and placebo effects should be meticulously addressed before study conception and design because they all may have substantial implications for our efforts to discover cognitive enhancing compounds for patients with schizophrenia.

REFERENCES

Adler, L. E., Hoffer, L. D., Wiser, A., & Freedman, R. (1993). Normalization of auditory physiology by cigarette smoking in schizophrenic patients. *American Journal of Psychiatry, 150*(12), 1856–1861.

Alloway, T. P., Bibile, V., & Lau, G. (2013). Computerized working memory training: Can it lead to gains in cognitive skills in students? *Computers in Human Behavior, 29*(3), 7.

Andrews, S. C., Hoy, K. E., Enticott, P. G., Daskalakis, Z. J., & Fitzgerald, P. B. (2011). Improving working memory: The effect of combining cognitive activity and anodal transcranial direct current stimulation to the left dorsolateral prefrontal cortex. *Brain Stimulation, 4*(2), 84–89.

Antal, A., Nitsche, M. A., & Paulus, W. (2006). Transcranial direct current stimulation and the visual cortex. *Brain Research Bulletin, 68*(6), 459–463.

Averbeck, B. B., Bobin, T., Evans, S., & Shergill, S. S. (2012). Emotion recognition and oxytocin in patients with schizophrenia. *Psychological Medicine, 42*(2), 259–266.

Barch, D. M., & Carter, C. S. (2005). Amphetamine improves cognitive function in medicated individuals with schizophrenia and in healthy volunteers. *Schizophrenia Research, 77*(1), 43–58.

Barr, M. S., Farzan, F., Rajji, T. K., Voineskos, A. N., Blumberger, D. M., Arenovich, T., et al. (2013). Can repetitive magnetic stimulation improve cognition in schizophrenia? Pilot data from a randomized controlled trial. *Biological Psychiatry, 73*(6), 510–517.

Bayley, A., Michalopoulou, P. G., Reichenberg, A., Wykes, T., Shergill, S. S., & Gilleen, J. (submitted). Modafinil combined with cognitive training improves neural efficiency during working memory: A randomised-controlled trial.

Bear, M. F., & Malenka, R. C. (1994). Synaptic plasticity: LTP and LTD. *Current Opinion in Neurobiology, 4*(3), 389–399.

Bell, M. D., Zito, W., Greig, T., & Wexler, B. E. (2008). Neurocognitive enhancement therapy with vocational services: Work outcomes at two-year follow-up. *Schizophrenia Research, 105*(1–3), 18–29.

Bobo, W. V., Woodward, N. D., Sim, M. Y., Jayathilake, K., & Meltzer, H. Y. (2011). The effect of adjunctive armodafinil on cognitive performance and psychopathology in antipsychotic-treated patients with schizophrenia/schizoaffective disorder: A randomized, double-blind, placebo-controlled trial. *Schizophrenia Research, 130*(1–3), 106–113.

Bowie, C. R., Depp, C., McGrath, J. A., Wolyniec, P., Mausbach, B. T., Thornquist, M. H., et al. (2010). Prediction of real-world functional disability in chronic mental disorders: A comparison of schizophrenia and bipolar disorder. *American Journal of Psychiatry, 167*(9), 1116–1124.

Breitenstein, C., Wailke, S., Bushuven, S., Kamping, S., Zwitserlood, P., Ringelstein, E. B., et al. (2004). D-Amphetamine boosts language learning independent of its cardiovascular and motor arousing effects. *Neuropsychopharmacology, 29*(9), 1704–1714.

Buchanan, R. W., Conley, R. R., Dickinson, D., Ball, M. P., Feldman, S., Gold, J. M., et al. (2008). Galantamine for the treatment of cognitive impairments in people with schizophrenia. *American Journal of Psychiatry, 165*(1), 82–89.

Buchanan, R. W., Javitt, D. C., Marder, S. R., Schooler, N. R., Gold, J. M., McMahon, R. P., et al. (2007). The Cognitive and Negative Symptoms in Schizophrenia Trial (CONSIST): The efficacy of glutamatergic agents for negative symptoms and cognitive impairments. *American Journal of Psychiatry, 164*(10), 1593–1602.

Buchanan, R. W., Keefe, R. S., Lieberman, J. A., Barch, D. M., Csernansky, J. G., Goff, D. C., et al. (2011). A randomized clinical trial of MK-0777 for the treatment of cognitive impairments in people with schizophrenia. *Biological Psychiatry, 69*(5), 442–449.

Buchanan, T., Heffernan, T. M., Parrott, A. C., Ling, J., Rodgers, J., & Scholey, A. B. (2010). A short self-report measure of problems with executive function suitable for administration via the Internet. *Behavior Research Methods, 42*(3), 709–714.

Burton, S. C. (2005). Strategies for improving adherence to second-generation antipsychotics in patients with schizophrenia by increasing ease of use. *Journal of Psychiatric Practice, 11*(6), 369–378.

Cacciotti-Saija, C., Langdon, R., Ward, P. B., Hickie, I. B., Scott, E. M., Naismith, S. L., et al. (2015). A double-blind randomized controlled trial of oxytocin nasal spray and social cognition training for young people with early psychosis. *Schizophrenia Bulletin, 41*(2), 483–493.

Canli, T., & Lesch, K. P. (2007). Long story short: The serotonin transporter in emotion regulation and social cognition. *Nature Neuroscience, 10*(9), 1103–1109.

Cella, M., Reeder, C., & Wykes, T. (2015). Lessons learnt? The importance of metacognition and its implications for cognitive remediation in schizophrenia. *Frontiers in Psychology, 6*, 1259.

Cervenka, S., Backman, L., Cselenyi, Z., Halldin, C., & Farde, L. (2008). Associations between dopamine D2-receptor binding and cognitive performance indicate functional compartmentalization of the human striatum. *Neuroimage, 40*(3), 1287–1295.

Chou, H. H., Talledo, J. A., Lamb, S. N., Thompson, W. K., & Swerdlow, N. R. (2013). Amphetamine effects on MATRICS Consensus Cognitive Battery performance in healthy adults. *Psychopharmacology (Berlin), 227*(1), 165–176.

Clarke, H. F., Dalley, J. W., Crofts, H. S., Robbins, T. W., & Roberts, A. C. (2004). Cognitive inflexibility after prefrontal serotonin depletion. *Science, 304*(5672), 878–880.

Cowen, P., & Sherwood, A. C. (2013). The role of serotonin in cognitive function: Evidence from recent studies and implications for understanding depression. *Journal of Psychopharmacology, 27*(7), 575–583.

Coyle, J. T. (1996). The glutamatergic dysfunction hypothesis for schizophrenia. *Harvard Review of Psychiatry, 3*(5), 241–253.

Cropley, V. L., Fujita, M., Innis, R. B., & Nathan, P. J. (2006). Molecular imaging of the dopaminergic system and its association with human cognitive function. *Biological Psychiatry, 59*(10), 898–907.

Dahlin, E., Neely, A. S., Larsson, A., Backman, L., & Nyberg, L. (2008). Transfer of learning after updating training mediated by the striatum. *Science, 320*(5882), 1510–1512.

Daniel, D. G., Weinberger, D. R., Jones, D. W., Zigun, J. R., Coppola, R., Handel, S., et al. (1991). The effect of amphetamine on regional cerebral blood flow during cognitive activation in schizophrenia. *Journal of Neuroscience, 11*(7), 1907–1917.

Davidson, M., Galderisi, S., Weiser, M., Werbeloff, N., Fleischhacker, W. W., Keefe, R. S., et al. (2009). Cognitive effects of antipsychotic drugs in first-episode schizophrenia and schizophreniform disorder: A randomized, open-label clinical trial (EUFEST). *American Journal of Psychiatry, 166*(6), 675–682.

Davis, M. C., Lee, J., Horan, W. P., Clarke, A. D., McGee, M. R., Green, M. F., et al. (2013). Effects of single dose intranasal oxytocin on social cognition in schizophrenia. *Schizophrenia Research, 147*(2–3), 393–397.

Demirtas-Tatlidede, A., Freitas, C., Cromer, J. R., Safar, L., Ongur, D., Stone, W. S., et al. (2010). Safety and proof of principle study of cerebellar vermal theta burst stimulation in refractory schizophrenia. *Schizophrenia Research, 124*(1–3), 91–100.

Dickinson, D., Ramsey, M. E., & Gold, J. M. (2007). Overlooking the obvious: A meta-analytic comparison of digit symbol coding tasks and other cognitive measures in schizophrenia. *Archives of General Psychiatry, 64*(5), 532–542.

D'Souza, D. C., Radhakrishnan, R., Perry, E., Bhakta, S., Singh, N. M., Yadav, R., et al. (2013). Feasibility, safety, and efficacy of the combination of D-serine and computerized cognitive retraining in schizophrenia: An international collaborative pilot study. *Neuropsychopharmacology, 38*(3), 492–503.

D'Souza, D. C., Singh, N., Elander, J., Carbuto, M., Pittman, B., Udo de Haes, J., et al. (2012). Glycine transporter inhibitor attenuates the psychotomimetic effects of ketamine in healthy males: Preliminary evidence. *Neuropsychopharmacology, 37*(4), 1036–1046.

Dyer, M. A., Freudenreich, O., Culhane, M. A., Pachas, G. N., Deckersbach, T., Murphy, E., et al. (2008). High-dose galantamine augmentation inferior to placebo on attention, inhibitory control and working memory performance in nonsmokers with schizophrenia. *Schizophrenia Research, 102*(1–3), 88–95.

Eack, S. M., Hogarty, G. E., Cho, R. Y., Prasad, K. M., Greenwald, D. P., Hogarty, S. S., et al. (2010). Neuroprotective effects of cognitive enhancement therapy against gray matter loss in early schizophrenia: Results from a 2-year randomized controlled trial. *Archives of General Psychiatry, 67*(7), 674–682.

Fatouros-Bergman, H., Cervenka, S., Flyckt, L., Edman, G., & Farde, L. (2014). Meta-analysis of cognitive performance in drug-naive patients with schizophrenia. *Schizophrenia Research, 158*(1–3), 156–162.

Feifel, D., Macdonald, K., Cobb, P., & Minassian, A. (2012). Adjunctive intranasal oxytocin improves verbal memory in people with schizophrenia. *Schizophrenia Research, 139*(1–3), 207–210.

Finke, K., Dodds, C. M., Bublak, P., Regenthal, R., Baumann, F., Manly, T., et al. (2010). Effects of modafinil and methylphenidate on visual attention capacity: A TVA-based study. *Psychopharmacology (Berlin), 210*(3), 317–329.

Floresco, S. B., Geyer, M. A., Gold, L. H., & Grace, A. A. (2005). Developing predictive animal models and establishing a preclinical trials network for assessing treatment effects on cognition in schizophrenia. *Schizophrenia Bulletin, 31*(4), 888–894.

Freudenreich, O., Henderson, D. C., Macklin, E. A., Evins, A. E., Fan, X., Cather, C., et al. (2009). Modafinil for clozapine-treated schizophrenia patients: A double-blind, placebo-controlled pilot trial. *Journal of Clinical Psychiatry, 70*(12), 1674–1680.

Friedman, J. I., Adler, D. N., Howanitz, E., Harvey, P. D., Brenner, G., Temporini, H., et al. (2002). A double blind placebo controlled trial of donepezil adjunctive treatment to risperidone for the cognitive impairment of schizophrenia. *Biological Psychiatry, 51*(5), 349–357.

Friedman, J. I., Carpenter, D., Lu, J., Fan, J., Tang, C. Y., White, L., et al. (2008). A pilot study of adjunctive atomoxetine treatment to second-generation antipsychotics for cognitive impairment in schizophrenia. *Journal of Clinical Psychopharmacology, 28*(1), 59–63.

Friedman, J. I., Harvey, P. D., Coleman, T., Moriarty, P. J., Bowie, C., Parrella, M., et al. (2001). Six-year follow-up study of cognitive and functional status across the lifespan in schizophrenia: A comparison with Alzheimer's disease and normal aging. *American Journal of Psychiatry, 158*(9), 1441–1448.

Fuller, R., Nopoulos, P., Arndt, S., O'Leary, D., Ho, B. C., & Andreasen, N. C. (2002). Longitudinal assessment of premorbid cognitive functioning in patients with schizophrenia through examination of standardized scholastic test performance. *American Journal of Psychiatry, 159*(7), 1183–1189.

Gibson, C. M., Penn, D. L., Smedley, K. L., Leserman, J., Elliott, T., & Pedersen, C. A. (2014). A pilot six-week randomized controlled trial of oxytocin on social cognition and social skills in schizophrenia. *Schizophrenia Research, 156*(2–3), 261–265.

Gilleen, J., Michalopoulou, P. G., Reichenberg, A., Drake, R., Wykes, T., Lewis, S. W., et al. (2014). Modafinil combined with cognitive training is associated with improved learning in healthy volunteers: A randomised controlled trial. *European Neuropsychopharmacology, 24*(4), 529–539.

Goff, D. C., & Coyle, J. T. (2001). The emerging role of glutamate in the pathophysiology and treatment of schizophrenia. *American Journal of Psychiatry, 158*(9), 1367–1377.

Goldberg, T. E., Bigelow, L. B., Weinberger, D. R., Daniel, D. G., & Kleinman, J. E. (1991). Cognitive and behavioral effects of the coadministration of dextroamphetamine and haloperidol in schizophrenia. *American Journal of Psychiatry, 148*(1), 78–84.

Goldberg, T. E., Keefe, R. S., Goldman, R. S., Robinson, D. G., & Harvey, P. D. (2010). Circumstances under which practice does not make perfect: A review of the practice effect literature in schizophrenia and its relevance to clinical treatment studies. *Neuropsychopharmacology, 35*(5), 1053–1062.

Gottlieb, J. D., Cather, C., Shanahan, M., Creedon, T., Macklin, E. A., & Goff, D. C. (2011). D-Cycloserine facilitation of cognitive behavioral therapy for delusions in schizophrenia. *Schizophrenia Research, 131*(1–3), 69–74.

Green, M. F. (1996). What are the functional consequences of neurocognitive deficits in schizophrenia? *American Journal of Psychiatry, 153*(3), 321–330.

Green, M. F., Kern, R. S., & Heaton, R. K. (2004). Longitudinal studies of cognition and functional outcome in schizophrenia: Implications for MATRICS. *Schizophrenia Research*, *72*(1), 41–51.

Guastella, A. J., Ward, P. B., Hickie, I. B., Shahrestani, S., Hodge, M. A., Scott, E. M., et al. (2015). A single dose of oxytocin nasal spray improves higher-order social cognition in schizophrenia. *Schizophrenia Research*, *168*(3), 628–633.

Hahn, B., Harvey, A. N., Concheiro-Guisan, M., Huestis, M. A., Holcomb, H. H., & Gold, J. M. (2013). A test of the cognitive self-medication hypothesis of tobacco smoking in schizophrenia. *Biological Psychiatry*, *74*(6), 436–443.

Harris, J. G., Kongs, S., Allensworth, D., Martin, L., Tregellas, J., Sullivan, B., et al. (2004). Effects of nicotine on cognitive deficits in schizophrenia. *Neuropsychopharmacology*, *29*(7), 1378–1385.

Harvey, P. D., Sacchetti, E., Galluzzo, A., Romeo, F., Gorini, B., Bilder, R. M., et al. (2008). A randomized double-blind comparison of ziprasidone vs. clozapine for cognition in patients with schizophrenia selected for resistance or intolerance to previous treatment. *Schizophrenia Research*, *105*(1–3), 138–143.

Hasan, A., Strube, W., Palm, U., & Wobrock, T. (2016). Repetitive noninvasive brain stimulation to modulate cognitive functions in schizophrenia: A systematic review of primary and secondary outcomes. *Schizophrenia Bulletin*, *42*(Suppl. 1), S95–S109.

Heaton, R. K., Gladsjo, J. A., Palmer, B. W., Kuck, J., Marcotte, T. D., & Jeste, D. V. (2001). Stability and course of neuropsychological deficits in schizophrenia. *Archives of General Psychiatry*, *58*(1), 24–32.

Heinrichs, R. W. (2005). The primacy of cognition in schizophrenia. *The American Psychologist*, *60*(3), 229–242.

Hjarthag, F., Helldin, L., Karilampi, U., & Norlander, T. (2010). Illness-related components for the family burden of relatives to patients with psychotic illness. *Social Psychiatry and Psychiatric Epidemiology*, *45*(2), 275–283.

Hoy, K. E., Arnold, S. L., Emonson, M. R., Daskalakis, Z. J., & Fitzgerald, P. B. (2014). An investigation into the effects of tDCS dose on cognitive performance over time in patients with schizophrenia. *Schizophrenia Research*, *155*(1–3), 96–100.

Hunter, M. D., Ganesan, V., Wilkinson, I. D., & Spence, S. A. (2006). Impact of modafinil on prefrontal executive function in schizophrenia. *American Journal of Psychiatry*, *163*(12), 2184–2186.

Ilieva, I. P., Hook, C. J., & Farah, M. J. (2015). Prescription stimulants' effects on healthy inhibitory control, working memory, and episodic memory: A meta-analysis. *Journal of Cognitive Neuroscience*, *27*(6), 1069–1089.

Jaeggi, S. M., Buschkuehl, M., Jonides, J., & Perrig, W. J. (2008). Improving fluid intelligence with training on working memory. *Proceedings of the National Academy of Sciences of the USA*, *105*(19), 6829–6833.

Kalechstein, A. D., De La Garza, R., 2nd, & Newton, T. F. (2010). Modafinil administration improves working memory in methamphetamine-dependent individuals who demonstrate baseline impairment. *American Journal of Addiction*, *19*(4), 340–344.

Kane, J. M., D'Souza, D. C., Patkar, A. A., Youakim, J. M., Tiller, J. M., Yang, R., et al. (2010). Armodafinil as adjunctive therapy in adults with cognitive deficits associated with schizophrenia: A 4-week, double-blind, placebo-controlled study. *Journal of Clinical Psychiatry*, *71*(11), 1475–1481.

Keefe, R. S., Bilder, R. M., Davis, S. M., Harvey, P. D., Palmer, B. W., Gold, J. M., et al. (2007). Neurocognitive effects of antipsychotic medications in patients with chronic schizophrenia in the CATIE trial. *Archives of General Psychiatry*, *64*(6), 633–647.

Keefe, R. S., Bilder, R. M., Harvey, P. D., Davis, S. M., Palmer, B. W., Gold, J. M., et al. (2006). Baseline neurocognitive deficits in the CATIE schizophrenia trial. *Neuropsychopharmacology*, *31*(9), 2033–2046.

Keefe, R. S., Buchanan, R. W., Marder, S. R., Schooler, N. R., Dugar, A., Zivkov, M., et al. (2013). Clinical trials of potential cognitive-enhancing drugs in schizophrenia: What have we learned so far? *Schizophrenia Bulletin*, *39*(2), 417–435.

Keefe, R. S., Malhotra, A. K., Meltzer, H. Y., Kane, J. M., Buchanan, R. W., Murthy, A., et al. (2008). Efficacy and safety of donepezil in patients with schizophrenia or schizoaffective disorder: Significant placebo/practice effects in a 12-week, randomized, double-blind, placebo-controlled trial. *Neuropsychopharmacology*, *33*(6), 1217–1228.

Keefe, R. S., Meltzer, H. A., Dgetluck, N., Gawryl, M., Koenig, G., Moebius, H. J., et al. (2015). Randomized, double-blind, placebo-controlled study of encenicline, an alpha7 nicotinic acetylcholine receptor agonist, as a treatment for cognitive impairment in schizophrenia. *Neuropsychopharmacology*, *40*(13), 3053–3060.

Keefe, R. S., Poe, M., Walker, T. M., Kang, J. W., & Harvey, P. D. (2006). The Schizophrenia Cognition Rating Scale: An interview-based assessment and its relationship to cognition, real-world functioning, and functional capacity. *American Journal of Psychiatry*, *163*(3), 426–432.

Keefe, R. S., Silva, S. G., Perkins, D. O., & Lieberman, J. A. (1999). The effects of atypical anti-psychotic drugs on neurocognitive impairment in schizophrenia: A review and meta-analysis. *Schizophrenia Bulletin*, *25*(2), 201–222.

Keefe, R. S., Sweeney, J. A., Gu, H., Hamer, R. M., Perkins, D. O., McEvoy, J. P., et al. (2007). Effects of olanzapine, quetiapine, and risperidone on neurocognitive function in early psychosis: A randomized, double-blind 52-week comparison. *American Journal of Psychiatry*, *164*(7), 1061–1071.

Keefe, R. S., Vinogradov, S., Medalia, A., Silverstein, S. M., Bell, M. D., Dickinson, D., et al. (2011). Report from the working group conference on multisite trial design for cognitive remediation in schizophrenia. *Schizophrenia Bulletin*, *37*(5), 1057–1065.

Kelly, D. (2015). *Effects of intranasal oxytocin or galantamine for primary enduring negative symptoms and cognitive impairments in people with schizophrenia.* Paper presented at the European College of Neuropsychopharmacology Congress. Amsterdam, The Netherlands.

Kelly, D. L., Buchanan, R. W., Boggs, D. L., McMahon, R. P., Dickinson, D., Nelson, M., et al. (2009). A randomized double-blind trial of atomoxetine for cognitive impairments in 32 people with schizophrenia. *Journal of Clinical Psychiatry*, *70*(4), 518–525.

Knecht, S., Breitenstein, C., Bushuven, S., Wailke, S., Kamping, S., Floel, A., et al. (2004). Levodopa: Faster and better word learning in normal humans. *Annals of Neurology*, *56*(1), 20–26.

Kumari, V., Aasen, I., ffytche, D., Williams, S. C., & Sharma, T. (2006). Neural correlates of adjunctive rivastigmine treatment to antipsychotics in schizophrenia: A randomized, placebo-controlled, double-blind fMRI study. *Neuroimage*, *29*(2), 545–556.

Lane, H. Y., Huang, C. L., Wu, P. L., Liu, Y. C., Chang, Y. C., Lin, P. Y., et al. (2006). Glycine transporter I inhibitor, *N*-methylglycine (sarcosine), added to clozapine for the treatment of schizophrenia. *Biological Psychiatry*, *60*(6), 645–649.

Lee, M. R., Wehring, H. J., McMahon, R. P., Linthicum, J., Cascella, N., Liu, F., et al. (2013). Effects of adjunctive intranasal oxytocin on olfactory identification and clinical symptoms in schizophrenia: Results from a randomized double blind placebo controlled pilot study. *Schizophrenia Research*, *145*(1–3), 110–115.

Lee, S. W., Lee, J. G., Lee, B. J., & Kim, Y. H. (2007). A 12-week, double-blind, placebo-controlled trial of galantamine adjunctive treatment to conventional antipsychotics for the cognitive impairments in chronic schizophrenia. *International Clinical Psychopharmacology*, *22*(2), 63–68.

Levkovitz, Y., Rabany, L., Harel, E. V., & Zangen, A. (2011). Deep transcranial magnetic stimulation add-on for treatment of negative symptoms and cognitive deficits of schizophrenia: A feasibility study. *International Journal of Neuropsychopharmacology*, *14*(7), 991–996.

Lewis, D. A., Cho, R. Y., Carter, C. S., Eklund, K., Forster, S., Kelly, M. A., et al. (2008). Subunit-selective modulation of GABA type A receptor neurotransmission and cognition in schizophrenia. *American Journal of Psychiatry*, *165*(12), 1585–1593.

Lieberman, J. A., Dunbar, G., Segreti, A. C., Girgis, R. R., Seoane, F., Beaver, J. S., et al. (2013). A randomized exploratory trial of an alpha-7 nicotinic receptor agonist (TC-5619) for cognitive enhancement in schizophrenia. *Neuropsychopharmacology*, *38*(6), 968–975.

Lieberman, J. A., Stroup, T. S., McEvoy, J. P., Swartz, M. S., Rosenheck, R. A., Perkins, D. O., et al. (2005). Effectiveness of antipsychotic drugs in patients with chronic schizophrenia. *New England Journal of Medicine*, *353*(12), 1209–1223.

Lindenmayer, J. P., & Khan, A. (2011). Galantamine augmentation of long-acting injectable risperidone for cognitive impairments in chronic schizophrenia. *Schizophrenia Research*, *125*(2–3), 267–277.

Mattay, V. S., Goldberg, T. E., Fera, F., Hariri, A. R., Tessitore, A., Egan, M. F., et al. (2003). Catechol *O*-methyltransferase val158–met genotype and individual variation in the brain response to amphetamine. *Proceedings of the National Academy of Sciences of the USA, 100*(10), 6186–6191.

McDonald, J. W., & Johnston, M. V. (1990). Nonketotic hyperglycinemia: Pathophysiological role of NMDA-type excitatory amino acid receptors. *Annals of Neurology, 27*(4), 449–450.

McGurk, S. R., Mueser, K. T., & Pascaris, A. (2005). Cognitive training and supported employment for persons with severe mental illness: One-year results from a randomized controlled trial. *Schizophrenia Bulletin, 31*(4), 898–909.

Melby-Lervag, M., & Hulme, C. (2013). Is working memory training effective? A meta-analytic review. *Developmental Psychology, 49*(2), 270–291.

Meltzer, H. Y., & Massey, B. W. (2011). The role of serotonin receptors in the action of atypical antipsychotic drugs. *Current Opinion in Pharmacology, 11*(1), 59–67.

Meltzer, H. Y., & McGurk, S. R. (1999). The effects of clozapine, risperidone, and olanzapine on cognitive function in schizophrenia. *Schizophrenia Bulletin, 25*(2), 233–255.

Meltzer, H. Y., & Sumiyoshi, T. (2008). Does stimulation of 5-HT(1A) receptors improve cognition in schizophrenia? *Behavioral Brain Research, 195*(1), 98–102.

Mesholam-Gately, R. I., Giuliano, A. J., Goff, K. P., Faraone, S. V., & Seidman, L. J. (2009). Neurocognition in first-episode schizophrenia: A meta-analytic review. *Neuropsychology, 23*(3), 315–336.

Michalopoulou, P. G., Lewis, S. W., Drake, R. J., Reichenberg, A., Emsley, R., Kalpakidou, A. K., et al. (2015). Modafinil combined with cognitive training: Pharmacological augmentation of cognitive training in schizophrenia. *European Neuropsychopharmacology, 25*(8), 1178–1189.

Michelson, D., Faries, D., Wernicke, J., Kelsey, D., Kendrick, K., Sallee, F. R., et al. (2001). Atomoxetine in the treatment of children and adolescents with attention-deficit/hyperactivity disorder: A randomized, placebo-controlled, dose–response study. *Pediatrics, 108*(5), E83.

Milev, P., Ho, B. C., Arndt, S., & Andreasen, N. C. (2005). Predictive values of neurocognition and negative symptoms on functional outcome in schizophrenia: A longitudinal first-episode study with 7-year follow-up. *American Journal of Psychiatry, 162*(3), 495–506.

Minzenberg, M. J., & Carter, C. S. (2008). Modafinil: A review of neurochemical actions and effects on cognition. *Neuropsychopharmacology, 33*(7), 1477–1502.

Minzenberg, M. J., & Carter, C. S. (2012). Developing treatments for impaired cognition in schizophrenia. *Trends in Cognitive Science, 16*(1), 35–42.

Muller, U., Steffenhagen, N., Regenthal, R., & Bublak, P. (2004). Effects of modafinil on working memory processes in humans. *Psychopharmacology (Berlin), 177*(1–2), 161–169.

Murthy, N. V., Mahncke, H., Wexler, B. E., Maruff, P., Inamdar, A., Zucchetto, M., et al. (2012). Computerized cognitive remediation training for schizophrenia: An open label, multi-site, multinational methodology study. *Schizophrenia Research, 139*(1–3), 87–91.

Narendran, R., Young, C. M., Valenti, A. M., Nickolova, M. K., & Pristach, C. A. (2002). Is psychosis exacerbated by modafinil? *Archives of General Psychiatry, 59*(3), 292–293.

Newhouse, P. A., Potter, A., & Singh, A. (2004). Effects of nicotinic stimulation on cognitive performance. *Current Opinion in Pharmacology, 4*(1), 36–46.

Nicoll, R. A., & Malenka, R. C. (1999). Expression mechanisms underlying NMDA receptor-dependent long-term potentiation. *Annals of the New York Academy of Sciences, 868*, 515–525.

Niemegeers, P., Dumont, G. J., Quisenaerts, C., Morrens, M., Boonzaier, J., Fransen, E., et al. (2014). The effects of nicotine on cognition are dependent on baseline performance. *European Neuropsychopharmacology, 24*(7), 1015–1023.

Nuechterlein, K. H., Green, M. F., Kern, R. S., Baade, L. E., Barch, D. M., Cohen, J. D., et al. (2008). The MATRICS Consensus Cognitive Battery, part 1: Test selection, reliability, and validity. *American Journal of Psychiatry, 165*(2), 203–213.

Olincy, A., Harris, J. G., Johnson, L. L., Pender, V., Kongs, S., Allensworth, D., et al. (2006). Proof-of-concept trial of an alpha7 nicotinic agonist in schizophrenia. *Archives of General Psychiatry, 63*(6), 630–638.

Owen, A. M., Hampshire, A., Grahn, J. A., Stenton, R., Dajani, S., Burns, A. S., et al. (2010). Putting brain training to the test. *Nature*, *465*(7299), 775–778.

Patel, A., Everitt, B., Knapp, M., Reeder, C., Grant, D., Ecker, C., et al. (2006). Schizophrenia patients with cognitive deficits: Factors associated with costs. *Schizophrenia Bulletin*, *32*(4), 776–785.

Pedersen, C. A., Gibson, C. M., Rau, S. W., Salimi, K., Smedley, K. L., Casey, R. L., et al. (2011). Intranasal oxytocin reduces psychotic symptoms and improves theory of mind and social perception in schizophrenia. *Schizophrenia Research*, *132*(1), 50–53.

Penades, R., Pujol, N., Catalan, R., Massana, G., Rametti, G., Garcia-Rizo, C., et al. (2013). Brain effects of cognitive remediation therapy in schizophrenia: A structural and functional neuroimaging study. *Biological Psychiatry*, *73*(10), 1015–1023.

Pierre, J. M., Peloian, J. H., Wirshing, D. A., Wirshing, W. C., & Marder, S. R. (2007). A randomized, double-blind, placebo-controlled trial of modafinil for negative symptoms in schizophrenia. *Journal of Clinical Psychiatry*, *68*(5), 705–710.

Pietrzak, R. H., Snyder, P. J., & Maruff, P. (2010). Amphetamine-related improvement in executive function in patients with chronic schizophrenia is modulated by practice effects. *Schizophrenia Research*, *124*(1–3), 176–182.

Prouteau, A., Verdoux, H., Briand, C., Lesage, A., Lalonde, P., Nicole, L., et al. (2005). Cognitive predictors of psychosocial functioning outcome in schizophrenia: A follow-up study of subjects participating in a rehabilitation program. *Schizophrenia Research*, *77*(2–3), 343–353.

Quisenaerts, C., Morrens, M., Hulstijn, W., de Bruijn, E., Timmers, M., Streffer, J., et al. (2014). The nicotinergic receptor as a target for cognitive enhancement in schizophrenia: Barking up the wrong tree? *Psychopharmacology (Berlin)*, *231*(3), 543–550.

Randall, D. C., Shneerson, J. M., & File, S. E. (2005). Cognitive effects of modafinil in student volunteers may depend on IQ. *Pharmacology, Biochemistry, and Behavior*, *82*(1), 133–139.

Reichenberg, A., Caspi, A., Harrington, H., Houts, R., Keefe, R. S., Murray, R. M., et al. (2010). Static and dynamic cognitive deficits in childhood preceding adult schizophrenia: A 30-year study. *American Journal of Psychiatry*, *167*(2), 160–169.

Reichenberg, A., Harvey, P. D., Bowie, C. R., Mojtabai, R., Rabinowitz, J., Heaton, R. K., et al. (2009). Neuropsychological function and dysfunction in schizophrenia and psychotic affective disorders. *Schizophrenia Bulletin*, *35*(5), 1022–1029.

Reichenberg, A., & Harvey, P. D. (2007). Neuropsychological impairments in schizophrenia: Integration of performance-based and brain imaging findings. *Psychological Bulletin*, 133(5), 833–858.

Reichenberg, A., Weiser, M., Rapp, M. A., Rabinowitz, J., Caspi, A., Schmeidler, J., et al. (2005). Elaboration on premorbid intellectual performance in schizophrenia: Premorbid intellectual decline and risk for schizophrenia. *Archives of General Psychiatry*, *62*(12), 1297–1304.

Revell, E. R., Neill, J. C., Harte, M., Khan, Z., & Drake, R. J. (2015). A systematic review and meta-analysis of cognitive remediation in early schizophrenia. *Schizophrenia Research*, *168*(1–2), 213–222.

Roth, B. L., Hanizavareh, S. M., & Blum, A. E. (2004). Serotonin receptors represent highly favorable molecular targets for cognitive enhancement in schizophrenia and other disorders. *Psychopharmacology (Berlin)*, *174*(1), 17–24.

Sacco, K. A., Termine, A., Seyal, A., Dudas, M. M., Vessicchio, J. C., Krishnan-Sarin, S., et al. (2005). Effects of cigarette smoking on spatial working memory and attentional deficits in schizophrenia: Involvement of nicotinic receptor mechanisms. *Archives of General Psychiatry*, *62*(6), 649–659.

Saeedi, H., Remington, G., & Christensen, B. K. (2006). Impact of haloperidol, a dopamine D2 antagonist, on cognition and mood. *Schizophrenia Research*, *85*(1–3), 222–231.

Scheidtmann, K., Fries, W., Muller, F., & Koenig, E. (2001). Effect of levodopa in combination with physiotherapy on functional motor recovery after stroke: A prospective, randomised, double-blind study. *Lancet*, *358*(9284), 787–790.

Schmiedek, F., Lovden, M., & Lindenberger, U. (2010). Hundred days of cognitive training enhance broad cognitive abilities in adulthood: Findings from the COGITO study. *Frontiers in Aging Neuroscience*, *2*, 27.

Schmitt, J. A., Wingen, M., Ramaekers, J. G., Evers, E. A., & Riedel, W. J. (2006). Serotonin and human cognitive performance. *Current Pharmaceutical Design*, *12*(20), 2473–2486.

Schubert, M. H., Young, K. A., & Hicks, P. B. (2006). Galantamine improves cognition in schizophrenic patients stabilized on risperidone. *Biological Psychiatry*, *60*(6), 530–533.

Scoriels, L., Barnett, J. H., Soma, P. K., Sahakian, B. J., & Jones, P. B. (2012). Effects of modafinil on cognitive functions in first episode psychosis. *Psychopharmacology (Berlin)*, *220*(2), 249–258.

Sevy, S., Rosenthal, M. H., Alvir, J., Meyer, S., Visweswaraiah, H., Gunduz-Bruce, H., et al. (2005). Double-blind, placebo-controlled study of modafinil for fatigue and cognition in schizophrenia patients treated with psychotropic medications. *Journal of Clinical Psychiatry*, *66*(7), 839–843.

Sharma, T., Reed, C., Aasen, I., & Kumari, V. (2006). Cognitive effects of adjunctive 24-weeks rivastigmine treatment to antipsychotics in schizophrenia: A randomized, placebo-controlled, double-blind investigation. *Schizophrenia Research*, *85*(1–3), 73–83.

Shipstead, Z., Redick, T. S., & Engle, R. W. (2012). Is working memory training effective? *Psychological Bulletin*, *138*(4), 628–654.

Spence, S. A., Green, R. D., Wilkinson, I. D., & Hunter, M. D. (2005). Modafinil modulates anterior cingulate function in chronic schizophrenia. *British Journal of Psychiatry*, *187*, 55–61.

Sumiyoshi, T. (2008). Possible dose–side effect relationship of antipsychotic drugs: Relevance to cognitive function in schizophrenia. *Expert Review of Clinical Pharmacology*, *1*(6), 791–802.

Sumiyoshi, T., Matsui, M., Nohara, S., Yamashita, I., Kurachi, M., Sumiyoshi, C., et al. (2001). Enhancement of cognitive performance in schizophrenia by addition of tandospirone to neuroleptic treatment. *American Journal of Psychiatry*, *158*(10), 1722–1725.

Sumiyoshi, T., Park, S., Jayathilake, K., Roy, A., Ertugrul, A., & Meltzer, H. Y. (2007). Effect of buspirone, a serotonin 1A partial agonist, on cognitive function in schizophrenia: A randomized, double-blind, placebo-controlled study. *Schizophrenia Research*, *95*(1–3), 158–168.

Swerdlow, N. R. (2012). Beyond antipsychotics: Pharmacologically-augmented cognitive therapies (PACTs) for schizophrenia. *Neuropsychopharmacology*, *37*(1), 310–311.

Takahashi, H., Kato, M., Hayashi, M., Okubo, Y., Takano, A., Ito, H., et al. (2007). Memory and frontal lobe functions; Possible relations with dopamine D2 receptors in the hippocampus. *Neuroimage*, *34*(4), 1643–1649.

Tandon, R., Nasrallah, H. A., & Keshavan, M. S. (2010). Schizophrenia, "just the facts" 5: Treatment and prevention—Past, present, and future. *Schizophrenia Research*, *122*(1–3), 1–23.

Terry, A. V., Jr., Buccafusco, J. J., & Wilson, C. (2008). Cognitive dysfunction in neuropsychiatric disorders: Selected serotonin receptor subtypes as therapeutic targets. *Behavioral Brain Research*, *195*(1), 30–38.

Thakurathi, N., Vincenzi, B., & Henderson, D. C. (2013). Assessing the prospect of donepezil in improving cognitive impairment in patients with schizophrenia. *Expert Opinion on Investigational Drugs*, *22*(2), 259–265.

Tsai, G., Lane, H. Y., Yang, P., Chong, M. Y., & Lange, N. (2004). Glycine transporter I inhibitor, *N*-methylglycine (sarcosine), added to antipsychotics for the treatment of schizophrenia. *Biological Psychiatry*, *55*(5), 452–456.

Turner, D. C., Clark, L., Pomarol-Clotet, E., McKenna, P., Robbins, T. W., & Sahakian, B. J. (2004). Modafinil improves cognition and attentional set shifting in patients with chronic schizophrenia. *Neuropsychopharmacology*, *29*(7), 1363–1373.

Tyson, P. J., Roberts, K. H., & Mortimer, A. M. (2004). Are the cognitive effects of atypical antipsychotics influenced by their affinity to 5HT-2A receptors? *International Journal of Neuroscience*, *114*(6), 593–611.

Velligan, D., Brenner, R., Sicuro, F., Walling, D., Riesenberg, R., Sfera, A., et al. (2012). Assessment of the effects of AZD3480 on cognitive function in patients with schizophrenia. *Schizophrenia Research*, *134*(1), 59–64.

Velligan, D. I., Mahurin, R. K., Diamond, P. L., Hazleton, B. C., Eckert, S. L., & Miller, A. L. (1997). The functional significance of symptomatology and cognitive function in schizophrenia. *Schizophrenia Research*, *25*(1), 21–31.

Vercammen, A., Rushby, J. A., Loo, C., Short, B., Weickert, C. S., & Weickert, T. W. (2011). Transcranial direct current stimulation influences probabilistic association learning in schizophrenia. *Schizophrenia Research, 131*(1–3), 198–205.

Vernaleken, I., Kumakura, Y., Cumming, P., Buchholz, H. G., Siessmeier, T., Stoeter, P., et al. (2006). Modulation of [^{18}F]fluorodopa (FDOPA) kinetics in the brain of healthy volunteers after acute haloperidol challenge. *Neuroimage, 30*(4), 1332–1339.

Veselinovic, T., Schorn, H., Vernaleken, I. B., Hiemke, C., Zernig, G., Gur, R., et al. (2013). Effects of antipsychotic treatment on cognition in healthy subjects. *Journal of Psychopharmacology, 27*(4), 374–385.

Vinogradov, S., Fisher, M., Holland, C., Shelly, W., Wolkowitz, O., & Mellon, S. H. (2009). Is serum brain-derived neurotrophic factor a biomarker for cognitive enhancement in schizophrenia? *Biological Psychiatry, 66*(6), 549–553.

Walker-Batson, D., Curtis, S., Natarajan, R., Ford, J., Dronkers, N., Salmeron, E., et al. (2001). A double-blind, placebo-controlled study of the use of amphetamine in the treatment of aphasia. *Stroke, 32*(9), 2093–2098.

Wallace, M. L., Frank, E., & Kraemer, H. C. (2013). A novel approach for developing and interpreting treatment moderator profiles in randomized clinical trials. *JAMA Psychiatry, 70*(11), 1241–1247.

Wallace, T. L., Ballard, T. M., Pouzet, B., Riedel, W. J., & Wettstein, J. G. (2011). Drug targets for cognitive enhancement in neuropsychiatric disorders. *Pharmacology, Biochemistry, and Behavior, 99*(2), 130–145.

Weiser, M., Heresco-Levy, U., Davidson, M., Javitt, D. C., Werbeloff, N., Gershon, A. A., et al. (2012). A multicenter, add-on randomized controlled trial of low-dose D-serine for negative and cognitive symptoms of schizophrenia. *Journal of Clinical Psychiatry, 73*(6), e728–e734.

Wexler, B. E., Anderson, M., Fulbright, R. K., & Gore, J. C. (2000). Preliminary evidence of improved verbal working memory performance and normalization of task-related frontal lobe activation in schizophrenia following cognitive exercises. *American Journal of Psychiatry, 157*(10), 1694–1697.

Wonnacott, S., Barik, J., Dickinson, J., & Jones, I. W. (2006). Nicotinic receptors modulate transmitter cross talk in the CNS: Nicotinic modulation of transmitters. *Journal of Molecular Neuroscience, 30*(1–2), 137–140.

Wykes, T., Brammer, M., Mellers, J., Bray, P., Reeder, C., Williams, C., et al. (2002). Effects on the brain of a psychological treatment: Cognitive remediation therapy—Functional magnetic resonance imaging in schizophrenia. *British Journal of Psychiatry, 181*, 144–152.

Wykes, T., Huddy, V., Cellard, C., McGurk, S. R., & Czobor, P. (2011). A meta-analysis of cognitive remediation for schizophrenia: Methodology and effect sizes. *American Journal of Psychiatry, 168*(5), 472–485.

Wykes, T., Reeder, C., Landau, S., Matthiasson, P., Haworth, E., & Hutchinson, C. (2009). Does age matter? Effects of cognitive rehabilitation across the age span. *Schizophrenia Research, 113*(2–3), 252–258.

Young, J. W., & Geyer, M. A. (2015). Developing treatments for cognitive deficits in schizophrenia: The challenge of translation. *Journal of Psychopharmacology, 29*(2), 178–196.

Zhu, W., Zhang, Z., Qi, J., Liu, F., Chen, J., Zhao, J., et al. (2014). Adjunctive treatment for cognitive impairment in patients with chronic schizophrenia: A double-blind, placebo-controlled study. *Neuropsychiatric Disease and Treatment, 10*, 1317–1323.

TEN

Cognitive Enhancement in Major Depressive Disorder

ANDRÉ F. CARVALHO, GILBERTO S. ALVES,

CRISTIANO A. KÖHLER,

AND ROGER S. MCINTYRE

INTRODUCTION

Major depressive disorder (MDD) affects approximately one in seven individuals in a lifetime and is associated with high rates of recurrence, non-recovery, and illness-associated burden.[1-3] Only approximately 30% of patients with MDD reach remission following an adequate trial with a first-line antidepressant, whereas the majority of individuals do not achieve long-term functional recovery.[4] The persistence of residual symptoms in MDD hinders the re-establishment of premorbid levels of psychosocial functioning and increases the risk for relapses and recurrences leading to chronicity.[5] It is noteworthy that even remitted MDD patients do not achieve full functional recovery.[3] Furthermore, impairments in psychosocial functioning, notably decrements in work productivity, significantly contribute to MDD-related societal costs.[6] Thus, it is important to identify which clinical features of depression correlate with functioning.

Self-perceived cognitive impairment is a widely recognized clinical manifestation of MDD. Consequently, current diagnostic criteria for depression of both the
10th revision of the *International Statistical Classification of Diseases and Related
Health Problems* (ICD-10) and the fifth edition of the *Diagnostic and Statistical
Manual of Mental Disorders* (DSM-5) list items such as "reduced concentration and
attention" and "diminished ability to think or concentrate," respectively. However,
self-reported cognitive deficits do not seem to correlate well with objectively measured neuropsychological impairments.[7,8]

It has been reported that approximately 25–50% of MDD patients exhibit cognitive deficits of at least 1 standard deviation (SD) below the mean on at least one
cognitive domain, and half of those presenting these deficits show scores 2 SD below
the mean.[9] Diverse cognitive domains are impaired in MDD, including attention,
memory, psychomotor speed, and executive function, which refers to the complex
cognitive activity required to coordinate several cognitive subprocesses to achieve a
particular goal.[10] Moderate deficits in attention and executive function may persist
even in remitted MDD patients.[11] Furthermore, several lines of evidence indicate that
cognitive dysfunction is an important mediator of functioning in MDD.[12–14] The relevance of cognitive dysfunction as a dimension of MDD at least in part independent
and dissociable from affective symptomatology fosters the routine assessment in
clinical practice of cognitive dysfunction in MDD and encourages the development
of novel treatment strategies targeting neuropsychological deficits in MDD.[15] In fact,
the achievement of cognitive remission has been proposed as a novel treatment aim
for MDD.[16]

A different taxonomy for cognitive impairment in MDD draws the distinction
between "hot" (emotional-laden) and "cold" (emotional-independent) cognitive dysfunction (Figure 10.1).[17,18] Whereas deficits in "hot" cognition in MDD refer to a
negative-biased pattern of response to stimuli on tasks of attention[19] and working
memory[20] in association with rumination and high levels of self-criticism,[21] "cold"
cognitive dysfunction refers to quantitative deficits on measures of memory, sustained attention, and executive function in both symptomatic and remitted states of
MDD.[22] Although useful for practical purposes, the distinction between "hot" and
"cold" cognitions is arbitrary. For example, aspects of "hot" cognition may influence
the performance on standard neuropsychological tests.[17]

Cognitive function in humans is mediated by interconnected neural circuits
encompassing the prefrontal cortex, thalamus, and basal ganglia.[23] For example,
response inhibition is attributed to circuits connecting the orbito-prefrontal cortex
with the ventromedial caudate. The hippocampus is pivotal for declarative learning
and memory, but it is also an area that is connected to several cortical structures

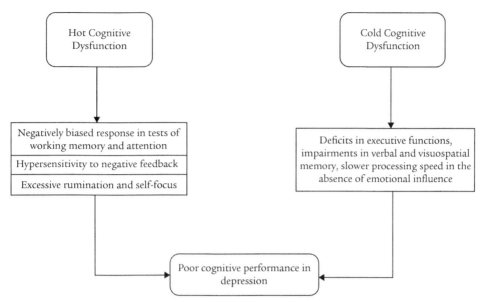

FIGURE 10.1 *Hot and cold cognitive dysfunction in major depressive disorder.*

and may be relevant for the integration of "hot" and "cold" cognitive processes.[23-25] These circuits are integrated with areas related to the pathophysiology of MDD, such as the hypothalamic–pituitary–adrenal (HPA) axis as well as the amygdala. The integrated functioning of these neurocircuits may underlie the relationship between mood disorders and cognition.[25]

Although some standard antidepressants may mitigate cognitive deficits in MDD, their effects are clinically unsatisfactory.[26-29] Furthermore, some preliminary evidence indicates that cognitive deficits in individuals with MDD may predict the failure to respond to selective serotonin reuptake inhibitors (SSRIs) or dual serotonergic–noradrenergic reuptake inhibitors (SNRIs), suggesting that impairments in some cognitive domains may stratify a subgroup of patients who would require additional treatment strategies.[30-32] Preclinical and clinical evidence indicates that the multimodal-acting antidepressant vortioxetine may have advantages compared to standard monoamine reuptake inhibitors for cognitive enhancement in MDD.[33-35]

In addition to antidepressant drug treatments, psychotherapeutic approaches for the treatment of depression have also been investigated. These strategies primarily involve cognitive remediation therapy. In brief, cognitive remediation therapy consists of the application of systematic instruction and structured experience to alter the functioning of neurocognitive systems with the aim of mitigating cognitive dysfunction in targeted domains.[36,37] Although the mechanisms underlying functional change remain poorly understood, repeated stimulation of impaired cognitive function through repetitive, targeted exercise has been shown to improve cognitive functioning across mental disorders, most notably schizophrenia.[37,38] Although cognitive remediation therapy has been less extensively investigated in MDD compared to schizophrenia, preliminary evidence indicates that this is an effective method to improve cognitive dysfunction in at least some domains, such as attention, verbal learning and memory, and executive function.[39–41] Synergistic effects for antidepressants and psychological treatments for depression have been suggested in recent neuropsychological models of antidepressant drug action.[42,43] It has been proposed that antidepressants enhance the relative balance of positive to negative emotional processing, which provides a framework for subsequent psychological and cognitive interventions.[44]

Noninvasive brain stimulation (NIBS) approaches, namely repeated transcranial magnetic stimulation (rTMS) and transcranial direct current stimulation (tDCS), have been investigated as therapeutic approaches for MDD. Although evidence supports the effectiveness of rTMS for the treatment of MDD,[45,46] the effectiveness of tDCS remains inconclusive.[47] Emerging data suggest that NIBS may improve cognitive performance in depression, but methodological inconsistencies across investigations limit the generalizability of these findings.[48]

The overarching aim of this chapter is to review available pharmacological, psychological, and neuromodulatory strategies for possible therapeutic effects on cognitive impairment in MDD. In addition, this chapter provides an overview of promising novel cognitive enhancers for MDD with primary mechanisms of action outside standard monoamine pathways. Finally, an integrative framework for the management of cognitive dysfunction in MDD is proposed.

COGNITIVE EFFECTS OF PHARMACOTHERAPY FOR DEPRESSION

The US Food and Drug Administration has not approved any pharmaceuticals for the treatment of cognitive impairment in MDD. Furthermore, clinical guidelines on this topic are lacking. Relatively few studies have primarily aimed to investigate the effect of standard antidepressants on cognitive performance in MDD.[15,29] Although evidence indicates that SSRIs or SNRIs may exert beneficial effects on cognitive dysfunction in MDD, these effects are suboptimal because a significant group of MDD patients may remain cognitively impaired in remission.[49] Furthermore, some data suggest that drugs targeting multiple neurotransmitter systems may be more effective than more selective agents (e.g., SSRI), although the exact clinical relevance of these findings remains to be established.[28,50] For instance, Herrera-Guzman et al.[28] evaluated cognitive function before treatment with escitalopram (SSRI) or duloxetine (SNRI), at the end of 24 weeks of treatment, and again at 24 weeks of unmedicated recovery. There were no significant differences in baseline cognitive function tests between the two treatment groups. Participants allocated to both treatment groups demonstrated improvement over baseline in verbal and visual episodic memory, working memory, and processing speed. However, those in the duloxetine group exhibited better improvement in working memory and episodic memory compared to those in the escitalopram group. Despite evidence of improvement, cognitive deficits remained.[28] After 24 weeks of treatment withdrawal, similar patterns of cognitive dysfunction persisted, and those in the SSRI group remained more impaired in episodic and working memory compared to participants from the SNRI group.[50] The clinical significance of these findings should be interpreted with caution because this study was not placebo-controlled, and it remained unclear to what extent cognitive improvement was secondary to treatment response. The same authors reported that 12 individuals who responded to bupropion (150 mg) for 8 weeks had lower baseline scores on tests of visual episodic memory and mental processing speed compared to those of 8 participants who did not respond to treatment.[31] Nevertheless, these results are limited by the small sample size and the lack of a placebo group. Furthermore, the 12 responders were significantly older and had more severe depressive symptoms at study intake.

A randomized, 8-week, controlled trial investigated the effects of duloxetine (60 mg/day; $n = 207$) versus placebo ($n = 104$) in older patients with MDD. At the end of the trial, participants allocated to the treatment group displayed significantly greater improvement on overall cognitive scores, primarily driven by improved verbal learning and memory.[51] Lam and colleagues[29] performed a systematic review of the effects of pharmacotherapy on cognitive performance in MDD. They found significant variations on overall methodological quality across different investigations. Standardized effect sizes (with 95% credible intervals) from placebo-controlled studies revealed that most results were not statistically significant. In the study by Raskin et al.,[51] duloxetine had a significant deleterious effect on mental processing speed compared to placebo. A clear limitation is that a uniformed and standardized neuropsychological battery is currently unavailable for clinical trials of participants with MDD.[15] Table 10.1 illustrates some neuropsychological tests as well as self-rated instruments commonly employed to measure cognition in MDD trials.

Since the publication of Lam et al.'s[29] systematic review, a few additional clinical trials have investigated the effects of antidepressants on cognitive dysfunction in MDD. An 8-week, randomized, double-blind study investigated the effects of bupropion (up to 450 mg/day; $n = 27$) or paroxetine (up to 37.5 mg/day; $n = 30$) on

TABLE 10.1 Common Neuropsychological Instruments and Subjective Measures of Cognitive Function Used across Studies in Major Depressive Disorder[a]

Instrument	Attention	Working Memory	Verbal Learning	Visuospatial Memory	Executive Functions	Processing Speed	Problem-Solving Reasoning	Social Cognition
CAS[b]								+
BRIEF-A[ba]		+			+			
SoCT[b]								+
CANTAB	+	+		+	+	+	+	+
DSST						+		
WCST	+	+			+	+		
RBANS	+	+	+	+				
CPT	+					+		
BAC-A	+	+	+			+	+	+
Cogtest	+	+	+	+	+	+	+	+
CVLT	+	+	+					
HVLT-R			+					
MCCB	+	+	+	+	+	+	+	+
TMT-A		+				+		
WAIS-R		+				+	+	
WMS	+	+	+					+

[a]Some instruments can be used for the assessment of different cognitive domains. Cognitive domains evaluated by instrument/test are indicated with a plus sign. The domain of executive functioning includes measures of abstraction, set shifting, planning, divided attention, decision-making, and response control.

[b]Available as a self-report cognitive measure/instrument.

CAS, Coping Attitude Scale; BRIEF-A, Behavior Rating Inventory of Executive Function; SoCT, Skills of Cognitive Therapy; CANTAB, Cambridge Neuropsychological Test Battery; DSST, Digit-Symbol Substitution Test; WCST, Wisconsin Card Sorting Test; RBANS, Repeatable Battery for the Assessment of Neuropsychological Status; CPT, Continuous Performance Task; BAC-A, Brief Assessment of Cognition for Affective Disorders; CVLT, California Verbal Learning Test; HVLT-R, Hopkins Verbal Learning Test–Revised; MCCB, MATRICS Consensus Cognitive Battery; TMT-A, Trail Making Test A; WAIS-R, Wechsler Adult Intelligence Scale–Revised; WMS, Wechsler Memory Scale.

cognition in suicidal participants with MDD. By the end of the trial, both treatments improved cognitive functioning in several domains.[52] Furthermore, a reduction in suicidal ideation occurred independently of memory improvement. In this study, suicidality was mitigated by the independent improvements in depressive symptomatology and verbal memory.

Soczynska and colleagues[53] investigated the effects of bupropion XL (up to 300 mg/day) and escitalopram (up to 20 mg/day) in a small ($N = 38$), 8-week, double-blind, randomized trial. By the end of the trial, both treatments significantly improved delayed verbal and nonverbal memory as well as global functioning and work productivity. Moreover, improvement in immediate verbal memory exerted a significant direct effect on psychosocial functioning amelioration.

Vortioxetine (Lu AA21004) is a multimodal antidepressant that exhibits 5-HT_3 and 5-HT_7 receptor antagonistic properties, 5-HT_{1B} receptor partial agonism, 5-HT_{1A} receptor agonism, and inhibition of the 5-HT transporter.[54] The antidepressant efficacy of vortioxetine has been well documented in adults with MDD;[55] a meta-analysis of 12 randomized controlled trials (RCTs) further supports its efficacy and safety despite the fact that the overall effect size for the primary outcome was small (-0.217).[56] Putative precognitive effects for vortioxetine have been demonstrated as a secondary outcome in a randomized, placebo-controlled trial on nondemented individuals with recurrent MDD ($N = 453$).[57] Improvements in learning and memory performance (as measured by the Rey Auditory Verbal Learning Test (RAVLT)), as well as processing speed (as measured by the Digit Symbol Substitution Test (DSST)), were largely a direct effect, independent from a reduction in depression symptoms' severity on the Hamilton Depression Rating Scale. A randomized, double-blind, placebo-controlled 8-week trial also evaluated vortioxetine's effect (10 or 20 mg) on cognitive performance in adults with MDD as the primary outcome.[34] This large-scale clinical trial revealed significant improvements in a composite score derived from measures of DSST and RAVLT. Significant improvement versus placebo was also observed on subjective patient-reported cognitive measures (i.e., the Perceived Deficits Questionnaire). Path analyses revealed that one-half to two-thirds of the pro-cognitive effects could not be attributed to overall antidepressant effects.[34] An 8-week RCT enrolled adult individuals with MDD to receive vortioxetine (10–20 mg/day; $n = 198$), duloxetine (60 mg/day; $n = 210$), or placebo ($n = 194$). By the end of the trial, the vortioxetine group had a significant improvement on the primary outcome measure (digit symbol processing speed test scores). Furthermore, a path analyses showed that these cognitive enhancing effects were largely independent of affective improvement.[58]

Lisdexamfetamine dimesylate (LDX) is a pharmacologically inactive pro-drug of D-amphetamine approved for treatment of attention deficit hyperactivity disorder in children, adolescents, and adults. The pro-cognitive properties of LDX in MDD have been documented in a randomized, double-blind, placebo-controlled study that evaluated its effects on cognitive dysfunction as a primary outcome in adults with MDD ($N = 143$). Augmentation therapy with LDX (20–70 mg/day) significantly improved executive dysfunction (as measured with the Behavior Rating Inventory of Executive Function–Adult Version (BRIEF-A) self-report global executive composite t score) from baseline to endpoint compared to placebo.[59] Another RCT with the primary objective to evaluate the effect of adjunctive LDX (20–50 mg/day) on residual symptoms and cognitive impairment in MDD adult patients partially responsive to SSRIs or SNRIs is currently under-way (ClinicalTrials.gov Identifier: NCT01148979).

NOVEL DRUG TARGETS FOR COGNITIVE DYSFUNCTION IN DEPRESSION

Moylan and colleagues[60] conceptualized MDD as a neuroprogressive disorder. Several concordant lines of evidence suggest that depressive episodes are neuro-toxic.[61–63] For example, a meta-analysis indicated that a difference in hippocampal volume between MDD patients and controls is evident only in patients with illness duration greater than 1 year and in those with more than one depressive episode.[62] Another meta-analysis indicated that the number of previous major depressive episodes is associated with a decrease in hippocampal volume.[64] MDD is also associated with a volumetric reduction in several other discrete brain structures, including, but not limited to, the frontal cortex, orbitofrontal cortex, cingulate cortex, and stria-tum.[65] Nevertheless, evidence for an association between the number of previous depressive episodes and volume reduction in these brain structures is less consis-tent.[66] In summary, studies to date indicate that an active neuroprogressive process may take place in recurring MDD[60,67,68] and that this may be a driver for cognitive impairment associated with this illness.

The depressive diathesis (i.e., vulnerability to MDD) varies across the life cycle. A genetic component has been demonstrated, with heritability estimates of up to 43%.[69] Early life stressors also significantly increase the risk for depression, includ-ing inadequate emotional contacts with parents and sexual abuse.[70–74] Hence, sev-eral lines of evidence indicate that multiple genes interact with early environmental insults to increase the risk for MDD.[75–77] In fact, it seems that a significant fraction of the depressive diathesis is laid down in early childhood.

Personality factors also play a role in the development of MDD. For example, neuroticism is a consistent risk factor for MDD.[74,78,79] Neuroticism may mediate the effects of early life events on the risk for developing MDD.[79] Individuals with more elevated neuroticism scores present with deficits in the perception of, and cognitive control over, negatively valenced emotional stimuli; this is similar to disturbances of "hot" cognition observed in MDD.[80]

Post[81] formulated the "kindling model" based on the fact that the repeated administration of subthreshold doses of convulsive substances leads to full-blown seizures; each seizure may increase the likelihood for subsequent seizures. Similarly, successive depressive episodes may be triggered by progressively weaker stressors.[73,82] The kindling phenomenon is apparent after exposure to a specific stressor, namely interpersonal loss.[73]

The brain does not always recover its structure and function after remission from a depressive episode. For example, hippocampal volume changes can persist after the resolution of depressive symptoms.[83] Furthermore, a reduced frontocingulate functional connectivity[84] as well as neurochemical abnormalities in the anterior cingulate and prefrontal cortices are observed even in remitted states.[85,86]

Chronic exposure to glucocorticoids is neurotoxic, and animal studies have shown that hippocampal granule cells are particularly sensitive to these effects.[87] Prolonged exposure to stress leads to enduring activation of the HPA axis, the main stress system in the brain. The hyperstimulation of glucocorticoid receptors triggers a cascade of events in part mediated by the overactivation of glutamatergic NMDA receptors.[88] These processes lead to several biochemical events, including the activation of calcium-dependent enzymes; the generation of reactive oxygen species; and a diminished production of brain-derived neurotrophic factor (BDNF), which provides support to neuronal structure and function. These events ultimately result in hippocampal granule cell death.[61] Consistent with these structural changes, prolonged exposure to either glucocorticoids or stress leads to a reduction in declarative memory in humans.[89,90]

Although the hippocampus is allegedly the brain area most sensitive to stress, other brain areas are also affected, including the prefrontal cortex (PFC).[91] For example, exposure to stress or glucocorticoids leads to neurodegenerative changes in the PFC, including microglial activation,[92] atrophy of pyramidal neurons,[93] and dendritic retraction.[94,95] These structural alterations translate into potential cognitive deficits in PFC-related tasks.[96,97]

Taken together, these findings suggest that a potential mechanism for structural brain abnormalities in depression is HPA axis-mediated glucocorticoid toxicity (Figure 10.2). Furthermore, there are reciprocal interactions between the HPA axis and pro-inflammatory cytokines (PICs). For example, interleukin-6 (IL-6), tumor

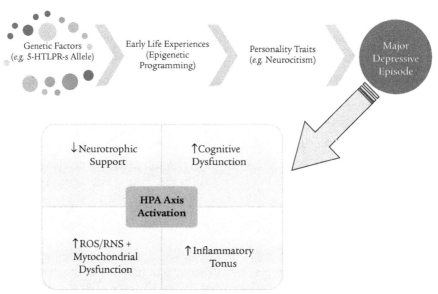

FIGURE 10.2 *Premorbid personality traits, exposure to early life insults, environmental risk factors (e.g., poor diet, sedentarism, smoking, physical inactivity, and vitamin D insufficiency), and genetic factors increase vulnerability to stress in part through epigenetic alteration in the glucocorticoid receptor (GR). The overactivation of the hypothalamic–pituitary–adrenal (HPA) axis leads to reciprocal interactions with the immune–inflammatory pathways (e.g., an increase in the production of pro-inflammatory cytokines and chemokines), mitochondrial dysfunction, oxidative and nitrosative stress (O&NS), as well as a decrease in neurotrophin (e.g., BDNF) signaling. Each subsequent major depressive episode activates this cascade of events, leading to neuroprogression and cognitive deterioration. RNS, reactive nitrogen species; ROS, reactive oxygen species.*

necrosis factor-α (TNF-α), interferon-γ (IFN-γ), and IL-1β activate the HPA axis.[60,98] Furthermore, glucocorticoid receptor resistance in depression may be mediated by IL-2 and IL-1β.[99] Although stress hormones such as glucocorticoids and catecholamines in physiological states diminish the production of T helper 1 (Th1) cytokines and increase the generation of Th2 (i.e., anti-inflammatory cytokines), evidence indicates that in depression, glucocorticoids may promote an increase in PICs such as TNF-α and IL-6.[100,101] Therefore, the cross-talk between the HPA axis and PICs may further contribute to neuroprogression and cognitive impairment in MDD.[68]

Overactivation of cell-mediated immunity in depression may also lead to a decrease in serotoninergic neurotransmission. Serotonin levels are to a large extent determined by the availability of its precursor, the tryptophan. Tryptophan is catabolized by indoleamine 2,3-dioxygenase (IDO) and the enzyme tryptophan 2,3-dioxygenase (TDO).[102] Pro-inflammatory cytokines such as IFN-γ, IL-1β, TNF-α, and IL-18 activate IDO, whereas TDO is primarily stimulated by cortisol but also by activation of the cAMP pathway in astrocytes. In MDD, neurotoxic tryptophan catabolites (TRYCATs) such as kynurenin and quinolinic acid are significantly increased, whereas the neuroprotective TRYCAT kynurenic acid is decreased in the periphery.[103,104] Furthermore, kynurenin is anxiogenic and depressogenic.[102] Activation of the TRYCAT pathway also leads to lowered melatonin levels, a neurotransmitter of significant relevance for MDD pathophysiology.[103] Thus, an overactivated TRYCAT pathway may partly mediate the neurotoxic effects of a hyperactive HPA axis and a heightened cell-mediated immunity in MDD, thus playing a role in depression-related cognitive impairment.

Depression is also accompanied by an increase in the generation of oxidative and nitrosative stress (O&NS).[105] Furthermore, MDD is associated with lowered levels of antioxidant molecules—namely zinc, coenzyme Q10, vitamin E, melatonin, and glutathione—which results in lipid peroxidation as well as damage to macromolecules such as DNA and mitochondrial dysfunction.[105] Figure 10.3 illustrates biological pathways leading to neuroprogression and cognitive deterioration in MDD.

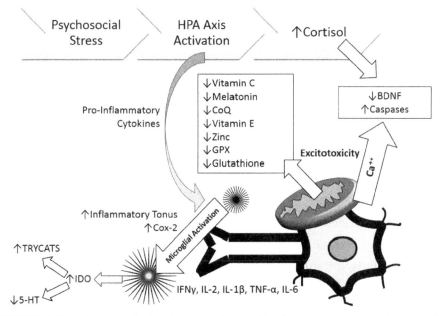

FIGURE 10.3 *Pathways involved in the progressive cognitive deterioration in major depressive disorder (MDD). Pathways include an overactive hypothalamic–pituitary–adrenal (HPA) axis; a decrease in neurotrophin (e.g., brain-derived neurotrophic factor (BDNF) signaling); excitotoxicity in part through overstimulation of glutamate NMDA receptors, which leads to an increase in intracellular calcium (Ca2+) and activation of pro-apoptotic caspases (e.g., caspase 3); an increase in the generation of reactive oxygen species (ROS) and reactive nitrogen species (RNS) along with lower levels of antioxidants and/or a decrease in the activity of antioxidant enzymes (e.g., glutathione peroxidase (GPX)), which ultimately results in oxidative and nitrosative stress (O&NS); mitochondrial dysfunction; and an increased production of inflammatory cytokines (e.g., tumor necrosis factor-α (TNF-α)). Inflammatory cytokines stimulate the enzyme indoleamine 2,3-dioxygenase (IDO), which metabolizes tryptophan, leading to a decrease in the production of serotonin and melatonin. Furthermore, some tryptophan catabolites are neurotoxic and depressogenic. Cyclooxygenase-2 (Cox-2) is increased in MDD. 5-HT, serotonin; CoQ, coenzyme Q; IFN-γ, interferon-γ; IL-1β, interleukin-1β; IL-2, interleukin-2; IL-6, interleukin-6; TRYCATS, tryptophan catabolites.*

Several non-monoaminergic drugs targeting the aforementioned pathways related to cognitive dysfunction in MDD may emerge as novel cognitive enhancers and/or neuroprotector agents for MDD. Carvalho and colleagues[106] provide an extensive list and discussion of candidate drugs. Several compounds are in relatively early stages of development and are beyond the scope of this chapter. Here, a selective overview of drugs that have been tested in clinical trials is presented, even though evidence in most circumstances is still preliminary.[106]

Erythropoietin

As mentioned previously, a downregulation in neurotrophic factors (e.g., BDNF) may play a role in MDD-related cognitive dysfunction. Systemically administered BDNF does not cross the blood–brain barrier (BBB). Thus, compounds that increase BDNF production in the central nervous system (CNS) following systemic administration offer novel opportunities for the amelioration of cognitive dysfunction in MDD. Erythropoietin (EPO) is a glycoprotein hormone primarily synthesized by the kidney, which regulates erythropoiesis. EPO and a specific EPO receptor (EPO-R) are expressed in the CNS of mammals, including humans.[107] Unlike BDNF, EPO crosses the BBB, and its neuroprotector, neurotrophic, and pro-cognitive properties have been demonstrated in more than 300 preclinical investigations; these effects are at least in part mediated by an upregulation of BDNF signaling pathways.[108] In healthy volunteers, EPO improved memory and executive function 1 week after a single high-dose administration (40,000 IU).[109,110] EPO was tested in an RCT involving 40 patients with treatment-resistant depression.[111] Although EPO did not improve the primary outcome measure (i.e., Hamilton Depression Rating Scale scores), this drug significantly improved verbal learning and memory.[111] Taken together, these findings suggest that EPO may have cognitive enhancing effects in MDD. Nevertheless, these interesting data require replication in a large-scale RCT.

S-Adenosylmethionine

S-Adenosylmethionine (SAMe), formed from methionine and ATP, is a natural component of all living cells, and it plays a key metabolic role as a major contributor of methyl groups for critical biochemical reactions. Methylation via SAMe is relevant for CNS function. SAMe regulates the biosynthesis of neurotransmitter molecules (e.g., dopamine, noradrenaline, and 5-HT). SAMe is also a precursor for reduced glutathione (GSH) and has antioxidant properties. Its pro-cognitive potential has been preliminary documented in a 6-week RCT on 40 SSRI-resistant outpatients with MDD. Participants allocated to SAMe therapy showed significant improvements in recall and word-finding scores on the self-rated Cognitive and Physical Symptoms Questionnaire (CPFQ) compared to placebo.[112]

Omega-3 Polyunsaturated Fatty Acids

Omega-3 polyunsaturated fatty acids (n-3 PUFAs) supplementation may be beneficial in the treatment of several mental disorders, including MDD. Preclinical evidence suggests that a diet rich in n-3 PUFAs (i.e., ethyl-eicosapentaenoic acid) may attenuate IL-1-induced memory impairment and block IL-1-induced increase in serum corticosterone.[113] Furthermore, n-3 PUFAs reduce the inflammatory response, limiting the production of pro-inflammatory mediators by microglial cells following ischemic insults.[114] In middle-aged to elderly healthy individuals (N = 40), n-3 PUFA supplementation (3 mg/day) significantly improved cognitive performance (i.e., working memory and attention) compared to placebo in a 5-week RCT.[115] Independent clinical trials and a meta-analysis of randomized controlled studies have also provided evidence of the superiority of n-3 PUFAs, namely eicosapentaenoic (EPA) and docosahexaenoic (DHA) acids, compared to placebo as adjunctive treatments for MDD.[116] However, few studies have investigated their effects on cognition, yielding inconclusive results to date. An RCT evaluating the effect of n-3 PUFA (1.5 g/day; EPA plus DHA) supplementation on mood and cognition in mildly to moderate depressed patients did not report any significant change in cognitive functions.[117] Conversely, in an RCT, supplementation with n-3 PUFA resulted in improving aspects of emotional information processing in individuals who recovered from MDD.[118] In addition, in a separate cross-sectional investigation on individuals who recovered from MDD (N = 132), plasmatic concentrations of n-3 PUFAs positively (and significantly) correlated with neurocognitive performance.[119] In conclusion, further investigation is needed to elucidate the effects of n-3 PUFAs on cognitive performance in MDD.

Anti-Inflammatory Drugs

Acetylsalicylic acid (aspirin) was tested in combination with fluoxetine in a sample of 70 patients with MDD.[120] Although aspirin combined with fluoxetine did not differ in efficacy to fluoxetine monotherapy, the authors found that aspirin plus fluoxetine significantly reduced superoxide dismutase, glutathione peroxidase, and catalase activities, in addition to reducing lipid peroxidation.[120] Aspirin also had antidepressant effects in the chronic unpredictable stress depression model, and it attenuated the microglial inflammatory response to lipopolysaccharide by triggering lipoxins and inhibiting activation of nitric oxide, IL-1, TNF-α, NF-κB, ERK, and MAP kinase.[121] A reduction in COX-2 and PGE$_2$ activities also contributes to aspirin's antidepressant-like effects in the chronic unpredictable stress model in rodents.[122] Furthermore, aspirin has neuroprotective effects via downregulation of the NF-κB signaling pathway in several experimental models.[123] However, a large RCT indicated that aspirin was of no benefit for improving cognitive function in middle-aged to elderly individuals at increased cardiovascular risk.[124]

Two meta-analyses support the efficacy of celecoxib, a selective COX-2 inhibitor, as an adjunctive agent for MDD.[125,126] Similarly, selective TNF-α antagonists may improve depressive symptoms in patients with inflammatory diseases such as psoriasis.[127] Furthermore, etanercept had antidepressant and anxiolytic-like behavioral effects in rodents.[128] Relatively recently, an RCT revealed that infliximab did not improve depressive symptoms in a sample of 60 patients with treatment-resistant depression.[129] However, infliximab was efficacious in patients with higher baseline levels of inflammatory markers (e.g., C-reactive protein).[129] Given the putative role of COX-2 and TNF-α on cognition,[130] future trials testing celecoxib and infliximab as pro-cognitive agents for MDD are needed. Furthermore, these agents may have a stratified benefit for MDD patients with elevated baseline levels of inflammatory mediators.

N-Acetylcysteine

N-Acetylcysteine (NAC), by supplying cysteine, increases the production of GSH, thereby reducing oxidative stress.[131] GSH is a tripeptide composed of glutamate, cysteine, and glycine. Glutamate–cysteine ligase (GCL) is the rate-limiting step for GSH generation: GCL ligates glutamate with cysteine to generate γ-glutamylcysteine, which is combined with glycine and catalyzed GSH synthase to form GSH.[131] Oral NAC prevents brain GSH depletion.[132] Furthermore, NAC may prevent oxidative damage by enhancing the expression of mitochondrial enzymes of type I electron transport chain.[133] NAC has antidepressant-like activities in animal models of depression.[134] In experimental models, NAC has cognitive enhancing effects. For instance, NAC prevented cadmium-induced memory deficits and decreased acetylcholinesterase activity and oxidative stress in rats.[135] Moreover, NAC reversed existing cognitive deficits in glutamate transporter type 3-deficient mice.[136] A relatively recent RCT did not indicate a beneficial effect of adjunctive NAC compared to placebo in patients with MDD on the primary outcome (i.e., depressive symptoms as evaluated with the Montgomery–Asberg Depression

Rating Scale).[137] NAC prevented cognitive dysfunction in an RCT involving US military personnel with acute sequelae of blast-induced mild traumatic brain injury.[138] However, adjunctive NAC did not enhance cognition in a proof-of-concept RCT involving bipolar disorder patients.[139] Taken together, evidence to date for NAC's cognitive enhancing effects is mixed and requires further investigation.

Creatine Monohydrate

Creatine is a nonessential dietary element found in meat and fish. It is primarily synthesized by the liver and kidneys. Exogenous creatine is available for dietary supplementation as creatine monohydrate. Creatine is the precursor of phosphorcreatine, which plays a pivotal role in brain metabolism. Furthermore, creatine has direct antioxidant effects.[140] Creatine supplementation presented significant neuroprotector effects in an animal model of transient cerebral ischemia.[141] Following a 24-hour sleep deprivation, creatine supplementation enhanced cognition in healthy volunteers.[142] Creatine monohydrate improved depressive symptoms in a case series of patients with treatment-resistant depression.[143] Taken together, creatine monohydrate holds promise as a repurposed cognitive enhancer for MDD.

Lithium

Lithium is an archetypal mood stabilizer and remains a first-line agent for the treatment of bipolar disorder.[144] Lithium is also an effective augmenting agent for treatment-resistant depression.[4] A meta-analysis indicated that lithium treatment may prevent a decrement in hippocampal volume in bipolar disorder.[145] Furthermore, epidemiological data and a few clinical trials indicate that lithium treatment may prevent dementia.[146] The pleiotropic actions of lithium may contribute to its putative neuroprotective effects. For example, lithium has antioxidant activities. Lithium also enhances the expression of proteins such as BDNF and Bcl-2, thereby improving neuroplasticity. Furthermore, lithium decreases apoptosis through inhibition of glycogen synthase kinase-3 and autophagy.[147] Therefore, lithium has therapeutic potential as a pro-cognitive and neuroprotector agent for MDD.

COGNITIVE REMEDIATION THERAPY

Although cognitive remediation therapy (CRT), also referred to as cognitive training, has been more extensively studied in schizophrenia with encouraging results, preliminary evidence has shown promise for MDD as well.[37,41] Several lines of evidence indicate that CRT may harness inherent neuroplastic capacities of the brain, targeting impaired brain networks across mental disorders, thus mitigating cognitive deficits. For example, in schizophrenia, CRT may decrease hypofrontality.[148] In addition, Wykes et al.[149] reported *a decrease* in frontal activation during performance of a working memory test, which was greatest for patients who derived significant benefits from the therapy. Vinogradov et al.[150] demonstrated a significant increase in BDNF levels following 50 hours of CRT in first-episode psychosis, with levels approaching those of healthy controls. Furthermore, CRT may even be neuroprotective. For example, Eack et al.[151] demonstrated that CRT in patients with schizophrenia or schizoaffective disorder preserved gray matter volumes in the left hippocampus, parahippocampal gyrus, and fusiform gyrus, along with volumetric increases in the left amygdala. Therefore, one would anticipate benefits for CRT for MDD as well.

To date, only a few published RCTs have investigated the benefits of CRT in MDD samples. Siegle and colleagues[152] investigated the effects of repeated practice in two tests that hypothetically activate the prefrontal cortex, namely the Paced Auditory Serial Addition Test and the Attention Control Training Intervention, a computerized modification of Wells' attention training technique.[153] The intervention aimed to increase "cognitive control." Nineteen patients with MDD received six 35-minute "cognitive control" training sessions during a 2-week period, and 7 patients received treatment as usual. The cognitive control group showed a significantly decreased self-rated depression score (Beck Depression Inventory) and a decreased incidence of rumination. In addition, 6 patients in the cognitive control group completed functional magnetic resonance imaging before and after treatment, showing evidence of a decrease in amygdala activity in an emotional sorting task and increased activity in the dorsolateral prefrontal cortex (DLPFC) in response to high working memory load. These investigations indicate that cognitive activation targeting frontal cognitive functions of the frontal lobes may have a positive effect on the outcome of MDD and prevent concomitant "hot" cognition changes (e.g., rumination).

Naismith et al.[40] randomized 16 patients with remitted MDD to receive a "neuropsychological educational approach to remediation" (NEAR) or to no additional treatment. The CRT intervention was performed with commercially available computer games, selected according to patients' strengths, 1 hour twice a week for 10 weeks. There was no significant effect on mood. However, a significant advantage of therapy compared with wait list in improving aspects of cognitive function, particularly verbal memory, was observed.

Another trial randomized 44 older patients with MDD to receive intervention (again based on NEAR) immediately or be wait listed. Forty-one patients took part in follow-up assessments. Patients had a lifetime history of major depression but were "stabilized on medication." Participants had very low depressive symptom scores at baseline (6.3 for active and 9.3 for wait list; Beck Depression Inventory). The intervention consisted of weekly 1-hour sessions of computerized cognitive training. In addition, there was a weekly 1-hour group session of psychoeducation. There were positive and significant effects on aspects of learning and memory, including verbal memory.[154]

Bowie and colleagues[155] performed an RCT on a form of CRT in treatment-resistant MDD. Treatment consisted of 15 hours of group treatment plus supplemental online computerized exercises completed at home. The treatment group (*n* = 17) had significantly greater improvements on attention/information processing speed and verbal memory domains compared with a wait-list control group (*n* = 16), and it also had a trend for larger improvements in real-world functioning.

As noted by Porter and colleagues,[156] the evidence for the effectiveness of CRT for MDD remains inconclusive due to the limited sample sizes of most investigations as well as methodological differences across trials (e.g., enrollment of remitted vs. symptomatic participants with MDD). Future research should shed light on the components of CRT that are more consistently associated with therapeutic benefits.

COGNITIVE EFFECTS OF NONINVASIVE BRAIN STIMULATION FOR DEPRESSION

NIBS techniques have gained increased attention in neuropsychiatry and neuropsychology during the past several years. The most extensively investigated NIBS techniques are rTMS and tDCS. These nonpharmacological therapeutic strategies aim to target specific brain areas to focally induce neuromodulatory effects, either increasing or decreasing baseline brain activity.[157]

The DLPFC plays a pivotal role in the cognitive dysfunction related to MDD. Therefore, stimulation of the DLPFC may enhance cognition in MDD. In fact, stimulation of the DLPFC has been extensively investigated as a target for both rTMS and tDCS in MDD.[47,158] A meta-analysis indicated a consistent positive effect of active versus sham NIBS in improving working memory performance in healthy as well as neuropsychiatric individuals.[159]

Recently, cognitive effects of NIBS techniques have been studied in samples with MDD. However, results thus far are inconsistent across studies. For example, Nadeau et al.[160] studied a sample of 48 patients with treatment-resistant MDD who were randomized to 5-Hz left- and right-side DLPFC rTMS and sham rTMS. These authors found that right stimulation of the DLPFC was associated with significant improvements in executive functions, which were independent of mood improvement.

Conversely, Januel and colleagues[161] studied a sample of 27 medication-free patients with MDD who were randomized to 16 sessions of rTMS to the right DLPFC or sham rTMS; these authors did not demonstrate cognitive improvement in the treatment group compared to the sham group.

Tortella et al.[48] conducted a comprehensive systematic review on the cognitive effects of NIBS techniques in patients with MDD. The authors emphasized that several shortcomings and methodological differences in the available studies limit the interpretation of the evidence, including differences in treatment protocols, poor statistical controlling for confounders, practice effects in cognitive measures, and the possibility that the improvement in cognition is an epiphenomenon secondary to the amelioration of depressive symptoms. In keeping with this view, the effects of NIBS on cognitive performance in MDD remain unknown.

COGNITIVE EFFECTS OF EXERCISE

The American College of Sports Medicine defines *physical activity* as "any body movement that is produced by the contraction of skeletal muscles that increases energy expenditure,"[162] whereas *exercise* refers to "a subset of physical activity that is planned, structured, and deliberate."[163] Physical activity has been recognized as a key component of a more holistic approach to recovery within mental health services, with potential benefits ranging from an improvement in symptoms to better service engagement and utilization.[164] In recent years, formal exercise has received increasing attention as both an alternative and an adjunctive strategy to usual care for MDD.[165] A meta-analysis supports the evidence that exercise has a moderate effect size for the amelioration of depressive symptoms (–0.62). However, this effect was considerably smaller when only methodologically robust RCTs were considered.[166]

Exercise may slow neuroprogressive changes through several mechanisms, including amelioration of cardiometabolic risk factors, an increase in neuroplasticity (e.g., BDNF expression), modulation of immune parameters, and alleviation of O&NS, as reviewed in detail by Knöchel and colleagues.[167] Although these mechanistic pathways are anticipated to have therapeutic benefits for physical activity and exercise upon neurocognition in MDD, evidence is limited because most studies have focused on specific psychopathological manifestations.[168]

OTHER INTERVENTIONS

Several biobehavioral interventions should be explored. Insomnia is a common complaint of MDD patients. Furthermore, specific variation in sleep architecture may precede depressive symptomatology in a subgroup of MDD patients (e.g., decreased slow-wave sleep and increased rapid eye movement density).[169] Sleep enhances neuroplasticity and facilitates the consolidation of memories learned before sleep as well as the acquisition of new memories to be learned after sleep.[170] Moreover, sleep may counteract the neurotoxic effects of MDD[171] by enhancing the clearance of neurotoxins.[172] Thus, proper sleep hygiene may mitigate cognitive deficits in MDD.

A Western-type diet may increase the risk for depression, whereas adherence to a healthy diet may lower the risk for incident depression.[173] A meta-analysis suggests that a Mediterranean diet is associated with a 30% reduction in the risk for incident depression and a 40% reduction in the risk for incident cognitive impairment.[174] Furthermore, a diet enriched with saturated fats is associated with greater risk of cognitive decline.[175] Taken together, these data suggest that healthy diet habits may alleviate cognitive deficits in MDD.

Loneliness may be associated with a greater risk for cognitive decline.[176,177] In fact, social isolation may overactivate the HPA axis, thereby promoting neurotoxicity and cognitive decline.[178] Therefore, strategies to engage MDD patients in social activities may mitigate cognitive impairment. Finally, although evidence for the beneficial effects of cognitive remediation therapies for depression is preliminary,[156] there are some encouraging but inconclusive results.[40,179]

CLINICAL IMPLICATIONS

The reliable clinical endpoints for MDD evolved initially from the classic concept of response (i.e., a 50% reduction in depressive symptoms from baseline) to remission.[4] Other experts advocate that the complex concept of functional recovery would be a proper target for MDD treatment.[3] Nevertheless, there is no unifying definition for recovery. The recognition that even after recovery from severe depressive episodes, MDD patients may still present with significant residual cognitive dysfunction[180] has led some authors to advocate a novel aim for MDD treatment, namely "cognitive remission."[16,49] Nevertheless, integration of multimodal approaches and the evolution of current treatment strategies (e.g., neuromodulation and novel cognitive enhancers) may be required before this outcome can be achieved. Figure 10.4 presents possible strategies to enhance cognitive function in MDD.

CONCLUSION

Although cognitive dysfunction has been understudied in MDD relative to schizophrenia and bipolar disorder, a growing body of evidence indicates that cognitive dysfunction in MDD is prevalent and may persist in a substantial subpopulation of

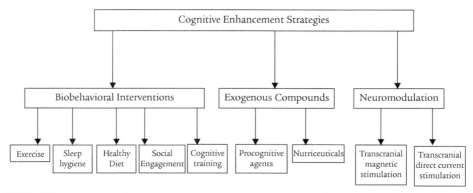

FIGURE 10.4 *Approaches to enhance cognitive function in major depressive disorder.*

patients even after full recovery from a major depressive episode. Furthermore, cognitive dysfunction may relate to several detrimental outcomes in MDD, including poor psychosocial functioning (e.g., diminished work productivity). Several measures for cognitive dysfunction, both self-report instruments and formal neuropsychological tests, have been employed across trials in MDD populations. However, a "gold standard" measure for the assessment of neurocognitive performance in MDD has not been identified. The identification of a gold standard would facilitate between-study comparisons and the establishment of a more consistent evidence base. Finally, although standard antidepressants may alleviate cognitive disturbances in MDD, the reported effects are far from optimum. Thus, proper assessment and management of cognitive dysfunction should be incorporated in the routine care of depressed patients.

REFERENCES

1. Kessler RC, Bromet EJ. The epidemiology of depression across cultures. *Annu Rev Public Health* 2013;34:119–138.
2. Alonso J, Vilagut G, Adroher ND, et al. Disability mediates the impact of common conditions on perceived health. *PLoS One* 2013;8(6):e65858.
3. Stotland NL. Recovery from depression. *Psychiatric Clin North Am* 2012;35(1):37–49.
4. Carvalho AF, Berk M, Hyphantis TN, et al. The integrative management of treatment-resistant depression: A comprehensive review and perspectives. *Psychother Psychosom* 2014;83(2):70–88.
5. Miller IW, Keitner GI, Schatzberg AF, et al. The treatment of chronic depression, Part 3: Psychosocial functioning before and after treatment with sertraline or imipramine. *J Clin Psychiatry* 1998;59(11):608–619.
6. Ekman M, Granstrom O, Omerov S, et al. The societal cost of depression: Evidence from 10,000 Swedish patients in psychiatric care. *J Affect Disord* 2013;150(3):790–797.
7. Lahr D, Beblo T, Hartje W. Cognitive performance and subjective complaints before and after remission of major depression. *Cogn Neuropsychiatry* 2007;12(1):25–45.
8. Rohling ML, Green P, Allen LM, 3rd, et al. Depressive symptoms and neurocognitive test scores in patients passing symptom validity tests. *Arch Clin Neuropsychol* 2002;17(3):205–222.
9. Gualtieri CT, Morgan DW. The frequency of cognitive impairment in patients with anxiety, depression, and bipolar disorder: An unaccounted source of variance in clinical trials. *J Clin Psychiatry* 2008;69(7):1122–1130.

10. Austin MP, Mitchell P, Goodwin GM. Cognitive deficits in depression: Possible implications for functional neuropathology. *Br J Psychiatry* 2001;178:200–206.

11. Rock PL, Roiser JP, Riedel WJ, et al. Cognitive impairment in depression: A systematic review and meta-analysis. *Psychol Med* 2013:1–12.

12. McIntyre RS, Cha DS, Soczynska JK, et al. Cognitive deficits and functional outcomes in major depressive disorder: Determinants, substrates, and treatment interventions. *Depression Anxiety* 2013;30(6):515–527.

13. Buist-Bouwman MA, Ormel J, de Graaf R, et al. Mediators of the association between depression and role functioning. *Acta Psychiatr Scand* 2008;118(6):451–458.

14. Jaeger J, Berns S, Uzelac S, et al. Neurocognitive deficits and disability in major depressive disorder. *Psychiatry Res* 2006;145(1):39–48.

15. Bortolato B, Carvalho AF, McIntyre RS. Cognitive dysfunction in major depressive disorder: A state-of-the-art clinical review. *CNS Neurol Disord Drug Targets* 2014;13(10):1804–1818.

16. McIntyre RS. Using measurement strategies to identify and monitor residual symptoms. *J Clin Psychiatry* 2013;74(Suppl 2):14–18.

17. Roiser JP, Sahakian BJ. Hot and cold cognition in depression. *CNS Spectrums* 2013;18(3):139–149.

18. Miskowiak KW, Carvalho AF. "Hot" cognition in major depressive disorder: A systematic review. *CNS Neurol Disord Drug Targets* 2014;13(10):1787–1803.

19. Gotlib IH, Joormann J. Cognition and depression: Current status and future directions. *Annu Rev Clin Psychol* 2010;6:285–312.

20. Joormann J, Gotlib IH. Updating the contents of working memory in depression: Interference from irrelevant negative material. *J Abnormal Psychol* 2008;117(1):182–192.

21. Chase HW, Frank MJ, Michael A, et al. Approach and avoidance learning in patients with major depression and healthy controls: Relation to anhedonia. *Psychol Med* 2010;40(3):433–440.

22. Snyder HR. Major depressive disorder is associated with broad impairments on neuropsychological measures of executive function: A meta-analysis and review. *Psychol Bull* 2013;139(1):81–132.

23. Millan MJ, Agid Y, Brune M, et al. Cognitive dysfunction in psychiatric disorders: Characteristics, causes and the quest for improved therapy. *Nat Rev Drug Discov* 2012;11(2):141–168.

24. Goosens KA. Hippocampal regulation of aversive memories. *Curr Opin Neurobiol* 2011;21(3):460–466.

25. Femenia T, Gomez-Galan M, Lindskog M, et al. Dysfunctional hippocampal activity affects emotion and cognition in mood disorders. *Brain Res* 2012;1476:58–70.

26. Biringer E, Lundervold A, Stordal K, et al. Executive function improvement upon remission of recurrent unipolar depression. *Eur Arch Psychiatry Clin Neurosci* 2005;255(6):373–380.

27. Behnken A, Schoning S, Gerss J, et al. Persistent non-verbal memory impairment in remitted major depression—Caused by encoding deficits? *J Affect Disord* 2010;122(1–2):144–148.

28. Herrera-Guzman I, Gudayol-Ferre E, Herrera-Guzman D, et al. Effects of selective serotonin reuptake and dual serotonergic–noradrenergic reuptake treatments on memory and mental processing speed in patients with major depressive disorder. *J Psychiatric Res* 2009;43(9):855–863.

29. Lam M, Collinson SL, Eng GK, et al. Refining the latent structure of neuropsychological performance in schizophrenia. *Psychol Med* 2014;44(16):3557–3570.

30. Dunkin JJ, Leuchter AF, Cook IA, et al. Executive dysfunction predicts nonresponse to fluoxetine in major depression. *J Affect Disord* 2000;60(1):13–23.

31. Herrera-Guzman I, Gudayol-Ferre E, Lira-Mandujano J, et al. Cognitive predictors of treatment response to bupropion and cognitive effects of bupropion in patients with major depressive disorder. *Psychiatry Res* 2008;160(1):72–82.

32. Gorlyn M, Keilp JG, Grunebaum MF, et al. Neuropsychological characteristics as predictors of SSRI treatment response in depressed subjects. *J Neural Transm* 2008;115(8):1213–1219.

33. Pehrson AL, Leiser SC, Gulinello M, et al. Treatment of cognitive dysfunction in major depressive disorder—A review of the preclinical evidence for efficacy of selective serotonin reuptake inhibitors, serotonin–norepinephrine reuptake inhibitors and the multimodal-acting antidepressant vortioxetine. *Eur J Pharmacol* 2015;753:19–31.

34. McIntyre RS, Lophaven S, Olsen CK. A randomized, double-blind, placebo-controlled study of vortioxetine on cognitive function in depressed adults. *Int J Neuropsychopharmacol* 2014;17(10):1557–1567.

35. Keefe RSE, Mahableshwarkar AR, Olsen CK. Clinical evidence for improvement in cognitive dysfunction in patients with major depressive disorder (MDD) after treatment with vortioxetine. *Eur Neuropsychopharmacol* 2013;23:S402–S403.

36. Robertson IH, Murre JM. Rehabilitation of brain damage: Brain plasticity and principles of guided recovery. *Psychol Bull* 1999;125(5):544–575.

37. Keshavan MS, Vinogradov S, Rumsey J, et al. Cognitive training in mental disorders: Update and future directions. *Am J Psychiatry* 2014;171(5):510–522.

38. Wykes T, Huddy V, Cellard C, et al. A meta-analysis of cognitive remediation for schizophrenia: Methodology and effect sizes. *Am J Psychiatry* 2011;168(5):472–485.

39. Elgamal S, McKinnon MC, Ramakrishnan K, et al. Successful computer-assisted cognitive remediation therapy in patients with unipolar depression: A proof of principle study. *Psychol Med* 2007;37(9):1229–1238.

40. Naismith SL, Redoblado-Hodge MA, Lewis SJ, et al. Cognitive training in affective disorders improves memory: A preliminary study using the NEAR approach. *J Affect Disord* 2010;121(3):258–262.

41. Porter RJ, Douglas K, Jordan J, et al. Psychological treatments for cognitive dysfunction in major depressive disorder: Current evidence and perspectives. *CNS Neurol Disord Drug Targets* 2014;13(10):1677–1692.

42. Pringle A, Browning M, Cowen PJ, et al. A cognitive neuropsychological model of antidepressant drug action. *Prog Neuropsychopharmacol Biol Psychiatry* 2011;35(7):1586–1592.

43. Antypa N, Calati R, Serretti A. The neuropsychological hypothesis of antidepressant drug action revisited. *CNS Neurol Disord Drug Targets* 2014;13(10):1722–1739.

44. Harmer CJ. Antidepressant drug action: A neuropsychological perspective. *Depression Anxiety* 2010;27(3):231–233.

45. Hovington CL, McGirr A, Lepage M, et al. Repetitive transcranial magnetic stimulation (rTMS) for treating major depression and schizophrenia: A systematic review of recent meta-analyses. *Ann Med* 2013;45(4):308–321.

46. Berlim MT, van den Eynde F, Tovar-Perdomo S, et al. Response, remission and drop-out rates following high-frequency repetitive transcranial magnetic stimulation (rTMS) for treating major depression: A systematic review and meta-analysis of randomized, double-blind and sham-controlled trials. *Psychol Med* 2014;44(2):225–239.

47. Shiozawa P, Fregni F, Bensenor IM, et al. Transcranial direct current stimulation for major depression: An updated systematic review and meta-analysis. *Int J Neuropsychopharmacol* 2014;17(9):1443–1452.

48. Tortella G, Selingardi PM, Moreno ML, et al. Does non-invasive brain stimulation improve cognition in major depressive disorder? A systematic review. *CNS Neurol Disord Drug Targets* 2014;13(10):1759–1769.

49. Trivedi MH, Greer TL. Cognitive dysfunction in unipolar depression: Implications for treatment. *J Affect Disord* 2014;152–154:19–27.

50. Herrera-Guzman I, Gudayol-Ferre E, Herrera-Abarca JE, et al. Major depressive disorder in recovery and neuropsychological functioning: Effects of selective serotonin reuptake inhibitor and dual inhibitor depression treatments on residual cognitive deficits in patients with major depressive disorder in recovery. *J Affect Disord* 2010;123(1–3):341–350.

51. Raskin J, Wiltse CG, Siegal A, et al. Efficacy of duloxetine on cognition, depression, and pain in elderly patients with major depressive disorder: An 8-week, double-blind, placebo-controlled trial. *Am J Psychiatry* 2007;164(6):900–909.

52. Gorlyn M, Keilp J, Burke A, et al. Treatment-related improvement in neuropsychological functioning in suicidal depressed patients: Paroxetine vs. bupropion. *Psychiatry Res* 2015;225(3):407–412.

53. Soczynska JK, Ravindran LN, Styra R, et al. The effect of bupropion XL and escitalopram on memory and functional outcomes in adults with major depressive disorder: Results from a randomized controlled trial. *Psychiatry Res* 2014;220(1–2):245–250.

54. Bang-Andersen B, Ruhland T, Jorgensen M, et al. Discovery of 1-[2-(2,4-dimethylphenylsulfanyl) phenyl]piperazine (Lu AA21004): A novel multimodal compound for the treatment of major depressive disorder. *J Med Chem* 2011;54(9):3206–3221.

55. Alvarez E, Perez V, Dragheim M, et al. A double-blind, randomized, placebo-controlled, active reference study of Lu AA21004 in patients with major depressive disorder. *Int J Neuropsychopharmacol* 2012;15(5):589–600.

56. Pae CU, Wang SM, Han C, et al. Vortioxetine: A meta-analysis of 12 short-term, randomized, placebo-controlled clinical trials for the treatment of major depressive disorder. *J Psychiatry Neurosci* 2014;39(6):140120.

57. Katona C, Hansen T, Olsen CK. A randomized, double-blind, placebo-controlled, duloxetine-referenced, fixed-dose study comparing the efficacy and safety of Lu AA21004 in elderly patients with major depressive disorder. *Int Clin Psychopharmacol* 2012;27(4):215–223.

58. Mahableshwarkar A ZJ, Jacobson W, Chen Y, et al. *Efficacy of vortioxetine on cognitive function in adult patients with major depressive disorder: Results of a randomized, double-blind, active-referenced, placebo-controlled trial* [Abstract]. Paper presented at the 29th CINP World Congress of Neuropsychopharmacology 2014; Vancouver, Canada.

59. Madhoo M, Keefe RS, Roth RM, et al. Lisdexamfetamine dimesylate augmentation in adults with persistent executive dysfunction after partial or full remission of major depressive disorder. *Neuropsychopharmacology* 2014;39(6):1388–1398.

60. Moylan S, Maes M, Wray NR, et al. The neuroprogressive nature of major depressive disorder: Pathways to disease evolution and resistance, and therapeutic implications. *Mol Psychiatry* 2013;18(5):595–606.

61. Sapolsky RM. The possibility of neurotoxicity in the hippocampus in major depression: A primer on neuron death. *Biol Psychiatry* 2000;48(8):755–765.

62. McKinnon MC, Yucel K, Nazarov A, et al. A meta-analysis examining clinical predictors of hippocampal volume in patients with major depressive disorder. *J Psychiatry Neurosci* 2009;34(1):41–54.

63. Catena-Dell'Osso M, Bellantuono C, Consoli G, et al. Inflammatory and neurodegenerative pathways in depression: A new avenue for antidepressant development? *Curr Med Chem* 2011;18(2):245–255.

64. Videbech P, Ravnkilde B. Hippocampal volume and depression: A meta-analysis of MRI studies. *Am J Psychiatry* 2004;161(11):1957–1966.

65. Arnone D, McIntosh AM, Ebmeier KP, et al. Magnetic resonance imaging studies in unipolar depression: Systematic review and meta-regression analyses. *Eur Neuropsychopharmacol* 2012;22(1):1–16.

66. Bora E, Fornito A, Pantelis C, et al. Gray matter abnormalities in major depressive disorder: A meta-analysis of voxel based morphometry studies. *J Affect Disord* 2012;138(1–2):9–18.

67. Myint AM, Kim YK. Cytokine–serotonin interaction through IDO: A neurodegeneration hypothesis of depression. *Med Hypotheses* 2003;61(5–6):519–525.

68. Maes M, Yirmyia R, Noraberg J, et al. The inflammatory & neurodegenerative (I&ND) hypothesis of depression: Leads for future research and new drug developments in depression. *Metab Brain Dis* 2009;24(1):27–53.

69. Flint J, Kendler KS. The genetics of major depression. *Neuron* 2014;81(3):484–503.

70. Willner P, Scheel-Kruger J, Belzung C. The neurobiology of depression and antidepressant action. *Neurosci Biobehav Rev* 2013;37(10 Pt 1):2331–2371.

71. Juruena MF. Early-life stress and HPA axis trigger recurrent adulthood depression. *Epilepsy Behav* 2014;38:148–159.

72. Roy A. Role of past loss in depression. *Arch Gen Psychiatry* 1981;38(3):301–302.

73. Slavich GM, Monroe SM, Gotlib IH. Early parental loss and depression history: Associations with recent life stress in major depressive disorder. *J Psychiatric Res* 2011;45(9):1146–1152.

74. Kendler KS, Gardner CO. Sex differences in the pathways to major depression: A study of opposite-sex twin pairs. *Am J Psychiatry* 2014;171(4):426–435.

75. Caspi A, Hariri AR, Holmes A, et al. Genetic sensitivity to the environment: The case of the serotonin transporter gene and its implications for studying complex diseases and traits. *Am J Psychiatry* 2010;167(5):509–527.

76. Klengel T, Mehta D, Anacker C, et al. Allele-specific FKBP5 DNA demethylation mediates gene–childhood trauma interactions. *Nat Neurosci* 2013;16(1):33–41.
77. Weaver IC, Cervoni N, Champagne FA, et al. Epigenetic programming by maternal behavior. *Nat Neurosci* 2004;7(8):847–854.
78. Christensen MV, Kessing LV. Do personality traits predict first onset in depressive and bipolar disorder? *Nordic J Psychiatry* 2006;60(2):79–88.
79. Fanous AH, Kendler KS. The genetic relationship of personality to major depression and schizophrenia. *Neurotoxicity Res* 2004;6(1):43–50.
80. Ormel J, Bastiaansen A, Riese H, et al. The biological and psychological basis of neuroticism: Current status and future directions. *Neurosci Biobehav Rev* 2013;37(1):59–72.
81. Post RM. Kindling and sensitization as models for affective episode recurrence, cyclicity, and tolerance phenomena. *Neurosci Biobehav Rev* 2007;31(6):858–873.
82. Stroud CB, Davila J, Hammen C, et al. Severe and nonsevere events in first onsets versus recurrences of depression: Evidence for stress sensitization. *J Abnorm Psychology* 2011;120(1):142–154.
83. Neumeister A, Wood S, Bonne O, et al. Reduced hippocampal volume in unmedicated, remitted patients with major depression versus control subjects. *Biol Psychiatry* 2005;57(8):935–937.
84. Aizenstein HJ, Butters MA, Wu M, et al. Altered functioning of the executive control circuit in late-life depression: Episodic and persistent phenomena. *Am J Geriatr Psychiatry* 2009;17(1):30–42.
85. Bhagwagar Z, Hinz R, Taylor M, et al. Increased 5-HT(2A) receptor binding in euthymic, medication-free patients recovered from depression: A positron emission study with [(11)C] MDL 100,907. *Am J Psychiatry* 2006;163(9):1580–1587.
86. Bhagwagar Z, Wylezinska M, Jezzard P, et al. Low GABA concentrations in occipital cortex and anterior cingulate cortex in medication-free, recovered depressed patients. *Int J Neuropsychopharmacol* 2008;11(2):255–260.
87. Raison CL, Miller AH. When not enough is too much: The role of insufficient glucocorticoid signaling in the pathophysiology of stress-related disorders. *Am J Psychiatry* 2003;160(9):1554–1565.
88. Gould E, McEwen BS, Tanapat P, et al. Neurogenesis in the dentate gyrus of the adult tree shrew is regulated by psychosocial stress and NMDA receptor activation. *J Neurosci* 1997;17(7):2492–2498.
89. de Quervain DJ, Roozendaal B, Nitsch RM, et al. Acute cortisone administration impairs retrieval of long-term declarative memory in humans. *Nat Neurosci* 2000;3(4):313–314.
90. Newcomer JW, Selke G, Melson AK, et al. Decreased memory performance in healthy humans induced by stress-level cortisol treatment. *Arch Gen Psychiatry* 1999;56(6):527–533.
91. McEwen BS, Morrison JH. The brain on stress: Vulnerability and plasticity of the prefrontal cortex over the life course. *Neuron* 2013;79(1):16–29.
92. Hinwood M, Tynan RJ, Charnley JL, et al. Chronic stress induced remodeling of the prefrontal cortex: Structural re-organization of microglia and the inhibitory effect of minocycline. *Cerebral Cortex* 2013;23(8):1784–1797.
93. Liu RJ, Aghajanian GK. Stress blunts serotonin- and hypocretin-evoked EPSCs in prefrontal cortex: Role of corticosterone-mediated apical dendritic atrophy. *Proc Natl Acad Sci USA* 2008;105(1):359–364.
94. Dias-Ferreira E, Sousa JC, Melo I, et al. Chronic stress causes frontostriatal reorganization and affects decision-making. *Science* 2009;325(5940):621–625.
95. McEwen BS. Stress, sex, and neural adaptation to a changing environment: Mechanisms of neuronal remodeling. *Ann N Y Acad Sci* 2010;1204(Suppl):E38–E59.
96. Miracle AD, Brace MF, Huyck KD, et al. Chronic stress impairs recall of extinction of conditioned fear. *Neurobiol Learn Mem* 2006;85(3):213–218.
97. Yuen EY, Wei J, Liu W, et al. Repeated stress causes cognitive impairment by suppressing glutamate receptor expression and function in prefrontal cortex. *Neuron* 2012;73(5):962–977.

98. Raison CL, Capuron L, Miller AH. Cytokines sing the blues: Inflammation and the pathogenesis of depression. *Trends Immunol* 2006;27(1):24–31.

99. Maes M, Bosmans E, Suy E, et al. Depression-related disturbances in mitogen-induced lymphocyte responses and interleukin-1 beta and soluble interleukin-2 receptor production. *Acta Psychiatr Scand* 1991;84(4):379–386.

100. Elenkov IJ, Chrousos GP. Stress system—Organization, physiology and immunoregulation. *Neuroimmunomodulation* 2006;13(5–6):257–267.

101. Heiser P, Lanquillon S, Krieg JC, et al. Differential modulation of cytokine production in major depressive disorder by cortisol and dexamethasone. *Eur Neuropsychopharmacol* 2008;18(12):860–870.

102. Maes M, Leonard BE, Myint AM, et al. The new "5-HT" hypothesis of depression: Cell-mediated immune activation induces indoleamine 2,3-dioxygenase, which leads to lower plasma tryptophan and an increased synthesis of detrimental tryptophan catabolites (TRYCATs), both of which contribute to the onset of depression. *Prog Neuropsychopharmacol Biol Psychiatry* 2011;35(3):702–721.

103. Anderson G, Maes M. Oxidative/nitrosative stress and immuno-inflammatory pathways in depression: Treatment implications. *Curr Pharm Des* 2014;20(23):3812–3847.

104. Maes M, Rief W. Diagnostic classifications in depression and somatization should include biomarkers, such as disorders in the tryptophan catabolite (TRYCAT) pathway. *Psychiatry Res* 2012;196(2–3):243–249.

105. Moylan S, Berk M, Dean OM, et al. Oxidative & nitrosative stress in depression: Why so much stress? *Neurosci Biobehav Rev* 2014;45:46–62.

106. Carvalho AF, Miskowiak KK, Hyphantis TN, et al. Cognitive dysfunction in depression—Pathophysiology and novel targets. *CNS Neurol Disord Drug Targets* 2014;13(10):1819–1835.

107. Marti HH, Wenger RH, Rivas LA, et al. Erythropoietin gene expression in human, monkey and murine brain. *Eur J Neurosci* 1996;8(4):666–676.

108. Sargin D, Friedrichs H, El-Kordi A, et al. Erythropoietin as neuroprotective and neuroregenerative treatment strategy: Comprehensive overview of 12 years of preclinical and clinical research. *Best Pract Res Clin Anaesthesiol* 2010;24(4):573–594.

109. Miskowiak K, Inkster B, O'Sullivan U, et al. Differential effects of erythropoietin on neural and cognitive measures of executive function 3 and 7 days post-administration. *Exp Brain Res* 2008;184(3):313–321.

110. Miskowiak K, O'Sullivan U, Harmer CJ. Erythropoietin enhances hippocampal response during memory retrieval in humans. *J Neurosci* 2007;27(11):2788–2792.

111. Miskowiak KW, Vinberg M, Christensen EM, et al. Recombinant human erythropoietin for treating treatment-resistant depression: A double-blind, randomized, placebo-controlled Phase 2 trial. *Neuropsychopharmacology* 2014;39(6):1399–1408.

112. Levkovitz Y, Alpert JE, Brintz CE, et al. Effects of *S*-adenosylmethionine augmentation of serotonin-reuptake inhibitor antidepressants on cognitive symptoms of major depressive disorder. *J Affect Disord* 2012;136(3):1174–1178.

113. Song C, Phillips AG, Leonard BE, et al. Ethyl-eicosapentaenoic acid ingestion prevents corticosterone-mediated memory impairment induced by central administration of interleukin-1beta in rats. *Mol Psychiatry* 2004;9(6):630–638.

114. Zhang W, Hu X, Yang W, et al. Omega-3 polyunsaturated fatty acid supplementation confers long-term neuroprotection against neonatal hypoxic–ischemic brain injury through anti-inflammatory actions. *Stroke* 2010;41(10):2341–2347.

115. Nilsson A, Radeborg K, Salo I, et al. Effects of supplementation with n-3 polyunsaturated fatty acids on cognitive performance and cardiometabolic risk markers in healthy 51 to 72 years old subjects: A randomized controlled cross-over study. *Nutr J* 2012;11:99.

116. Grosso G, Pajak A, Marventano S, et al. Role of omega-3 fatty acids in the treatment of depressive disorders: A comprehensive meta-analysis of randomized clinical trials. *PLoS One* 2014;9(5):e96905.

117. Rogers PJ, Appleton KM, Kessler D, et al. No effect of n-3 long-chain polyunsaturated fatty acid (EPA and DHA) supplementation on depressed mood and cognitive function: A randomised controlled trial. *Br J Nutr* 2008;99(2):421–431.

118. Antypa N, Smelt AH, Strengholt A, et al. Effects of omega-3 fatty acid supplementation on mood and emotional information processing in recovered depressed individuals. *J Psychopharmacol* 2012;26(5):738–743.

119. Chiu CC, Frangou S, Chang CJ, et al. Associations between n-3 PUFA concentrations and cognitive function after recovery from late-life depression. *Am J Clin Nutr* 2012;95(2):420–427.

120. Galecki P, Szemraj J, Bienkiewicz M, et al. Oxidative stress parameters after combined fluoxetine and acetylsalicylic acid therapy in depressive patients. *Hum Psychopharmacol* 2009;24(4):277–286.

121. Wang YP, Wu Y, Li LY, et al. Aspirin-triggered lipoxin A4 attenuates LPS-induced pro-inflammatory responses by inhibiting activation of NF-κB and MAPKs in BV-2 microglial cells. *J Neuroinflammation* 2011;8:95.

122. Wang Y, Yang F, Liu YF, et al. Acetylsalicylic acid as an augmentation agent in fluoxetine treatment resistant depressive rats. *Neurosci Lett* 2011;499(2):74–79.

123. Kim SW, Jeong JY, Kim HJ, et al. Combination treatment with ethyl pyruvate and aspirin enhances neuroprotection in the postischemic brain. *Neurotox Res* 2010;17(1):39–49.

124. Price JF, Stewart MC, Deary IJ, et al. Low dose aspirin and cognitive function in middle aged to elderly adults: Randomised controlled trial. *Br Med J* 2008;337:a1198.

125. Na KS, Lee KJ, Lee JS, et al. Efficacy of adjunctive celecoxib treatment for patients with major depressive disorder: A meta-analysis. *Prog Neuropsychopharmacol Biol Psychiatry* 2014;48:79–85.

126. Faridhosseini F, Sadeghi R, Farid L, et al. Celecoxib—A new augmentation strategy for depressive mood episodes: A systematic review and meta-analysis of randomized placebo-controlled trials. *Hum Psychopharmacol* 2014;29(3):216–223.

127. Krishnan R, Cella D, Leonardi C, et al. Effects of etanercept therapy on fatigue and symptoms of depression in subjects treated for moderate to severe plaque psoriasis for up to 96 weeks. *Br J Dermatol* 2007;157(6):1275–1277.

128. Bayramgurler D, Karson A, Ozer C, et al. Effects of long-term etanercept treatment on anxiety- and depression-like neurobehaviors in rats. *Physiol Behav* 2013;119:145–148.

129. Raison CL, Rutherford RE, Woolwine BJ, et al. A randomized controlled trial of the tumor necrosis factor antagonist infliximab for treatment-resistant depression: The role of baseline inflammatory biomarkers. *JAMA* 2013;70(1):31–41.

130. Galecki P, Talarowska M, Bobinska K, et al. COX-2 gene expression is correlated with cognitive function in recurrent depressive disorder. *Psychiatry Res* 2014;215(2):488–490.

131. Berk M, Malhi GS, Gray LJ, et al. The promise of *N*-acetylcysteine in neuropsychiatry. *Trends Pharmacol Sci* 2013;34(3):167–177.

132. Dodd S, Dean O, Copolov DL, et al. *N*-acetylcysteine for antioxidant therapy: Pharmacology and clinical utility. *Expert Opin Biol Ther* 2008;8(12):1955–1962.

133. Nicoletti VG, Marino VM, Cuppari C, et al. Effect of antioxidant diets on mitochondrial gene expression in rat brain during aging. *Neurochem Res* 2005;30(6–7):737–752.

134. Smaga I, Pomierny B, Krzyzanowska W, et al. *N*-acetylcysteine possesses antidepressant-like activity through reduction of oxidative stress: Behavioral and biochemical analyses in rats. *Prog Neuropsychopharmacol Biol Psychiatry* 2012;39(2):280–287.

135. Goncalves JF, Fiorenza AM, Spanevello RM, et al. *N*-acetylcysteine prevents memory deficits, the decrease in acetylcholinesterase activity and oxidative stress in rats exposed to cadmium. *Chem Biol Interact* 2010;186(1):53–60.

136. Cao L, Li L, Zuo Z. *N*-acetylcysteine reverses existing cognitive impairment and increased oxidative stress in glutamate transporter type 3 deficient mice. *Neuroscience* 2012;220:85–89.

137. Berk M, Dean OM, Cotton SM, et al. The efficacy of adjunctive *N*-acetylcysteine in major depressive disorder: A double-blind, randomized, placebo-controlled trial. *J Clin Psychiatry* 2014;75(6):628–636.

138. Hoffer ME, Balaban C, Slade MD, et al. Amelioration of acute sequelae of blast induced mild traumatic brain injury by *N*-acetyl cysteine: A double-blind, placebo controlled study. *PLoS One* 2013;8(1):e54163.

139. Dean OM, Bush AI, Copolov DL, et al. Effects of *N*-acetyl cysteine on cognitive function in bipolar disorder. *Psychiatry Clin Neurosci* 2012;66(6):514–517.

140. Nierenberg AA, Kansky C, Brennan BP, et al. Mitochondrial modulators for bipolar disorder: A pathophysiologically informed paradigm for new drug development. *Aust N Z J Psychiatry* 2013;47(1):26–42.

141. Adcock KH, Nedelcu J, Loenneker T, et al. Neuroprotection of creatine supplementation in neonatal rats with transient cerebral hypoxia–ischemia. *Dev Neurosci* 2002;24(5):382–388.

142. McMorris T, Harris RC, Swain J, et al. Effect of creatine supplementation and sleep deprivation, with mild exercise, on cognitive and psychomotor performance, mood state, and plasma concentrations of catecholamines and cortisol. *Psychopharmacology* 2006;185(1):93–103.

143. Roitman S, Green T, Osher Y, et al. Creatine monohydrate in resistant depression: A preliminary study. *Bipolar Disord* 2007;9(7):754–758.

144. Yatham LN, Kennedy SH, Parikh SV, et al. Canadian Network for Mood and Anxiety Treatments (CANMAT) and International Society for Bipolar Disorders (ISBD) collaborative update of CANMAT guidelines for the management of patients with bipolar disorder: Update 2013. *Bipolar Disord* 2013;15(1):1–44.

145. Hajek T, Kopecek M, Hoschl C, et al. Smaller hippocampal volumes in patients with bipolar disorder are masked by exposure to lithium: A meta-analysis. *J Psychiatry Neurosci* 2012;37(5):333–343.

146. Mauer S, Vergne D, Ghaemi SN. Standard and trace-dose lithium: A systematic review of dementia prevention and other behavioral benefits. *Aust N Z J Psychiatry* 2014;48(9):809–818.

147. Malhi GS, Tanious M, Das P, et al. Potential mechanisms of action of lithium in bipolar disorder: Current understanding. *CNS Drugs* 2013;27(2):135–153.

148. Penades R, Boget T, Lomena F, et al. Could the hypofrontality pattern in schizophrenia be modified through neuropsychological rehabilitation? *Acta Psychiatr Scand* 2002;105(3):202–208.

149. Wykes T, Brammer M, Mellers J, et al. Effects on the brain of a psychological treatment: Cognitive remediation therapy—Functional magnetic resonance imaging in schizophrenia. *Br J Psychiatry* 2002;181:144–152.

150. Vinogradov S, Fisher M, Holland C, et al. Is serum brain-derived neurotrophic factor a biomarker for cognitive enhancement in schizophrenia? *Biol Psychiatry* 2009;66(6):549–553.

151. Eack SM, Hogarty GE, Cho RY, et al. Neuroprotective effects of cognitive enhancement therapy against gray matter loss in early schizophrenia: Results from a 2-year randomized controlled trial. *Arch Gen Psychiatry* 2010;67(7):674–682.

152. Siegle GJ, Ghinassi F, Thase ME. Neurobehavioral therapies in the 21st century: Summary of an emerging field and an extended example of cognitive control training for depression. *Cognit Ther Res* 2007;31(2):235–262.

153. Wells A. The attention training technique: Theory, effects, and a metacognitive hypothesis on auditory hallucinations. *Cognit Behav Pract* 2007;14(2):134–138.

154. Naismith SL, Diamond K, Carter PE, et al. Enhancing memory in late-life depression: The effects of a combined psychoeducation and cognitive training program. *Am J Geriatr Psychiatry* 2011;19(3):240–248.

155. Bowie CR, Gupta M, Holshausen K, et al. Cognitive remediation for treatment-resistant depression: Effects on cognition and functioning and the role of online homework. *J Nerv Ment Dis* 2013;201(8):680–685.

156. Porter RJ, Bowie CR, Jordan J, et al. Cognitive remediation as a treatment for major depression: A rationale, review of evidence and recommendations for future research. *Aust N Z J Psychiatry* 2013;47(12):1165–1175.

157. Di Lazzaro V. Biological effects of non-invasive brain stimulation. *Handbook Clin Neurol* 2013;116:367–374.

158. Berlim MT, Van den Eynde F, Jeff Daskalakis Z. Clinically meaningful efficacy and acceptability of low-frequency repetitive transcranial magnetic stimulation (rTMS) for treating primary major depression: A meta-analysis of randomized, double-blind and sham-controlled trials. *Neuropsychopharmacology* 2013;38(4):543–551.

159. Brunoni AR, Vanderhasselt MA. Working memory improvement with non-invasive brain stimulation of the dorsolateral prefrontal cortex: A systematic review and meta-analysis. *Brain Cognit* 2014;86:1–9.

160. Nadeau SE, Bowers D, Jones TL, et al. Cognitive effects of treatment of depression with repetitive transcranial magnetic stimulation. *Cognit Behav Neurol* 2014;27(2):77–87.

161. Januel D, Dumortier G, Verdon CM, et al. A double-blind sham controlled study of right prefrontal repetitive transcranial magnetic stimulation (rTMS): Therapeutic and cognitive effect in medication free unipolar depression during 4 weeks. *Prog Neuropsychopharmacol Biol Psychiatry* 2006;30(1):126–130.

162. Garber CE, Blissmer B, Deschenes MR, et al. American College of Sports Medicine position stand: Quantity and quality of exercise for developing and maintaining cardiorespiratory, musculoskeletal, and neuromotor fitness in apparently healthy adults: Guidance for prescribing exercise. *Med Sci Sports Exercise* 2011;43(7):1334–1359.

163. Thompson PD, Buchner D, Pina IL, et al. Exercise and physical activity in the prevention and treatment of atherosclerotic cardiovascular disease: A statement from the Council on Clinical Cardiology (Subcommittee on Exercise, Rehabilitation, and Prevention) and the Council on Nutrition, Physical Activity, and Metabolism (Subcommittee on Physical Activity). *Circulation* 2003;107(24):3109–3116.

164. Richardson CR, Faulkner G, McDevitt J, et al. Integrating physical activity into mental health services for persons with serious mental illness. *Psychiatr Serv* 2005;56(3):324–331.

165. Rethorst CD, Trivedi MH. Evidence-based recommendations for the prescription of exercise for major depressive disorder. *J Psychiatr Pract* 2013;19(3):204–212.

166. Cooney GM, Dwan K, Greig CA, et al. Exercise for depression. *Cochrane Database Syst Rev* 2013;9:CD004366.

167. Knöchel C, Oertel-Knöchel V, O'Dwyer L, et al. Cognitive and behavioural effects of physical exercise in psychiatric patients. *Prog Neurobiol* 2012;96(1):46–68.

168. Wolff E, Gaudlitz K, von Lindenberger BL, et al. Exercise and physical activity in mental disorders. *Eur Arch Psychiatry Clin Neurosci* 2011;261(Suppl 2):S186–S191.

169. Kudlow PA, Cha DS, Lam RW, et al. Sleep architecture variation: A mediator of metabolic disturbance in individuals with major depressive disorder. *Sleep Med* 2013;14(10):943–949.

170. Diekelmann S. Sleep for cognitive enhancement. *Front Syst Neurosci* 2014;8:46.

171. Gorwood P, Corruble E, Falissard B, et al. Toxic effects of depression on brain function: Impairment of delayed recall and the cumulative length of depressive disorder in a large sample of depressed outpatients. *Am J Psychiatry* 2008;165(6):731–739.

172. Xie L, Kang H, Xu Q, et al. Sleep drives metabolite clearance from the adult brain. *Science* 2013;342(6156):373–377.

173. Lai JS, Hiles S, Bisquera A, et al. A systematic review and meta-analysis of dietary patterns and depression in community-dwelling adults. *Am J Clin Nutr* 2014;99(1):181–197.

174. Psaltopoulou T, Sergentanis TN, Panagiotakos DB, et al. Mediterranean diet, stroke, cognitive impairment, and depression: A meta-analysis. *Ann Neurol* 2013;74(4):580–591.

175. Okereke OI, Rosner BA, Kim DH, et al. Dietary fat types and 4-year cognitive change in community-dwelling older women. *Ann Neurol* 2012;72(1):124–134.

176. Conroy RM, Golden J, Jeffares I, et al. Boredom-proneness, loneliness, social engagement and depression and their association with cognitive function in older people: A population study. *Psychol Health Med* 2010;15(4):463–473.

177. Tilvis RS, Kahonen-Vare MH, Jolkkonen J, et al. Predictors of cognitive decline and mortality of aged people over a 10-year period. *J Gerontol Ser A Biol Sci Med Sci* 2004;59(3):268–274.

178. Cacioppo JT, Hawkley LC, Norman GJ, et al. Social isolation. *Ann N Y Acad Sci* 2011;1231:17–22.
179. Lee RS, Redoblado-Hodge MA, Naismith SL, et al. Cognitive remediation improves memory and psychosocial functioning in first-episode psychiatric out-patients. *Psychol Med* 2013;43(6):1161–1173.
180. Boeker H, Schulze J, Richter A, et al. Sustained cognitive impairments after clinical recovery of severe depression. *J Nerv Ment Dis* 2012;200(9):773–776.

ELEVEN

Cognitive Enhancement in Bipolar Disorder

KATIE MAHON, MANUELA RUSSO,

AND M. MERCEDES PEREZ-RODRIGUEZ

INTRODUCTION

Bipolar disorder (BD) is a chronic and disabling condition characterized by notable mood changes interspersed with periods of symptom remission (euthymic state). Along with mood abnormalities, other clinical phenomena, such as emotion dysregulation (e.g., hyperreactivity to life events), impulsivity, substance abuse, sleep and circadian abnormalities, and prominent deficits in neurocognition, characterize the disorder. Neurocognitive dysfunction has recently been recognized as a core feature of the illness and an important target for intervention in BD.

This chapter describes the clinical presentation and cognitive profile of BD. Next, potential targets for the pharmacological treatment of cognitive impairment are discussed. Finally, recommendations for clinical trial design with regard to neurocognitive enhancement in BD are proposed.

Classification of Bipolar Disorder

The term *bipolar disorder* refers to a group of psychiatric disorders whose clinical course is defined by alternating depressive and hypomanic, manic, or mixed episodes. A diagnosis of BD is determined by the presence of one or more manic or hypomanic episodes. The majority of individuals with BD also experience depressive episodes. Based on the type and the duration of the mood episode(s), the fifth edition of the *Diagnostic and Statistical Manual of Mental Disorders* (DSM-5)[1] categorizes BD into different subtypes: BD type I (BD I; assigned when criteria for a history of at least one major depressive episode (MDE) and at least one full manic episode are met); BD type II (BD II; assigned to individuals with a history of MDE and at least one hypomanic episode but no full manic episodes); cyclothymic disorder (assigned when criteria for a BD I or BD II are not met, but there is a history of mood cycling over a 2-year period); substance/medication-induced bipolar and related disorder; bipolar and related disorder due to another medical condition; other specified bipolar and related disorder; and unspecified bipolar and related disorder. In contrast to the classification in the fourth edition, text revision, of the DSM (DSM-IV-TR), the DSM-5 classification provides a list of specifiers for current or most recent mood episode aiming to describe the intrinsic features of the episode (i.e., with anxious distress, mixed features, rapid cycling, melancholic features, atypical features, mood-congruent/-incongruent psychotic features, catatonia, peripartum onset, and seasonal pattern).

Prevalence and Clinical Correlates of Bipolar Disorder

Bipolar disorder is the sixth leading cause of disability among all diseases,[2] and its socioeconomic burden in the United States is estimated at approximately $150 billion.

The lifetime prevalence of BD in the general population is 2.4%.[3] Prevalence rates vary slightly across the different BD subtypes (0.6% for BD I, 0.4% for BD II, and 1.4% for other BD disorders)[3]. The mean age of illness onset is 25 years for BD I, whereas it is slightly later for BD II. Research in pediatric samples suggests that the disorder has a prevalence rate similar to that of adults (2.5% based on a sample of 10,123 adolescents aged between 13 and 18 years).[3] Because of the severity of the clinical presentation of BD, it is a major cause of psychiatric hospitalizations, partially due to the higher level of suicidality in patients with BD compared to the general population. Annual rates of attempts and completed suicides are 3.9% and 1.4%, respectively.[4]

Family and twin studies indicate a strong genetic component to the disorder, with heritability being estimated between 80% and 85%.[5] In addition to a genetic factor, there are several risk factors that may influence the clinical course of the disorder, thus making the diagnostic process, as well as its treatment, a challenge for mental health professionals. Environmental adverse events such as childhood trauma represent a common risk factor with very high prevalence (~50%) in patients with BD. Current data suggest that childhood trauma may modulate the clinical expression of the disorder.[6] Indeed, patients with BD and a history of childhood trauma present with an overall worse clinical picture (higher impulsiveness, earlier onset, rapid cycling, higher rates of suicidal behaviors, more severe symptoms, more mood episodes, and a higher number of comorbid psychiatric disorders) compared to patients with BD without such a history. Moreover, high rates of comorbidity with other psychiatric conditions contribute to further increase the clinical complexity of BD. Data show that BD usually overlaps with other disorders, particularly anxiety disorders (namely panic attacks (49.8%) and specific phobia (30.1%)), behavior disorder (44.8%), and substance abuse (34.2% for alcohol abuse and 17.8% for drug abuse).[3]

Given the complexity of the clinical presentation in individuals with BD, it is not surprising that the levels of misdiagnosis are high, with estimates between 30% and approximately 70%.[7] The ascertainment of diagnosis and its stability are often impeded by the intrinsic features of BD, which require not only a cross-sectional evaluation but also a retrospective evaluation of symptoms in order to identify the alternation between mood episodes. Another major challenge in clinical practice is the discrimination between BD I or BD II from unipolar depression, particularly for patients presenting to psychiatric services during a depressive episode or for those with an unclear history of mania or hypomania.[8] Moreover, the occurrence of psychotic features poses an additional obstacle to diagnostic assignment, contributing to intercategorical misclassification, particularly with schizoaffective disorder due to the overlapping affective symptomatology.[9] Taken together, these factors make the treatment particularly challenging during the early stages of the illness and contribute to a lag between the illness onset and the diagnosis of BD.[10]

Functional Disability in Bipolar Disorder

Although BD has been generally regarded as having a better level of functioning compared to other chronic psychiatric disorders such as schizophrenia (SZ),[11–14] data suggest that even when a euthymic state is achieved, the premorbid level of functioning is rarely fully re-established.[15] Longitudinal data indicate that patients with BD, even early in the course of the illness, have high levels of subthreshold symptomatology despite treatment.[16] It has also been demonstrated that individuals with BD are socially disadvantaged compared to the healthy population. Only 22.5% of BD patients are married or cohabiting.[17] Between 57% and 65% are unemployed, and only half of those who were employed had returned to their premorbid work level, thus suggesting that approximately 80% of BD patients are at least partially vocationally disabled. Finally, only 42% of BD patients live independently, whereas 58% live with one or both of their parents.[18]

It has been suggested that residual symptomatology and psychosocial variables can account for functional disability in BD;[19–22] however, growing evidence demonstrates that specific cognitive dysfunctions[23] are the major contributors of functional disability in BD.[24–27] In particular, it appears that processing speed deficits are associated with a poorer global level of functioning, whereas a lower performance in verbal memory is predictive of impairment in occupational functioning.[25] The importance of intact cognitive ability in real-world functioning in individuals with BD is highlighted by the finding that neurocognitive deficits are strong predictors of community and household activities, whereas their effect on work functioning and interpersonal behavior is mediated by social and adaptive competencies.[24]

COGNITIVE DYSFUNCTION IN BIPOLAR DISORDER

Although general cognitive ability (as measured by IQ) tends to fall within the normal range during euthymia,[28] persistent deficits in attention, verbal learning, and executive function[29–31] have been demonstrated in individuals with BD, with performance falling 0.75 to 1 standard deviation below that of healthy controls.

Cross-sectional studies show that individuals with BD in manic or depressed states present with profound and extensive neurocognitive impairment comparable to that in individuals with SZ.[32] Although some of the impairment seen during acute episodes may improve along with mood symptoms with effective treatment, many patients demonstrate deficits regardless of the presence of active mood symptomatology,[29,33,34] thus suggesting that cognitive dysfunctions are a critical feature of BD that persists during euthymia.[33]

A meta-analysis[35] suggested that neurodevelopmental factors might play a role in BD because neurocognitive deficits are found to be present from the very early stages of the illness. Patients as early as the first episode underperformed compared to healthy controls across all major cognitive domains, with prominent deficits in processing speed (Cohen's $d = 0.61$), verbal memory ($d = 0.63$), and attention ($d = 0.80$). Compared to participants with first-episode schizophrenia, participants with BD demonstrated better performance in the domains of processing speed, verbal fluency, verbal memory, and working memory, whereas there were no significant differences in reasoning, sustained attention, and visual memory.

Executive Functions

Executive functioning refers to high-level abilities responsible for planning, abstract reasoning, and organizing thoughts and behaviors while considering alternative strategies. The most commonly used tasks to measure this domain are Digit Span, Trail Making Test B (TMT-B), the Wisconsin Card Sorting Test (WCST), verbal fluency, and the Stroop interference test.[28,36] Impairments in executive functioning in BD are consistently reported across studies. The data suggest deficits in subcomponents of executive functioning, including set shifting,[34,37–39] planning,[39] and verbal fluency.[39,40] However, whereas some studies have reported stable deficits in executive functioning,[41,42] other studies have suggested that such deficits improve during remission.[43,44] Meta-analytic studies report an overall moderate to large effect size for executive functioning, with particularly large effects in Digit Span Backwards, TMT-B, category fluency, and the WCST.[28,29,45] However, Robinson et al.[45] highlighted that not all measures of executive functioning were impaired at the same level: Whereas large effect sizes ($d > 0.8$) were reported for category fluency and mental manipulation (Digit Span Backwards), medium effect sizes were reported for response inhibition (Stroop test) and set shifting (WCST and TMT-B).

Verbal Learning and Memory

Verbal learning and memory refer to the ability to encode, retain, and retrieve verbal information. The California Verbal Learning Test (CVLT), the Rey Auditory Verbal Learning Test (RAVLT), and the Hopkins Verbal Learning Test (HVLT) are the most widely used tests to measure verbal learning and memory.[28,36] Impairment in verbal memory has been detected in this domain at the onset of the illness and in pediatric BD samples.[46,47] Meta-analytic data suggest that impairment is more pronounced in total learning (learning a list of words after a series of repetitions) rather than recall after both short and long delays.[28,45] With regard to the stability of impairment over time, whereas some studies report that deficits are stable and do not progress,[42] others suggest that dysfunction (particularly in verbal recall) has a progressive course that cannot be explained by clinical or treatment variables.[48] Visual memory, although less investigated than verbal memory, has been found to be impaired in euthymic BD patients, with performance falling below the mean of healthy populations.[49–51]

Data suggest that the presence of substance misuse can further worsen impairment on visual learning.[52]

Attention and Processing Speed

Attention and processing speed are directly related to each other and refer to the ability to maintain the focus on a target and to process and understand a task requiring a motor response. Evaluation of these functions is commonly pursued through the Trail Making Test A (TMT-A), the Continuous Performance Test (CPT), and the Digit Symbol test.[28,36] Convergent data suggest that deficits in speed of processing and attention appear to be trait-like in BD, with findings demonstrating persistent impairment.[44,53,54] However, there are data that indicate that impairments in sustained attention are associated with manic[55] or psychotic symptoms.[56,57] The effect size of impairments in these domains appears to be moderate to large in magnitude,[28,35,53] as well as relatively stable over time.[54,58]

Social Cognition

Social cognition refers to the ability to recognize, understand, and appropriately respond to socioemotional stimuli, such as emotions, intentions, and dispositions of the self and of others.[59] Social cognition is crucial to maintain appropriate social relationships;[60] therefore, dysfunctions in this area can contribute to impaired social and global levels of everyday functioning. The evidence to date suggests that BD patients tend to demonstrate subtle but persistent deficits in social cognition, with impairment also present in subjects at risk of developing BD.[61]

Social cognition is considered a multidimensional construct composed of five different components: theory of mind (ToM; the ability to represent others' mental states and to make inferences about others' intentions), emotion recognition (the ability to identify emotions by facial expressions and/or vocal prosody), social perception (the capacity to infer social roles as well as rules in complex and/or ambiguous situations from nonverbal and paraverbal social cues), social knowledge (the awareness of rules and behaviors that are expected in social situations and/or interactions), and causal attributional style (the tendency to attribute causality to events in life to internal or external reality).[59]

The majority of the research in social cognition in BD has been focused on emotion recognition/processing and ToM. Data on emotion processing suggest that deficits in this area are persistent in BD patients,[62,63] specifically in facial emotion recognition,[64–67] emotional decision-making,[68,69] and affective response inhibition.[63]

The evidence suggests that a trait-like decision-making dysfunction is present during all phases of the illness, with an increased salience toward negative outcomes during depressive states,[68] whereas there are more inconsistent choices during manic states.[70,71] A recent meta-analysis on social cognition in euthymic BD reported a small but significant effect size ($d = 0.35$) for impairments in facial emotion perception.[72] There were no significant differences for the effect sizes between any of the six most commonly presented emotions in these tasks (happiness, fear, disgust, anger, sadness, and surprise).[72] ToM (also referred to as mentalization) is also abnormal in BD, with data showing that, during euthymia, patients tend to hypomentalize[30] and that the severity of the deficits may be related to the number of previous (hypo)manic episodes.[73] Although some evidence suggests that there are no differences in deficits in BD patients across mood phases and euthymia,[74] other data suggest that symptomatic patients perform worse than remitted patients on tasks measuring ToM.[75,76] However, regardless of mood states, BD patients tend to underperform on ToM tasks compared to healthy controls.[74–76]

Cognitive Heterogeneity in Bipolar Disorder

The cognitive performance of patients with BD is usually reported as being at an intermediate level between that of healthy subjects and that of individuals with SZ.[49,57,77] However, a recent development in our understanding of cognitive dysfunction in BD is the acknowledgment of substantial cognitive heterogeneity within the disorder.[78] Indeed, data suggest that approximately 30–50% of BD patients perform at the same level as healthy controls during periods of euthymia,[79,80,81] which is in contrast to the relative homogeneity of cognitive impairment reported in SZ.

Burdick et al.[82] demonstrated that from a sample of 136 affectively stable BD patients, three discrete cognitive subgroups emerged based on their cognitive performance. Using the Measurement and Treatment Research to Improve Cognition in Schizophrenia (MATRICS) Consensus Cognitive Battery (MCCB),[83] the authors identified a subgroup of BD patients with normal cognitive functioning (31.6% of the sample) who did not differ from demographically matched healthy controls; a subgroup of BD patients whose cognitive profile was consistent with selective impairments (28.7% of the sample), with modest deficits on only a subset of the seven cognitive domains versus healthy controls; and a subgroup of BD patients (39.7% of the sample) with severe impairments across all cognitive domains that were qualitatively and quantitatively similar to the performance of a comparison SZ patient group.

The presence of such considerable cognitive heterogeneity in BD may be due to numerous clinical factors, such as bipolar subtype, number of mood episode, a positive history of psychosis, age at onset, and duration of illness.[81,84]

Data regarding the magnitude of cognitive impairment between BD I and BD II are inconsistent. Whereas some data suggest that individuals with BD I exhibit more severe deficits compared to those with BD II,[85] other data demonstrate that patients with BD I and those with BD II have equal levels of cognitive impairment.[86] In a study comparing BD I, BD II, and unipolar depression during a depressive state, Xu et al.[44] showed that greater cognitive impairment characterized BD I in almost all cognitive domains (particularly in verbal memory and executive functions) compared to the BD II and unipolar depression groups. However, when in remission, the BD I and BD II groups displayed similar levels of cognitive impairments, with both groups demonstrating major deficits in processing speed and visual memory.[44]

Convergent data support that a history of psychosis can in part account for different degrees of deficit in cognition across bipolar subtypes. Psychotic symptoms are reported in approximately 50% of individuals with BD I during acute affective episodes; psychosis is reported much less frequently in patients with BD II (based on the DSM-IV-TR). Some studies suggest that individuals with BD who have psychotic features perform worse compared to BD patients who have never experienced such symptoms in the domains of verbal learning and memory, executive functions,[81,87,88] verbal fluency, response inhibition, and set shifting.[88] Although with small to moderate effect sizes, a meta-analytic study suggested that the presence of psychosis worsens the cognitive performance of BD patients in a number of cognitive domains (processing speed, executive functions, and verbal memory).[89]

Several lines of evidence suggest that the number of lifetime mood episodes is related to cognitive deficits in BD. Specifically, the number of manic episodes is strongly correlated with dysfunction in verbal memory and executive functioning, whereas the number of depressive episodes appears to be associated, although with weaker correlation, with spatial working memory and visual memory.[84] These findings are corroborated by an investigation that focused on the progression of cognitive dysfunctions in SZ and BD and demonstrated that whereas individuals with SZ tend to exhibit cognitive deficits even before the onset of the illness and then demonstrate a relatively stable, nonprogressive course as the illness progresses, cognitive deterioration in BD coincides with illness onset and then increases gradually with the occurrence of mood episodes.[90] A longer duration of illness and an earlier age at onset were found to be associated with greater cognitive impairment, namely in psychomotor speed and verbal memory.[30]

NEUROCHEMICAL TARGETS FOR PHARMACOLOGICAL TREATMENT OF COGNITIVE IMPAIRMENT IN BIPOLAR DISORDER

One of the major challenges in identifying pharmacological agents with which to treat cognitive impairment in BD is that the neurobiological mechanisms associated with cognitive impairment in BD are not known. Given this, it is sensible to identify targets based on known neurobiological abnormalities in BD that may have some relevance to cognition as well as neurobiological systems that are known to be involved in cognition that are likely to be relevant to the pathophysiology of BD. Neurochemical targets that are likely to be important in cognition include dopamine, glutamate, acetylcholine, and nodes within the hypothalamus–pituitary–adrenal (HPA) axis. Systems subserving these targets have been found to be altered in BD, and they are discussed later.

Dopamine

The dopaminergic system is integral to healthy cognitive functioning, with a wealth of preclinical and human data suggesting correlations between dopamine (DA) and cognition (e.g., in animals and humans, DA has been found to be integral to aspects of cognition such as working memory, attention, set shifting, learning, processing speed, and executive functioning[91–95]). Although it is clear that DA is critical to cognitive functioning, the nature of the relationship between this neurotransmitter and cognition is not well understood. It is clear from studies of patients with Parkinson's disease (PD) that as less DA becomes available in the brain, cognition tends to decline somewhat predictably.[96] However, it is also the case that too much DA has adverse consequences for cognition; this complex relationship is likely to be highly individualized and can be best represented by an inverted U-shaped curve, with too little or too much DA resulting in adverse cognitive effects.[97]

The DA system has long been hypothesized to play a central role in the pathophysiology of BD. Early appreciation for the similarities between the manic BD state and the behavioral effects of amphetamines, which increase dopamine within the brain, suggested a role for DA in mania. Similarly, the relatively high percentage of patients with PD who experience depression[98] suggested that perhaps a decrease in DA may be associated with this mood state in BD.

Evidence from structural neuroimaging studies of BD also suggests the presence of aberrations in brain regions known to be rich in DA projections and receptors.[99] These regions, including anterior cingulate, dorsolateral, orbital, and subgenual cortex,[100–102] as well as the basal ganglia,[103] have also demonstrated abnormal activation in BD during cognitive tasks using functional neuroimaging.[104,105]

Given that DA is integral to cognition, it is perhaps unsurprising that increasing levels of DA via agents such as pergolide, a D1 agonist,[106] or bromocriptine, a D2 agonist,[107,108] improves cognition in healthy individuals, particularly in cognitive domains linked to prefrontal cortex (PFC) functions. Nevertheless, very few trials of DA agonists as potential cognitive enhancers have been conducted in BD. More often, DA agonists have been studied in BD as potential treatments for depression, but very few cognitive data have been collected in these trials. One such agent, pramipexole, a DA agonist that may hold promise as a potential cognitive enhancer, is discussed next.

Pramipexole

Pramipexole (Mirapex) is a US Food and Drug Administration (FDA)-approved medication for PD and restless leg syndrome. Several independent neurochemical investigations using human receptors have confirmed that pramipexole binds selectively and completely to DA D2-like receptors and has the greatest affinity for D3 receptors.[109–111] This has also been demonstrated in vivo using positron emission tomography (PET). Ishibashi et al.[112] showed that low-dose pramipexole (0.25 mg) binds to D2/D3 receptors in the PFC, amygdala, and thalamus within 1–1.5 hours of administration. In early PD patients, 6 weeks of pramipexole (1.5 mg) was found to decrease striatal levels of the DA transporter,[113] which resulted in increased DA transmission. In nonhuman primates, PET revealed decreased regional cerebral blood flow in the bilateral orbitofrontal cortex, thalamus, insula, operculum, and cingulate cortex[114] after pramipexole administration. These findings are consistent with known D3 efferents originating in the striatum.

Pramipexole has been investigated as an adjunctive treatment for BD depression, with two randomized controlled trials suggesting that this agent is effective in reducing depressive symptoms.[115,116] Secondary analyses indicated that a subset of patients improved not only in depressive symptomatology but also in the cognitive domain; in particular, patients demonstrated an improvement in attention and processing speed.[117] These analyses led to a larger study comprising the first randomized controlled trial of pramipexole's effect on cognition in affectively stable individuals with BD.[118] This study suggested that euthymic individuals who evidenced cognitive impairment at baseline demonstrated improvements in cognition (specifically, on the Digit Span Backwards and Stroop Color tasks) after 8 weeks of adjunctive pramipexole.[118]

Modafinil

Modafinil (Provigil) is a wake-promoting drug that has demonstrated efficacy in reducing daytime sleepiness, leading to its FDA approval for sleep disorders that are characterized by chronic phase shift disruptions (e.g., shift work disorder). Modafinil exerts primary dopaminergic and serotonergic effects, with secondary effects on GABA, glutamate, and histamine.[119] In healthy volunteers, modafinil has been found to improve cognition in domains such as working memory, spatial planning, and stop-signal reaction time after a single administration of the drug.[120] A study by Grady et al.[121] demonstrated that modafinil offset performance decrements resulting from a 25-day forced desynchrony period in 9 healthy adults randomized to receive daily modafinil compared to 9 healthy adults receiving placebo. Effects were most pronounced on measures of processing speed and sustained attention. Cognitive improvements associated with modafinil have also been demonstrated in patients with SZ, particularly in the domain of executive functioning and attention,[122] and in patients with major depressive disorder (MDD) in the Stroop Interference Test.[123]

Several clinical trials have demonstrated the safety and efficacy of modafinil or armodafinil in treating depression in BD,[124,125] but this agent has not been investigated as a treatment for cognitive impairment in BD. The first double-blind, randomized, placebo-controlled trial of adjunctive modafinil to treat circadian dysfunction and cognitive impairment in BD is now underway (Clinicaltrials.gov Identifier: NCT01965925).

Potential Risks of Dopaminergic Agents in Bipolar Disorder

Due to the risk that DA agonist and stimulants may precipitate a (hypo)manic episode, and also due to the increased risk of rapid cycling and suicidality,[126,127] clinicians and researchers have been slow to adopt these drugs compared to more traditional treatment of BD. However, there is increasing interest in the potential antidepressant effect of DA agonist (pramipexole) and stimulants/stimulant-like drugs (modafinil, armodafinil, and methylphenidate) in bipolar depression. Studies investigating the antidepressant effect of adjunctive pramipexole in the treatment of bipolar depressed patients have shown an overall favorable psychiatric tolerability of pramipexole, with very low rates of discontinuation due to the development of hypomanic[116,128–130] or manic symptoms.[130,131] A similarly good level of somatic tolerability was found (nausea, sedation, and restlessness were reported as the most common adverse effects).[118,128,130–133] However, evidence regarding the level of tolerability during long-term treatments is limited, and further investigation with larger samples and longer follow-up is warranted.[134] In fact, although there were no reports of dis-inhibited behaviors nor any increase in mania among 50 BD participants receiving pramipexole in an 8-week clinical trial of the drug targeting cognitive impairment in BD,[118] an analysis of participants' performance on the Iowa Gambling Task indicated a deleterious effect of pramipexole on reward processing.[135] Specifically, compared to baseline performance, participants who received pramipexole demonstrated an increase in high-risk/high-reward choices after active treatment that was not seen in the placebo group.[135]

There is only limited data regarding the safety and efficacy of dopaminergic stimulants in the treatment of BD, with very few studies testing methylphenidate and amphetamine in this population.[136,137] In an open 12-week trial involving 14 BD patients, El-Mallakh[136] found that methylphenidate added to a stable (at least 1-month) mood-stabilizer regimen ameliorated psychiatric symptoms, although there was no significant change in depressive symptomatology and 1 patient had a manic switch. Another study that retrospectively evaluated 8 BD patients treated (open label) with either methylphenidate or amphetamine as adjunctive antidepressant agents found improvement in overall bipolar illness and no signs of stimulant-induced switching or abuse.[137] A case report study[138] evaluating the clinical benefit of methylphenidate and dexamphetamine (as a monotherapy or as an augmentation to existing treatment) in a sample of 50 unipolar or bipolar depression patients found that 34% of the patients reported distinct improvement (comparable across unipolar or bipolar depression), 30% some improvement, and 36% no improvement and/or side effects. Mild side effects were reported in 18% of the sample. The relative safety of methylphenidate was also reported by Lydon and El-Mallekh,[139] who performed a retrospective case review of 16 depressed BD patients in whom methylphenidate was used as an adjunctive to mood stabilizers, which resulted in an improvement in depressive symptoms, with no exacerbation of (hypo)manic symptoms or substance abuse. Another potential agent of interest is dihydrexidine, a full D1 receptor agonist that has recently been shown to improve working memory in individuals with schizotypal personality disorder.[140] Future work with these and other DA-enhancing medications is warranted.

Taken together, these data are promising with regard to the potential adoption of DA agonist and stimulants as adjunctive treatment in bipolar depression; nevertheless, a paucity of controlled trials (especially for pramipexole) and lack of longer follow-up and larger sample sizes limit the deep understanding of the efficacy and safety of these compounds and their role in the neurobiological mechanisms underpinning BD. Future research addressing these points needs to be pursued.

Glutamate

Glutamate is the main excitatory neurotransmitter in the brain and is strongly implicated in learning and memory. In particular, glutamate binds with the *N*-methyl-
D-aspartate (NMDA) receptor to achieve long-term potentiation; this process is
understood to be a critical component in the cellular basis of learning and memory.[141,142] Moreover, disruption of NMDA receptor functioning results in prominent
impairment in cognition in both mice and humans.[143]

Abnormalities in the glutamatergic system have been reported in BD.[144] Serum
levels of glutamate have been found to be increased in individuals with BD,[145,146]
and postmortem analysis of the PFC has also demonstrated increases in glutamate in
individuals with BD.[147] A meta-analysis of proton magnetic resonance spectroscopy
studies examining glutamate in BD found increased levels of this neurotransmitter
in frontal regions in patients compared to healthy controls; this increase was found
in medicated as well as unmedicated individuals with BD.[144] As with dopaminergic agents, very few agents targeting glutamate have been investigated as potential
cognitive enhancers in BD; nevertheless, several agents may hold promise and are
discussed next.

D-Serine/D-Cycloserine

D-Serine is an endogenous NMDA co-agonist that has received much attention
recently with regard to the treatment of cognitive symptoms in schizophrenia. Several
randomized, double-blind, controlled studies investigating the effect of adjunctive
D-serine on positive, negative, and cognitive symptoms in schizophrenia have been
conducted, with some studies reporting improvements in all symptom domains.[148–150]
Note, however, that cognition was assessed either subjectively or using only one or a
few cognitive tasks in these trials. Relatively recently, a large multisite trial of adjunctive D-serine did not find any effect of this agent on negative or cognitive symptoms
in schizophrenia.[151] Recent data from a randomized, placebo-controlled, crossover
study showed that D-serine administration in a sample of 35 healthy individuals had a
beneficial effect on mood and cognition.[152] Specifically, it was found that the level of
anxiety and sadness decreased after D-serine administration; similarly, there was also
an effect of treatment on cognitive performance, specifically in attention and verbal
memory.[152] Preclinical data suggest the involvement of D-serine on cognitive deficits subsequent to induced acute stress in mice.[153] Results suggest that although the
acute stress reduced the level of D-serine in the prefrontal cortex and that of glycine
(endogenous NMDA co-agonist) in the hippocampus, the peripheral administration

of D-serine prevented the effects of acute stress in recognition memory.[153] This result is particularly relevant to psychiatric disorders, especially BD, given the higher prevalence of stressful events (e.g., childhood trauma) compared to healthy population.

A 26-week randomized clinical trial investigating the utility of combining D-cycloserine and cognitive remediation therapy in approximately 40 BD patients is currently underway (Clinicaltrials.gov Identifier: NCT01934972). The study aims to explore the changes in both general cognition (assessed with the MCCB)[83] and specific cognitive domains, as well as functional outcomes.

Memantine

Memantine is an NMDA receptor antagonist that is FDA-approved for the treatment of Alzheimer's disease. A meta-analysis of memantine augmentation trials in schizophrenia reported a significant effect on improving Mini-Mental State Examination scores.[154] However, a trial of memantine in schizophrenia that included a neuropsychological assessment failed to detect any effect of this agent on cognition,[155] and in a trial involving MDD, no changes in cognition were detected between pre- and post-treatment.[156] To date, two case studies have been reported that suggest memantine may improve depressive and cognitive symptoms in patients with BD;[157,158] however, the cognitive symptoms were assessed subjectively in both reports. A recent randomized, double-blind, placebo-controlled trial of adjunctive memantine as an augmentation treatment to lamotrigine failed to find any statistically significant effects of memantine on symptoms of depression in BD;[159] however, there was an indication that memantine may have improved depressive symptoms in the first half of the 8-week trial. Cognition was not assessed in this trial. An open-label trial of memantine for the treatment of mania suggested that the drug was well tolerated in patients and may have some efficacy, although, again, cognition was not examined in this trial. Given the current lack of data on memantine's effects on cognition in BD, as well as the apparent safety of the drug, randomized, double-blind, placebo-controlled trials of memantine for the treatment of cognitive impairment in BD are warranted.

Lamotrigine

Lamotrigine is a commonly used anticonvulsant medication that is FDA-approved for the treatment of both epilepsy and BD. Although the precise mechanism of action of lamotrigine is unknown, the main effect of the drug in BD appears to be to inhibit the presynaptic release of glutamate.[160] Given that too much glutamate may result in excitatory neurotoxicity, this inhibition may be neuroprotective. The potential cognitive effects of lamotrigine, however, have not been rigorously studied in BD. Several clinical trials of lamotrigine as a treatment for BD depression have reported on some limited, generally self-reported cognitive outcomes;[161,162] these data have been positive and suggest that lamotrigine may have some cognitive benefits for patients with BD. Daban et al.[163] investigated the effects of lamotrigine on cognition in 15 patients with BD II compared to 18 patients receiving valproate or carbamazepine and found that patients receiving lamotrigine performed better on a test of phonemic verbal fluency, part of a comprehensive neuropsychological battery that was administered to all participants. All other cognitive results were equivocal among the groups, although the statistical power to detect differences between the groups was low. Moreover, the groups were not matched on potentially relevant clinical variables, such as number of mood episodes or BD subtype.

As is the case with dopaminergic agents, there are several glutamatergic agents that may hold promise as potential cognitive enhancing agents in BD. Large, rigorous clinical trials with comprehensive neuropsychological batteries are required to further investigate the potential utility of these agents as cognitive enhancers in BD.

Acetylcholinergic Agents

Acetylcholinesterase inhibitors (AChEIs) are a class of agents that increase the amount of available acetylcholine in the brain. Acetylcholine has long been associated with cognitive functioning; in particular, it is believed to play an important role in both the encoding and the maintenance of novel information.[164,165] Several AChEIs, including galantamine, donepezil, and rivastigmine, are FDA-approved medications for the treatment of cognitive impairment in Alzheimer's disease. There is evidence that the cholinergic system is altered in mood disorders;[166] targeting this system is thus a natural step in seeking to identify cognitive enhancers in BD.

Galantamine

An early case series of four patients suggested that two of the patients experienced improvement in cognition after augmentation treatment with galantamine; however, this retrospective chart review included only the Clinical Global Impression scale as a measure of cognitive response.[167] Galantamine in MDD failed to result in any improvement in cognition,[168] with the exception of a potential protective factor against impaired memory during electroconvulsive therapy.[169]

Two trials of galantamine as a potential treatment for cognitive impairment in BD have been conducted to date.[170] Iosifescu et al.[170] conducted a 16-week, open-label trial of adjunctive galantamine in 19 affectively stable patients with BD. Baseline and post-treatment cognitive evaluations focused on attention, executive functioning, and verbal learning and memory as assessed by the Conners Continuous Performance Test (Connors CPT), the WCST, and the CVLT, respectively. Healthy subjects were assessed at baseline and at a 16-week follow-up appointment. Results indicated that patients improved significantly in both attention and verbal learning after 16 weeks of treatment with galantamine. Patients also reported subjective improvement in cognition by week 12 of the study. Baseline and post-treatment proton magnetic resonance spectroscopy revealed a post-treatment decrease in choline in the left hippocampus in patients that was similar to baseline levels in healthy volunteers.

Ghaemi et al.[171] conducted a small randomized, double-blind, placebo-controlled trial of 12 weeks of galantamine augmentation in affectively stable patients with BD. Sixteen patients completed the study, with 10 of those patients having received galantamine. Neuropsychological assessments conducted at baseline and post-treatment included the CVLT, WCST, and the Delis Kaplan Executive Functioning System (DKEFS). Despite the low power of the study, results indicated that patients who received galantamine demonstrated post-treatment improvements in verbal learning as assessed by the CVLT. However, patients in the placebo group demonstrated improvements on the DKEFS, suggesting that practice effects may have played a role in the final outcome.[171]

Donepezil

Donepezil is an AChEI that has been shown to have some beneficial effect on cognition in schizophrenia.[172,173] Two randomized clinical trials were conducted in elderly depressed patients, and whereas one study reported amelioration in memory,[174] the other suggested that donepezil did not have a clear benefit in preventing progression to mild cognitive impairment in those patients with intact cognitive functioning.[175] A 12-week, open-label study of adjunctive donepezil in elderly patients with BD did not find any improvements in cognitive or daily living outcome measures.[176] To date, only one randomized, placebo-controlled trial of donepezil has been conducted in BD;[177] the target of this trial was treatment-resistant mania, and cognition was not evaluated. The group receiving donepezil did not improve and, in fact, reported higher scores on the Young Mania Rating Scale by the end of the study compared to the placebo group; two patients experienced abrupt manic switches within hours of starting the medication. An association between donepezil and manic switching or new or worsening mania has also been described in several case reports,[178–180] suggesting that this agent may not be appropriate for use in BD.

Rivastigmine

Rivastigmine is the third FDA-approved AChEI agent used to treat cognitive impairment in Alzheimer's disease. To date, this agent has not been investigated in BD, although there is evidence that it may improve memory in patients with schizophrenia.[181]

Hypothalamus–Pituitary–Adrenal Axis Dysfunction

The HPA axis is involved in initiating, maintaining, and regulating the body's physiological response to stress. When stressed, the hypothalamus releases corticotropin-releasing factor (CRF), which then stimulates the release of adrenocorticotropin (ACTH), which in turn triggers the release of glucocorticoids from the adrenal cortex.[182] This system is regulated in part by circulating corticoids, which bind to two main subtypes of receptors in the brain: glucocorticoid receptors and mineralocorticoid receptors.[183] The HPA axis plays an integral role in memory; for example, it has been demonstrated that acute[184] and chronic[185] administration of glucocorticoids impairs memory retrieval as well as working memory.[182]

HPA axis abnormalities have been described in BD, including aberrant corticoid receptors in the hippocampus in postmortem samples,[186] decreased mRNA expression of mineralocorticoid receptors in the dorsolateral PFC,[187] and alterations in mRNA expression of selected glucocorticoid receptors in the orbital frontal cortex.[188,189] Abnormal results from the dexamethasone suppression test, a test of glucocorticoid receptor function, have also been reported in BD,[190–192] and an association has been described between abnormal glucocorticoid receptor and impaired memory in BD.[193] Given the abnormalities in glucocorticoid receptor function, and the association between these abnormalities and neurocognition in BD, it is possible that glucocorticoid receptor antagonists may serve to normalize the function of these receptors, perhaps resulting in improved HPA axis functioning and cognition.

Mifepristone

Mifepristone is a synthetic steroid that acts as a progesterone receptor antagonist as well as a glucocorticoid receptor antagonist.[194,195] As such, it can serve to lower the level of cortisol, and it is used for this purpose to treat hypercortisolism in endocrine disorders such as Cushing's syndrome. Relatively recently, mifepristone has been explored as potential adjunctive treatment in neuropsychiatric disorders.[194] In addition to potential beneficial effects on depression, antipsychotic-induced weight gain, and post-traumatic stress disorder, mifepristone may act as a cognitive enhancer in disorders such as BD.

In a double-blind, crossover design,[196] 600 mg/day of mifepristone or placebo was administered for 1 week to 20 patients with BD who were experiencing some residual depressive symptoms but were generally affectively stable. A comprehensive neuropsychological battery was completed at baseline and after each week of treatment with either mifepristone or placebo, for a total of three assessments. Results indicated that mifepristone was associated with a mild but statistically significant improvement in spatial working memory, spatial recognition, and verbal fluency. Depressive symptoms also improved after mifepristone administration.

In a larger, randomized, placebo-controlled trial in which 600 mg/day of mifepristone was administered for 1 week to 60 individuals with BD depression, results demonstrated that the drug led to improvements in female participants in spatial working memory—an effect not seen in males; these improvements were evident at 7 weeks post-treatment. Participants were also assessed at 3 weeks post-treatment; however, there were no significant changes in cognition compared to baseline at this time point. No other cognitive domains were improved by mifepristone. The level of cortisol response to mifepristone after 1 week of treatment was correlated with spatial working memory performance at 3 and 7 weeks post-treatment in both males and females. The gender difference in improvement may be due to lower baseline performance in spatial working memory in female participants compared to male participants; it may also have implications for the neurobiological mechanism through which mifepristone may contribute to cognitive improvement in this domain. In particular, the authors suggest that improvements in spatial working memory associated with mifepristone may be mediated by progesterone antagonism. Further work is needed to clarify the efficacy of mifepristone in improving cognition and to understand the mechanisms by which any improvements may be occurring.

Role of Inflammation

HPA axis dysregulation in BD may be closely related to evidence of abnormal levels of inflammation in this disorder.[197] Patients with BD have been found to have increased levels of interleukin-1 (IL-1), soluble IL-2 receptor, IL-6, tumor necrosis factor-α-2 (TNF-α), and C-reactive protein (CRP) and low IL-4 in different phases of BD—a profile that is only partially ameliorated by medication.[198] It is possible that increased pro-inflammatory cytokines may contribute to glucocorticoid resistance and receptor dysfunction, ultimately resulting in hypercortisolism and lower peripheral brain-derived neurotrophic factor (BDNF) levels. It is also possible that a more primary glucocorticoid receptor dysfunction in BD leads to increased inflammation.[199,200] Although the directionality of the abnormalities in both the HPA axis and inflammatory markers is not currently known, it is reasonable to seek treatment options that might target each system.

Just as there is evidence that HPA axis dysfunction may be related to cognitive impairment in BD, there are also limited data demonstrating that increased levels of inflammatory markers are associated with cognitive functioning. Barbosa et al.[201] evaluated executive functioning in 25 euthymic BPD patients and 25 matched controls. They measured plasma levels of BDNF, TNF-α, soluble tumor necrosis factor receptor 1 (sTNFR1), and sTNFR2 using enzyme-linked immunosorbent assay and correlated levels with performance on executive tasks. BD patients demonstrated impaired executive functioning and increased plasma BDNF levels compared to controls. A significant correlation between TNF-α and inhibitory control performance ($r = 0.50$; $p = 0.02$) was found in the BD subjects, indicating a relationship between higher cytokine levels and neurocognitive impairment. No relationship was noted between BDNF levels and cognitive performance in BD patients, which is consistent with at least one prior report.[202] Increased levels of CRP, another marker of inflammation, have also been reported in BD; moreover, a significant negative correlation between CRP levels and neurocognitive performance on the Repeatable Battery for the Assessment of Neuropsychological Status (RBANS) has been described in a sample of patients with BD.[203]

To date, there have not been any published trials of the potential effects on cognition of anti-inflammatory agents in BD. Increasing evidence suggests that anti-inflammatory agents such as omega-3 fatty acids and *N*-acetylcysteine may have some benefit for both depressive and manic symptoms in patients with BD;[204] however, it is currently unknown whether these agents or other anti-inflammatory agents such as curcumin may improve cognition as well.

Other Agents and Targets

Erythropoietin

Erythropoietin (EPO) is a non-immunological cytokine that plays a key role in stimulating red blood cell production. Exogenous EPO is an FDA-approved treatment for anemia, and it has also been used as a (generally illegal) performance-enhancing drug in athletes. Relatively recently, EPO has been investigated as a treatment for cognitive impairment due to its neuroprotective and potential neuroregenerative effects in patients with neuropsychiatric disorders.[205,206] In particular, a randomized, double-blind, placebo-controlled trial of recombinant human EPO in patients with schizophrenia demonstrated that participants receiving the drug infusion improved significantly on a comprehensive neuropsychological battery compared to controls.[207] Similar improvements have been demonstrated in patients with treatment-resistant depression.[208]

A randomized, double-blind, placebo-controlled trial of recombinant human EPO in patients with BD demonstrated that this treatment is associated with cognitive improvement in this population as well.[209] In this study, 23 patients diagnosed with BD were administered eight weekly infusions of EPO, and 20 patients received placebo. Comprehensive neurocognitive assessments were conducted at baseline, week 9, and week 14. Although the main outcome measure of verbal memory (as assessed by the RAVLT) did not differ between active drug and placebo, participants receiving EPO demonstrated significant post-treatment improvements in sustained attention and visual processing speed. Subsequent analyses of these data suggest that EPO is associated with a reversal of hippocampal volume loss in patients with treatment-resistant depression and BD and that this gain in hippocampal volume is correlated with improvements in memory.[210] Based on the limited but increasing amount of data available on the role and use of EPO in treating cognitive impairment, this agent holds particular promise as a potential cognitive enhancer and requires further study.

Targeting Social Cognition with Oxytocin

Evidence from a range of studies demonstrates that many patients with BD have measurable impairments in aspects of social cognition such as facial emotion perception, ToM, and attributional style.[211,212] Although the neurochemical mechanisms underlying impaired social cognition are unknown, oxytocin is an endogenous hormone that may be administered exogenously to improve social cognition in disorders such as autism and schizophrenia.[211] To date, no studies have examined the potential efficacy of oxytocin as a treatment for social cognitive impairments in BD.

Cognitive Remediation in Bipolar Disorder

Nonpharmacological strategies for treating cognitive impairment in neuropsychiatric disorders have focused largely on cognitive remediation. However, the vast majority of studies on cognitive remediation have focused on schizophrenia. These studies demonstrate that cognitive remediation may take many forms and that, in general, it is an effective means of improving cognition in patients with schizophrenia.[213] Nevertheless, this nonpharmacological approach to improving cognition has not been thoroughly investigated in BD. To date, no randomized, double-blind, placebo-controlled trials of cognitive remediation have been conducted in BD. One published report of an open trial of a cognitive rehabilitation treatment in BD demonstrated significant improvements in executive functioning.[214] A large, multisite trial of functional rehabilitation—a novel treatment approach composed of ecological training in strategies designed to enhance real-world performance in domains such as memory, planning, attention, multitasking, and problem-solving in BD—found this treatment to be effective in improving functional outcomes, although there were no differences in post-treatment neurocognitive functioning associated with active treatment compared to either a control treatment or placebo.[215]

Several clinical trials of cognitive remediation in BD are currently underway, including a trial that includes adjunctive D-cycloserine in addition to traditional, computer-based cognitive remediation.[216] Combined pharmacological and either psychosocial or computer-based treatments targeting cognition are an intriguing next step in potentially optimizing the cognitive enhancing properties of either treatment alone.

Clinical Trial Design for Neurocognitive Enhancement in Bipolar Disorder

Given the persuasive converging evidence supporting cognitive impairment as a core symptom and therapeutic target in BD,[58,81,217–220] it is increasingly important to test potential cognitive enhancement treatments in clinical trials. However, the design of these trials poses several challenges, some of which are specifically related to the nature of BD, whereas others are shared more broadly by all neurocognitive enhancement clinical trials.[221]

Surprisingly, there is a dearth of formal guidelines to guide the design of cognitive enhancement clinical trials in BD—in contrast to the ones available for other disorders such as schizophrenia. The MATRICS initiative—a collaboration among academia, the FDA, and the pharmaceutical industry—led to the development of a consensus battery to assess cognition in clinical trials in patients with schizophrenia and also a set of recommendations to optimize study design.[222] A recently published consensus statement[221] represents the first similar effort in BD, providing the first comprehensive set of best practice recommendations for the design and conduct of treatment trials targeting neurocognition in BD.

Challenges specific to BD research include the episodic nature of the illness with fluctuating mood states over time, the substantial heterogeneity in illness subtype and course (e.g., type I vs. type II and rapid cycling), the high rate of diverse comorbid conditions, and frequent use of polypharmacy.[221] Moreover, unlike in schizophrenia, there appears to be significant cognitive heterogeneity in BD, with patients ranging from unimpaired to very impaired.[82,221]

TABLE 11.1 Summary of the Consensus Statement on Challenges and Recommendations for Cognitive Enhancement Trial Design in Bipolar Disorder

Challenges/Confounds	Recommendations
Diagnostic issues	
Bipolar subtype (bipolar I/bipolar II)	Include both subtypes, with cognitive impairment threshold.
Substance use disorder comorbidity	Allow remote history of substance use disorder.
	Exclude history of substance use disorder within 3 months.
	Test for illicit substances at time of assessment to rule out intoxication or very recent use.
	Include standardized measures of substance use, even of legal substances such as alcohol and tobacco, that may affect cognitive measures.
Anxiety disorder comorbidity	Allow history of anxiety disorder diagnosis.
	Evaluate current state and rule out subjects with current syndromal anxiety symptoms.
ADHD comorbidity	Allow subjects diagnosed with ADHD in adulthood (after the onset of BD) but exclude those diagnosed and treated in childhood, before the onset of BD.
Clinical issues	
Mood symptoms (state)	Only include patients who are stable.
	Define thresholds for both acute depression and mania symptoms that would result in exclusion from the trial, but allow subsyndromal symptoms.
	Assess mood symptom severity at baseline and on cognitive testing days, and include mood symptom scores as covariates in statistical models.
	Stratify randomization based on baseline mood symptom severity.
Concomitant medications	
Specific medication restrictions	The following treatments should not be allowed: high-dose anticholinergics; topiramate; clozapine; tricyclic antidepressants; benzodiazepines within 6 hours of testing; and ECT within past 6 months.
Effect of polypharmacy	Exclude subjects taking more than three psychotropic medications.
	Dosing limitations and "medication load" quantification might be useful.
Cognitive heterogeneity within BD	Select only those participants with objective evidence of significant cognitive impairment using a pre-screening battery.
	Threshold recommended at 0.5 to 1 SD below normative performance.

TABLE 11.1 Continued

Challenges/Confounds	Recommendations
Sample size	Should be large enough to detect an effect size around Cohen's d = 0.5, which likely represents the threshold for a meaningful effect on cognition.
	Given the cognitive heterogeneity in BD, large samples may be needed to show an effect; alternatively, smaller, narrowly defined subgroups of homogeneous patients may be targeted.
Measurement issues	
Choice of neurocognitive outcome measures	There is no consensus cognitive battery designed for clinical trials of cognitive enhancement interventions in BD.
	A single cognitive test or a global neurocognitive composite (which may be required for FDA approval of a cognitive enhancement indication) may be chosen.
	The measures should be sensitive enough to detect meaningful change, easy to implement, with minimal practice effects, and objective (not based on patient self-report).
	The MCCB is suggested as a core battery.
	Other measures may be added as needed to enhance sensitivity, assess the affective processing domain, or tap into the specific mechanism of the drug.
Functional outcome measures	Sensitive enough to capture partial disability.
	Based on objective information and an external informant whenever possible.
	The University of California at San Diego Performance-Based Skills Assessment (UPSA), the Sheehan Disability Scale, and the Functioning Assessment Short Test (FAST) are examples of useful measures.
Overall trial design	
Mood fluctuation	Choose the shortest possible trial duration that allows for cognitive improvement.
Frequency of assessments	Add-on trial design with mandatory concurrent treatment with a mood stabilizer.
Carryover effects of medications and practice effects in cognitive outcome measures	Test cognitive outcome measures at baseline and at least at two other time points to avoid losing all data for a given subject in case of attrition.
	Always include a placebo arm.
	Avoid crossover designs.
	Choose cognitive outcome measures tasks with minimal practice effects.

ADHD, *attention deficit hyperactivity disorder; ECT, electroconvulsive therapy; MCCB, Measurement and Treatment Research to Improve Cognition in Schizophrenia (MATRICS) Consensus Cognitive Battery; SD, standard deviation.*
Source: *Modified from Burdick et al.*[221]

Given the very limited clinical trial data available on cognitive enhancement interventions in BD, the following recommendations by Burdick and colleagues[221] are largely based on broader expertise of the consensus panel and extrapolation of the guidelines available in schizophrenia. Based on the MATRICS recommendations for schizophrenia, the optimal approach suggested in the consensus statement is a randomized, double-blind, placebo-controlled, add-on trial design.

The number of previous mood episodes, age of onset, duration of illness, and history of psychosis need to be addressed as part of the study design.[49] Table 11.1 describes the current challenges in the design and conduct of treatment trials targeting cognition in BD and provides the consensus recommendations for addressing these challenges.[221]

CONCLUSION

Neurocognitive impairments are now recognized as core features of BD with significant deficits in attention, verbal memory, and executive function. These cognitive deficits have been shown to directly contribute to the poor level of everyday functioning in BD. Given the negative impact of these deficits on overall clinical presentation and on quality of life of individuals with BD, cognitive impairment represents an important target for intervention. Because the neurobiological mechanisms associated with the deficits are not fully understood, the field is still in its infancy with regard to direct attempts to intervene. Nonetheless, there are several potential pharmacological agents that have been investigated for pro-cognitive effects in BD and several ongoing efforts to expand on prior findings. Future research will be critical for gaining a deep understanding of the efficacy and safety of pharmacological compounds/nonpharmacological interventions and to elucidate their role in the neurobiological mechanisms underpinning cognition in BD.

REFERENCES

1. American Psychiatric Association. *Diagnostic and statistical manual of mental disorders*. 5 ed. Arlington, VA: American Psychiatric Publishing; 2013.
2. Murray CJ, Lopez AD. Evidence-based health policy—Lessons from the Global Burden of Disease Study. *Science* 1996;274(5288):740–743.
3. Merikangas KR, Jin R, He J-P, et al. Prevalence and correlates of bipolar spectrum disorder in the world mental health survey initiative. *Arch Gen Psychiatry* 2011;68(3):241–251. doi:10.1001/archgenpsychiatry.2011.12
4. Baldessarini RJ, Pompili M, Tondo L. Suicide in bipolar disorder: Risks and management. *CNS Spectr* 2006;11(6):465–471.
5. Bienvenu OJ, Davydow DS, Kendler KS. Psychiatric "diseases" versus behavioral disorders and degree of genetic influence. *Psychol Med* 2011;41(1):33–40. doi:10.1017/S003329171000084X

6. Garno JL, Goldberg JF, Ramirez PM, et al. Impact of childhood abuse on the clinical course of bipolar disorder. *Br J Psychiatry J Ment Sci* 2005;186:121–125. doi:10.1192/bjp.186.2.121

7. Leboyer M, Kupfer DJ. Bipolar disorder: New perspectives in health care and prevention. *J Clin Psychiatry* 2010;71(12):1689–1695. doi:10.4088/JCP.10m06347yel

8. Phillips ML, Kupfer DJ. Bipolar disorder diagnosis: Challenges and future directions. *Lancet* 2013;381(9878):1663–1671. doi:10.1016/S0140-6736(13)60989-7

9. Bromet EJ, Kotov R, Fochtmann LJ, et al. Diagnostic shifts during the decade following first admission for psychosis. *Am J Psychiatry* 2011;168(11):1186–1194. doi:10.1176/appi.ajp.2011.11010048

10. Baldessarini RJ, Tondo L, Baethge CJ, et al. Effects of treatment latency on response to maintenance treatment in manic-depressive disorders. *Bipolar Disord* 2007;9(4):386–393. doi:10.1111/j.1399-5618.2007.00385.x

11. Green MF. What are the functional consequences of neurocognitive deficits in schizophrenia? *Am J Psychiatry* 1996;153(3):321–330. doi:10.1176/ajp.153.3.321

12. McClure MM, Bowie CR, Patterson TL, et al. Correlations of functional capacity and neuropsychological performance in older patients with schizophrenia: Evidence for specificity of relationships? *Schizophr Res* 2007;89(1–3):330–338. doi:10.1016/j.schres.2006.07.024

13. Perlick DA, Rosenheck RA, Kaczynski R, et al. Association of symptomatology and cognitive deficits to functional capacity in schizophrenia. *Schizophr Res* 2008;99(1–3):192–199. doi:10.1016/j.schres.2007.08.009

14. Shamsi S, Lau A, Lencz T, et al. Cognitive and symptomatic predictors of functional disability in schizophrenia. *Schizophr Res* 2011;126(1–3):257–264. doi:10.1016/j.schres.2010.08.007

15. Tohen M, Hennen J, Zarate CM, et al. Two-year syndromal and functional recovery in 219 cases of first-episode major affective disorder with psychotic features. *Am J Psychiatry* 2000;157(2):220–228.

16. Tohen M, Zarate CA, Hennen J, et al. The McLean–Harvard First-Episode Mania Study: Prediction of recovery and first recurrence. *Am J Psychiatry* 2003;160(12):2099–2107.

17. Abood Z, Sharkey A, Webb M, et al. Are patients with bipolar affective disorder socially disadvantaged? A comparison with a control group. *Bipolar Disord* 2002;4(4):243–248.

18. Kupfer DJ, Frank E, Grochocinski VJ, et al. Demographic and clinical characteristics of individuals in a bipolar disorder case registry. *J Clin Psychiatry* 2002;63(2):120–125.

19. Judd LL, Akiskal HS, Schettler PJ, et al. Psychosocial disability in the course of bipolar I and II disorders: A prospective, comparative, longitudinal study. *Arch Gen Psychiatry* 2005;62(12):1322–1330. doi:10.1001/archpsyc.62.12.1322

20. Kennedy N, Foy K, Sherazi R, et al. Long-term social functioning after depression treated by psychiatrists: A review. *Bipolar Disord* 2007;9(1–2):25–37. doi:10.1111/j.1399-5618.2007.00326.x

21. Michalak EE, Yatham LN, Maxwell V, et al. The impact of bipolar disorder upon work functioning: A qualitative analysis. *Bipolar Disord* 2007;9(1–2):126–143. doi:10.1111/j.1399-5618.2007.00436.x

22. Pope M, Dudley R, Scott J. Determinants of social functioning in bipolar disorder. *Bipolar Disord* 2007;9(1–2):38–44. doi:10.1111/j.1399-5618.2007.00323.x

23. McGurk SR, Mueser KT. Cognitive and clinical predictors of work outcomes in clients with schizophrenia receiving supported employment services: 4-Year follow-up. *Adm Policy Ment Health* 2006;33(5):598–606. doi:10.1007/s10488-006-0070-2

24. Bowie CR, Depp C, McGrath JA, et al. Prediction of real-world functional disability in chronic mental disorders: A comparison of schizophrenia and bipolar disorder. *Am J Psychiatry* 2010;167(9):1116–1124. doi:10.1176/appi.ajp.2010.09101406

25. Burdick KE, Goldberg JF, Harrow M. Neurocognitive dysfunction and psychosocial outcome in patients with bipolar I disorder at 15-year follow-up. *Acta Psychiatr Scand* 2010;122(6):499–506. doi:10.1111/j.1600-0447.2010.01590.x

26. Sanchez-Moreno J, Martinez-Aran A, Tabarés-Seisdedos R, et al. Functioning and disability in bipolar disorder: An extensive review. *Psychother Psychosom* 2009;78(5):285–297. doi:10.1159/000228249

27. Tabarés-Seisdedos R, Balanzá-Martínez V, Sánchez-Moreno J, et al. Neurocognitive and clinical predictors of functional outcome in patients with schizophrenia and bipolar I disorder at one-year follow-up. *J Affect Disord* 2008;109(3):286–299. doi:10.1016/j.jad.2007.12.234

28. Torres IJ, Boudreau VG, Yatham LN. Neuropsychological functioning in euthymic bipolar disorder: A meta-analysis. *Acta Psychiatr Scand Suppl* 2007;(434):17–26. doi:10.1111/j.1600-0447.2007.01055.x

29. Arts B, Jabben N, Krabbendam L, et al. Meta-analyses of cognitive functioning in euthymic bipolar patients and their first-degree relatives. *Psychol Med* 2008;38(6):771–785. doi:10.1017/S0033291707001675

30. Bora E, Yucel M, Pantelis C. Cognitive endophenotypes of bipolar disorder: A meta-analysis of neuropsychological deficits in euthymic patients and their first-degree relatives. *J Affect Disord* 2009;113(1–2):1–20. doi:10.1016/j.jad.2008.06.009

31. Torres IJ, DeFreitas VG, DeFreitas CM, et al. Neurocognitive functioning in patients with bipolar I disorder recently recovered from a first manic episode. *J Clin Psychiatry* 2010;71(9):1234–1242. doi:10.4088/JCP.08m04997yel

32. Daban C, Martinez-Aran A, Torrent C, et al. Specificity of cognitive deficits in bipolar disorder versus schizophrenia: A systematic review. *Psychother Psychosom* 2006;75(2):72–84. doi:10.1159/000090891

33. Malhi GS, Ivanovski B, Hadzi-Pavlovic D, et al. Neuropsychological deficits and functional impairment in bipolar depression, hypomania and euthymia. *Bipolar Disord* 2007;9(1–2):114–125. doi:10.1111/j.1399-5618.2007.00324.x

34. Martínez-Arán A, Vieta E, Colom F, et al. Cognitive impairment in euthymic bipolar patients: Implications for clinical and functional outcome. *Bipolar Disord* 2004;6(3):224–232. doi:10.1111/j.1399-5618.2004.00111.x

35. Bora E, Pantelis C. Meta-analysis of cognitive impairment in first-episode bipolar disorder: Comparison with first-episode schizophrenia and healthy controls. *Schizophr Bull* 2015;41(5):1095–1104. doi:10.1093/schbul/sbu198

36. Spreen O, Strauss E. *A compendium of neuropsychological tests: Administration, norms, and commentary.* 2 ed. New York, NY: Oxford University Press; 1998.

37. Clark L, Iversen SD, Goodwin GM. Sustained attention deficit in bipolar disorder. *Br J Psychiatry J Ment Sci* 2002;180:313–319.

38. Coffman JA, Bornstein RA, Olson SC, et al. Cognitive impairment and cerebral structure by MRI in bipolar disorder. *Biol Psychiatry* 1990;27(11):1188–1196.

39. Ferrier IN, Stanton BR, Kelly TP, et al. Neuropsychological function in euthymic patients with bipolar disorder. *Br J Psychiatry J Ment Sci* 1999;175:246–251.

40. Atre-Vaidya N, Taylor MA, Seidenberg M, et al. Cognitive deficits, psychopathology, and psychosocial functioning in bipolar mood disorder. *Neuropsychiatry Neuropsychol Behav Neurol* 1998;11(3):120–126.

41. Bearden CE, Shih VH, Green MF, et al. The impact of neurocognitive impairment on occupational recovery of clinically stable patients with bipolar disorder: A prospective study. *Bipolar Disord* 2011;13(4):323–333. doi:10.1111/j.1399-5618.2011.00928.x

42. Mur M, Portella MJ, Martínez-Arán A, et al. Long-term stability of cognitive impairment in bipolar disorder: A 2-year follow-up study of lithium-treated euthymic bipolar patients. *J Clin Psychiatry* 2008;69(5):712–719.

43. Burdick KE, Goldberg JF, Harrow M, et al. Neurocognition as a stable endophenotype in bipolar disorder and schizophrenia. *J Nerv Ment Dis* 2006;194(4):255–260. doi:10.1097/01.nmd.0000207360.70337.7e

44. Xu G, Lin K, Rao D, et al. Neuropsychological performance in bipolar I, bipolar II and unipolar depression patients: A longitudinal, naturalistic study. *J Affect Disord* 2012;136(3):328–339. doi:10.1016/j.jad.2011.11.029

45. Robinson LJ, Thompson JM, Gallagher P, et al. A meta-analysis of cognitive deficits in euthymic patients with bipolar disorder. *J Affect Disord* 2006;93(1–3):105–115. doi:10.1016/j.jad.2006.02.016

46. Pavuluri MN, West A, Hill SK, et al. Neurocognitive function in pediatric bipolar disorder: 3-Year follow-up shows cognitive development lagging behind healthy youths. *J Am Acad Child Adolesc Psychiatry* 2009;48(3):299–307. doi:10.1097/CHI.0b013e318196b907

47. Schretlen DJ, Cascella NG, Meyer SM, et al. Neuropsychological functioning in bipolar disorder and schizophrenia. *Biol Psychiatry* 2007;62(2):179–186. doi:10.1016/j.biopsych.2006.09.025

48. Santos JL, Aparicio A, Bagney A, et al. A five-year follow-up study of neurocognitive functioning in bipolar disorder. *Bipolar Disord* 2014;16(7):722–731. doi:10.1111/bdi.12215

49. Burdick KE, Goldberg TE, Cornblatt BA, et al. The MATRICS Consensus Cognitive Battery in patients with bipolar I disorder. *Neuropsychopharmacology* 2011;36(8):1587–1592. doi:10.1038/npp.2011.36

50. Rubinsztein JS, Michael A, Paykel ES, et al. Cognitive impairment in remission in bipolar affective disorder. *Psychol Med* 2000;30(5):1025–1036.

51. Van Rheenen TE, Rossell SL. An empirical evaluation of the MATRICS Consensus Cognitive Battery in bipolar disorder. *Bipolar Disord* 2014;16(3):318–325. doi:10.1111/bdi.12134

52. Marshall DF, Walker SJ, Ryan KA, et al. Greater executive and visual memory dysfunction in comorbid bipolar disorder and substance use disorder. *Psychiatry Res* 2012;200(2–3):252–257. doi:10.1016/j.psychres.2012.06.013

53. Clark L, Kempton MJ, Scarnà A, et al. Sustained attention-deficit confirmed in euthymic bipolar disorder but not in first-degree relatives of bipolar patients or euthymic unipolar depression. *Biol Psychiatry* 2005;57(2):183–187. doi:10.1016/j.biopsych.2004.11.007

54. Harmell AL, Mausbach BT, Moore RC, et al. Longitudinal study of sustained attention in outpatients with bipolar disorder. *J Int Neuropsychol Soc* 2014;20(2):230–237. doi:10.1017/S1355617713001422

55. Fleck DE, Shear PK, Strakowski SM. Processing efficiency and sustained attention in bipolar disorder. *J Int Neuropsychol Soc* 2005;11(1):49–57. doi:10.1017/S1355617705050071

56. Liu SK, Chiu C-H, Chang C-J, et al. Deficits in sustained attention in schizophrenia and affective disorders: Stable versus state-dependent markers. *Am J Psychiatry* 2002;159(6):975–982.

57. Seidman LJ, Kremen WS, Koren D, et al. A comparative profile analysis of neuropsychological functioning in patients with schizophrenia and bipolar psychoses. *Schizophr Res* 2002;53(1–2):31–44.

58. Lim CS, Baldessarini RJ, Vieta E, et al. Longitudinal neuroimaging and neuropsychological changes in bipolar disorder patients: Review of the evidence. *Neurosci Biobehav Rev* 2013;37(3):418–435. doi:10.1016/j.neubiorev.2013.01.003

59. Ochsner KN. The social–emotional processing stream: Five core constructs and their translational potential for schizophrenia and beyond. *Biol Psychiatry* 2008;64(1):48–61. doi:10.1016/j.biopsych.2008.04.024

60. Eisenberg N, Miller PA. The relation of empathy to prosocial and related behaviors. *Psychol Bull* 1987;101(1):91–119.

61. Samamé C. Social cognition throughout the three phases of bipolar disorder: A state-of-the-art overview. *Psychiatry Res* 2013;210(3):1275–1286. doi:10.1016/j.psychres.2013.08.012

62. Bora E, Harrison BJ, Yücel M, et al. Cognitive impairment in euthymic major depressive disorder: A meta-analysis. *Psychol Med* 2013;43(10):2017–2026. doi:10.1017/S0033291712002085

63. Gopin CB, Burdick KE, Derosse P, et al. Emotional modulation of response inhibition in stable patients with bipolar I disorder: A comparison with healthy and schizophrenia subjects. *Bipolar Disord* 2011;13(2):164–172. doi:10.1111/j.1399-5618.2011.00906.x

64. George MS, Huggins T, McDermut W, et al. Abnormal facial emotion recognition in depression: Serial testing in an ultra-rapid-cycling patient. *Behav Modif* 1998;22(2):192–204.

65. Guyer AE, McClure EB, Adler AD, et al. Specificity of facial expression labeling deficits in childhood psychopathology. *J Child Psychol Psychiatry* 2007;48(9):863–871. doi:10.1111/j.1469-7610.2007.01758.x

66. Lennox BR, Jacob R, Calder AJ, et al. Behavioural and neurocognitive responses to sad facial affect are attenuated in patients with mania. *Psychol Med* 2004;34(5):795–802.

67. Venn HR, Gray JM, Montagne B, et al. Perception of facial expressions of emotion in bipolar disorder. *Bipolar Disord* 2004;6(4):286–293. doi:10.1111/j.1399-5618.2004.00121.x

68. Adida M, Jollant F, Clark L, et al. Trait-related decision-making impairment in the three phases of bipolar disorder. *Biol Psychiatry* 2011;70(4):357–365. doi:10.1016/j.biopsych.2011.01.018

69. Brambilla P, Cerruti S, Bellani M, et al. Shared impairment in associative learning in schizophrenia and bipolar disorder. *Prog Neuropsychopharmacol Biol Psychiatry* 2011;35(4):1093–1099. doi:10.1016/j.pnpbp.2011.03.007

70. Adida M, Clark L, Pomietto P, et al. Lack of insight may predict impaired decision making in manic patients. *Bipolar Disord* 2008;10(7):829–837. doi:10.1111/j.1399-5618.2008.00618.x

71. Yechiam E, Hayden EP, Bodkins M, et al. Decision making in bipolar disorder: A cognitive modeling approach. *Psychiatry Res* 2008;161(2):142–152. doi:10.1016/j.psychres.2007.07.001

72. Samamé C, Martino DJ, Strejilevich SA. Social cognition in euthymic bipolar disorder: Systematic review and meta-analytic approach. *Acta Psychiatr Scand* 2012;125(4):266–280. doi:10.1111/j.1600-0447.2011.01808.x

73. Montag C, Ehrlich A, Neuhaus K, et al. Theory of mind impairments in euthymic bipolar patients. *J Affect Disord* 2010;123(1–3):264–269. doi:10.1016/j.jad.2009.08.017

74. Wolf F, Brüne M, Assion H-J. Theory of mind and neurocognitive functioning in patients with bipolar disorder. *Bipolar Disord* 2010;12(6):657–666.

75. Bazin N, Brunet-Gouet E, Bourdet C, et al. Quantitative assessment of attribution of intentions to others in schizophrenia using an ecological video-based task: A comparison with manic and depressed patients. *Psychiatry Res* 2009;167(1–2):28–35. doi:10.1016/j.psychres.2007.12.010

76. Kerr N, Dunbar RIM, Bentall RP. Theory of mind deficits in bipolar affective disorder. *J Affect Disord* 2003;73(3):253–259.

77. Zanelli J, Reichenberg A, Morgan K, et al. Specific and generalized neuropsychological deficits: A comparison of patients with various first-episode psychosis presentations. *Am J Psychiatry* 2010;167(1):78–85. doi:10.1176/appi.ajp.2009.09010118

78. Lee RSC, Hickie IB, Hermens DF. Letter to the editor: Neuropsychological subgroups are evident in both mood and psychosis spectrum disorders. *Psychol Med* 2014;44(9):2015. doi:10.1017/S0033291714001019

79. Martino DJ, Strejilevich SA, Scápola M, et al. Heterogeneity in cognitive functioning among patients with bipolar disorder. *J Affect Disord* 2008;109(1–2):149–156. doi:10.1016/j.jad.2007.12.232

80. Reichenberg A, Harvey PD, Bowie CR, et al. Neuropsychological function and dysfunction in schizophrenia and psychotic affective disorders. *Schizophr Bull* 2009;35(5):1022–1029. doi:10.1093/schbul/sbn044

81. Martinez-Aran A, Torrent C, Tabares-Seisdedos R, et al. Neurocognitive impairment in bipolar patients with and without history of psychosis. *J Clin Psychiatry* 2008;69(2):233–239.

82. Burdick KE, Russo M, Frangou S, et al. Empirical evidence for discrete neurocognitive subgroups in bipolar disorder: Clinical implications. *Psychol Med* 2014;44(14):3083–3096. doi:10.1017/S0033291714000439

83. Nuechterlein KH, Green MF, Kern RS, et al. The MATRICS Consensus Cognitive Battery, Part 1: Test selection, reliability, and validity. *Am J Psychiatry* 2008;165(2):203–213. doi:10.1176/appi.ajp.2007.07010042

84. Robinson LJ, Ferrier IN. Evolution of cognitive impairment in bipolar disorder: A systematic review of cross-sectional evidence. *Bipolar Disord* 2006;8(2):103–116. doi:10.1111/j.1399-5618.2006.00277.x

85. Simonsen C, Sundet K, Vaskinn A, et al. Neurocognitive profiles in bipolar I and bipolar II disorder: Differences in pattern and magnitude of dysfunction. *Bipolar Disord* 2008;10(2):245–255. doi:10.1111/j.1399-5618.2007.00492.x

86. Dittmann S, Hennig-Fast K, Gerber S, et al. Cognitive functioning in euthymic bipolar I and bipolar II patients. *Bipolar Disord* 2008;10(8):877–887. doi:10.1111/j.1399-5618.2008.00640.x

87. Glahn DC, Bearden CE, Barguil M, et al. The neurocognitive signature of psychotic bipolar disorder. *Biol Psychiatry* 2007;62(8):910–916. doi:10.1016/j.biopsych.2007.02.001

88. Simonsen C, Sundet K, Vaskinn A, et al. Neurocognitive dysfunction in bipolar and schizophrenia spectrum disorders depends on history of psychosis rather than diagnostic group. *Schizophr Bull* 2011;37(1):73–83. doi:10.1093/schbul/sbp034

89. Bora E, Yücel M, Pantelis C. Neurocognitive markers of psychosis in bipolar disorder: A meta-analytic study. *J Affect Disord* 2010;127(1–3):1–9. doi:10.1016/j.jad.2010.02.117

90. Lewandowski KE, Cohen BM, Ongur D. Evolution of neuropsychological dysfunction during the course of schizophrenia and bipolar disorder. *Psychol Med* 2011;41(2):225–241. doi:10.1017/S0033291710001042

91. Bäckman L, Nyberg L, Lindenberger U, et al. The correlative triad among aging, dopamine, and cognition: Current status and future prospects. *Neurosci Biobehav Rev* 2006;30(6):791–807. doi:10.1016/j.neubiorev.2006.06.005

92. Seamans JK, Yang CR. The principal features and mechanisms of dopamine modulation in the prefrontal cortex. *Prog Neurobiol* 2004;74(1):1–58. doi:10.1016/j.pneurobio.2004.05.006

93. El-Ghundi M, O'Dowd BF, George SR. Insights into the role of dopamine receptor systems in learning and memory. *Rev Neurosci* 2007;18(1):37–66.

94. Nakajima S, Gerretsen P, Takeuchi H, et al. The potential role of dopamine D3 receptor neurotransmission in cognition. *Eur Neuropsychopharmacol* 2013;23(8):799–813. doi:10.1016/j.euroneuro.2013.05.006

95. Takahashi H, Yamada M, Suhara T. Functional significance of central D1 receptors in cognition: beyond working memory. *J Cereb Blood Flow Metab* 2012;32(7):1248–1258. doi:10.1038/jcbfm.2011.194

96. Halliday GM, Leverenz JB, Schneider JS, et al. The neurobiological basis of cognitive impairment in Parkinson's disease. *Mov Disord* 2014;29(5):634–650. doi:10.1002/mds.25857

97. Cools R, D'Esposito M. Inverted-U-shaped dopamine actions on human working memory and cognitive control. *Biol Psychiatry* 2011;69(12):e113–e125. doi:10.1016/j.biopsych.2011.03.028

98. Lieberman A. Depression in Parkinson's disease—A review. *Acta Neurol Scand* 2006;113(1):1–8. doi:10.1111/j.1600-0404.2006.00536.x

99. Cousins DA, Butts K, Young AH. The role of dopamine in bipolar disorder. *Bipolar Disord* 2009;11(8):787–806. doi:10.1111/j.1399-5618.2009.00760.x

100. Drevets WC, Öngür D, Price JL. Neuroimaging abnormalities in the subgenual prefrontal cortex: Implications for the pathophysiology of familial mood disorders. *Mol Psychiatry* 1998;3(3):190–191, 220–226.

101. López-Larson MP, DelBello MP, Zimmerman ME, et al. Regional prefrontal gray and white matter abnormalities in bipolar disorder. *Biol Psychiatry* 2002;52(2):93–100.

102. Strakowski SM, DelBello MP, Adler C, et al. Neuroimaging in bipolar disorder. *Bipolar Disord* 2000;2(3 Pt 1):148–164.

103. Womer FY, Wang L, Alpert KI, et al. Basal ganglia and thalamic morphology in schizophrenia and bipolar disorder. *Psychiatry Res* 2014;223(2):75–83. doi:10.1016/j.pscychresns.2014.05.017

104. Blumberg HP, Stern E, Martinez D, et al. Increased anterior cingulate and caudate activity in bipolar mania. *Biol Psychiatry* 2000;48(11):1045–1052.

105. Gonul AS, Coburn K, Kula M. Cerebral blood flow, metabolic, receptor, and transporter changes in bipolar disorder: The role of PET and SPECT studies. *Int Rev Psychiatry Abingdon Engl* 2009;21(4):323–335. doi:10.1080/09540260902962131

106. Kimberg DY, D'Esposito M. Cognitive effects of the dopamine receptor agonist pergolide. *Neuropsychologia* 2003;41(8):1020–1027.

107. Kimberg DY, D'Esposito M, Farah MJ. Effects of bromocriptine on human subjects depend on working memory capacity. *Neuroreport* 1997;8(16):3581–3585.

108. Luciana M, Collins PF, Depue RA. Opposing roles for dopamine and serotonin in the modulation of human spatial working memory functions. *Cereb Cortex* 1998;8(3):218–226.

109. Mierau J, Schneider FJ, Ensinger HA, et al. Pramipexole binding and activation of cloned and expressed dopamine D2, D3 and D4 receptors. *Eur J Pharmacol* 1995;290(1):29–36.

110. Piercey MF. Pharmacology of pramipexole, a dopamine D3-preferring agonist useful in treating Parkinson's disease. *Clin Neuropharmacol* 1998;21(3):141–151.

111. Piercey MF, Hoffmann WE, Smith MW, et al. Inhibition of dopamine neuron firing by pramipexole, a dopamine D3 receptor-preferring agonist: Comparison to other dopamine receptor agonists. *Eur J Pharmacol* 1996;312(1):35–44. doi:10.1016/0014-2999(96)00454-2

112. Ishibashi K, Ishii K, Oda K, et al. Binding of pramipexole to extrastriatal dopamine D2/D3 receptors in the human brain: A positron emission tomography study using 11C-FLB 457. *PLoS One* 2011;6(3):e17723. doi:10.1371/journal.pone.0017723

113. Guttman M, Stewart D, Hussey D, et al. Influence of L-DOPA and pramipexole on striatal dopamine transporter in early PD. *Neurology* 2001;56(11):1559–1564.

114. Black KJ, Hershey T, Koller JM, et al. A possible substrate for dopamine-related changes in mood and behavior: Prefrontal and limbic effects of a D3-preferring dopamine agonist. *Proc Natl Acad Sci USA* 2002;99(26):17113–17118. doi:10.1073/pnas.012260599

115. Goldberg JF, Burdick KE, Endick CJ. Preliminary randomized, double-blind, placebo-controlled trial of pramipexole added to mood stabilizers for treatment-resistant bipolar depression. *Am J Psychiatry* 2004;161(3):564–566.

116. Zarate CA, Payne JL, Singh J, et al. Pramipexole for bipolar II depression: A placebo-controlled proof of concept study. *Biol Psychiatry* 2004;56(1):54–60. doi:10.1016/j.biopsych.2004.03.013

117. Burdick KE, Braga RJ, Goldberg JF, Malhotra AK. Cognitive dysfunction in bipolar disorder: Future place of pharmacotherapy. *CNS Drugs* 2007;21(12):971–981.

118. Burdick KE, Braga RJ, Nnadi CU, et al. Placebo-controlled adjunctive trial of pramipexole in patients with bipolar disorder: Targeting cognitive dysfunction. *J Clin Psychiatry* 2012;73(1):103–112. doi:10.4088/JCP.11m07299

119. Minzenberg MJ, Carter CS. Modafinil: A review of neurochemical actions and effects on cognition. *Neuropsychopharmacology* 2008;33(7):1477–1502. doi:10.1038/sj.npp.1301534

120. Turner DC, Robbins TW, Clark L, et al. Cognitive enhancing effects of modafinil in healthy volunteers. *Psychopharmacology (Berlin)* 2003;165(3):260–269. doi:10.1007/s00213-002-1250-8

121. Grady S, Aeschbach D, Wright KP, et al. Effect of modafinil on impairments in neurobehavioral performance and learning associated with extended wakefulness and circadian misalignment. *Neuropsychopharmacology* 2010;35(9):1910–1920. doi:10.1038/npp.2010.63

122. Morein-Zamir S, Turner DC, Sahakian BJ. A review of the effects of modafinil on cognition in schizophrenia. *Schizophr Bull* 2007;33(6):1298–1306. doi:10.1093/schbul/sbm090

123. DeBattista C, Lembke A, Solvason HB, et al. A prospective trial of modafinil as an adjunctive treatment of major depression. *J Clin Psychopharmacol* 2004;24(1):87–90. doi:10.1097/01.jcp.0000104910.75206.b9

124. Calabrese JR, Ketter TA, Youakim JM, et al. Adjunctive armodafinil for major depressive episodes associated with bipolar I disorder: A randomized, multicenter, double-blind, placebo-controlled, proof-of-concept study. *J Clin Psychiatry* 2010;71(10):1363–1370. doi:10.4088/JCP.09m05900gry

125. Frye MA, Grunze H, Suppes T, et al. A placebo-controlled evaluation of adjunctive modafinil in the treatment of bipolar depression. *Am J Psychiatry* 2007;164(8):1242–1249. doi:10.1176/appi.ajp.2007.06060981

126. Yatham LN, Torres IJ, Malhi GS, et al. The International Society for Bipolar Disorders–Battery for Assessment of Neurocognition (ISBD-BANC). *Bipolar Disord* 2010;12(4):351–363. doi:10.1111/j.1399-5618.2010.00830.x

127. Grunze HCR. Switching, induction of rapid cycling, and increased suicidality with antidepressants in bipolar patients: Fact or overinterpretation? *CNS Spectr* 2008;13(9):790–795.

128. Sporn J, Ghaemi SN, Sambur MR, et al. Pramipexole augmentation in the treatment of unipolar and bipolar depression: A retrospective chart review. *Ann Clin Psychiatry* 2000;12(3):137–140.

129. Lattanzi L, Dell'Osso L, Cassano P, et al. Pramipexole in treatment-resistant depression: A 16-week naturalistic study. *Bipolar Disord* 2002;4(5):307–314.

130. Cassano P, Lattanzi L, Soldani F, et al. Pramipexole in treatment-resistant depression: An extended follow-up. *Depress Anxiety* 2004;20(3):131–138. doi:10.1002/da.20038

131. Goldberg JF, Burdick KE, Endick CJ. Preliminary randomized, double-blind, placebo-controlled trial of pramipexole added to mood stabilizers for treatment-resistant bipolar depression. *Am J Psychiatry* 2004;161(3):564–566.

132. Perugi G, Toni C, Ruffolo G, et al. Adjunctive dopamine agonists in treatment-resistant bipolar II depression: An open case series. *Pharmacopsychiatry* 2001;34(4):137–141. doi:10.1055/s-2001-15872

133. El-Mallakh RS, Penagaluri P, Kantamneni A, et al. Long-term use of pramipexole in bipolar depression: A naturalistic retrospective chart review. *Psychiatr Q* 2010;81(3):207–213. doi:10.1007/s11126-010-9130-6

134. Dell'Osso B, Ketter TA, Cremaschi L, et al. Assessing the roles of stimulants/stimulant-like drugs and dopamine-agonists in the treatment of bipolar depression. *Curr Psychiatry Rep* 2013;15(8):378. doi:10.1007/s11920-013-0378-z

135. Burdick KE, Braga RJ, Gopin CB, et al. Dopaminergic influences on emotional decision making in euthymic bipolar patients. *Neuropsychopharmacology* 2014;39(2):274–282. doi:10.1038/npp.2013.177

136. El-Mallakh RS. An open study of methylphenidate in bipolar depression. *Bipolar Disord* 2000;2(1):56–59.

137. Carlson PJ, Merlock MC, Suppes T. Adjunctive stimulant use in patients with bipolar disorder: Treatment of residual depression and sedation. *Bipolar Disord* 2004;6(5):416–420. doi:10.1111/j.1399-5618.2004.00132.x

138. Parker G, Brotchie H. Do the old psychostimulant drugs have a role in managing treatment-resistant depression? *Acta Psychiatr Scand* 2010;121(4):308–314. doi:10.1111/j.1600-0447.2009.01434.x

139. Lydon E, El-Mallakh RS. Naturalistic long-term use of methylphenidate in bipolar disorder. *J Clin Psychopharmacol* 2006;26(5):516–518. doi:10.1097/01.jcp.0000236655.62920.dc

140. Rosell DR, Zaluda LC, McClure MM, et al. Effects of the D1 dopamine receptor agonist dihydrexidine (DAR-0100A) on working memory in schizotypal personality disorder. *Neuropsychopharmacology* 2015;40(2):446–453. doi:10.1038/npp.2014.192

141. Collingridge G. Synaptic plasticity: The role of NMDA receptors in learning and memory. *Nature* 1987;330(6149):604–605. doi:10.1038/330604a0

142. Cotman CW, Monaghan DT, Ganong AH. Excitatory amino acid neurotransmission: NMDA receptors and Hebb-type synaptic plasticity. *Annu Rev Neurosci* 1988;11:61–80. doi:10.1146/annurev.ne.11.030188.000425

143. Shapiro M. Plasticity, hippocampal place cells, and cognitive maps. *Arch Neurol* 2001;58(6):874–881.

144. Gigante AD, Bond DJ, Lafer B, et al. Brain glutamate levels measured by magnetic resonance spectroscopy in patients with bipolar disorder: A meta-analysis. *Bipolar Disord* 2012;14(5):478–487. doi:10.1111/j.1399-5618.2012.01033.x

145. Altamura CA, Mauri MC, Ferrara A, et al. Plasma and platelet excitatory amino acids in psychiatric disorders. *Am J Psychiatry* 1993;150(11):1731–1733.

146. Pålsson E, Jakobsson J, Södersten K, et al. Markers of glutamate signaling in cerebrospinal fluid and serum from patients with bipolar disorder and healthy controls. *Eur Neuropsychopharmacol* 2015;25(1):133–140. doi:10.1016/j.euroneuro.2014.11.001

147. Hashimoto K, Sawa A, Iyo M. Increased levels of glutamate in brains from patients with mood disorders. *Biol Psychiatry* 2007;62(11):1310–1316. doi:10.1016/j.biopsych.2007.03.017

148. Heresco-Levy U, Javitt DC, Ebstein R, et al. D-Serine efficacy as add-on pharmacotherapy to risperidone and olanzapine for treatment-refractory schizophrenia. *Biol Psychiatry* 2005;57(6):577–585. doi:10.1016/j.biopsych.2004.12.037

149. Kantrowitz JT, Malhotra AK, Cornblatt B, et al. High dose D-serine in the treatment of schizophrenia. *Schizophr Res* 2010;121(1–3):125–130. doi:10.1016/j.schres.2010.05.012

150. Tsai G, Yang P, Chung LC, et al. D-Serine added to antipsychotics for the treatment of schizophrenia. *Biol Psychiatry* 1998;44(11):1081–1089.

151. Weiser M, Heresco-Levy U, Davidson M, et al. A multicenter, add-on randomized controlled trial of low-dose D-serine for negative and cognitive symptoms of schizophrenia. *J Clin Psychiatry* 2012;73(6):e728–e734. doi:10.4088/JCP.11m07031

152. Levin R, Dor-Abarbanel AE, Edelman S, et al. Behavioral and cognitive effects of the *N*-methyl-D-aspartate receptor co-agonist D-serine in healthy humans: Initial findings. *J Psychiatr Res* 2015;61:188–195. doi:10.1016/j.jpsychires.2014.12.007

153. Guercio GD, Bevictori L, Vargas-Lopes C, et al. D-Serine prevents cognitive deficits induced by acute stress. *Neuropharmacology* 2014;86:1–8. doi:10.1016/j.neuropharm.2014.06.021

154. Kishi T, Iwata N. NMDA receptor antagonists interventions in schizophrenia: Meta-analysis of randomized, placebo-controlled trials. *J Psychiatr Res* 2013;47(9):1143–1149. doi:10.1016/j.jpsychires.2013.04.013

155. Lee JG, Lee SW, Lee BJ, et al. Adjunctive memantine therapy for cognitive impairment in chronic schizophrenia: A placebo-controlled pilot study. *Psychiatry Investig* 2012;9(2):166–173. doi:10.4306/pi.2012.9.2.166

156. Muhonen LH, Lönnqvist J, Juva K, et al. Double-blind, randomized comparison of memantine and escitalopram for the treatment of major depressive disorder comorbid with alcohol dependence. *J Clin Psychiatry* 2008;69(3):392–399.

157. Strzelecki D, Tabaszewska A, Barszcz Z, et al. A 10-week memantine treatment in bipolar depression—A case report: Focus on depressive symptomatology, cognitive parameters and quality of life. *Psychiatry Investig* 2013;10(4):421–424. doi:10.4306/pi.2013.10.4.421

158. Teng CT, Demetrio FN. Memantine may acutely improve cognition and have a mood stabilizing effect in treatment-resistant bipolar disorder. *Rev Bras Psiquiatr* 2006;28(3):252–254.

159. Anand A, Gunn AD, Barkay G, et al. Early antidepressant effect of memantine during augmentation of lamotrigine inadequate response in bipolar depression: A double-blind, randomized, placebo-controlled trial. *Bipolar Disord* 2012;14(1):64–70. doi:10.1111/j.1399-5618.2011.00971.x

160. Ketter TA, Manji HK, Post RM. Potential mechanisms of action of lamotrigine in the treatment of bipolar disorders. *J Clin Psychopharmacol* 2003;23(5):484–495. doi:10.1097/01.jcp.0000088915.02635.e8

161. Kaye NS, Graham J, Roberts J, et al. Effect of open-label lamotrigine as monotherapy and adjunctive therapy on the self-assessed cognitive function scores of patients with bipolar I disorder. *J Clin Psychopharmacol* 2007;27(4):387–391.

162. Khan A, Ginsberg LD, Asnis GM, et al. Effect of lamotrigine on cognitive complaints in patients with bipolar I disorder. *J Clin Psychiatry* 2004;65(11):1483–1490.

163. Daban C, Martínez-Arán A, Torrent C, et al. Cognitive functioning in bipolar patients receiving lamotrigine: Preliminary results. *J Clin Psychopharmacol* 2006;26(2):178–181. doi:10.1097/01.jcp.0000204332.64390.f3

164. Hasselmo ME. The role of acetylcholine in learning and memory. *Curr Opin Neurobiol* 2006;16(6):710–715. doi:10.1016/j.conb.2006.09.002

165. Hasselmo ME, Stern CE. Mechanisms underlying working memory for novel information. *Trends Cogn Sci* 2006;10(11):487–493. doi:10.1016/j.tics.2006.09.005

166. Hannestad JO, Cosgrove KP, DellaGioia NF, et al. Changes in the cholinergic system between bipolar depression and euthymia as measured with [123I]5IA single photon emission computed tomography. *Biol Psychiatry* 2013;74(10):768–776. doi:10.1016/j.biopsych.2013.04.004

167. Schrauwen E, Ghaemi SN. Galantamine treatment of cognitive impairment in bipolar disorder: Four cases. *Bipolar Disord* 2006;8(2):196–199. doi:10.1111/j.1399-5618.2006.00311.x

168. Elgamal S, MacQueen G. Galantamine as an adjunctive treatment in major depression. *J Clin Psychopharmacol* 2008;28(3):357–359. doi:10.1097/JCP.0b013e318172756c

169. Matthews JD, Siefert CJ, Blais MA, et al. A double-blind, placebo-controlled study of the impact of galantamine on anterograde memory impairment during electroconvulsive therapy. *J ECT.* 2013;29(3):170–178. doi:10.1097/YCT.0b013e31828b3523

170. Iosifescu DV, Moore CM, Deckersbach T, et al. Galantamine-ER for cognitive dysfunction in bipolar disorder and correlation with hippocampal neuronal viability: A proof-of-concept study. *CNS Neurosci Ther* 2009;15(4):309–319. doi:10.1111/j.1755-5949.2009.00090.x

171. Ghaemi SN, Gilmer WS, Dunn RT, et al. A double-blind, placebo-controlled pilot study of galantamine to improve cognitive dysfunction in minimally symptomatic bipolar disorder. *J Clin Psychopharmacol* 2009;29(3):291–295. doi:10.1097/JCP.0b013e3181a497d7

172. Choi K-H, Wykes T, Kurtz MM. Adjunctive pharmacotherapy for cognitive deficits in schizophrenia: Meta-analytical investigation of efficacy. *Br J Psychiatry J Ment Sci* 2013;203(3):172–178. doi:10.1192/bjp.bp.111.107359

173. Erickson SK, Schwarzkopf SB, Palumbo D, et al. Efficacy and tolerability of low-dose donepezil in schizophrenia. *Clin Neuropharmacol* 2005;28(4):179–184.

174. Pelton GH, Harper OL, Tabert MH, et al. Randomized double-blind placebo-controlled donepezil augmentation in antidepressant-treated elderly patients with depression and cognitive impairment: A pilot study. *Int J Geriatr Psychiatry* 2008;23(7):670–676. doi:10.1002/gps.1958

175. Reynolds CF, Butters MA, Lopez O, et al. Maintenance treatment of depression in old age: A randomized, double-blind, placebo-controlled evaluation of the efficacy and safety of donepezil combined with antidepressant pharmacotherapy. *Arch Gen Psychiatry* 2011;68(1):51–60. doi:10.1001/archgenpsychiatry.2010.184

176. Gildengers AG, Butters MA, Chisholm D, et al. A 12-week open-label pilot study of donepezil for cognitive functioning and instrumental activities of daily living in late-life bipolar disorder. *Int J Geriatr Psychiatry* 2008;23(7):693–698. doi:10.1002/gps.1962

177. Eden Evins A, Demopulos C, Nierenberg A, et al. A double-blind, placebo-controlled trial of adjunctive donepezil in treatment-resistant mania. *Bipolar Disord* 2006;8(1):75–80. doi:10.1111/j.1399-5618.2006.00243.x

178. Benazzi F. Mania associated with donepezil. *Int J Geriatr Psychiatry* 1998;13(11):814–815.

179. Leung JG. Donepezil-induced mania. *Consult Pharm J Am Soc Consult Pharm* 2014;29(3):191–195. doi:10.4140/TCP.n.2014.191

180. Wicklund S, Wright M. Donepezil-induced mania. *J Neuropsychiatry Clin Neurosci* 2012;24(3):E27. doi:10.1176/appi.neuropsych.11070160

181. Stip E, Sepehry AA, Chouinard S. Add-on therapy with acetylcholinesterase inhibitors for memory dysfunction in schizophrenia: A systematic quantitative review, Part 2. *Clin Neuropharmacol* 2007;30(4):218–229. doi:10.1097/WNF.0b013e318059be76

182. Wingenfeld K, Wolf OT. HPA axis alterations in mental disorders: Impact on memory and its relevance for therapeutic interventions. *CNS Neurosci Ther* 2011;17(6):714–722. doi:10.1111/j.1755-5949.2010.00207.x

183. Tsigos C, Chrousos GP. Hypothalamic–pituitary–adrenal axis, neuroendocrine factors and stress. *J Psychosom Res* 2002;53(4):865–871.

184. Het S, Ramlow G, Wolf OT. A meta-analytic review of the effects of acute cortisol administration on human memory. *Psychoneuroendocrinology* 2005;30(8):771–784. doi:10.1016/j.psyneuen.2005.03.005

185. Young AH, Sahakian BJ, Robbins TW, et al. The effects of chronic administration of hydrocortisone on cognitive function in normal male volunteers. *Psychopharmacology (Berlin)* 1999;145(3):260–266.

186. Knable MB, Barci BM, Webster MJ, et al; Stanley Neuropathology Consortium. Molecular abnormalities of the hippocampus in severe psychiatric illness: Postmortem findings from the Stanley Neuropathology Consortium. *Mol Psychiatry* 2004;9(6):609–620, 544. doi:10.1038/sj.mp.4001471

187. Xing G-Q, Russell S, Webster MJ, et al. Decreased expression of mineralocorticoid receptor mRNA in the prefrontal cortex in schizophrenia and bipolar disorder. *Int J Neuropsychopharmacol* 2004;7(2):143–153. doi:10.1017/S1461145703004000

188. Sinclair D, Webster MJ, Fullerton JM, et al. Glucocorticoid receptor mRNA and protein isoform alterations in the orbitofrontal cortex in schizophrenia and bipolar disorder. *BMC Psychiatry* 2012;12:84. doi:10.1186/1471-244X-12-84

189. Young AH. The effects of HPA axis function on cognition and its implications for the pathophysiology of bipolar disorder. *Harv Rev Psychiatry* 2014;22(6):331–333. doi:10.1097/HRP.0000000000000020

190. Rybakowski JK, Twardowska K. The dexamethasone/corticotropin-releasing hormone test in depression in bipolar and unipolar affective illness. *J Psychiatr Res* 1999;33(5):363–370.
191. Schmider J, Lammers CH, Gotthardt U, et al. Combined dexamethasone/corticotropin-releasing hormone test in acute and remitted manic patients, in acute depression, and in normal controls: I. *Biol Psychiatry* 1995;38(12):797–802. doi:10.1016/0006-3223(95)00064-X
192. Watson S, Gallagher P, Ritchie JC, et al. Hypothalamic–pituitary–adrenal axis function in patients with bipolar disorder. *Br J Psychiatry J Ment Sci* 2004;184:496–502.
193. Watson S, Thompson JM, Ritchie JC, et al. Neuropsychological impairment in bipolar disorder: The relationship with glucocorticoid receptor function. *Bipolar Disord* 2006;8(1):85–90. doi:10.1111/j.1399-5618.2006.00280.x
194. Howland RH. Mifepristone as a therapeutic agent in psychiatry. *J Psychosoc Nurs Ment Health Serv* 2013;51(6):11–14.
195. Mahajan DK, London SN. Mifepristone (RU486): A review. *Fertil Steril* 1997;68(6):967–976.
196. Young AH, Gallagher P, Watson S, et al. Improvements in neurocognitive function and mood following adjunctive treatment with mifepristone (RU-486) in bipolar disorder. *Neuropsychopharmacology* 2004;29(8):1538–1545. doi:10.1038/sj.npp.1300471
197. Rosenblat JD, Cha DS, Mansur RB, et al. Inflamed moods: A review of the interactions between inflammation and mood disorders. *Prog Neuropsychopharmacol Biol Psychiatry* 2014;53:23–34. doi:10.1016/j.pnpbp.2014.01.013
198. Goldstein BI, Kemp DE, Soczynska JK, et al. Inflammation and the phenomenology, pathophysiology, comorbidity, and treatment of bipolar disorder: A systematic review of the literature. *J Clin Psychiatry* 2009;70(8):1078–1090. doi:10.4088/JCP.08r04505
199. Bauer IE, Pascoe MC, Wollenhaupt-Aguiar B, et al. Inflammatory mediators of cognitive impairment in bipolar disorder. *J Psychiatr Res* 2014;56:18–27. doi:10.1016/j.jpsychires.2014.04.017
200. Silverman MN, Sternberg EM. Glucocorticoid regulation of inflammation and its functional correlates: From HPA axis to glucocorticoid receptor dysfunction. *Ann N Y Acad Sci* 2012;1261:55–63. doi:10.1111/j.1749-6632.2012.06633.x
201. Barbosa IG, Rocha NP, Huguet RB, et al. Executive dysfunction in euthymic bipolar disorder patients and its association with plasma biomarkers. *J Affect Disord* 2012;137(1–3):151–155. doi:10.1016/j.jad.2011.12.034
202. Dias VV, Brissos S, Frey BN, et al. Cognitive function and serum levels of brain-derived neurotrophic factor in patients with bipolar disorder. *Bipolar Disord* 2009;11(6):663–671. doi:10.1111/j.1399-5618.2009.00733.x
203. Dickerson F, Stallings C, Origoni A, et al. Elevated C-reactive protein and cognitive deficits in individuals with bipolar disorder. *J Affect Disord* 2013;150(2):456–459. doi:10.1016/j.jad.2013.04.039
204. Ayorech Z, Tracy DK, Baumeister D, et al. Taking the fuel out of the fire: Evidence for the use of anti-inflammatory agents in the treatment of bipolar disorders. *J Affect Disord* 2015;174C:467–478. doi:10.1016/j.jad.2014.12.015
205. Sargin D, Friedrichs H, El-Kordi A, et al. Erythropoietin as neuroprotective and neuroregenerative treatment strategy: Comprehensive overview of 12 years of preclinical and clinical research. *Best Pract Res Clin Anaesthesiol* 2010;24(4):573–594. doi:10.1016/j.bpa.2010.10.005
206. Sirén A-L, Fasshauer T, Bartels C, et al. Therapeutic potential of erythropoietin and its structural or functional variants in the nervous system. *Neurother J Am Soc Exp Neurother* 2009;6(1):108–127. doi:10.1016/j.nurt.2008.10.041
207. Ehrenreich H, Hinze-Selch D, Stawicki S, et al. Improvement of cognitive functions in chronic schizophrenic patients by recombinant human erythropoietin. *Mol Psychiatry* 2007;12(2):206–220. doi:10.1038/sj.mp.4001907
208. Miskowiak KW, Vinberg M, Christensen EM, et al. Recombinant human erythropoietin for treating treatment-resistant depression: A double-blind, randomized, placebo-controlled Phase 2 trial. *Neuropsychopharmacology* 2014;39(6):1399–1408. doi:10.1038/npp.2013.335

209. Miskowiak KW, Ehrenreich H, Christensen EM, et al. Recombinant human erythropoietin to target cognitive dysfunction in bipolar disorder: A double-blind, randomized, placebo-controlled Phase 2 trial. *J Clin Psychiatry* 2014;75(12):1347–1355. doi:10.4088/JCP.13m08839

210. Miskowiak KW, Vinberg M, Macoveanu J, et al. Effects of erythropoietin on hippocampal volume and memory in mood disorders. *Biol Psychiatry* 2015;15;78(4):270–277. doi:10.1016/j.biopsych.2014.12.013

211. Mercedes Perez-Rodriguez M, Mahon K, Russo M, et al. Oxytocin and social cognition in affective and psychotic disorders. *Eur Neuropsychopharmacol* 2015;25(2):265–282. doi:10.1016/j.euroneuro.2014.07.012

212. Samamé C, Martino DJ, Strejilevich SA. Social cognition in euthymic bipolar disorder: Systematic review and meta-analytic approach. *Acta Psychiatr Scand* 2012;125(4):266–280. doi:10.1111/j.1600-0447.2011.01808.x

213. Barlati S, Deste G, De Peri L, et al. Cognitive remediation in schizophrenia: Current status and future perspectives. *Schizophr Res Treat* 2013;2013:156084. doi:10.1155/2013/156084

214. Deckersbach T, Nierenberg AA, Kessler R, et al. RESEARCH: Cognitive rehabilitation for bipolar disorder: An open trial for employed patients with residual depressive symptoms. *CNS Neurosci Ther* 2010;16(5):298–307. doi:10.1111/j.1755-5949.2009.00110.x

215. Torrent C, Bonnin C del M, Martínez-Arán A, et al. Efficacy of functional remediation in bipolar disorder: A multicenter randomized controlled study. *Am J Psychiatry* 2013;170(8):852–859. doi:10.1176/appi.ajp.2012.12070971

216. Breitborde NJ, Dawson SC, Woolverton C, et al. A randomized controlled trial of cognitive remediation and D-cycloserine for individuals with bipolar disorder. *BMC Psychol* 2014;2(1):41. doi:10.1186/s40359-014-0041-4

217. Olvet DM, Burdick KE, Cornblatt BA. Assessing the potential to use neurocognition to predict who is at risk for developing bipolar disorder: A review of the literature. *Cognit Neuropsychiatry* 2013;18(1–2):129–145. doi:10.1080/13546805.2012.724193

218. Vieta E, Popovic D, Rosa AR, et al. The clinical implications of cognitive impairment and allostatic load in bipolar disorder. *Eur Psychiatry* 2013;28(1):21–29. doi:10.1016/j.eurpsy.2011.11.007

219. Manove E, Levy B. Cognitive impairment in bipolar disorder: An overview. *Postgrad Med.* 2010;122(4):7–16. doi:10.3810/pgm.2010.07.2170

220. Harvey PD, Wingo AP, Burdick KE, et al. Cognition and disability in bipolar disorder: Lessons from schizophrenia research. *Bipolar Disord* 2010;12(4):364–375. doi:10.1111/j.1399-5618.2010.00831.x

221. Burdick KE, Ketter TA, Goldberg JF, et al. Assessing cognitive function in bipolar disorder: Challenges and recommendations for clinical trial design. *J Clin Psychiatry* 2015;76(3):e342–e350. doi:10.4088/JCP.14cs09399

222. Buchanan RW, Davis M, Goff D, et al. A summary of the FDA–NIMH–MATRICS workshop on clinical trial design for neurocognitive drugs for schizophrenia. *Schizophr Bull* 2005;31(1):5–19. doi:10.1093/schbul/sbi020

TWELVE

Autism, Attention Deficit Hyperactivity Disorder, and Cognitive Enhancement

IULIA DUD, LOUISE BRENNAN, AND DENE ROBERTSON

INTRODUCTION

This chapter considers two common neurodevelopmental disorders: attention deficit hyperactivity disorder (ADHD) and autism spectrum disorder (ASD). The latter includes childhood autism, high-functioning autism, Asperger's syndrome, atypical autism, and pervasive developmental disorder not otherwise specified. The chapter also discusses the postulated underlying etiological factors and associated cognitive deficits, and it reviews the interventions available to enhance cognitive functioning and ameliorate the difficulties associated with these disorders.

The spectrum of cognitive enhancements for neurodevelopmental disorders includes medical interventions, psychosocial interventions, as well as improvements of external technological and institutional structures that support cognition.

Michael Rutter's extensive work on neurodevelopment and cognitive processing described continuities, as well as discontinuities, in the span of behavioral variation from normality to psychopathology. Currently, there is little understanding of the neurobiological basis of ADHD and ASD. Lack of such knowledge prevents the definition of biological criteria that can validate the diagnoses.[1] The diagnoses of neurodevelopmental disorders are currently based on schedules that examine behaviors that lie along spectra. ADHD is often characterized by a triad of attentional, hyperactive, and impulsive symptom clusters[2] that impair function in the home and school. ASD is characterized by qualitative impairments in two core domains: social communication and restricted interests and repetitive behaviors.[2] Clinical heterogeneity is prominent, and symptom severity may vary across the life span.

Comorbidity among individuals with neurodevelopmental disorders is common. There are often accompanying complex medical and psychiatric disorders including intellectual disabilities, affective disorders, anxiety symptoms, and atypical sensory processing. Intellectual disability is the most commonly associated condition in people with ASD; approximately 50% have a comorbid intellectual disability.[3] However, intellectual functioning in individuals with ASD can range from those with disability to the superior range. Core autistic symptoms vary independently of IQ measures and can be equally severe in those with average and above-average IQ.[4] Cognitive profiling of individuals with neurodevelopmental disorders is typically uneven, with areas of both strength and deficit.

Cognitive deficits seen in neurodevelopmental disorders may operate in both direct and indirect ways, resulting in the characteristic behaviors that underpin diagnostic schedules for these conditions. Autism constitutes an example of hypothesized direct effects.[5] Early behavioral manifestations of ASD typically occur within the first year of life and include the social communication skills of eye contact and joint attentional behaviors. The acquisition of such skills has significant consequences for later social and language competence.[6,7]

A wide variety of cognitive deficits may underlie autistic individuals' failure to engage in normal reciprocal responsive social interchanges that constitute the social incapacity that defines the disorder.[8] ASD is the prototypical social dysfunction disorder, but deficits in social behavior are present in a number of other disorders, such as schizophrenia. Similarly, it has been argued that attentional deficits may constitute the core of both hyperkinetic disorders[9] and schizophrenia,[10] with the specific type of attentional problems not quite the same in the two conditions.[11] Possible indirect effects of cognitive deficits are exemplified by the relatively strong and well-documented associations between language retardation and psychiatric disorder[12] and between reading disabilities and conduct disorders.[13] There is much to be understood about the mechanisms involved in these associations, but it is generally presumed that in some manner cognitive development plays a crucial role in psychiatric disorders.

There are two-way interactions between cognition and emotion. Affective states also influence cognitive processing, as the evidence on the effects of mood on memory and concentration shows.[14] It would be unwise to suppose that either cognition or affect was primary; development involves an integrated organization of the two.[15] It seems reasonable to suppose that if cognitive processing is so important in people's appraisal of and response to experiences, then abnormalities or limitations in the ability to undertake such cognitive processing might have profound implications for the risk of psychiatric disorder. The empirical evidence suggests that this is indeed the case, although the mechanisms by which the psychiatric risk comes about remain unclear.

ATTENTION DEFICIT HYPERACTIVITY DISORDER

Attention deficit hyperactivity disorder is the most common developmental disorder of childhood, affecting 3–7% of children and often continuing into adulthood.[16] The long-term consequences of childhood ADHD include lower educational and vocational outcomes and increased risk for antisocial disorders and drug abuse in adulthood.[17]

Cognitive deficits, particularly impairments in attention and executive function, are an important component of ADHD.[18-24] ADHD was initially regarded as primarily a hyperactive disorder;[25] however, during the past two decades there has been a growing emphasis on the associated cognitive dysfunction,[26,27] with increased appreciation of the long-term influence that cognitive deficits in ADHD may have on morbidity. The attentional cluster of symptoms of ADHD includes inattention, distractibility, shifting activities, forgetfulness, poor attention to detail, poor follow through, and organizational difficulties. Highlighting the critical importance of core cognitive symptoms in ADHD are consistent findings that these deficits persist,[28,29] despite reductions in hyperactivity and impulsive symptoms over time.[30] In keeping with this, the evidence shows that the presence of cognitive dysfunction is particularly common in adolescents and adults with ADHD, with greater than 90% of adults seeking treatment for ADHD manifesting cognitive dysfunction.[30] Moreover, individuals with pronounced cognitive deficits in ADHD (e.g., particular learning disabilities or dysfunction on multiple tests of neuropsychological functioning) are at heightened risk for more academic and occupational difficulties.[31]

The reduction in ADHD symptoms across the life span may result from noncortical neural dysfunction that persists throughout life but is compensated for by more complex, later developed prefrontally mediated executive and other higher order cortical functions.[32,33] The extent to which these higher cortical functions compensate for the primary dysfunction accounts for the degree of reduction in symptom intensity and hence the recovery from ADHD. This hypothesis also implies the idea that the prefrontal cortex (PFC) and other cortical functions are more involved with the recovery from illness rather than its etiology.

This hypothesis is consistent with data suggesting that trajectories of cortical development throughout middle childhood might be closely linked to ADHD outcomes[34] and that lower reaction time variability is associated with increased activation of the prefrontal circuit (prefrontal cortex and caudate) in children with ADHD.[35] This latter finding may be interpreted as prefrontal compensation for a more primary motor deficiency. In addition, functional magnetic resonance imaging (fMRI) findings indicate that PFC activation in response to inhibition, in adolescents with childhood ADHD, corresponds to the persistence of symptoms such that those who are less symptomatic appear more like never-ADHD controls.[36] Finally, longitudinal data[37] from studies examining neurocognitive functioning in adults who had ADHD in childhood indicate that only those in whom ADHD has persisted differ from controls on measures of executive functions such as working memory, sustained attention, and inhibitory control.

The hypothesized developmentally related compensation for earlier deficits may also be related to changes in functional connectivity in the brain that occur during development. For example, Dosenbach et al.[38] described two distinct "top-down" functional control networks in adults—a frontoparietal network involved in adaptive online task control and a cingulo-opercular network involved in more stable set control. When compared across groups of children, adolescents, and adults, a clear pattern of developmentally related differences emerged such that short-range connections associated with these networks decreased and long-range connections increased across development.[39] These findings suggest greater segregation between networks as well as improved integration within networks with increased age. It is possible that these developmental processes that support the maturation of this dual-network control system play a critical role in the hypothesized compensation for earlier deficits in youth with ADHD. Notably, this pattern of developmental decreases in local connectivity and increases in long-range connectivity does not appear limited to these specific neural systems. Rather, it appears to be a more general developmental principle that operates throughout the brain.[40]

AUTISM SPECTRUM DISORDER

Autism spectrum disorder effects 1 in 68 individuals in the United States.[41] Deficits in social cognition manifest in behaviors that vary across the life span as social demands change. Prognosis in individuals with ASD is poor in terms of functioning.[42] Most adults with ASD live dependent lives with their parents or in supported living. Fewer than one-third are employed, and they are often paid less than a living wage.[43] Levy and Perry[43] found that across studies, 90–95% of individuals with ASD were unable to establish long-term meaningful romantic or platonic relationships. There has been an increase in the diagnosed incidence of ASD,[44] with implications for individuals, families, and services. Therefore, the provision of timely, effective, evidenced-based interventions to improve core deficits in social skills and communication, limit the impact of repetitive behaviors and restricted interests, optimize quality of life, and increase functioning is of paramount importance.[45]

There are several cognitive models for ASD. The temporal primacy hypothesis postulates that a single deficit in a cognitive domain gives rise to additional deficits as the brain matures. The neural system hypothesis suggests that deficits arise because of abnormalities in a particular cortical region or network. Candidate networks include the executive function or dorsolateral PFC network and the theory of mind or medial frontal network. Another postulated mechanism underlying autism is altered connectivity, with intact simple local processing but impaired complex distributed processing.[46]

Brain circuits involved in social behaviors, verbal communication, and nonverbal communication are hierarchical in nature and dependent on lower level sensory, motor, and homeostatic regulatory components.[47] Neuroimaging studies have shown that the paracingulate gyrus of the medial PFC, the temporoparietal junction of the superior temporal sulcus, and the temporal poles show decreased activity in individuals in ASD during mentalizing tasks.[48] The medial frontal region is utilized when individuals reflect on internal mental states, whereas the inferior orbital region shows activation when responding to emotional states. The right temporoparietal junction is integral to the representations of the beliefs of others.[49]

The posterior superior temporal sulcus is central in the perception of intentionality in human action and also the perception of biological motion. Biological motion detection arises in the first days of life and is separate from the development of the visual system. It facilitates complex attributions about identity, activity, and emotional states,[50] and it shows reduced activity in individuals with ASD.[51] Activity in the fusiform face area is diminished in individuals with ASD,[52] but less so when the faces presented are familiar.[53] The preference for attending to faces seen in neurotypical individuals from 3 months[54] of age is absent in those with ASD.[55] Other differences in visual attention are also present, including a tendency to fixate on the mouth instead of the eyes.[56]

Other regions of interest in the social brain include the amygdala and limbic system, which are involved in the perception of emotional states and emotional experience, as well as the evaluation of social and nonsocial information for signs of danger. The action-perception system of the inferior frontal gyrus and inferior parietal lobe and the extrastriate body area in the lateral occipitotemporal area are also important in social behavior.

COGNITIVE DEFICITS

Attention Deficit Hyperactivity Disorder

Cognitive models of ADHD posit executive,[57] motivational,[58] inhibitory control,[59] cognitive-energetic,[60] and reward-related[61] deficits as being central to the etiology of ADHD. Recent research has focused on multiple causal pathways that lead to the development of ADHD during childhood.[62,63]

Executive Functions

Deficits in executive functioning are thought to be at the core of cognitive dysfunction in ADHD. Pennington defines executive function as "the ability to maintain an appropriate problem solving set for attainment of a future goal including selecting the option that is most appropriate for that specific set of circumstances."[57,64]

Specific dimensions of executive functions vary to some extent between studies. Separable dimensions of executive functions have typically included the ability to inhibit maladaptive behaviors (response inhibition/inhibitory control), hold and manipulate information in memory (working memory), shift back and forth between two simultaneous tasks (set shifting), and suppress attention to extraneous information in the environment to increase focus on a target (interference control). Some cognitive theories of ADHD suggest an association with a more focal weakness in a specific domain of executive functions, such as response inhibition, than a global executive functions deficit.[65] Interindividual variation in the magnitude of these impairments in ADHD has also become evident.

Research shows that the primary neural circuit involved includes the thalamus, basal ganglia, cerebellum, and PFC; however, several distributed neural networks appear to play a role in executive functions.[57,64] Studies using structural MRI to measure the volume of different brain regions found that groups with ADHD consistently have smaller volumes in the area of PFC that is most closely involved in executive functions,[66] and several fMRI studies have reported differences in brain activity in these regions when groups with and without ADHD are completing an executive functions task.[67,68] Weaknesses in these prefrontal regions are thought to interact with dysfunction in subcortical regions, including striatal regions and the cerebellum, to produce executive functions deficits in ADHD patients.[69] Previous theoretical models of ADHD often invoked the notion of "executive control" as a single unified construct. However, exploratory and confirmatory factor analyses of executive functions tasks and results from fMRI studies suggest that executive functions may be more accurately described as a collection of related but separable abilities.[70,71]

Processing Speed

Although no theoretical models of ADHD explicitly propose slow cognitive processing speed as the primary neuropsychological weakness in ADHD, deficits in this domain are among the most robust predictors of ADHD symptoms.[72] Slow processing speed has been reported in groups with ADHD on a range of measures that require both verbal and nonverbal responses.[73] The overall effect size for processing speed is the largest effect in meta-analyses of studies of both children and adults with ADHD.[74] The neurophysiology of slow processing speed is not well understood, but generalized low cortical arousal is one potential explanation.

Reward Sensitivity

A neural circuit that includes ventromedial PFC, the amygdala, and other limbic structures plays an essential role in coordinating the interface between motivation and cognition during decision-making processes.[75] Damage to this network often leads to difficulty learning from mistakes, delaying gratification, and monitoring subtle shifts in reward and punishment probabilities to maximize the short- and long-term benefits of a choice. Two studies report a correlation between reduced ventromedial prefrontal cortex volume and ADHD.[76]

Several slightly varying models suggest that ADHD is attributable to a dysfunctional response to reward and punishment contingencies.[77,78] Delay aversion is a special variant of the dysfunctional reward sensitivity model that suggests that children with ADHD have a motivational style that leads them to find delay extremely aversive.[79]

Response Variability

Compared to healthy controls, children, adolescents, and adults with ADHD present with a higher variability of reaction time (RT) across a wide set of neurocognitive tasks.[80–82] The overall effect size of the group difference is medium to large in magnitude, and it is similar to the effects observed for response inhibition and working memory tasks.[83] One theory proposes that a slower overall reaction time in conjunction with measurement error gives rise to the characteristic difficulties of ADHD; consistent findings seem to support this theory.[84] However, the difference in response variability between groups with and without ADHD is not eliminated when mean RT is controlled, and more complex statistical models of RT distributions suggest that increased response variability may be due to a relatively small number of trials with extremely long RTs rather than systematically greater response variability across all trials.[85] One theoretical model suggests that these slow trials reflect attentional lapses due to chronic underarousal or inconsistent regulation of arousal during lengthy tasks and that these attentional lapses are related to compromises in the functional connectivity between anterior cingulate and precuneal regions.[86,87] Another theoretical account of reaction time abnormalities suggests that greater response variability could result from dysfunction in short-duration timing mechanisms that are largely mediated by cerebellar circuits.[88,89]

Social Interaction and Social Cognition

Many children with ADHD have difficulties with social interaction, affecting relationships with parents, family, friends, and other significant adults such as teachers. These difficulties can be severe. Although medication can help in the management of core behavioral symptoms, it is not designed to address skills deficits. Pervasive social difficulties have an implicit impact on academic performance and achievement. How much of the academic achievement is actually modulated by social cognitive deficits (i.e., impairments in face perception, theory of mind, reduced empathy, and emotional prosody perception[90]) remains unknown, and it is very likely that the behavioral symptoms of ADHD bear a considerable weight. To this effect, some studies examining group differences in IQ level and academic performance argue that the neuropsychological deficits associated with ADHD are likely to explain this,[91–93] whereas others consider ADHD symptoms to have a direct impact on participants' performance on standardized tests, resulting in poor scores.[94]

Autism Spectrum Disorder

Postulated deficits in three principal neuropsychological domains have attracted attention as the key cognitive impairment underlying the autistic phenotype: central coherence, executive dysfunction, and social cognition. When the diversity of behaviors across domains and subtypes in ASD is considered, these theories may be complementary rather than competitive.

Weak Central Coherence

Modifications of the weak central coherence theory, originally proposed by Firth,[95] propose a superiority in local or detail-focused information processing in individuals with ASD rather than a core deficit in central processing preventing extraction of global form and meaning. Weak central coherence can be overcome in tasks with explicit demands in global processing.[96] Suggesting central coherence is a continuum with individual differences in the default balance between weak and strong central coherence, difficulty may arise in shifting between modes of processing, reflecting executive functioning deficits. Global integrative processing skills are predominantly mediated by the right hemispheric areas, whereas local featural processing is associated with left hemisphere functioning.[97] The weak central coherence theory is attractive in that it also explains areas of cognitive strength seen in approximately 1 in 10 individuals with ASD.

Enhanced Perceptual Functioning

This model of autism was originally proposed as an alternative to the weak central coherence theory. This model suggests higher order processing is inadequate for the perceptual flow of information. This imbalance in higher and lower order processing disrupts the development of other behaviors and abilities.[98] The mandatory higher order processing seen in neurotypical individuals is in contrast to that in individuals with ASD, in whom higher order control is not mandatory if it interferes with task processing. In the enhanced perceptual functioning model, restricted interests are an adaptation rooted in perceptual processing superiority.

Multisensory Processing and Integration

Sensory inputs processed in modality-specific areas are integrated with other modalities in dedicated association areas. Abnormal sensitivity to temperature, pain, and auditory or visual stimuli can be present in ASD.[99] Abnormalities in sensory processing often give rise to symptoms within the first 2 years of life in individuals with ASD.[100] The diagnostically relevant behaviors that arise depend on whether an individual is sensory seeking or sensory avoidant, a reflection of hypo- or hyperreactivity to stimuli that may persist throughout the life span.[101,102]

Motion Perception

There is neuroimaging evidence of abnormal visual perception processing underlying a number of symptoms of social cognition, such as processing of faces and facial expression, as well as nontriadic symptoms. Bertone et al.[103] suggest that deficits in this processing domain can be separated into positive (e.g., preoccupation with flickering or spinning objects) and negative (e.g., absence of eye contact) symptoms, and they can also give rise to nontriadic symptoms. These authors found that individuals with autism and normal intelligence process motion stimuli, which require additional neural processing, less efficiently at the perceptual level and possibly at higher levels as well.

Diminished Processing of Complexity

In this theory, it is suggested that high processing demands are common to all areas of impairment and that these deficits give rise to the core symptoms and associated difficulties, such as those involving memory, motor functioning, sensory processing, the postural control system, and the oculomotor system.[104–106] It is hypothesized that intact or enhanced abilities involve low-level cognitive or neurologic processes. It is argued that symptoms are most prominent in domains that place the highest demands on higher order processing and integration of information—the social, communication, and reasoning areas.

Right Hemisphere Dysfunction

Increased right hemisphere activity is seen with global tasks and in suppressing repetitive stereotyped behavior. Right hemisphere damage can give rise to difficulties in visuospatial constructional abilities that are similar to those seen in individuals with weak central coherence,[107] with the maintenance of details from local processing but deficits in global processing abilities. Individuals with this type of damage also struggle with integrating verbal information and extracting gist.[108] However, to date, there is little evidence of right hemisphere damage in individuals with ASD.

Executive Dysfunction

Individuals with autism have difficulty with several cognitive skills that are mediated by the PFC, such as response inhibition, working memory, cognitive flexibility, planning, and fluency.[57,109–111] Deficits in these functions can appear as impairments in planning and managing a task, monitoring task performance, keeping multiple tasks in working memory, shifting attention, and the ability to disengage from a task.[112] These difficulties may underlie the repetitive and inflexible core behaviors seen in ASD.

There is increasing evidence for comorbidity between ADHD and ASD.[113–115] The predominant executive functioning deficit seen in ADHD is poor motor response inhibition, which is less consistently seen in individuals with ASD.[116,117] Poor inhibitory control may manifest as impulsiveness in ADHD and motor stereotypies in ASD.[118] Executive attention regulation, involving attention control and inhibitory control, underlies joint attention development, which is diminished in children with ASD.[119,120]

Executive dysfunction in ASD results in poor flexibility, generativity, and planning. The cognitive functions of working memory and cognitive flexibility are central to these tasks. Cognitive flexibility involves both switching and reward reversal learning, with deficits linked to repetitive behaviors in ASD.[121] Switching tasks involve a number of regions of the frontal lobes, including the inferior frontal cortex, dorsolateral prefrontal cortex, anterior cingulate cortex (ACC), as well as the parietal lobe and anterior striatum.[122–128] Reward reversal learning tasks involve assessment of the emotional valence of the reward and punishment present. These tasks involve the medial prefrontal cortex, medial orbitofrontal cortex, ACC,[152–157][129–134] as well as ventral striatal regions involved in reward-related habitual learning and stimulus–response associations.[131,135,136]

Social Cognition

Social cognition relates to how people process, store, and apply information about other people and social interactions, with a particular emphasis on the role of thought processes. The social perception and information processing group of theories of ASD includes the social motivation hypothesis and theory of mind. Social theories adequately explain social communication deficits but struggle to describe the origins of repetitive behaviors and restricted interests, as well as areas of cognitive strength, sensory processing difficulties, intellectual disabilities, and comorbid psychiatric illness seen in ASD.

Theory of Mind

Theory of mind (ToM) is the capacity to attribute subjective mental states to others and oneself in order to explain and predict behavior.[137] Deficits in mentalizing spontaneously affect the ability to discern the emotions, knowledge, beliefs, desires, and intentions of others, impacting on social behavior. Difficulties with ToM are seen in multiple psychiatric conditions, including ASD and ADHD.[138,139]

Theory of mind may represent a single integrated ability or two separate or related constructs, namely social reasoning and intrapersonal reasoning—the ability to reason about others' and one's own mental states, respectively. There has been recent support for the differentiated functional multilinear socialization model, in which, for children with ASD, weaknesses in social ToM are more pronounced than interpersonal reasoning deficits. This disparity between social and interpersonal reasoning is more exaggerated in children with the more severe form of ASD (childhood autism) compared to those with less severe forms (e.g., Asperger's syndrome).[140] Proposed underlying mechanisms of ToM deficits include the social–affective hypothesis[141] and specific developmental delays in joint attentional behaviors.[142]

Social Motivation

The social motivation hypothesis proposes that the primary deficit in ASD is reduced motivation to engage in social activities such as joint attention and eye gaze because these activities are less rewarding for those with ASD compared to neurotypical individuals.[143] This decreases motivation to engage in social interaction and avail of learning opportunities, with subsequent social cognition and social skills deficits. It is argued that social motivation represents an evolutionary adaptation that serves to enhance the individual's fitness in collaborative environments.

Of the brain regions involved in social motivation, the amygdala is central in guiding attention to visual social stimuli such as the eyes, face, and biological motion.[144] The ventral striatum is important in computing salience of social stimuli alongside the orbitofrontal cortex.[145] The latter is also important in transforming reward inputs from the amygdala and ventral striatum into subjective hedonic value that guides goal-directed action and executive systems. Reduced activation in reward centers in response to social stimuli for ASD individuals[146,147] may reflect a general reward processing deficit.[148,149]

COGNITIVE ENHANCEMENT

Treatments for neurodevelopmental disorders should be tailored to alleviate the impact of core impairments and associated symptoms as well as improve functional capacity and quality of life of both individuals and their carers.[150] These chronic conditions require sustained intervention over time commencing as early as possible in the course, with consolidation of any therapeutic gains. Traditionally, treatments have focused on the control of problem behaviors and have not targeted possible underlying cognitive difficulties.

The evidence base for treatment interventions in neurodevelopmental disorders, particularly ASD, is limited and should be interpreted with caution. First, studies are prone to type I errors due to multiple comparisons in individual studies, including symptom cluster subscores, across separate domains and using different assessment tools. Second, small sample sizes and short follow-up increase the risk of type II errors. Third, many studies involve clinical heterogeneous samples and fail to separate individuals with higher and lower intellectual capabilities. Fourth, studies often lack consistency in how outcomes are measured, leading to an inability to assess pooled effects.

A wide range of treatment interventions have been developed that may potentially enhance cognition, including behavioral, educational, medical, allied health, and complementary treatments.

Attention Deficit Hyperactivity Disorder

Research on the neurochemistry of ADHD indicates that there is not a single neurotransmitter abnormality that is responsible for the symptoms of ADHD.[151] Dopamine and norepinephrine have attracted the most attention, largely due to the positive therapeutic effects of psychostimulants. Imbalance between these two systems may result in symptoms of ADHD.[152] Support derives from neuroimaging studies, which reveal anatomical changes in dopamine-rich brain regions such as the globus pallidus and frontal cortex in children with ADHD.[153] Subjects with ADHD also display reduced frontal and striatal activity during relevant cognitive tasks,[154,155] which may be related to reduced dopaminergic tone. Other changes observed in individuals with ADHD include reduced noradrenergic activity, altered dopamine reuptake, and changes in the dopamine D_4 receptor.[156]

Autism Spectrum Disorder

As with ADHD, there is no overwhelming indication of a causative role for a single neurotransmitter abnormality in ASD. There is evidence of a role for serotonin in the pathogenesis of both conditions.[157,158] Serotonin is involved in multiple neurobiological pathways, including those that mediate mood, social interaction, sleep, obsessive–compulsive behaviors, and aggression. It is an obvious candidate for manipulation by pharmacological means to alleviate the symptoms associated with ASD. There are reports of lower platelet serotonin levels in ADHD children compared to controls;[159] in contrast, 30% of individuals with ASD have enhanced platelet serotonin levels.[160] There is widespread dysfunction in the serotonin system of individuals with ASD, as evidenced by abnormal 5-hydroxytryptamine (5-HT) synthesis[161] and reduced binding to the 5-HT reuptake transporter and 5-HT2A receptors in the frontal lobe and posterior cingulate cortex, with the latter having been linked to poor social communication.[162,163] The increase in serotonin levels may therefore counteract the decreased receptor binding.[162] Serotonin functioning is central to executive functioning, including motor inhibition,[164] verbal working memory,[165,166] and cognitive flexibility, which may be disrupted in individuals with ASD. Other neurotransmitters that are implicated in the pathogenesis of ASD include the GABAergic system[167] and glutamate,[168] which have been postulated to result in an excitatory/inhibitory balance.[169]

Pharmacological Interventions for ADHD

Stimulant Medications

Current treatments for ADHD consist mainly of psychostimulants (e.g., methylphenidate and amphetamine), which are thought to exert their effects by increasing both dopaminergic and noradrenergic neurotransmission.[170] Stimulant medications have been well demonstrated to significantly reduce ADHD symptoms, as measured by both parent and teacher ratings. These effects include reductions on ratings of activity levels, hyperactivity/impulsivity, and inattention.[171] In addition, psychostimulant treatment has been shown to improve "non-ADHD" symptoms such as teacher-reported social skills,[172] and aggressive behavior in the school setting, contributing to improvements in classroom performance.[170,172]

The exact mechanisms by which psychostimulants produce improvements in ADHD symptoms remain unclear. It is also not entirely certain which dopaminergic system(s) is involved or how it regulates behavior. Recent neuroimaging studies suggest blockade of presynaptic dopamine in the striatum,[173,174] with significant increases in extracellular dopamine levels and possibly even more affinity for blockade of the norepinephrine transporter.[175] Moreover, psychostimulants have greater effects on overt behavioral features of the disorder as measured by observer-rated behavior checklists than on cognitive domains measured in the laboratory.[171] The reduction of motor activity associated with administration of psychostimulants also follows a different dose–response curve than that for the effects on cognition (i.e., sustained attention).[176]

Studies of normal volunteers indicate that psychostimulants improve performance on a broad array of tasks and that these improvements are not specific to individuals with ADHD.[175] Extensive work examining the effects of stimulants on attentional and executive processes has not found consistent evidence that stimulants enhance or ameliorate ADHD cognitive deficits.[177,178] Although reaction times are significantly reduced, performance on tasks with increased attentional or executive demands is not consistently improved by stimulants.[179] Furthermore, although short-term improvements in academic achievement scores have been demonstrated with stimulant treatment, stimulant medications do not normalize long-term academic achievement in children with ADHD and improvement was shown not to be sustained at follow-up.[180] Similarly, although largely unknown, available evidence suggests that deficits in social cognition are not restored with stimulant treatment and emotional regulation is minimally improved, but still impaired, compared to that of the healthy population.[181]

Nonstimulant Medications

ATOMOXETINE

Atomoxetine is the most widely used nonstimulant for treatment of ADHD. Although of a lower efficacy compared to stimulant drugs,[182] atomoxetine has been well established as effectively treating ADHD during the past two decades,[183] often preferred due to its lower addictive potential.[184,185] Atomoxetine's mechanism of action is described by increasing the levels of norepinephrine through its uptake inhibition, mainly in the PFC,[186,187] in a dose-dependent manner.[188] It has been found to have an inhibitory effect on binding of both serotonin and dopamine, with a similar preference for the PFC.[186] Recent studies have also put forward the hypothesis of possible antihistaminic and cholinergic implications; however, these theories require much more research to be fully understood.[211–213189–191]

There is little literature to date on the effects of atomoxetine on cognitive function in ADHD, and more evidence is required to reach any robust conclusions. Early research suggests that it may have a beneficial effect on specific deficits such as visuospatial memory and inhibitory control in children with ADHD and reading disorder;[192] a set of executive functions including set shifting, spatial short-term memory, sustained attention, inhibitory control, spatial working memory, spatial planning, and problem-solving;[193] and regulation of alertness and modulation of emotion and working memory.[194]

CLONIDINE AND GUANFACINE

Clonidine and guanfacine are α_2 agonists and usually prescribed as second-line therapies. This may be in the context of stimulant intolerance, combined with stimulant medication or comorbid tic disorder. The α_2 agonists mimic norepinephrine actions in the PFC through the stimulation of α_{2A} receptors on PFC neurons.[195] In humans, research on the effects of α_2 agonists on cognition has shown considerable inconsistencies and is difficult to interpret in the context of ADHD. One randomized control trial of guanfacine in individuals with ADHD and tic disorder showed that guanfacine improved cognitive performance on measures of sustained attention and response inhibition on a Continuous Performance Task.[196]

ANTIDEPRESSANTS

Antidepressants (tricyclic antidepressants, monoamine oxidase inhibitors (MAOI), and bupropion) have been used as treatment alternatives in ADHD.[197,198] There is little understanding of how antidepressants might impact cognitive function in ADHD; however, a number of studies have shown a more general beneficial effect on cognition in depression (improving learning and memory)[199,200] and schizophrenia (improving set shifting and reaction time variability).[201] Rubinstein et al.[202] described the effects of selegiline on ADHD symptoms in a placebo-controlled study, indicating that it improved cognitive deficits such as sustained attention and learning of novel information.

The side effect profile of tricyclic and MAOI antidepressants remains an impediment for widely prescribing these drugs to ADHD—a population of mainly children and young adults.

NICOTINIC AGENTS

A large literature demonstrates the bidirectional overlap of ADHD and cigarette smoking/nicotine use.[203] Nicotinic cholinergic neurotransmission plays an important role in attention and executive function processes, and nicotine has demonstrated pro-cognitive effects in a number of animal studies, with emerging data regarding efficacy in the ADHD population. A substantial literature has also identified cognitive improvements associated with nicotine administration in human non-ADHD subjects,[204,205] from improved visual information processing[206] to reaction time[207] and vigilance.[208] Beneficial cognitive enhancing effects of nicotine have been described in other conditions associated with cognitive impairment, such as Alzheimer's disease[209] and schizophrenia.[210]

In ADHD, modest effects on cognition have been shown, particularly when nicotine was administered in a patch form as part of a combined therapy with methylphenidate.[211,212] The considerable side effect profile and concern regarding cardiovascular and gastrointestinal toxicity have precluded the widespread prescribing of nicotine.[213] A small number of nicotinic agonists have been approved for administration to humans and tested in samples of individuals with ADHD. ABT-418, which preferentially targets the $\alpha_4\beta_2$ receptor, has been shown to improve memory in preclinical studies.[214] Although ABT-418 was found to improve ADHD symptoms in a randomized crossover trial in adults with ADHD,[215] its effects on cognitive performance were not assessed. More recently, another agonist targeting the $\alpha_4\beta_2$ receptor, ABT-089, was evaluated in a small sample of adults with ADHD.[216] In that study, ABT-089 resulted in dose-dependent improvements in working memory and response inhibition. Whereas other nicotinic agonists have been tested in Alzheimer's disease and other patient populations, no data on their effects in ADHD patients are currently available. Considerable further research is needed before therapeutic interventions using nicotinic agents can be used as mainstream prescribing to enhance cognitive function in ADHD.

CHOLINESTERASE INHIBITORS/N-METHYL-D-ASPARTATE ANTAGONISTS

Although this class has been widely studied and discussed for its pro-cognitive properties in dementing syndromes such as Alzheimer's disease, less evidence has been gathered to date for ADHD.[217–220] There are currently no systematic reviews and no studies evaluating combined therapy (i.e., cholinesterase inhibitors + N-methyl-D-aspartate (NMDA) antagonists). Donepezil showed modest results in improving functioning in children with ADHD and pervasive developmental disorders or tics;[219,220] however, it had little or no impact on cognitive functioning/dysexecutive syndrome of ADHD.[217,218] Galantamine showed equally disappointing results in a placebo-controlled, double-blind study,[221] with no statistically relevant effects on any of the cognitive measures. Similarly, the NMDA antagonist memantine, which has good cognitive enhancing properties in dementia,[222] showed only modest, dose-dependent improvements in ADHD symptoms in a population of pediatric patients with ADHD.[223]

MODAFINIL

There is controversy regarding this versatile stimulant-like agent and its use as a cognitive enhancer. Some effects on working memory (e.g., digit span, digit sequencing, and pattern recognition) have been recognized in the healthy population; however, results related to spatial memory, executive function, and attention are more ambiguous.[224–226] Modafinil is an effective treatment for ADHD,[227,228] with a comparable effect on symptomatology as that of methylphenidate.[229] However, due to its side effect profile and concerns of the risk of Stevens–Johnson syndrome, its use in a pediatric population has not been approved by the US Food and Drug Administration.

POLYSATURATED FATTY ACIDS

Essential fatty acids are polyunsaturated fatty acids (PUFAs) that must be taken in dietary form because the body cannot produce them. PUFAs are necessary for normal neural and immune system development and functioning.[230] Previous studies showed that children and adolescents with ADHD have significantly lower plasma and blood concentrations of PUFAs and, in particular, lower levels of omega-3 PUFA.[231,232] A systematic review[233] examined the available randomized controlled trials (RCTs) that have investigated the effectiveness of PUFA supplementation and found very few of high quality. The authors concluded that there is little evidence that PUFA supplementation provides any benefit for the symptoms of ADHD in children and adolescents. The majority of data showed no benefit of PUFA supplementation. Three trials showed improvement when combined omega-3 and omega-6 supplementation was given, including improvement in parent-rated total ADHD symptoms and teacher ratings of attention.

Pharmacological Interventions for Autism Spectrum Disorder

There are currently no approved pharmacological treatments for ASD. Educational and behavioral interventions are the bedrock of treatment to address the core social and communication deficits.[234] Interventions targeting social symptoms are aimed at improving social and communication skills and usually involve skills-based teaching programs.[235] However, psychotropic medications are often prescribed for comorbid psychiatric conditions and the most severe challenging behaviors. Antidepressants are the most commonly prescribed psychotropic medications in individuals with ASD. Recent studies show that neuroleptics and stimulants are also being prescribed.[236,237] There is a limited evidence base for pharmacological treatments of the core features of ASD, but there is preliminary evidence for medications showing potential benefit in the treatment of challenging behaviors as well as repetitive behaviors and hyperactivity.

Selective Serotonin Reuptake Inhibitors and Tricyclic Antidepressants

Selective serotonin reuptake inhibitors (SSRIs) have shown some efficacy in alleviating core symptoms in both ADHD and ASD. Fluoxetine has demonstrated improvements in inattention and hyperactivity in children with comorbid ASD and ADHD,[238–240] as well as mild ameliorating deficits in social interaction, communication, and stereotyped behaviors in children with ASD.[241–243] Chronic fluoxetine administration has been shown to result in increased metabolic activity in prefrontal areas, with associated improvements in ASD behaviors.[244–246] A series of studies examined the association between acute dose of fluoxetine and brain activation in ADHD and ASD. The studies documented disorder-specific abnormalities, particularly in the frontal lobes, during tasks examining motor inhibition,[247] working memory,[248] and reward reversal,[267247] which reflect cognitive flexibility. Fluoxetine showed normalizing effects on individuals with ASD and ADHD in many of the tasks but through opposite effects.

However, a systematic review of SSRI treatment for core symptoms of ASD in children[249] reported no evidence of effectiveness for citalopram, fenfluramine, or fluoxetine and suggested emerging evidence of harm. A single crossover RCT of fluoxetine showed benefit for repetitive behavior that was driven primarily by the second arm of the study.[250] Another RCT of citalopram[251] revealed no benefit for repetitive behavior but possible improvement in challenging behavior. All of the studies included in the systematic reviews, examining children or adults, used behaviorally based rating scales with few cognitive items.

The evidence base for the clinical effectiveness of tricyclic antidepressants (TCAs) in ASD is even more limited. Only three studies, involving small numbers of patients, withstood sufficient scrutiny to be included in a systematic review.[252] Two studies examined the use of clomipramine,[253,254] and one examined the use of tianeptine.[255] One of the clomipramine trials involved children and young adults (aged 10–36 years),[253] whereas the other two trials enrolled only children (aged 4–15 years). The use of TCAs in children is limited by concerns about a narrow therapeutic index and high potential for side effects, including sedation, impaired cognition, weight gain, and cardiac conduction abnormalities.

In the tianeptine study,[255] parents and teachers reported reductions in irritability, hyperactivity, inadequate eye contact, and what is termed inappropriate speech. These findings were not supported by clinician ratings. Significant adverse effects were reported, including increased drowsiness and reduced activity levels. The findings of the clomipramine studies are contradictory. In one of the studies, there was evidence of statistically significant improvements in autistic symptoms such as withdrawal, rhythmic motion, abnormal object relationships, unspontaneous relation to examiner, and underproductive speech.[254] Irritability and obsessive–compulsive disorder-type symptoms were also reduced. However, there was conflicting evidence in relation to hyperactivity across the two studies, and no significant changes were found regarding inappropriate speech. There were also adverse effects reported with the use of clomipramine, with significant dropout rates in the clomipramine arm of one study. Clomipramine did show statistically significant superiority to placebo on the Clinical Global Impression scale.

Therefore, although there is accumulating evidence for both abnormalities in serotonin metabolism in neurodevelopmental disorders and the possible mediating effect on underlying cognitive functioning, there is currently no robust evidence base for a treatment effect for medications that enhance the functioning of the serotonergic system, such as SSRIs and TCAs.

Antipsychotic Medications

The evidence to support use of antipsychotic medications for challenging behaviors, hyperactivity, and repetitive behaviors in children with ASD is strongest for aripiprazole and moderate for risperidone.[256] There is little evidence to support their use in adolescents and young adults with ASD.[257] Because of the adverse effects associated with these medications, combined with their limited effects on repetitive and challenging behaviors, the risk–benefit ratio only weighs in favor of medication for those who are severely impaired or at risk of injury. None of the trials have studied cognitive outcomes.

One RCT recruited 124 children aged 4–14 years, with 49 children in the intervention group.[258] The effect of the addition of a risperidone to parent-training program on adaptive behavior and communication and socialization skills was measured. At follow-up at 24 weeks, children in the intervention group showed improved scores on the Home Situations Questionnaire and the Aberrant Behavior Checklist subscales for irritability, stereotypic behavior, and hyperactivity. Children in the combined intervention group also showed greater improvements in scores on Vineland socialization and adaptive composite standard scores and on Vineland noncompliance, socialization, and communication age equivalent scores. However, at 1-year follow-up of 87 participants, the differences in Home Situations Questionnaire and Aberrant Behavior Checklist were not sustained. The Vineland was not measured at the follow-up.

Stimulants

Research Units on Pediatric Psychopharmacology (RUPP) Autism Network trials examined the use of methylphenidate in children with pervasive developmental disorders and hyperactivity.[259] This was a double-blind, 4-week crossover trial with placebo and increasing doses of methylphenidate given in random order each for 1 week, with a subsequent open-label continuation phase. The primary outcome measure was hyperactivity/noncompliance. The ABC parent and teacher-rated hyperactivity subscales and Clinical Global Impression of Improvement scale detected mean effects of all methylphenidate doses that were statistically superior to placebo.

Subsequent secondary analyses[260] examined social communication and self-regulation, including emotional regulation, in 33 children. The children included in these secondary analyses had an additional inclusion criterion of a mental age younger than 9 years and were engaged in semistructured tasks of joint attention and caregiver–child interactions. This study showed a significant positive effect of methylphenidate on use of joint attention initiations, response to bids for joint attention, self-regulation, and regulated affective states. The authors concluded that there was no clear dose–response relationship in improvements in joint attentional behaviors but that lower doses showed a larger impact on these skills. They argued that higher doses of methylphenidate have been associated with greater parent ratings of "irritability" and "social withdrawal" in previous analyses.[261] They further suggested that future directions of research should include more extensive examination of the impact of methylphenidate on joint attention, the subsequent impact (if any) on language development, and the effect of methylphenidate on joint attention in individuals with ASD without comorbid ADHD.

Oxytocin

A number of small-sample, pilot, crossover trials have examined the effects of short-term administration of intranasal oxytocin in individuals with ASD. A review of six RCTs by Preti et al.[262] found that the most reproducible findings were of improvements in emotion recognition and eye gaze.[263,264] Anagnostou et al.[265] demonstrated persistence in these improvements in social cognition with short-term administration of oxytocin during a 6-week period. However, there was no distal effect on global clinical status. Any decreases in repetitive behaviors that were seen acutely did not persist. Most improvements were of medium effect size, and the quality of evidence was found to be moderate at best, with a medium to high risk of bias. These short-term trials documented only mild side effects. However, evidence from the animal literature has raised concern about the longer term effects of oxytocin administration. In prairie voles, which are often utilized in animal models of social behavior, oxytocin administration initially leads to increases in social behaviors, but repeated administration leads to deficits in partner preference behavior.[266]

Polysaturated Fatty Acids

Two RCTs have examined omega-3 fatty acid supplementation in children with ASD.[267,268] There was no improvement in social interaction, inappropriate speech, or stereotypies detected, although the number of participants was small—37 children across both trials—and the duration of follow-up was short at 6–12 weeks. Secondary outcomes of hyperactivity and irritability also remained unchanged.

Nonpharmacological Interventions for ADHD

Cognitive Training

Cognitive training incorporates the teaching of techniques such as self-regulating (self-instructional training, self-monitoring, and self-reinforcement) as well as cognitive modeling and interpersonal problem-solving.[269,270] The central goal in ADHD is the development of self-control skills and reflective problem-solving strategies, both of which are presumed to be deficient in children with ADHD and to account for difficulties in regulating attentive, impulsive, and interpersonal behaviors. The expectation is that the enhancement and internalization of self-regulating cognitive skills will facilitate more appropriate behavioral regulation, as well as academic functioning.

One neuropsychological test, the Matching Familiar Figures Test (MFFT), is used in several studies evaluating cognitive training. The MFFT is a match-to-standard procedure that requires participants to choose from among a set of highly similar variants the one that is an identical match to the standard stimulus picture. The test purportedly assesses reflection impulsivity or cognitive tempo. There is little evidence that cognitive training has an advantageous effect.[271–273]

Except for scattered instances of improvement, there is no compelling evidence that cognitive training differentially enhances attentional (e.g., as measured using the Continuous Performance Test) or memory (e.g., as measured using Paired Associates Test or Digit Span) processes in ADHD children. An exception to these negative findings are those reported by Reid and Borkowski.[274] The authors used a treatment approach that combined cognitive self-control training, specific strategy training to enhance associative and sorting skills, and attributional training that focused on coping with failure and success experiences. Compared to children who had only the self-control or strategy training, those in the combined treatment group significantly improved and maintained their performance on associative and sorting tasks and also showed increased "metamemory" (i.e., general knowledge about strategic task behavior) 10 months after the end of training. Note that the 77 hyperactive children in the study constituted a nonclinical sample chosen solely on the basis of their scores on the Conners Teacher Rating Scale (CTRS)[275] and that 35 (45%) had scores below 1.5, the typical clinical cut-off score for hyperactivity on the CTRS. It is unknown whether clinically diagnosed youngsters with ADHD would demonstrate similar benefit with this treatment approach.

A number of studies have evaluated the efficacy of cognitive training in combination with psychostimulant medication. None of these studies provide any support for the adjunctive efficacy of cognitive training in improving the cognitive functioning of stimulant-treated samples. Considering this body of negative findings, it should be noted that the improvements in cognitive test performance commonly found with medication[276] may create ceiling effects, thereby limiting the opportunity to detect any additive effects of training.

Educational Interventions, Cognitive Training, and Academic Performance

Attempts to enhance the academic functioning of children with ADHD have included a variety of strategies, including stimulant medication and educational interventions, either singly or in combination. Although there is mounting evidence that stimulants improve academic productivity and task performance,[277,278] medication's impact on academic skill acquisition and achievement has not been established, and evidence of the efficacy of educational interventions in combination with medication in academically impaired children with ADHD is equivocal.[279,280] Several studies[281–283] showed that in medication-free ADHD participants, cognitive training had some beneficial effect on academic performance: Benefits were evident for mathematic abilities and overall productivity, but less so for reading performance.

Computer-Based Working Memory Training

Working memory training has shown promise in enhancing cognitive deficits among patients with ADHD, with concomitant beneficial effects on the core symptoms of the disorder. Klingberg et al.[284,285] used cognitive computer training for several weeks, with those in the intervention group showing lasting improvements on outcome measures of working memory, response inhibition, and parent-rated inattentive symptoms. The same training protocol was shown to produce increases in brain activation[286] and changes in the density of prefrontal and parietal dopamine D_1 receptor binding potential, indicating neural plasticity that arises as a result of the training.[287]

Neurofeedback

Neurofeedback is derived from the principles of biofeedback, in which the participant is provided with a representation of his or her performance while consciously attempting to alter response. In ADHD, a computerized video game format representing electroencephalograph activity by proxy is presented to the subject while positive reinforcement is given as an attempt to increase fast wave activity.[220,288,289] A number of studies have examined the effects of neurofeedback on a range of outcome measures, and in general they have detected large effects on parent- and teacher-rated ADHD symptoms.[220] Cognitive outcomes have shown more variable effects.[220] Although controversial, the literature on neurofeedback continues to grow, and recent studies have begun to address some of the methodological problems raised in earlier work.[289] Additional research is needed to establish an impact on cognition.

Social Skills Interventions

Social skills training focuses on techniques that aim to improve and maintain the individual's social skills. The children are taught how to adjust their verbal and nonverbal behavior in their social interactions. It also includes efforts to change the children's cognitive assessment of the "social world." There is substantial emphasis on teaching children how to pick up on routine social cues and build on a to-and-for interaction, consciously compensating for their urge to constantly change topics or skip the queue, while building more awareness on recognizing emotional reactions/ expressions in others.[290] Social skills training also includes teaching social norms, social "rules," and expectations of others.[291] It can be delivered on a one-to-one basis or through group work. Social skills training is also referred to as "cognitive–behavioral training," and it often consists of role play, exercises, and games, as well as homework; it may include parents and sometimes teachers.

Although two previous meta-analyses investigating the efficacy of social skills and psychosocial training for children with ADHD found a significant effect for social skills and psychosocial treatment,[292,293] one did not find any significant effect.[294] However, serious methodological limitations have been highlighted. A systematic review[295] investigated a wide range of social skills interventions. The results showed no statistically significant treatment effects on social skills competences, the teacher-rated general behavior, or the ADHD symptoms. The authors discuss the need for further research in this field because there is little evidence to date to support or indeed refute the efficacy of social skills training for children and adolescents with ADHD.

Non-Pharmalogical Interventions for Autism Spectrum Disorder

Cognitive Training

SOCIAL SKILLS AND THEORY OF MIND TRAINING

Social skills training programs for individuals with ASD incorporate skills to improve emotional recognition and regulation, social competency, social problem-solving, and social communication skills. These programs are often utilized for individuals with higher functioning ASD and can include individual, peer-led, and group-based training. Most studies include children aged 7–12 years. There is insufficient evidence to support individual or group-based social skills training for children with ASD.[296] However, some gains in overall social competencies and friendship quality and reductions in loneliness have been detected for children, adolescents, and young adults.[297]

Computer-based social skills training programs are largely acceptable to individuals with ASD. However, there is insufficient evidence to support their use for children. Studies are few, of short follow-up periods, and often the diagnostic approach and treatment fidelity are poorly described. There is one report of improved emotional recognition in testing, but this did not generalize.[298]

Theory of mind training includes teaching components of, or precursors to, ToM. Specific skills include recognizing emotions, understanding differences between fantasy and reality, perspective taking, joint attention and communication, imitation, and reasoning about other people's mental states. These studies are often of low or very low quality, with associated multiple sources of potential bias. Interventions to address ToM deficits show gains in language abilities, nonverbal intelligence, and some emotional awareness skills in children.[299] Overall, analyses of these interventions in children show positive effects on emotional recognition, imitation abilities, and ToM skills between control and intervention groups. However, there is a lack of application of learned skills to novel situations and stimuli.[300]

In a review of psychosocial interventions for adults with ASD, more studies described social cognition training interventions than those based on applied behavioral analysis (ABA) techniques.[301] The majority of these studies were designed to address deficits in ToM functioning. Overall, there were documented significant improvements in included measures, such as facial emotion recognition. Many of the programs utilized computer-based interventions. Turner-Brown et al.[302] utilized a group-based three-phase intervention focusing on emotion training, figuring out situations, and integration of skills designed to improve social–cognitive functioning. There was significant improvement in ToM skills in the intervention group and trend-level improvement in social communication skills detected. Although ToM skills can be taught to people with ASD, they remain effortful and error-prone. There is little evidence of skill maintenance, generalization to other settings, or developmental effects on related skills.[300]

Early Intensive Behavioral and Developmental Interventions

Early intensive behavioral and developmental interventions have their basis in or draw from principles of ABA. ABA-based interventions all share similar principles and techniques to assess, treat, and prevent challenging behaviors and to teach new skills and promote their generalization. These interventions include the manualized interventions, University of California, Los Angeles (UCLA)/Lovaas model[303,304] and the Early Start Denver Model (ESDM); nonmanualized approaches that are similar to the UCLA/Lovaas model; and parent-mediated interventions. They focus on key or foundation skills and behaviors such as initiating or organizing activity or core communication skills.

There is moderate evidence that high-intensity ABA-based approaches delivered over extended time frames are associated with improvement in cognitive functioning and language skills in some groups of young children with ASD relative to community controls. However, it is unclear which groups benefit from these high-cost interventions and what moderates these effects.[296] A review of ABA-based interventions in adults based on five single case studies described interventions to reduce instances of undesirable behaviors or increase instances of a desirable behavior.[307] Although all studies had positive outcomes, maintenance of effects varied, and the quality of evidence was poor.

Early intensive behavioral intervention (EIBI) is a highly structured manualized teaching approach for children, usually younger than 5 years old, with ASD. The origins of EIBI are based in the UCLA/Lovaas model. The core elements involve a specific teaching procedure referred to as discrete trial training, which is delivered on an individual basis initially and then systematically transferred to other settings.[306,307]Parental involvement is central. EIBI is individualized, examining the core deficits and current behavioral repertoires with a functional approach to challenging behaviors.

A meta-analysis[308] of four controlled clinical trials[309–312] of EIBI in young children with ASD showed improved adaptive behavior, expressive and receptive language, everyday communication skills, everyday social competence, and daily living skills. Improvements in IQ were the most substantial and equivalent to 11 points for those in the EIBI treatment arms. Additional measures of psychopathology and quality of life were reported, but meta-analyses were not conducted due to the variety of measurement tools used across the studies. The quality of the evidence was rated as low due to the risk of bias.

A review of 37 papers involving 25 different studies of early intensive behavioral and developmental interventions suggested that the evidence for their impact on core ASD symptoms is limited and mixed, and it found that long-term follow-up studies are not available.[296] The authors suggested that improvements in adaptive behavior may be due to pretreatment child characteristics, such as cognitive or language skills and severity of core ASD symptoms.

Early parent-mediated training programs have attracted increasing attention.[296] These lower intensity interventions aim to augment social communication skills. They have been shown to be successful in modifying parenting behaviors and improving parent–child interaction in terms of joint attention and parent synchrony.[313] However, data on their ability to improve developmental skills are limited. Language comprehension gains have been demonstrated for some children, but there is inconsistent evidence for gains in other areas, such as core symptoms of ASD, adaptive behaviors, and cognition. Stavropoulos and Carver.[314] propose that adding oxytocin to behavioral interventions that increase joint attention may be beneficial and help to overcome lack of intrinsic motivation that appears to decrease the long-term success of these interventions.

A review of enhanced school-based interventions examined ABA modalities,[296] including general ABA,[315,316] individual UCLA/Lovaas-based behavioral intervention,[317] Treatment and Education of Autistic and Communication Related Handicapped Children (TEACCH)[318] or Learning Experiences and Alternative Program for Pre-schoolers and Their Parents (LEAP) programs,[319,320] and a mix of behaviorally based operant conditioning techniques.[321] Studies reported mixed results, with some[317,318,321] showing greater gains in cognitive outcomes and parent-reported adaptive skills in the enhanced intervention group. This contrasted with findings of other studies,[319–321] which showed improvements in cognitive, adaptive, and ASD symptom measures across all groups. Boyd et al.[319] examined a TEACCH intervention that utilizes an educational framework with an emphasis on structuring class environments through visual cueing, communication routines, and individual tasks. This project aims to increase children's independence, focusing on enhancing existing strengths rather than focusing on weaknesses. The study demonstrated that the efficacy of a TEACCH intervention was associated with baseline cognitive scores, with greater improvements seen in those individuals with lower scores.

Play and Joint Attention-Based Interventions

Studies of play or interaction-based approaches examine interventions that address joint attention, parent–child communication, imitation behaviors, or pretend play. Analyses show that joint attention interventions may demonstrate positive outcomes in preschool-aged children with ASD when targeting joint attention skills but with limited effects on play skills, language and social skills, adaptive behaviors, or cognition.[296] Children receiving these play interventions very often receive early intervention in addition to play interventions.

Cognitive–Behavioral Therapy

Studies examining the effects of cognitive–behavioral therapy (CBT) on ASD have reported positive results in older children with IQs ≥70,[296] and the quality of evidence is high. Positive effects on socialization have also been shown. One RCT that included 57 children demonstrated improvements in executive function in the CBT treatment group compared to the control group receiving social skills intervention.[322] The CBT group improved significantly more on measures of problem-solving, cognitive flexibility, and parent- and teacher-rated executive function measures. Higher baseline scores predicted greater improvements in measurements of flexible thinking, social tasks, executive function shift, and planning/organization measures as rated by parents and teachers. Higher IQ levels predicted greater improvements in flexible thinking and the challenge task plan measurements.

Neurofeedback

There is limited evidence for the impact of neurofeedback in ASD. In a nonrandomized trial including 14 high-functioning children with pervasive developmental disorder not otherwise specified, 40 sessions of neurofeedback resulted in improvement on executive function measures, including auditory selective attention, inhibition of verbal responses and impulsive tendencies, cognitive flexibility, and goal setting, compared to the control group.[323] An RCT that included 10 children with ASD showed improved social behavior, especially reciprocal social interaction, compared to controls. There were also gains in the treatment group on the Children's Communication Checklist and on the set-shifting domain of executive function. Scores on other domains of executive function were equivalent between groups.

Six-month follow-up showed continued improvement of the intervention group in set-shifting measures and parent-rated core symptoms.[324]

Social Interventions for ADHD

The revolutionary work of Hebb and Rosenweig[325–327] in the 1950s and 1960s has brought to the fore the concept of environmental influences on neurodevelopment and neural plasticity and also on behavior and cognition. During the following decades, the accumulated data, mainly from animal studies, have facilitated better understanding of these influences at the molecular and neural levels.

Environmental enrichment studies have been criticized for their manipulation strategy, precision, and duration of interventions. Most rodent studies focusing on environmental enrichment employ a combination of social (e.g., multiple animals in a cage), cognitive (e.g., toys and tunnels), and motor (e.g., running wheels) stimuli. As such, it is difficult to determine the extent to which any one of these contributes to positive outcome. However, invaluable results were obtained from these studies, demonstrating the positive effect of environmental enrichment on increasing neuronal size, dendritic branching and spine number, synaptic density, and overall neurotransmission in the neocortex.[328–331] Environmental enrichment also enhances neurogenesis,[332,333] long-term potentiation,[334] neurotrophin levels,[335,336] dendritic spine growth and branching,[337,338] synaptophysin levels,[339] and nerve growth factor mRNA and CREB gene expression[340,341] in the dentate gyrus of the hippocampus. Consistent with the effects of environmental enrichment on neurodevelopment, numerous studies have shown that it significantly improves performance on an array of spatial and nonspatial memory tasks in rats[325,333] and mice.[341]

Physical exercise has a central effect on brain development in rodent studies, showing increased levels of synaptic proteins[342] and glutamate receptors[343] and the availability of brain-derived neurotrophic factor (BDNF)[344] and insulin-like growth factor-1, all of which can enhance neural plasticity. Neural changes are accompanied by behavioral changes such that physical exercise enhances spatial learning and passive avoidance memory. Physical exercise has also been reported to increase BDNF levels,[345,346] enhance cognitive performance,[347] and promote brain health[348] in human adults.

Shim et al.[349] showed that ADHD children express higher levels of BDNF and an inverse correlation for BDNF with neuropsychological performance. However, BDNF change in response to exercise was not assessed. Exercise and environmental enhancements also have been shown to have a positive effect on outcome in several animal models of neurodevelopmental disorders. Another study showed that chronic exercise blunted the developmental rise of blood pressure while increasing glutamic acid decarboxylase mRNA in the caudal hypothalamus in spontaneously hypertensive rats, which are commonly used as an animal model for ADHD.[350]

Two studies have examined exercise regimes in children with ADHD, with one reporting a blunted catecholamine response[351] and the other showing changes in eye blink responses and reductions in motor impersistence that were specific to boys.[352] However, neither study examined clinical response nor brain-related changes following exercise. Thus, although the literature on children is sparse, the extensive body of animal research suggests that environmental enrichment could play a key role in the treatment, and possibly even the amelioration, of ADHD symptomatology through improving the core neural deficits associated with the disorder. Future controlled trials are necessary to test this hypothesis.

Social Interventions for Autism Spectrum Disorder

Vocational Interventions

Levy and Perry[43] found across studies that an average of 50–60% of adults with ASD leave school without educational or vocational credentials. Less than 50% of adults with ASD, including high-functioning individuals, will maintain employment, but these rates can be improved by structured supports to gain and sustain employment.[353,354]

Studies of employment in individuals with ASD have shown an improvement in quality of life outcomes.[355] Individuals who participate in supported employment programs have better scores on assessments of ASD symptoms, which remain stable during follow-up periods.[356] This contrasts with a worsening over time in ASD symptoms in individuals in sheltered workshops.

García-Villamisar and Hughes[357] examined cognitive outcomes in 44 individuals with ASD and compared those in supported employment with a group participating in vocational activities in sheltered workshops. The two groups were nonrandomly distributed but were similar at baseline in terms of autism symptoms, IQ, vocabulary, and measures of cognition. Individuals in the supported employment program showed an improvement in 8 of 12 cognitive tests from baseline to follow-up, including on tests of executive functions. This was in contrast to those in the sheltered workshop group, who demonstrated no change during the follow-up period of up to 30 months. However, the quality of this study was poor due to the nonrandom assignment and nonmasking of assessors. A number of aspects of the study were not fully described, including rates of attrition, the full nature of the intervention, treatment fidelity, and any concomitant medical or psychological interventions.

Complementary Therapies for Autism Spectrum Disorder

A wide range of "alternative" therapies, including diet, vitamins, and auditory and sensory integration, have been used in the treatment of ASD. One study reported that 74% of children with ASD try complementary and alternative medicines.[358] There is little robust evidence for many of these interventions, and ongoing use may lead to harm.

Acupuncture

Acupuncture is increasingly used in Western cultures.[359] Acupuncture is viewed as a relatively safe intervention, although it has been associated with adverse effects. Research on medical acupuncture paradigms shows that the acupoints are closely related to neural tissues, and interventions have been shown to lead to direct stimulation of neural pathways and the release of neurotransmitters such as serotonin[360] and endocannabinoids.[361] Postulated mechanisms of action in the alleviation of symptoms in ASD include regulation of glutamate[362] and GABA[363,364] or modulation of neuroinflammatory responses.[365]

A systematic review of acupuncture in ASD detected some benefits for acupuncture plus conventional treatment compared to conventional treatments alone or with the addition of sham acupuncture.[366] There were recorded improvements in core autistic features; speech; cognitive functioning; self-care; and social, cognitive, and global functioning. However, overall examination of results suggests that robust recommendations cannot be made.

Auditory Integration Training and Other Sound Therapies

Bérard developed auditory integration training (AIT) as a result of the observation that individuals with behavioral and learning difficulties had abnormal sensitivity or insensitivity to a range of sound frequencies but normal hearing.[367] He suggested that AIT would bring about a "re-education" of the hearing process. His techniques have been utilized in a wide range of conditions, including ASD, depression, hyperactivity, and learning difficulties.

AIT uses filtering to dampen the peak frequencies to which the individual is hypersensitive. The device delivers electronically modified music through headphones and consists of sounds modulated by random dampening of high and low frequencies and intensities.[368] The therapy consists of twice-daily half-hour sessions for 10 days. Two other sound therapies have been developed: Tomatis sound therapy, which uses electronically modified human voice and music, and Samonas therapy, in which filtered music, voice, and sounds of nature are delivered through headphones under a therapist's direction. Often, these interventions are modified by therapists on an individual basis, thus limiting comparisons. Systematic analyses of trials utilizing these interventions show inconsistent findings in terms of overall behavioral outcomes.[369] Two trials examined cognitive outcomes as measured by Leiter International Performance Scale and Vineland Adaptive Behavior Scores after treatment with AIT, and findings were contradictory.[370,371]

Music Therapy

Music therapy is "a systematic process of intervention wherein the therapist helps the client to promote health, using musical experiences and the relationships that develop through them as dynamic forces of change."[372] There is a wide variety of possible modes of therapy, including individual or group sessions, peer-mediated groups, and family involvement. Interventions can take the form of structured or improvised singing or vocalizations, as well as listening to prerecorded or live music.

A systematic review examined studies of music therapy and found moderate to large effect sizes for social interaction outside the therapy setting.[373] There was a moderate effect for nongeneralized, nonverbal communication skills when examining observed behavior but no effect when using standardized tools. The effect size for verbal communication skills for music therapy was small to moderate, but the evidence was considered to be of low quality, as was that for nonverbal generalized communication skills. The effect size for initiating behaviors was close to large, and it was large for social reciprocity. No adverse effects were recorded. There were small to moderate effects on social adaptation. Effects on quality of life and family relationships were not reliable. No data were collected on other cognitive outcomes or effects on hyperacusis.

CONCLUSION

This chapter reviewed the evidence base for treatments to enhance cognition in two common neurodevelopmental disorders: ADHD and ASD. There is currently only limited evidence for efficacy of either pharmacological or behavioral interventions for the treatment of the cognitive deficits associated with these disorders. Controlled trials including pragmatic, cost-effective interventions, applying outcomes that are assessed using standardized objective measures and over long periods of follow-up, are necessary.

REFERENCES

1. Vaidya CJ, Austin G, Kirkorian G, et al. Selective effects of methylphenidate in attention deficit hyperactivity disorder: A functional magnetic resonance study. *Proc Natl Acad Sci USA* 1998;95(24):14494–14499.

2. American Psychiatric Association. *Diagnostic and statistical manual of mental disorders* (4th ed.) Washington, DC: American Psychiatric Association; 1994.

3. Nishiyama T, Taniai H, Miyachi T, et al. Genetic correlation between autistic traits and IQ in a population-based sample of twins with autism spectrum disorders (ASD). *J Hum Genet* 2009;54(1):56–61.

4. Joseph RM, Tager-Flusberg H, Lord C. Cognitive profiles and social-communicative functioning in children with autism spectrum disorder. *J Child Psychol Psychiatry* 2002;43(6):807–821.

5. Rutter, M. Cognitive deficits in the pathogenesis of autism. *J Child Psychol Psychiatry* 1983;24:513–531.

6. Bakeman R, Adamson LB. Coordinating attention to people and objects in mother–infant and peer–infant interaction. *Child Dev* 1984;55(4):1278–1289.

7. Van Hecke AV, Stevens S, Carson AM, et al. Measuring the plasticity of social approach: A randomized controlled trial of the effects of the PEERS intervention on EEG asymmetry in adolescents with autism spectrum disorders. *J Autism Dev Disord* 2015;45(2):316–335.

8. Fein D, Pennington B, Markowitz P, et al. Toward a neuropsychological model of infantile autism: Are the social deficits primary? *J Am Acad Child Psychiatry* 1986;25:198–212.

9. Douglas VI. Attentional and cognitive problems. In Rutter M (Ed.), *Developmental neuropsychiatry*. New York, NY: Guilford; 1983:280–329.

10. Nuechterlein KH, Dawson ME. Information processing and attentional functioning in the developmental cause of schizophrenic disorders. *Schizophrenia Bull* 1984;10:160–203.

11. Nuechterlein KH. Signal detection in vigilance tasks and behavioural attributes among offspring of schizophrenic mothers and among hyperactive children. *J Abnorm Psychol* 1983;92:428.

12. Howlin P, Rutter M. The consequences of language delay for other aspects of development. In Yule W, Rutter M (Eds.), *Language development and disorders*. London: MacKeith/Blackwell; 1987.

13. Yule W, Rutter M. Reading and other learning difficulties. In Rutter M, Hersov L (Eds.), *Child and adolescent psychiatry: Modern approaches* (2nd ed.). Oxford, UK: Blackwell; 1985.

14. Bower GN. Mood and memory. *American Psychologist* 1981;36:129–148.

15. Sroufe LA. The coherence of individual development. *American Psychologist* 1979;34:834–841.

16. Barkley RA. *Attention deficit hyperactivity disorder: A handbook for diagnosis and treatment.* New York, NY: Guilford; 1990.

17. Mannuzza S, Klein RG, Bessler A, et al. Educational and occupational outcome of hyperactive boys grown up. *Am Acad Child Adolesc Psychiatry* 1997;36:1222–1227.

18. Denckla MB. Executive function, the overlap zone between attention deficit hyperactivity disorder and learning disabilities. *Int Pediatr* 1989;4:155–160.

19. Barkley RA. Behavioral inhibition, sustained attention, and executive functions: Constructing a unifying theory of ADHD. *Psychol Bull* 1997;121:65–94.

20. Chelune GJ, Ferguson W, Koon R, et al. Frontal lobe disinhibition in attention deficit disorder. *Child Psychiatry Hum Dev* 1986;16:221–234.

21. Clark C, Prior M, Kinsella G. The relationship between executive function abilities, adaptive behaviour, and academic achievement in children with externalising behaviour problems. *J Child Psychol Psychiatry* 2002;43:785–796.

22. Sergeant J. A theory of attention: An information processing perspective. In Lyon G, Krasnegor K (Eds.), *Attention, memory, and executive function*. Baltimore, MD: Brooks; 1996:57–71.

23. Sergeant J, Geurts H, Oosterlaan J. How specific is a deficit of executive functioning for attention deficit hyperactivity disorder? *Behav Brain Res* 2002;130:3–28.

24. Douglas VI. Stop, look and listen: The problem of sustained attention and impulse control in hyperactive and normal children. *Can J Behav Sci* 1972;4:259–282.

25. Deuel RK. Minimal brain dysfunction, hyperkinesis, learning disabilities, attention deficit disorder. *J Pediatr* 1981;98:912–915.
26. Lahey BB, Carlson CL. Validity of a diagnostic category of attention deficit disorder without hyperactivity. *J Learn Disabil* 1991;24(2):110–112.
27. Lahey BB, Applegate B, McBurnett K, et al. DSM-IV field trials for attention deficit hyperactivity disorder in children and adolescents. *Am J Psychiatry* 1994;151(11):1673–1685.
28. Seidman J, Biederman J, Faraone S, et al. *Neuropsychological findings in ADHD children: Findings from a sample of ADHD children* [Abstract]. Paper presented at the 44th Annual Meeting of the American Academy of Child & Adolescent Psychiatry, 1997.
29. Fischer M, Barkley RA, Edelbrock CS, et al. The adolescent outcome of hyperactive children diagnosed by research criteria: II. Academic, attentional, and neuropsychological status. *J Consult Clin Psychol* 1990;58:580–588.
30. Millstein RB, Wilens TE, Biederman J, et al. Presenting ADHD symptoms and subtypes in clinically referred adults with ADHD. *J Atten Disord* 1997;2:159–166.
31. Faraone SV, Biederman J, Monuteaux M, et al. Attention deficit hyperactivity disorder and learning disability: A prospective four-year follow-up study. *J Atten Disord* 2001;3:23–25.
32. Halperin, JM, Schulz KP. Revisiting the role of the prefrontal cortex in the pathophysiology of attention-deficit/hyperactivity disorder. *Psychol Bull* 2006;132:560–581.
33. Halperin JM, Marks DJ, Schulz KP. Neuropsychological perspectives of ADHD. In Morgan JE, Ricker JH (Eds.), *Handbook of clinical neuropsychology*. Lisse, the Netherlands: Swets & Zeitlinger; 2008a:333–345
34. Shaw P, Lerch J, Greenstein D, et al. Longitudinal mapping of cortical thickness and clinical outcome in children and adolescents with attention-deficit/hyperactivity disorder. *Arch Gen Psychiatry* 2006;63:540–549.
35. Supekar K, Musen M, Menon V. Development of large-scale functional brain networks in children. *PLoS Biol* 2009;7:e1000157.
36. Schulz KP, Newcorn JH, Fan J, et al. Brain activation gradients in ventrolateral prefrontal cortex related to persistence of ADHD in adolescence. *J Am Acad Child Adolescent Psychiatry* 2005;44:47–54.
37. Halperin JM, Trampush JT, Miller CJ, et al. Neuropsychological outcome in adolescents/young adults with childhood ADHD: Profiles of persisters, remitters and controls. *J Child Psychol Psychiatry* 2008;49:958–966.
38. Dosenbach NU, Fair DA, Miezin FM, et al. Distinct brain networks for adaptive and stable task control in humans. *Proc Natl Acad Sci USA* 2007;104:11073–11078.
39. Fair DA, Dosenbach NU, Church JA, et al. Development of distinct control networks through segregation and integration. *Proc Natl Acad Sci USA* 2007;104:13507–13512.
40. Fair DA, Cohen AL, Power JD, et al. Functional brain networks develop from a "local to distributed" organization. *PLoS Comput Biol* 2009;5:e1000381.
41. Community Report from the Autism and Developmental Disabilities Monitoring (ADDM) Network. *A snapshot of autism spectrum disorder among 8-year-old children in multiple communities across the United States in 2010.* Atlanta, GA: Centers for Disease Control and Prevention, US Department of Health and Human Services; 2014.
42. Seltzer MM, Shattuck P, Abbeduto L, et al. Trajectory of development in adolescents and adults with autism. *Ment Retard Dev Disabil Res Rev* 2004;10(4):234–247.
43. Levy A, Perry A. Outcomes in adolescents and adults with autism: A review of the literature. *Res Autism Spectrum Disorders* 2011;5(4):1271–1282.
44. Williams E, Thomas K, Sidebotham H, et al. Prevalence and characteristics of autistic spectrum disorders in the ALSPAC cohort. *Dev Med Child Neurol* 2008;50(9):672–677.
45. Myers SM, Johnson CP. Management of children with autism spectrum disorders. *Pediatrics* 2007;120(5):1162–1182.
46. McPartland JC, Coffman M, Pelphrey KA. Recent advances in understanding the neural bases of autism spectrum disorder. *Curr Opin Pediatr* 2011;23(6):628–632.

47. Geschwind DH, Levitt P. Autism spectrum disorders: Developmental disconnection syndromes. *Curr Opin Neurobiol* 2007;17:103–111.
48. Castelli F, Frith C, Happé F, et al. Autism, Asperger syndrome and brain mechanisms for the attribution of mental states to animated shapes. *Brain* 2002;125(Pt 8):1839–1849.
49. Lombardo MV, Chakrabarti B, Bullmore ET, et al.; MRC AIMS Consortium. Specialization of right temporo-parietal junction for mentalizing and its relation to social impairments in autism. *Neuroimage* 2011;56(3):1832–1838.
50. Dittrich WH, Troscianko T, Lea SE, et al. Action categories and the perception of biological motion. *Perception* 1996;22:15–22.
51. Kaiser M, Hudac CM, Shultz S, et al. Neural signatures of autism. *Proc Natl Acad Sci USA* 2010;107(49):21223–21228.
52. Schultz RT. Developmental deficits in social perception in autism: The role of the amygdala and fusiform face area. *Int J Dev Neurosci* 2005;23(2-3):125–141.
53. Pierce K, Haist F, Sedaghat F, et al. The brain response to personally familiar faces in autism: Findings of fusiform activity and beyond. *Brain* 2004;127(Pt 12):2703–2716.
54. de Haan M, Johnson MH, Halit H. Development of face-sensitive event-related potentials during infancy: A review. *Int J Psychophysiol* 2003;51(1):45–58.
55. Maestro S, Muratori F, Cavallaro MC, et al. Attentional skills during the first 6 months of age in autism spectrum disorder. *J Am Acad Child Adolesc Psychiatry* 2002;41(10):1239–1245.
56. Dalton KM, Nacewicz BM, Johnstone T, et al. Gaze fixation and the neural circuitry of face processing in autism. *Nat Neurosci* 2005;8(4):519–526.
57. Pennington BF, Ozonoff S. Executive functions and developmental psychopathology. *J Child Psychol Psychiatry* 1996;37:51–87.
58. Sonuga-Barke EJ, Williams E, Hall M, et al. Hyperactivity and delay aversion: III. The effect on cognitive style of imposing delay after errors. *J Child Psychol Psychiatry* 1996;37:189–194.
59. Werry JS, Elkind GS, Reeves JC. Attention deficit, conduct, oppositional, and anxiety disorders in children: III. Laboratory differences. *J Abnorm Child Psychol* 1987;15:409–428.
60. Sergeant JA, Oosterlaan J, van der Meere J. Information processing and energetic factors in attention-deficit/hyperactivity disorder. In Quay HQ, Hogan AE (Eds.), *Handbook of disruptive behavior disorders.* New York, NY: Kluwer/Plenum; 1999:75–104.
61. Sagvolden T, Johansen EB, Aase H, et al. A dynamic developmental theory of attention-deficit/hyperactivity disorder (ADHD) predominantly hyperactive/impulsive and combined subtypes. *Behav Brain Sci* 2005;28:397–419.
62. Sonuga-Barke EJ, Halperin JM. Developmental phenotypes and causal pathways in attention deficit/hyperactivity disorder: Potential targets for early intervention? *J Child Psychol Psychiatry* 2010;51(4):368–389.
63. Sonuga-Barke EJ. Psychological heterogeneity in AD/HD—A dual pathway model of behaviour and cognition. *Behav Brain Res* 2002;130:29–36.
64. Pennington BF. *The development of psychopathology.* New York, NY: Guilford; 2002.
65. Barkley RA. Differential diagnosis of adults with ADHD: The role of executive function and self-regulation. *J Clin Psychiatry* 2010;71:e17.
66. Seidman LJ, Valera EM, Makris N. Structural brain imaging of attention-deficit/hyperactivity disorder. *Biol Psychiatry* 2005;57:1263–1272.
67. Banich MT, Burgess GC, Depue BE, et al. The neural basis of sustained and transient attentional control in young adults with ADHD. *Neuropsychologia* 2009;47:3095–3104.
68. Ernst M, Kimes AS, London ED, et al. Neural substrates of decision making in adults with attention deficit hyperactivity disorder. *Am J Psychiatry* 2003;160:1061–1070.
69. Halperin JM, Schulz KP. Revisiting the role of the prefrontal cortex in the pathophysiology of attention-deficit/hyperactivity disorder. *Psychol Bull* 2006;132:560–581.
70. Friedman NP, Miyake A, Corley RP, et al. Not all executive functions are related to intelligence. *Psychol Sci* 2006;17:172–179.
71. Collette F, Hogge M, Salmon E, et al. Exploration of the neural substrates of executive functioning by functional neuroimaging. *Neuroscience* 2006;139:209–221.

72. Willcutt EG, Pennington BF, Olson RK, et al. Neuropsychological analyses of comorbidity between reading disability and attention deficit hyperactivity disorder: In search of the common deficit. *Dev Neuropsychol* 2005;27:35–78.

73. Shanahan MA, Pennington BF, Yerys BE, et al. Processing speed deficits in attention deficit/ hyperactivity disorder and reading disability. *J Abnorm Child Psychol* 2006;34:585–602.

74. Willcutt EG, Bidwell LC. Etiology of ADHD: Implications for assessment and treatment. In Hoza B, Evans SW (Eds.), *Treating attention deficit hyperactivity disorder*. Kingston, NJ: Civic Research Institute; 2011.

75. Bechara A. The role of emotion in decision-making: Evidence from neurological patients with orbitofrontal damage. *Brain Cogn* 2004;55:30–40.

76. Carmona S, Proal E, Hoekzema EA, et al. Ventro-striatal reductions underpin symptoms of hyperactivity and impulsivity in attention deficit/hyperactivity disorder. *Biol Psychiatry* 2009;66:972–977.

77. Hartung CM, Milich R, Lynam DR, et al. Understanding the relations among gender, disinhibition, and disruptive behavior in adolescents. *J Abnorm Psychol* 2002;111:659–664.

78. Luman M, Oosterlaan J, Sergeant JA. The impact of reinforcement contingencies on ADHD: A review and theoretical appraisal. *Clin Psychol Rev* 2005;25:183–213.

79. Sonuga-Barke EJ, Sergeant JA, Nigg J, et al. Executive dysfunction and delay aversion in attention deficit hyperactivity disorder: Nosologic and diagnostic implications. *Child Adolesc Psychiatr Clin North Am* 2008;17:367–384.

80. Castellanos FX, Sonuga-Barke EJ, Scheres A, et al. Varieties of attention-deficit/hyperactivity disorder-related intra-individual variability. *Biol Psychiatry* 2005;57:1416–1423.

81. Leth-Steensen C, Elbaz ZK, Douglas VI. Mean response times, variability, and skew in the responding of ADHD children: A response time distributional approach. *Acta Psychol (Amst)* 2000;104:167–190.

82. Sergeant JA, Geurts H, Huijbregts S, et al. The top and the bottom of ADHD: A neuropsychological perspective. *Neurosci Biobehav Rev* 2003;27:583–592.

83. Willcutt EG, Pennington BF, Olson RK, et al. Neuropsychological analyses of comorbidity between reading disability and attention deficit hyperactivity disorder: In search of the common deficit. *Dev Neuropsychol* 2005;27:35–78.

84. Klein C, Wendling K, Huettner P, et al. Intra-subject variability in attention-deficit hyperactivity disorder. *Biol Psychiatry* 2006;60:1088–1097.

85. Hervey AS, Epstein JN, Curry JF, et al. Reaction time distribution analysis of neuropsychological performance in an ADHD sample. *Child Neuropsychol* 2006;12:125–140.

86. Castellanos FX, Margulies DS, Kelly C, et al. Cingulate–precuneus interactions: A new locus of dysfunction in adult attention-deficit/hyperactivity disorder. *Biol Psychiatry* 2008;63:332–337.

87. Sonuga-Barke EJ, Castellanos FX. Spontaneous attentional fluctuations in impaired states and pathological conditions: A neurobiological hypothesis. *Neurosci Biobehav Rev* 2007;31:977–986.

88. Toplak ME, Tannock R. Tapping and anticipation performance in attention deficit hyperactivity disorder. *Percept Mot Skills* 2005;100:659–675.

89. Castellanos FX, Tannock R. Neuroscience of attention-deficit/hyperactivity disorder: The search for endophenotypes. *Nat Rev Neurosci* 2002;3:617–628.

90. Uekermann J, Kraemer M, Abdel-Hamid M, et al. Social cognition in attention-deficit hyperactivity disorder (ADHD). *Neurosci Biobehav Rev* 2009;34:734–743.

91. Bidwell LC, Dew RE, Kollins SH. Alpha-2 adrenergic receptors and attention-deficit/hyperactivity disorder. *Curr Psychiatry Rep* 2010;12:366–373.

92. Lahey BB, Pelham WE, Stein MA, et al. Validity of DSM-IV attention-deficit/hyperactivity disorder for younger children. *J Am Acad Child Adolesc Psychiatry* 1998;37:695–702.

93. Werry JS, Elkind GS, Reeves JC. Attention deficit, conduct, oppositional, and anxiety disorders in children: III. Laboratory differences. *J Abnorm Child Psychol* 1987;15:409–428.

94. Barkley RA. Behavioral inhibition, sustained attention, and executive functions: Constructing a unifying theory of ADHD. *Psychol Bull* 1997;121:65–94.

95. Frith U. (1989). A new look at language and communication in autism. *Br J Disord Commun* 24(2):123–150.

96. Happé F, Frith U. The weak coherence account: Detail-focused cognitive style in autism spectrum disorders. *J Autism Dev Disord* 2006;36(1):5–25.

97. Losh M, Adolphs R, Poe MD, et al. Neuropsychological profile of autism and the broad autism phenotype. *Arch Gen Psychiatry* 2009;66(5):518–526.

98. Mottron L, Dawson M, Soulières I, et al. Enhanced perceptual functioning in autism: An update, and eight principles of autistic perception. *J Autism Dev Disord* 2006;36(1):27–43.

99. Klintwall L, Holm A, Eriksson M, et al. (2011). Sensory abnormalities in autism: A brief report *Res Dev Disabil* 2011;32(2):795–800.

100. Dahlgren SO, Gillberg C. Symptoms in the first two years of life: A preliminary population study of infantile autism. *Eur Arch Psychiatry Neurol Sci* 1989;238(3):169–174.

101. Greenspan SI, Wieder S. Developmental patterns and outcomes in infants and children with disorders in relating and communicating: A chart review of 200 cases of children with autistic spectrum diagnoses. *J Dev Learning Disord* (1997;1:87–141.

102. O'Neill M, Jones RS. Sensory–perceptual abnormalities in autism: A case for more research? *J Autism Dev Disord* 1997;27(3):283–293.

103. Bertone A, Mottron L, Jelenic P, et al. Motion perception in autism: A "complex" issue. *J Cogn Neurosci* 2003;15(2):218–225.

104. Williams DL, Minshew NJ, Goldstein G. Further understanding of complex information processing in verbal adolescents and adults with autism spectrum disorders. *Autism* 2015;19(7):859–867.

105. Minshew NJ, Goldstein G. Autism as a disorder of complex information processing. *Mental Retardation Dev Disabil Res Rev* 1998;4(2), 129–136.

106. Minshew NJ, Goldstein G, Siegel DJ. Neuropsychologic functioning in autism: Profile of a complex information processing disorder. *J Int Neuropsychol Soc* 1997;3(4):303–316.

107. Robertson LC, Lamb MR. Neuropsychological contribution to theories of part/whole organization. *Cognit Psychol* 1991;23:299–330.

108. Benowitz LI, Moya KL, Levine DN. Impaired verbal reasoning and constructional apraxia in subjects with right hemisphere damage. *Neuropsychologia* 1990;23:231–241.

109. Geurts HM, Verté S, Oosterlaan J, et al. How specific are executive functioning deficits in attention deficit hyperactivity disorder and autism? *J Child Psychol Psychiatry* 2004;45(4):836–854.

110. Hill EL. Executive dysfunction in autism. *Trends Cogn Sci* 2004;8(1):26–32.

111. Edgin JO, Pennington BF. Spatial cognition in autism spectrum disorders: Superior, impaired, or just intact? *J Autism Dev Disord* 2005;35(6):729–745.

112. Williams DL, Goldstein G, Minshew NJ. Neuropsychological functioning in children with autism: Further evidence for disordered complex information processing. *Child Neuropsychol* 2006;12(4-5):279–298.

113. Rommelse NN, Geurts HM, Franke B, et al. A review on cognitive and brain endophenotypes that may be common in autism spectrum disorder and attention-deficit/hyperactivity disorder and facilitate the search for pleiotropic genes. *Neurosci Biobehav Rev* 2011;35: 1363–1396.

114. Simonoff E, Pickles A, Charman T, et al. Psychiatric disorders in children with autism spectrum disorders: Prevalence, comorbidity, and associated factors in a population-derived sample. *J Am Acad Child Adolesc Psychiatry* 2008;47(8):921–929.

115. Van der Meer JMJ, Oerlemans AM, van Steijn DJ, et al. Are autism spectrum disorder and attention-deficit/hyperactivity disorder different manifestations of one overarching disorder? Cognitive and symptom evidence from a clinical and population-based sample. *J Am Acad Child Adolesc Psychiatry* 2012;51(11):1160–1172.

116. Ozonoff S, Strayer D. Inhibitory function in nonretarded children with autism. *J Autism Dev Disord* 1997;27(1):59–77.

117. Raymaekers R, Antrop I, van der Meere JJ, et al. HFA and ADHD: A direct comparison on state regulation and response inhibition. *J Clin Exp Neuropsychol* 2007;29(4):418–427.

118. Langen M, Durston S, Kas MJ, et al. The neurobiology of repetitive behavior: . . . and men. *Neurosci Biobehav Rev* 2011;35(3):356–365.

119. Vaughan Van Hecke A, Mundy PC, Acra CF, et al. Infant joint attention, temperament, and social competence in preschool children. *Child Dev* 2007;78(1):53–69.

120. Yerys BE, Wallace GL, Sokoloff JL, et al. Attention deficit/hyperactivity disorder symptoms moderate cognition and behavior in children with autism spectrum disorders. *Autism Res* 2009;2(6):322–333.

121. D'Cruz A-M, Ragozzino ME, Mosconi MW, et al. Reduced behavioral flexibility in autism spectrum disorders. *Neuropsychology* 2013;27(2):152–160.

122. Schmitz N, Rubia K, Daly E, et al. Neural correlates of executive function in autistic spectrum disorders. *Biol Psychiatry* 2006;59(1):7–16.

123. Solomon M, Ozonoff SJ, Ursu S, et al. The neural substrates of cognitive control deficits in autism spectrum disorders. *Neuropsychologia* 2009;47(12):2515–2526.

124. Christakou A, Halari R, Smith AB, et al. Sex-dependent age modulation of frontostriatal and temporo-parietal activation during cognitive control. *Neuroimage* 2009;48(1):223–236.

125. Schmitz N, Rubia K, Daly E, et al. Neural correlates of executive function in autistic spectrum disorders. *Biol Psychiatry* 2006;59(1):7–16.

126. Christakou A, Murphy CM, Chantiluke K, et al. Disorder-specific functional abnormalities during sustained attention in youth with attention deficit hyperactivity disorder (ADHD) and with autism. *Mol Psychiatry* 2013;18(2):236–244.

127. O'Doherty J, Kringelbach ML, Rolls ET, et al. Abstract reward and punishment representations in the human orbitofrontal cortex. *Nat Neurosci* 2001;4(1):95–102.

128. O'Doherty J, Critchley H, Deichmann R, et al. Dissociating valence of outcome from behavioral control in human orbital and ventral prefrontal cortices. *J Neurosci* 2003;23(21):7931–7939.

129. Cools R, Clark L, Owen AM, et al. Defining the neural mechanisms of probabilistic reversal learning using event-related functional magnetic resonance imaging. *J Neurosci* 2002;22(11):4563–4567.

130. Remijnse PL, Nielen MM, Uylings HB, et al. Neural correlates of a reversal learning task with an affectively neutral baseline: An event-related fMRI study. *Neuroimage* 2005;26(2):609–618.

131. Cohen MX, Elger CE, Weber B. Amygdala tractography predicts functional connectivity and learning during feedback-guided decision-making. *Neuroimage* 2008;39(3):1396–1407.

132. Kehagia AA, Murray GK, Robbins TW. Learning and cognitive flexibility: Frontostriatal function and monoaminergic modulation. *Curr Opin Neurobiol* 2010;20(2):199–204.

133. Packard MG, Knowlton BJ. Learning and memory functions of the basal ganglia. *Annu Rev Neurosci* 2002;25(1):563–593.

134. Tsuchida A, Doll BB, Fellows LK. Beyond reversal: A critical role for human orbitofrontal cortex in flexible learning from probabilistic feedback. *J Neurosci* 2010;30(50):16868–16875.

135. Yin HH, Knowlton BJ. The role of the basal ganglia in habit formation. *Nat Rev Neurosci* 2006;7(6):464–476.

136. Baron-Cohen S, Ring HA, Bullmore ET, et al. The amygdala theory of autism. *Neurosci Biobehav Rev* 2000;24(3):355–364.

137. Baron-Cohen S, Leslie AM, Frith U. Does the autistic child have a "theory of mind?" *Cognition* 1985;21(1):37–46.

138. Brüne M. "Theory of mind" in schizophrenia: A review of the literature. *Schizophrenia Bull* 2005;31(1):21–42.

139. Dahlgren S, Sandberg AD, Hjelmquist E. The non-specificity of theory of mind deficits: Evidence from children with communicative disabilities. *Eur J Cogn Psychol* 2003;15(1):129–155.

140. Tine M, Lucariello J. Unique theory of mind differentiation in children with autism and Asperger syndrome. *Autism Res Treat* 2012;2012:505393.

141. Hobson RP. *Autism and the development of mind.* Hove, UK: Psychology Press; 1995.

142. Baron-Cohen S. Precursors to a theory of mind: Understanding attention in others. In Whiten A (Ed.), *Natural theories of mind: Evolution, development, and simulation of everyday mindreading.* Cambridge, MA: Blackwell; 1991:233–251.

143. Chevallier C, Kohls G, Troiani V, et al. The social motivation theory of autism. *Trends Cogn Sci* 2012;16(4):231–239.

144. Adolphs R, Spezio M. Role of the amygdala in processing visual social stimuli. *Prog Brain Res* 2006;156:363–378.

145. Klein JT, Shepherd SV, Platt ML. Social attention and the brain. *Curr Biol* 2009;19(20):R958–R962.

146. Zeeland SV, Ashley A, Dapretto M, et al. Reward processing in autism. *Autism Res* 2010;3(2):53–67.

147. Kohls G, Schulte-Rüther M, Nehrkorn B, et al. Reward system dysfunction in autism spectrum disorders. *Soc Cogn Affect Neurosci* 2013;8(5):565–572.

148. Dichter GS, Felder JN, Green SR, et al. Reward circuitry function in autism spectrum disorders. *Soc Cogn Affect Neurosci* 2012;7(2):160–172.

149. Dichter GS, Richey JA, Rittenberg AM, et al. Reward circuitry function in autism during face anticipation and outcomes. *J Autism Dev Disord* 2012;42(2):147–160.

150. Myers SM, Johnson CP. Management of children with autism spectrum disorders. *Pediatrics* 2007;120(5):1162–1182.

151. Zametkin AJ, Rapoport JL. Neurobiology of attention deficit disorder with hyperactivity: Where have we come in 50 years? *J Am Acad Child Adolescent Psychiatry* 1987;26:676–686.

152. Solanto MV, Conners CK. A dose–response and time–action analysis of autonomic and behavioral effects of methylphenidate in attention deficit disorder with hyperactivity. *Psychophysiology* 1982;19:658–667.

153. Castellanos FX. Neuroimaging studies of ADHD. In Solanto MV, Arnsten AF, Castellanos FX (Eds.), *Stimulant drugs and ADHD: Basic and clinical neuroscience*. New York, NY: Oxford University Press; 2001:243–258.

154. Dougherty DD, Bonab AA, Spencer TJ, et al. Dopamine transporter density in patients with attention deficit hyperactivity disorder. *Lancet* 1999;354:2132–2133.

155. Krause KH, Dresel SH, Krause J, et al. Increased striatal dopamine transporter in adult patients with attention deficit hyperactivity disorder: Effects of methylphenidate as measured by single photon emission computed tomography. *Neurosci Lett* 2000;285:107–110.

156. Cook EH, Stein MA, Krasowski MD, et al. Association of attention-deficit disorder and the dopamine transporter gene. *Am J Hum Genet* 1995;56:993–998.

157. Oades RD. Role of the serotonin system in ADHD: Treatment implications. *Expert Rev Neurother* 2007;7(10):1357–1374.

158. Zafeiriou DI, Ververi A, Vargiami E. The serotonergic system: Its role in pathogenesis and early developmental treatment of autism. *Curr Neuropharmacol* 2009;7(2):150.

159. Spivak B, Vered Y, Yoran-Hegesh R, et al. Circulatory levels of catecholamines, serotonin and lipids in attention deficit hyperactivity disorder. *Acta Psychiatr Scand* 1999;99(4):300–304.

160. Mulder EJ, Anderson GM, Kema IP, et al. Platelet serotonin levels in pervasive developmental disorders and mental retardation: Diagnostic group differences, within-group distribution, and behavioral correlates. *J Am Acad Child Adolesc Psychiatry* 2004;43(4):491–499.

161. Chugani DC, Muzik O, Rothermel R, et al. Altered serotonin synthesis in the dentatothalamocortical pathway in autistic boys. *Ann Neurol* 1997;42(4):666–669.

162. Murphy DG, Daly E, Schmitz N, et al. Cortical serotonin 5-HT 2A receptor binding and social communication in adults with Asperger's syndrome: An in vivo SPECT study. *Am J Psychiatry* 2006;163(5):934–936.

163. Nakamura K, Sekine Y, Ouchi Y, et al. Brain serotonin and dopamine transporter bindings in adults with high-functioning autism. *Arch Gen Psychiatry* 2010;67(1):59–68.

164. Robbins TW, Crockett MJ. Role of central serotonin in impulsivity and compulsivity: Comparative studies in experimental animals and humans. *Handbook Behav Neurosci* 2010;21:415–427.

165. Allen PP, Cleare AJ, Lee F, et al. Effect of acute tryptophan depletion on prefrontal engagement. *Psychopharmacology* 2006;187(4):486–497.

166. Robbins TW, Roberts AC. Differential regulation of fronto-executive function by the mono-amines and acetylcholine. *Cerebral Cortex* 2007;17(Suppl 1):i151–i160.

167. Coghlan S, Horder J, Inkster B, et al. GABA system dysfunction in autism and related disorders: From synapse to symptoms. *Neurosci Biobehav Rev* 2012;36:2044–2055.

168. Fatemi SH. The hyperglutamatergic hypothesis of autism. *Prog Neuropsychopharmacol Biol Psychiatry* 2008;32:911.

169. Rubenstein JLR, Merzenich MM. Model of autism: Increased ratio of excitation/inhibition in key neural systems. *Genes Brain Behav* 2003;2:255–267.

170. Mercugliano M. What is attention-deficit/hyperactivity disorder? *Pediatr Clin North Am* 1999;46(5):831–843.

171. MTA Cooperative Group. A 14 month randomized clinical trial of treatment strategies of attention-deficit/hyperactivity disorder. *Arch Gen Psychiatry* 1999;56:1073–1086.

172. Porrino LJ, Rapoport JL, Behar D, et al. A naturalistic assessment of the motor activity of hyperactive boys: II. Stimulant drug effects. *Arch Gen Psychiatry* 1983;40:688–693.

173. Volkow ND, Fowler JS, Wang G, et al. Mechanism of action of methylphenidate: Insights from PET imaging studies. *J Atten Disord* 2002;6(Suppl 1):S31–S43.

174. Volkow ND, Wang GJ, Fowler JS, et al. Relationship between blockade of dopamine transporters by oral methylphenidate and the increases in extracellular dopamine: Therapeutic implications. *Synapse* 2002;43:181–187.

175. Hannestad J, Gallezot JD, Planeta-Wilson B, et al. Clinically relevant doses of methylphenidate significantly occupy norepinephrine transporters in humans in vivo. *Biol Psychiatry* 2010;68:854–860.

176. Solanto MV, Conners CK. A dose–response and time–action analysis of autonomic and behavioral effects of methylphenidate in attention deficit disorder with hyperactivity. *Psychophysiology* 1982;19:658–667.

177. Swanson J, Baler RD, Volkow ND. Understanding the effects of stimulant medications on cognition in individuals with attention-deficit hyperactivity disorder: A decade of progress. *Neuropsychopharmacology* 2011;36:207–226.

178. Advokat C. What are the cognitive effects of stimulant medications? Emphasis on adults with attention-deficit/hyperactivity disorder (ADHD). *Neurosci Biobehav Rev* 2010;34:1256–1266.

179. Doyle RL, Frazier J, Spencer TJ, et al. Donepezil in the treatment of ADHD-like symptoms in youths with pervasive developmental disorder: A case series. *J Atten Disord* 2006;9:543–549.

180. Jensen PS, Arnold LE, Swanson JM, et al. 3-year follow-up of the NIMH MTA study. *J Am Acad Child Adolesc Psychiatry* 2007;46:989–1002.

181. Williams LM, Hermens DF, Palmer D, et al. Misinterpreting emotional expressions in attention-deficit/hyperactivity disorder: Evidence for a neural marker and stimulant effects. *Biol Psychiatry* 2008;63:917–926.

182. Gibson AP, Bettinger TL, Patel NC, et al. Atomoxetine versus stimulants for treatment of attention deficit/hyperactivity disorder. *Ann Pharmacother* 2006;40:1134–1142.

183. Michelson D, Faries D, Wernicke J, et al. Atomoxetine in the treatment of children and adolescents with attention-deficit/hyperactivity disorder: A randomized, placebo-controlled, dose–response study. *Pediatrics* 2001;108:E83.

184. Wee S, Woolverton WL. Evaluation of the reinforcing effects of atomoxetine in monkeys: Comparison to methylphenidate and desipramine. *Drug Alcohol Depend* 2004;75:271–276.

185. Heil SH, Holmes HW, Bickel WK, et al. Comparison of the subjective, physiological, and psychomotor effects of atomoxetine and methylphenidate in light drug users. *Drug Alcohol Depend* 2002;67:149–156.

186. Bymaster FP, Katner JS, Nelson DL, et al. Atomoxetine increases extracellular levels of norepinephrine and dopamine in prefrontal cortex of rat: A potential mechanism for efficacy in attention deficit/hyperactivity disorder. *Neuropsychopharmacology* 2002;27:699–711.

187. Wong DT, Threlkeld PG, Best KL, et al. A new inhibitor of norepinephrine uptake devoid of affinity for receptors in rat brain. *J Pharmacol Exp Ther* 1982;222:61–65.

188. Seneca N, Gulyas B, Varrone A, et al. Atomoxetine occupies the norepinephrine transporter in a dose-dependent fashion: A PET study in nonhuman primate brain using (S,S)-(18F)FMeNER-D2. *Psychopharmacology (Berl)* 2006;188:119–127.

189. Logan J, Wang GJ, Telang F, et al. Imaging the norepinephrine transporter in humans with (S,S)-(11C)O-methyl reboxetine and PET: Problems and progress. *Nucl Med Biol* 2007;34:667–679.

190. Liu LL, Yang J, Lei GF, et al. Atomoxetine increases histamine release and improves learning deficits in an animal model of attention-deficit hyperactivity disorder: The spontaneously hypertensive rat. *Basic Clin Pharmacol Toxicol* 2008;102:527–532.

191. Tzavara ET, Bymaster FP, Overshiner CD, et al. Procholinergic and memory enhancing properties of the selective norepinephrine uptake inhibitor atomoxetine. *Mol Psychiatry* 2006;11:187–195.

192. de Jong CG, Van De Voorde S, Roeyers H, et al. Differential effects of atomoxetine on executive functioning and lexical decision in attention-deficit/hyperactivity disorder and reading disorder. *J Child Adolesc Psychopharmacol* 2009;19:699–707.

193. Gau SS, Shang CY. Improvement of executive functions in boys with attention deficit hyperactivity disorder: An open-label follow-up study with once-daily atomoxetine. *Int J Neuropsychopharmacol* 2010;13:243–256.

194. Brown TE, Holdnack J, Saylor K, et al. Effect of atomoxetine on executive function impairments in adults with ADHD. *J Atten Disord* 2011;15:130–138.

195. Ramos BP, Stark D, Verduzco L, et al. Alpha2A-adrenoceptor stimulation improves prefrontal cortical regulation of behavior through inhibition of cAMP signalling in aging animals. *Learn Mem* 2006;13:770–776.

196. Scahill L, Chappell PB, Kim YS, et al. A placebo controlled study of guanfacine in the treatment of children with tic disorders and attention deficit hyperactivity disorder. *Am J Psychiatry* 2001;158:1067–1074.

197. Verbeeck W, Tuinier S, Bekkering GE. Antidepressants in the treatment of adult attention deficit hyperactivity disorder: A systematic review. *Adv Ther* 2009;26:170–184.

198. Pliszka S. Practice parameter for the assessment and treatment of children and adolescents with attention-deficit/hyperactivity disorder. *J Am Acad Child Adolesc Psychiatry* 2007;46:894–921.

199. Herrera-Guzman I, Gudayol-Ferre E, Lira-Mandujano J, et al. Cognitive predictors of treatment response to bupropion and cognitive effects of bupropion in patients with major depressive disorder. *Psychiatry Res* 2008;160:72–82.

200. Doraiswamy PM, Krishnan KR, Oxman T, et al. Does antidepressant therapy improve cognition in elderly depressed patients? *J Gerontol A Biol Sci Med Sci* 2003;58:M1137–M1144.

201. Evins AE, Cather C, Deckersbach T, et al. A double-blind placebo-controlled trial of bupropion sustained-release for smoking cessation in schizophrenia. *J Clin Psychopharmacol* 2005;25:218–225.

202. Rubinstein S, Malone MA, Roberts W, et al. Placebo-controlled study examining effects of selegiline in children with attention-deficit/hyperactivity disorder. *Child Adolesc Psychopharmacol* 2006;16:404–415.

203. Wilens TE, Decker MW. Neuronal nicotinic receptor agonists for the treatment of attention-deficit/hyperactivity disorder: Focus on cognition. *Biochem Pharmacol* 2007;74:1212–1223.

204. Levin ED, McClernon FJ, Rezvani AH. Nicotinic effects on cognitive function: Behavioural characterization, pharmacological specification, and anatomic localization. *Psychopharmacology (Berl)* 2006;184:523–539.

205. Lambert NM, Hartsough CS. Prospective study of tobacco smoking and substance dependencies among samples of ADHD and non-ADHD participants. *J Learn Disabil* 1998;31:533–544.

206. Wesnes K, Warburton D. The effects of cigarettes of varying yield on rapid information processing performance. *Psychopharmacology* 1984;82:338–342.

207. Bekker EM, Bocker KBE, Van Hunsel F, et al. Acute effects of nicotine on attention and response inhibition. *Pharmacol Biochem Behav* 2005;82:539–548.

208. Wesnes K, Warburton DM. Smoking, nicotine, and human performance. *Pharmacol Ther* 1983;21:189–208.

209. Newhouse P, Sunderland T, Tariot P, et al. Intravenous nicotine in Alzheimer's disease: A pilot study. *Psychopharmacology* 1988;95:171–175.

210. Harris JG, Kongs S, Allensworth D, et al. Effects of nicotine on cognitive deficits in schizophrenia. *Neuropsychopharmacology* 2004;29:1378–1385.

211. Potter AS, Newhouse PA. Effects of acute nicotine administration on behavioural inhibition in adolescents with attention-deficit/hyperactivity disorder. *Psychopharmacology (Berl)* 2004;176:182–194.

212. Gehricke J-G, Whalen CK, Jamner LD, et al. The reinforcing effects of nicotine and stimulant medication in the everyday lives of adult smokers with ADHD: A preliminary examination. *Nicotine Tobacco Res* 2006;8:37–47.

213. Gehricke JG, Hong N, Whalen CK, et al. Effects of transdermal nicotine on symptoms, moods, and cardiovascular activity in the everyday lives of smokers and nonsmokers with attention-deficit/hyperactivity disorder. *Psychol Addict Behav* 2009;23:644–655.

214. Levin ED, Conners CK, Sparrow E, et al. Nicotine effects on adults with attention-deficit/hyperactivity disorder. *Psychopharmacology (Berl)* 1996;123:55–63.

215. Wilens TE, Biederman J, Spencer TJ, et al. A pilot controlled clinical trial of ABT-418, a cholinergic agonist, in the treatment of adults with attention deficit hyperactivity disorder. *Am J Psychiatry* 1999;156:1931–1937.

216. Wilens TE, Verlinden MH, Adler LA, et al. ABT-089, a neuronal nicotinic receptor partial agonist, for the treatment of attention-deficit/hyperactivity disorder in adults: Results of a pilot study. *Biol Psychiatry* 2006;59:1065–1070.

217. Wilens TE, Biederman J, Wong J, et al. Adjunctive donepezil in attention deficit hyperactivity disorder youth: Case series. *J Child Adolesc Psychopharmacol* 2000;10:217–222.

218. Wilens TE, Waxmonsky J, Scott M, et al. An open trial of adjunctive donepezil in attention-deficit/hyperactivity disorder. *J Child Adolesc Psychopharmacol* 2005;15:947–955.

219. Cubo E, Fernandez Jaen A, Moreno C, et al. Donepezil use in children and adolescents with tics and attention-deficit/hyperactivity disorder: An 18-week, single-center, dose-escalating, prospective, open-label study. *Clin Ther* 2008;30:182–189.

220. Toplak ME, Connors L, Shuster J, et al. Review of cognitive, cognitive behavioral, and neural-based interventions for attention-deficit/hyperactivity disorder (ADHD). *Clin Psychol Rev* 2008;28:801–823.

221. Biederman J, Mick E, Faraone S, et al. A double blind comparison of galantamine hydrogen bromide and placebo in adults with attention-deficit/hyperactivity disorder: A pilot study. *J Clin Psychopharmacol* 2006;26:163–166.

222. McKeage K. Memantine: A review of its use in moderate to severe Alzheimer's disease. *CNS Drugs* 2009;23:881–897.

223. Findling RL, McNamara NK, Stansbrey RJ, et al. A pilot evaluation of the safety, tolerability, pharmacokinetics, and effectiveness of memantine in pediatric patients with attention-deficit/hyperactivity disorder combined type. *J Child Adolesc Psychopharmacol* 2007;17:19–33.

224. Minzenberg MJ, Carter CS. Modafinil: A review of neurochemical actions and effects on cognition. *Neuropsychopharmacology* 2008;33:1477–1502.

225. Turner DC, Clark L, Dowson J, et al. Modafinil improves cognition and response inhibition in adult attention-deficit/hyperactivity disorder. *Biol Psychiatry* 2004;55:1031–1040.

226. Finke K, Dodds CM, Bublak P, et al. Effects of modafinil and methylphenidate on visual attention capacity: A TVA-based study. *Psychopharmacology (Berl)* 2010;210:317–329.

227. Greenhill LL, Biederman J, Boellner SW, et al. A randomized, double-blind, placebo-controlled study of modafinil film-coated tablets in children and adolescents with attention-deficit/hyperactivity disorder. *J Am Acad Child Adolesc Psychiatry* 2006;45:503–511.

228. Swanson JM, Greenhill LL, Lopez FA, et al. Modafinil filmcoated tablets in children and adolescents with attention-deficit/hyperactivity disorder: Results of a randomized, double-blind, placebo-controlled, fixed-dose study followed by abrupt discontinuation. *J Clin Psychiatry* 2006;67:137–147.

229. Amiri S, Mohammadi MR, Mohammadi M, et al. Modafinil as a treatment for attention-deficit/ hyperactivity disorder in children and adolescents: A double blind, randomized clinical trial. *Prog Neuropsychopharmacol Biol Psychiatry* 2008;32:145–149.

230. Yehuda S, Rabinovitz S, Mostofsky DI. Essential fatty acids and the brain: From infancy to aging. *Neurobiol Aging* 2005;26(1):98–102.

231. Stevens L, Zhang W, Peck L, et al. EFA supplementation in children with inattention, hyperactivity, and other disruptive behaviors. *Lipids* 2003;38(10):1007–1021.

232. Chen J-R, Hsu S-F, Hsu C-D, et al. Dietary patterns and blood fatty acid composition in children with attention-deficit hyperactivity disorder in Taiwan. *J Nutr Biochem* 2004;15(8):467–472.

233. Gillies D, Sinn JKH, Lad SS, et al. Polyunsaturated fatty acids (PUFA) for attention deficit hyperactivity disorder (ADHD) in children and adolescents. *Cochrane Database Syst Rev* 2012;2012(7):CD007986.

234. National Institute for Health and Care Excellence (NICE). *Autism spectrum disorder in adults: Diagnosis and management.* NICE guideline CG142. London: NICE; 2012.

235. Maglione MA, Gans D, Das L, et al. Nonmedical interventions for children with ASD: Recommended guidelines and further research needs. *Pediatrics* 2012;130(Suppl 2):S169–S178.

236. Mandell DS, Morales KH, Marcus SC, et al. Psychotropic medication use among Medicaid-enrolled children with autism spectrum disorders. *Pediatrics* 2008;121(3):e441–e448.

237. Rosenberg RE, Mandell DS, Farmer JE, et al. Psychotropic medication use among children with autism spectrum disorders enrolled in a national registry, 2007–2008. *J Autism Dev Disord* 2010;40(3):342–351.

238. Barrickman L, Noyes R, Kuperman S, et al. Treatment of ADHD with fluoxetine: A preliminary trial. *J Am Acad Child Adolesc Psychiatry* 1991;30(5):762–767.

239. Gammon GD, Brown TE. Fluoxetine and methylphenidate in combination for treatment of attention deficit disorder and comorbid depressive disorder. *J Child Adolesc Psychopharmacol* 1993;3(1):1–10.

240. Quintana H, Butterbaugh GJ, Purnell W, et al. Fluoxetine monotherapy in attention-deficit/ hyperactivity disorder and comorbid non-bipolar mood disorders in children and adolescents. *Child Psychiatry Hum Dev* 2007;37(3):241–253.

241. DeLong GR, Ritch CR, Burch S. Fluoxetine response in children with autistic spectrum disorders: Correlation with familial major affective disorder and intellectual achievement. *Dev Med Child Neurol* 2002;44(10):652–659.

242. DeLong GR, Teague LA, Kamran MM. Effects of fluoxetine treatment in young children with idiopathic autism. *Dev Med Child Neurol* 1998;40(8):551–562.

243. Hollander E, Phillips A, Chaplin W, et al. A placebo controlled crossover trial of liquid fluoxetine on repetitive behaviors in childhood and adolescent autism. *Neuropsychopharmacology* 2005;30(3):582–589.

244. Buchsbaum MS, Hollander E, Haznedar MM, et al. Effect of fluoxetine on regional cerebral metabolism in autistic spectrum disorders: A pilot study. *Int J Neuropsychopharmacol* 2001;4(2):119–125.

245. Makkonen I, Riikonen R, Kokki H, et al. Serotonin and dopamine transporter binding in children with autism determined by SPECT. *Dev Med Child Neurol* 2008;50(8):593–597.

246. Nakamura K, Sekine Y, Ouchi Y, et al. Brain serotonin and dopamine transporter bindings in adults with high-functioning autism. *Arch Gen Psychiatry* 2010;67(1):59–68.

247. Chantiluke K, Barrett N, Giampietro V, et al. Inverse effect of fluoxetine on medial prefrontal cortex activation during reward reversal in ADHD and autism. *Cerebral Cortex* 2015;25(7):1757–1770.

248. Chantiluke K, Barrett N, Giampietro V, et al. Disorder-dissociated effects of fluoxetine on brain function of working memory in attention deficit hyperactivity disorder and autism spectrum disorder. *Psychol Med* 2015;45:1195–1205.

249. Williams K, Wheeler DM, Silvone N, et al. Selective serotonin reuptake inhibitors (SSRIs) for autism spectrum disorders (ASD). *Cochrane Database Syst Rev* 2010;2010(8):CD004677.

250. Hollander E, Phillips A, Chaplin W, et al. A placebo controlled crossover trial of liquid fluoxetine on repetitive behaviors in childhood and adolescent autism. *Neuropsychopharmacology* 2005;30(3):582–589.

251. King BH, Hollander E, Sikich L, et al. Lack of efficacy of citalopram in children with autism spectrum disorders and high levels of repetitive behavior: Citalopram ineffective in children with autism. *Arch Gen Psychiatry* 2009;66(6):583–590.

252. Hurwitz R, Blackmore R, Hazell P, et al. Tricyclic antidepressants for autism spectrum disorders (ASD) in children and adolescents. *Cochrane Database Syst Rev* 2012;2012(3):CD008372.

253. Remington G, Sloman L, Konstantareas M, et al. Clomipramine versus haloperidol in the treatment of autistic disorder: A double-blind, placebo-controlled, crossover study. *J Clin Psychopharmacol* 2001;21(4):440–444.

254. Gordon CT, State RC, Nelson JE, et al. A double-blind comparison of clomipramine, desipramine and placebo in the treatment of autistic disorder. *Arch Gen Psychiatry* 1993;50(6):441–447.

255. Niederhofer H, Staffen W, Mair A. Tianeptine: A novel strategy of psychopharmacological treatment of children with autistic disorder. *Hum Psychopharmacol Clin Exp* 2003;18:389–393.

256. McPheeters ML, Warren Z, Sathe N, et al. A systematic review of medical treatments for children with autism spectrum disorders. *Pediatrics* 2011;127(5):e1312–e1321.

257. Taylor JL, Dove D, Veenstra-VanderWeele J, et al. *Interventions for adolescents and young adults with autism spectrum disorders*. Comparative Effectiveness Review No. 65. AHRQ Publication No. 12-EHC063-EF. Rockville, MD: Agency for Healthcare Research and Quality; 2012.

258. Arnold LE, Aman MG, Li X, et al. Research Units of Pediatric Psychopharmacology (RUPP) Autism Network randomized clinical trial of parent training and medication: One-year follow-up. *J Am Acad Child Adolesc Psychiatry* 2012;51(11):1173–1184.

259. Autism P. Randomized, controlled, crossover trial of methylphenidate in pervasive developmental disorders with hyperactivity. *Arch Gen Psychiatry* 2005;62:1266–1274.

260. Jahromi LB, Kasari CL, McCracken JT, et al. Positive effects of methylphenidate on social communication and self-regulation in children with pervasive developmental disorders and hyperactivity. *J Autism Dev Disord* 2009;39(3):395–404.

261. Posey DJ, Aman MG, McCracken JT, et al. Positive effects of methylphenidate on inattention and hyperactivity in pervasive developmental disorders: An analysis of secondary measures. *Biol Psychiatry* 2007;61(4):538–544.

262. Preti A, Melis M, Siddi S, et al. Oxytocin and autism: A systematic review of randomized controlled trials. *J Child Adolesc Psychopharmacol* 2014;24(2):54–68.

263. Elsabbagh M, Mercure E, Hudry K, et al.; the BASIS Team. Infant neural sensitivity to dynamic eye gaze is associated with later emerging autism. *Curr Biol* 2012;22(4):338–342.

264. Sucksmith E, Allison C, Baron-Cohen S, et al. Empathy and emotion recognition in people with autism, first-degree relatives, and controls. *Neuropsychologia* 2013;51(1):98–105.

265. Anagnostou E, Soorya L, Chaplin W, et al. Intranasal oxytocin versus placebo in the treatment of adults with autism spectrum disorders: A randomized controlled trial. *Mol Autism* 2012;3(1):16.

266. Bales KL, Perkeybile AM. Developmental experiences and the oxytocin receptor system. *Horm Behav* 2012;61(3):313–319.

267. Amminger GP, Berger GE, Schäfer MR, et al. Omega-3 fatty acids supplementation in children with autism: A double-blind randomized, placebo-controlled pilot study. *Biol Psychiatry* 2007;61(4):551–553.

268. Bent S, Bertoglio K, Hendren RL. Omega-3 fatty acids for autistic spectrum disorder: A systematic review. *J Autism Dev Disord* 2009;39(8):1145–1154.

269. Meichenbaum DH. *Cognitive–behavior modification: An integrative approach*. New York, NY: Plenum; 1977.

270. Douglas VI. Treatment and training approaches to hyperactivity: Establishing internal or external control. In Whalen C, Henker B (Eds.), *Hyperactive children: The social ecology of identification and treatment*. New York: Academic Press; 1980:283–317.

271. Kagan J, Rosman BL, Day D, et al. Information processing in the child: Significance of analytic and reflective attitudes. *Psychol Monogr* 1964;78:1–37.

272. Douglas VI, Parry P, Marton P, et al. Assessment of a cognitive training program for hyperactive children. *J Abnorm Child Psychol* 1976;4:389–410.

273. Moore SF, Cole SD. Cognitive self-mediation training with hyperkinetic children. *Bull Psychonom Soc* 1978;12:18–20.

274. Reid MK, Borkowski JG. Causal attributions of hyperactive children: Implications for teaching strategies and self-control. *J Educ Psychol* 1987;79:296–307.

275. Conners CK. A teacher rating scale for use in drug studies with children *Am J Psychiatry* 1969;126:884–888.

276. Horn WF, Chatoor I, Conners CK. Additive effects of Dexedrine and self-control training: A multiple assessment. *Behav Modif* 1983;7:383–402.

277. Douglas VI, Ban RG, O'Neill ME, et al. Short term effects of methylphenidate on the cognitive, learning and academic performance of children with attention deficit disorder in the laboratory and the classroom. *J Child Psychol Psychiatry* 1986;27:191–211.

278. Pelham WE Jr. The effects of psychostimulant drugs on learning and academic achievement in children with attention-deficit disorders and learning disabilities. In Torgesen JK, Wong BYL (Eds.), *Psychological and educational perspectives on learning disabilities.* New York, NY: Academic Press; 1986:259–295.

279. Conrad WG, Dworkin ES, Shai A, et al. Effects of amphetamine therapy and prescriptive tutoring on the behavior and achievement of lower class hyperactive children. *J Learn Disabil* 1971;4:45–53.

280. Richardson E, Kupietz SS, Winsberg BG, et al. Effects of methylphenidate dosage in hyperactive reading-disabled children: II. Reading achievement. *J Am Acad Child Adolesc Psychiatry* 1988;27:78–87.

281. Kirby EA. *Durable and generalized effects of cognitive behavior modification with attention deficit disorder children.* Paper presented at the annual meeting of the American Psychological Association, Toronto, Ontario, Canada, August 1984.

282. Cameron ME, Robinson VMJ. Effects of cognitive training on academic and on task behavior of hyperactive children. *J Abnorm Child Psychol* 1980;8:405–420.

283. Varni JW, Henker B. A self-regulation approach to the treatment of three hyperactive boys. *Child Behav Ther* 1979;1:171–192.

284. Klingberg T, Forssberg H, Westerberg H. Training of working memory in children with ADHD. *J Clin Exp Neuropsychol* 2002;24:781–791.

285. Klingberg T, Fernell E, Olesen PJ, et al. Computerized training of working memory in children with ADHD—A randomized, controlled trial. *J Am Acad Child Adolesc Psychiatry* 2005;44:177–186.

286. Olesen PJ, Westerberg H, Klingberg T. Increased prefrontal and parietal activity after training of working memory. *Nat Neurosci* 2004;7:75–79.

287. McNab F, Varrone A, Farde L, et al. Changes in cortical dopamine D1 receptor binding associated with cognitive training. *Science* 2009;323:800–802.

288. Butnik SM. Neurofeedback in adolescents and adults with attention deficit hyperactivity disorder. *J Clin Psychol* 2005;61:621–625.

289. Heinrich H, Gevensleben H, Strehl U. Annotation: neurofeedback—Train your brain to train behaviour. *J Child Psychol Psychiatry* 2007;48:3–16.

290. Fohlmann AH. Social skills training [Social færdighedstræning [Danish]]. In Nordentoft M, Melau M, Iversen T, et al. (Eds.), *Psychosis in the young. Symptoms, treatment and the future [Psykose hos unge. Symptomer, behandling og fremtid [Danish]].* Copenhagen, Denmark: Psykiatrifondens Forlag, 2009:161–189.

291. Liberman RP. Social skills training. In Liberman RP (Ed.), *Psychiatric rehabilitation of chronic mental patients.* Washington, DC: American Psychiatric Press; 1988.

292. Majewicz-Hefley A, Carlson JS. A meta-analysis of combined treatments for children diagnosed with ADHD. *J Atten Disord* 2007;10(3):239–250.

293. Boo de GM, Prins PJM. Social incompetence in children with ADHD: Possible moderators and mediators in social skills training. *Clin Psychol Rev* 2007;27(1):78–97.

294. van der Oord S, Prins PJM, Oosterlaan J, et al. Does brief, clinically based, intensive multi-modal behaviour therapy enhance the effects of methylphenidate in children with ADHD? *Eur Child Adolesc Psychiatry* 2007;16(1):48–57.

295. Storebø OJ, Skoog M, Damm D, et al. Social skills training for attention deficit hyper-activity disorder (ADHD) in children aged 5 to18 years. *Cochrane Database Syst Rev* 2011;2011(12):CD008223.

296. Weitlauf AS, McPheeters ML, Peters B, et al. (2014). *Therapies for children with autism spec-trum disorder: Behavioral interventions update.* Comparative Effectiveness Review No. 137. (Prepared by the Vanderbilt Evidence-based Practice Center under Contract No. 290-2012-00009-I.) AHRQ Publication No. 14-EHC036-EF. Rockville, MD: Agency for Healthcare Research and Quality; 2014.

297. Reichow B, Steiner AM, Volkmar F. Social skills groups for people aged 6 to 21 with autism spectrum disorders (ASD). *Cochrane Database Syst Rev* 2012;2012(7):CD008511.

298. Williams BT, Gray KM, Tonge BJ. Teaching emotion recognition skills to young children with autism: A randomised controlled trial of an emotion training programme. *J Child Psychol Psychiatry* 2012;53(12):1268–1276.

299. Begeer S, Gevers C, Clifford P, et al. Theory of mind training in children with autism: A ran-domized controlled trial. *J Autism Dev Disord* 2011;41(8):997–1006.

300. Fletcher-Watson S, McConnell F, Manola E, et al. Interventions based on the theory of mind cognitive model for autism spectrum disorder (ASD). *Cochrane Database Syst Rev* 2014;2014(3):CD008785.

301. Bishop-Fitzpatrick L, Minshew NJ, Eack SM. A systematic review of psychosocial interven-tions for adults with autism spectrum disorders. In Volkmar FR, Reichow B, McPartland J (Eds.), *Adolescents and adults with autism spectrum disorders.* New York, NY: Springer; 2014:315–327.

302. Turner-Brown LM, Perry TD, Dichter GS, et al. Brief report: Feasibility of social cogni-tion and interaction training for adults with high functioning autism. *J Autism Dev Disord* 2008;38(9):1777–1784.

303. Lovaas OI. *Teaching developmentally disabled children: The me book.* Baltimore, MD: University Park Press; 1981.

304. Lovaas OI. Behavioral treatment and normal educational and intellectual functioning in young autistic children. *J Consult Clin Psychol* 1987;55(1):3.

305. Bishop-Fitzpatrick L, Minshew NJ, Eack SM. A systematic review of psychosocial interven-tions for adults with autism spectrum disorders. *J Autism Dev Disord* 2013;43(3):687–694.

306. Eikeseth S, Hayward D, Gale C, et al. Intensity of supervision and outcome for preschool aged children receiving early and intensive behavioral interventions: A preliminary study. *Res Autism Spectrum Disord* 2009;3(1):67–73.

307. Smith IM, Koegel RL, Koegel LK, et al. Effectiveness of a novel community-based early intervention model for children with autistic spectrum disorder. *Am J Intellect Dev Disabil* 2010;115(6):504–523.

308. Reichow B, Barton EE, Boyd BA, et al. Early intensive behavioral intervention (EIBI) for young children with autism spectrum disorders (ASD). *Cochrane Database Syst Rev* 2012;2012(10):CD009260.

309. Howard JS, Sparkman CR, Cohen HG, et al. A comparison of intensive behavior analytic and eclectic treatments for young children with autism. *Res Dev Disabil* 2005;26(4):359–383.

310. Cohen H, Amerine-Dickens M, Smith T. Early intensive behavioral treatment: Replication of the UCLA model in a community setting. *J Dev Behav Pediatr* 2006;27(2):S145–S155.

311. Magiati I, Charman T, Howlin P. A two-year prospective follow-up study of community-based early intensive behavioural intervention and specialist nursery provision for children with autism spectrum disorders. *J Child Psychol Psychiatry* 2007;48(8):803–812.

312. Remington B, Hastings RP, Kovshoff H, et al. Early intensive behavioral intervention: Outcomes for children with autism and their parents after two years. *Am J Mental Retardation* 2007;112(6):418–438.

313. Oono IP, Honey EJ, McConachie H. Parent-mediated early intervention for young children with autism spectrum disorders (ASD). *Cochrane Database Syst Rev* 2013;2013(4):CD009774.

314. Stavropoulos KMK, Carver LJ. Research review: Social motivation and oxytocin in autism—Implications for joint attention development and intervention. *J Child Psychol Psychiatry* 2013;54(6):603–618.

315. Itzchak EB, Zachor DA. Who benefits from early intervention in autism spectrum disorders? *Res Autism Spectrum Disord* 2011;5(1):345–350.

316. Zachor DA, Itzchak EB. Treatment approach, autism severity and intervention outcomes in young children. *R Autism Spectrum Disord* 2010;4(3):425–432.

317. Peters-Scheffer N, Didden R, Mulders M, et al. Low intensity behavioral treatment supplementing preschool services for young children with autism spectrum disorders and severe to mild intellectual disability. *Res Dev Disabil* 2010;31(6):1678–1684.

318. Eikeseth S, Klintwall L, Jahr E, et al. Outcome for children with autism receiving early and intensive behavioral intervention in mainstream preschool and kindergarten settings. *Res Autism Spectrum Disord* 2012;6(2):829–835.

319. Boyd BA, Hume K, McBee MT, et al. Comparative efficacy of LEAP, TEACCH and non-model-specific special education programs for preschoolers with autism spectrum disorders. *J Autism Dev Disord* 2014;44(2):366–368.

320. Strain PS, Bovey EH. Randomized, controlled trial of the LEAP model of early intervention for young children with autism spectrum disorders. *Topics Early Childhood Special Educ* 2011;31(3):133–154.

321. Eldevik S, Hastings RP, Jahr E, et al. Outcomes of behavioral intervention for children with autism in mainstream pre-school settings. *J Autism Dev Disord* 2012;42(2):210–220.

322. Kenworthy L, Anthony LG, Naiman DQ, et al. Randomized controlled effectiveness trial of executive function intervention for children on the autism spectrum. *J Child Psychol Psychiatry* 2014;55(4):374–383.

323. Kouijzer MEJ, de Moor JMH, Gerrits BJL, et al. Neurofeedback improves executive functioning in children with autism spectrum disorders. *Res Autism Spectrum Disord* 2009;3(1):145–162.

324. Oberman LM, Ramachandran VS, Pineda JA. Modulation of mu suppression in children with autism spectrum disorders in response to familiar or unfamiliar stimuli: The mirror neuron hypothesis. *Neuropsychologia* 2008;46:1558–1565.

325. Hebb DO. *The organization of behavior: A neuropsychological theory*. New York, NY: Wiley; 1949:335.

326. Rosenzweig MR, Bennett EL. Effects of differential environments on brain weights and enzyme activities in gerbils, rats, and mice. *Dev Psychobiol* 1969;2:87–95.

327. Globus A, Rosenzweig MR, Bennett EL, et al. Effects of differential experience on dendritic spine counts in rat cerebral cortex. *J Comp Physiol Psychol* 1973;82:175–181.

328. Diamond MC, Krech D, Rosenzweig MR. The effects of an enriched environment on the histology of the rat cerebral cortex. *J Comp Neurol* 1964;123:111–120.

329. Green EJ, Greenough WT, Schlumpf BE. Effects of complex or isolated environments on cortical dendrites of middle-aged rats. *Brain Res* 1983;264:233–240.

330. Greenough WT, Volkmar FR. Pattern of dendritic branching in occipital cortex of rats reared in complex environments. *Exp Neurol* 1973;40:491–504.

331. Leggio MG, Mandolesi L, Federico F, et al. Environmental enrichment promotes improved spatial abilities and enhanced dendritic growth in the rat. *Behav Brain Res* 2005;163:78–90.

332. Kempermann G, Kuhn HG, Gage FH. Experience-induced neurogenesis in the senescent dentate gyrus. *J Neurosci* 1998;18:3206–3212.

333. Nilsson M, Perfilieva E, Johansson U, et al. Enriched environment increases neurogenesis in the adult rat dentate gyrus and improves spatial memory. *J Neurobiol* 1999;39:569–578.

334. Duffy SN, Craddock KJ, Abel T, et al. Environmental enrichment modifies the PKA-dependence of hippocampal LTP and improves hippocampus-dependent memory. *Learn Mem* 2001;8:26–34.

335. Ickes BR, Pham TM, Sanders LA, et al. Long-term environmental enrichment leads to regional increases in neurotrophin levels in rat brain. *Exp Neurol* 2000;164:45–52.

336. Pham TM, Winblad B, Granholm AC, et al. Environmental influences on brain neurotrophins in rats. *Pharmacol Biochem Behav* 2002;73:167–175.

337. Faherty CJ, Kerley D, Smeyne RJ. A Golgi–Cox morphological analysis of neuronal changes induced by environmental enrichment. *Brain Res Dev Brain Res* 2003;141:55–61.

338. Rampon C, Tang YP, Goodhouse J, et al. Enrichment induces structural changes and recovery from nonspatial memory deficits in CA1 NMDAR1-knockout mice. *Nat Neurosci* 2000;3:238–244.

339. Frick KM, Fernandez SM. Enrichment enhances spatial memory and increases synaptophysin levels in aged female mice. *Neurobiol Aging* 2003;24:615–626.

340. Torasdotter M, Metsis M, Henriksson BG, et al. Environmental enrichment results in higher levels of nerve growth factor mRNA in the rat visual cortex and hippocampus. *Behav Brain Res* 1998;93:83–90.

341. Williams BM, Luo Y, Ward C, et al. Environmental enrichment: Effects on spatial memory and hippocampal CREB immunoreactivity. *Physiol Behav* 2001;73:649–658.

342. Vaynman SS, Ying Z, Yin D, et al. Exercise differentially regulates synaptic proteins associated to the function of BDNF. *Brain Res.* 2006;1070:124–130.

343. Farmer J, Zhao X, van Praag H, et al. Effects of voluntary exercise on synaptic plasticity and gene expression in the dentate gyrus of adult male Sprague–Dawley rats in vivo. *Neuroscience* 2004;124:71–79.

344. Berchtold NC, Chinn G, Chou M, et al. Exercise primes amolecular memory for brain-derived neurotrophic factor protein induction in the rat hippocampus. *Neuroscience* 2005;133:853–861.

345. Seifert T, Brassard P, Wissenberg M, et al. Endurance training enhances BDNF release from the human brain. *Am J Physiol Regul Integr Comp Physiol* 2010;298:R372–R377.

346. Strohle A, Stoy M, Graetz B, et al. Acute exercise ameliorates reduced brain-derived neurotrophic factor in patients with panic disorder. *Psychoneuroendocrinology* 2010;35:364–368.

347. Baker LD, Frank LL, Foster-Schubert K, et al. Effects of aerobic exercise on mild cognitive impairment: A controlled trial. *Arch Neurol* 2010;67:71–79.

348. Colcombe SJ, Erickson KI, Raz N, et al. Aerobic fitness reduces brain tissue loss in aging humans. *J Gerontol A Biol Sci Med Sci* 2003;58:176–180.

349. Shim SH, Hwangbo Y, Kwon YJ, et al. Increased levels of plasma brain-derived neurotrophic factor (BDNF) in children with attention deficit-hyperactivity disorder (ADHD). *Prog Neuropsychopharmacol Biol Psychiatry* 2008;32:1824–1828.

350. Neeper SA, Gomez-Pinilla F, Choi J, et al. Physical activity increases mRNA for brain-derived neurotrophic factor and nerve growth factor in rat brain. *Brain Res* 1996;726:49–56.

351. Wigal T, Greenhill L, Chuang S, et al. Safety and tolerability of methylphenidate in preschool children with ADHD. *J Am Acad Child Adolesc Psychiatry* 2006;45:1294–1303.

352. Tantillo M, Kesick CM, Hynd GW, et al. The effects of exercise on children with attention-deficit hyperactivity disorder. *Med Sci Sports Exerc* 2002;34:203–212.

353. Howlin P, Alcock J, Burkin C. An 8 year follow-up of a specialist supported employment service for high-ability adults with autism or Asperger syndrome. *Autism* 2005;9(5):533–549.

354. Lawer L, Brusilovskiy E, Salzer MS, et al. Use of vocational rehabilitative services among adults with autism. *J Autism Dev Disord* 2009;39(3):487–494.

355. García-Villamisar D, Wehman P, Navarro MD. Changes in quality of life of autistic people's life that work in supported and sheltered employment: A 5-year follow-up study. *J Vocat Rehab* 2002;17(4):309–312-

356. García-Villamisar D, Ross D, Wehman P. Clinical differential analysis of persons with autism in a work setting: A follow-up study. *J Vocat Rehab* 2000;14(3):183–185.

357. García-Villamisar D, Hughes C. Supported employment improves cognitive performance in adults with autism. *J Intellect Disali Res* 2007;51(Pt 2):142–150.
358. Hanson E, Kalish LA, Bunce E, et al. Use of complementary and alternative medicine among children diagnosed with autism spectrum disorder. *J Autism Dev Disord* 2007;37(4):628–636.
359. NIH Consensus Conference. Acupuncture. *JAMA* 1998;280:1518–1524.
360. Moazzami A, Tjen-A-Looi SC, Guo ZL, et al. Serotonergic projection from nucleus raphe pallidus to rostral ventrolateral medulla modulates cardiovascular reflex responses during acupuncture. *J Appl Physiol* 2010;108:1336–1346.
361. Wang Q, Peng Y, Chen S, et al. Pretreatment with electroacupuncture induces rapid tolerance to focal cerebral ischemia through regulation of endocannabinoid system. *Stroke* 2009;40(6):2157–2164.
362. Lee GJ, Yin CS, Choi SK, et al. Acupuncture attenuates extracellular glutamate level in global ischemia model of rat. *Neurol Res* 2010;32(Suppl 1):79–83.
363. Fu LW, Longhurst JC. Electroacupuncture modulates vlPAG release of GABA through presynaptic cannabinoid CB1 receptors. *J Appl Physiol* 2009;106(6):1800–1809.
364. Yoon SS, Kim H, Choi KH, et al. Acupuncture suppresses morphine self-administration through the GABA receptors. *Brain Res Bull* 2010;81(6):625–630.
365. Yang EJ, Jiang JH, Lee SM, et al. Electroacupuncture reduces neuroinflammatory responses in symptomatic amyotrophic lateral sclerosis model. *J Neuroimmunol* 2010;223(1):84–91.
366. Cheuk DK, Wong V, Chen WX. Acupuncture for autism spectrum disorders (ASD). *Cochrane Database Syst Rev* 2011;7(9):CD007849.
367. Bérard G. Audition égale comportement. *Maisonneuve* 1982.
368. Bérard G. *Hearing equals behaviour*. New Canaan, CT: Keats; 1993.
369. Sinha Y, Silove N, Hayen A, et al. Auditory integration training and other sound therapies for autism spectrum disorders (ASD). *Cochrane Database Syst Rev* 2011;7(12):CD003681.
370. Bettison S. The long-term effects of auditory training on children with autism. *J Autism Dev Disord* 1996;26(3):361–374.
371. Mudford OC, Cross BA, Breen S, et al. Auditory integration training for children with autism: No behavioral benefits detected. *Am J Mental Retardation* 2000;105(2):118–129.
372. Bruscia KE. *Defining music therapy*. New Braunfels, TX: Barcelona Publishers; 1998.
373. Geretsegger M, Elefant C, Mössler KA, et al. Music therapy for people with autism spectrum disorder. *Cochrane Database Syst Rev* 2014;17(6):CD004381.

THIRTEEN

Targeted Treatment for Cognitive Impairment Associated with Cancer and Cancer Treatment

SHELLI R. KESLER AND JEFFREY S. WEFEL

INTRODUCTION

Cognitive difficulty is one of the most common quality-of-life complaints among cancer patients and survivors.[1] These impairments significantly extend disease-related disability by disrupting educational, occupational, home, and social functioning.[2,3] Cancer-related cognitive impairment (CRCI) is also associated with reduced medication adherence and overall survival.[4–6] The incidence of these impairments is estimated to be 78% or higher in non-central nervous system (CNS) cancers[7–9] and nearly ubiquitous in CNS cancers. Although some patients treated for non-CNS cancers improve within 1 or 2 years following treatment completion, approximately 30–40% show persistent and/or worsening cognitive difficulties.[10,11] In fact, some studies suggest that non-CNS cancer and its therapies may be associated with increased risk for dementia.[12–14] These findings highlight the importance of developing interventions to prevent and/or reduce the effects of CRCI. Although currently there is no standardized, effective management strategy for this syndrome, many promising, evidence-based approaches are emerging. This chapter describes CRCI in further detail, including putative pathophysiologic mechanisms, and then discusses potential approaches for enhancing cognitive outcome.

CENTRAL NERVOUS SYSTEM CANCER

Primary brain tumor patients frequently exhibit impaired cognitive function at the time of initial diagnosis. More than 90% of primary brain tumor patients have been reported to exhibit cognitive dysfunction prior to surgical intervention.[15,16] The most common domains of cognition affected are memory and executive function, which reflects the tendency for primary brain tumors to arise in the frontal or temporal regions. Lesions caused by brain tumors produce deficits that track with the expected behavioral neuroanatomy (e.g., left hemisphere lesions frequently cause difficulties with verbal learning and memory and language functions).[17] However, cognitive dysfunction in brain tumor patients has been documented to be more subtle and diffuse compared to cognitive dysfunction observed in sudden-onset neurological conditions such as stroke.[18] The differences in cognitive presentation between these two neurologic illnesses are due in part to differences in pathophysiology, with tumors frequently having a slower rate of lesion onset, pathologically invading the brain in a more diffuse manner, which causes compression and displacement of adjacent normal tissue, edema, vascular changes, and disconnection of distant sites within the brain, known as diaschisis. Furthermore, molecular genetic subtypes of brain tumors (i.e., IDH1-mutated vs. wild-type glioma) have been demonstrated to be associated with differing rates of lesion growth, which in turn have been found to produce dramatic differences in the frequency and severity of cognitive impairments despite similar lesion volume within the brain.[19] Connectivity analyses using magnetoencephalography and functional magnetic resonance imaging (fMRI) have demonstrated disrupted organization of widespread brain networks even for "focal" tumors and also between tumors that vary by grade and molecular subtype.[20–24]

NON-CENTRAL NERVOUS SYSTEM CANCER

It is perhaps easy to accept that CNS cancer may result in cognitive changes given that neuropathologic damage associated with a brain tumor, for example, can be seen with the naked eye on radiologic images. However, most cancers originate outside the CNS, and CRCI associated with non-CNS cancer has historically been controversial. One potential reason for this controversy is that most systemic chemotherapy regimens have restricted direct access to the brain due to the blood–brain barrier and therefore a mechanism for CRCI in these patients was not readily apparent.

Other factors include the discrepancy between patient-reported cognitive outcomes and findings from objective testing. Whereas patients tend to endorse significant cognitive decline, objective testing can indicate normal or average performance. In addition, CRCI has commonly been referred to as "chemobrain," but studies show cognitive changes prior to adjuvant therapy.[25]

Fortunately, during approximately the past decade, there has been a significant increase in empirical attention regarding CRCI in non-CNS cancer. A search of "cognit* and breast cancer" in PubMed, for example, indicates a 123% increase in the number of studies since the year 2000 (Figure 13.1). Thus far, most studies have focused on breast cancer, which has become an initial model for investigating CRCI in adult-onset, non-CNS cancer. This is due in part to breast cancer's high incidence and survival rate, and multiple studies have demonstrated significant CRCI in breast cancer.[26]

Cognitive decline is also associated with other non-CNS cancers. Specifically, CRCI is associated with prostate cancer,[27] ovarian cancer,[28–30] hematologic cancers,[31] colorectal cancer,[32–34] and lung cancer,[35,36] among others. Adult survivors of pediatric leukemia also show significant CRCI.[14,37,38] Results from animal studies indicate that systemic chemotherapies have direct effects on neural progenitor cells, disrupting neurogenesis even after an initial dose, with repetitive doses causing persistent suppression of cell division.[39] Suppression of cell proliferation is equivalent for agents that do not actively cross the blood–brain barrier compared to those that do.[40] Methods involving objective testing have improved, with recommendations from the International Cognition and Cancer Task Force that include a common core battery of neuropsychological measures as well as standard definitions of impairment.[41] In

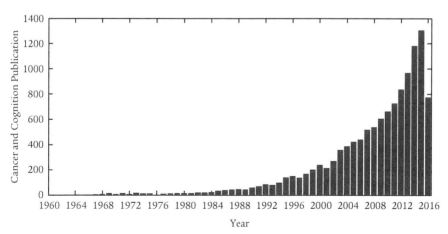

FIGURE 13.1 *Number of publications related to breast cancer and cognition between 1960 and 2016.*

addition, prospective, longitudinal studies have provided essential insights regarding individual patient trajectories of cognitive decline and recovery.

These studies reveal that executive function, memory, processing speed, and attention are the most commonly affected cognitive domains. CRCI tends to be mild to moderate in severity but can also be characterized by an intact ability to complete various cognitive tasks in the context of requiring significantly more time, effort, and/or alternate strategies. Thus, although mean cognitive outcome can be within the psychometrically defined normal range across patients, it is often significantly lower than the patient's previous baseline and/or the performance of matched healthy controls. Moreover, a subset of patients demonstrate markedly lower cognitive performance. Older patients and individuals with lower cognitive reserve tend to be more vulnerable to CRCI.[42] In addition, patients with certain genetic variations may show increased risk for CRCI.[43-45]

PATHOPHYSIOLOGIC MECHANISMS OF CRCI

In addition to the adverse effects of the brain tumor itself on cognition, many therapies used to manage the disease can have either off-target toxicity (e.g., incidental exposure of normal healthy brain to radiation) or on-target, off-tumor toxicity (e.g., targeted chemotherapies that operate on a single pathway overexpressed on tumor cells but also expressed on normal brain cells). Surgery is frequently used to treat CNS neoplasms and is a critical intervention to establish a tissue diagnosis, to reduce symptoms due to mass effect and increased intracranial pressure, and to increase overall survival. However, surgery can also cause damage to functioning brain regions,[15] causing a worsening of cognitive function in some cases.[15,46] Reports of patients assessed before and after surgical resection have observed improvement in 24–84% and decline in 36–38% of patients. Preoperative cognitive test results in domains of memory and language are associated with increased risk for postoperative cognitive decline in those domains in patients with high-grade glioma.[15,47,48] Postoperative cognitive impairment particularly in domains of executive functioning and attention has been associated with survival time in patients with newly diagnosed glioblastoma.[49]

Many primary and metastatic brain tumor patients receive cranial radiation in an effort to control tumor growth. Despite many advances in radiation delivery techniques, off-target toxicity remains common. A number of risk factors for radiation toxicity have been identified, including age younger than 5 years or older than

60 years, greater than 2 Gy dose per fraction, higher total dose, hyperfractionated schedules, shorter overall treatment time, the presence of comorbid vascular risk factors, concomitant or subsequent treatment with chemotherapy, greater total volume of brain irradiated, and radiation exposure to the bilateral hippocampi.[50–52] Several mechanisms have been proposed to account for the off-target adverse effects of radiation, including reactive oxidative stress, sustained activation of microglia and neuroinflammation, decreased neurogenesis and neuronal function, vascular injury, and gliosis.[53–55]

Adverse effects of chemotherapy in patients with brain tumor have been difficult to disentangle from the other CNS-directed therapies that often precede or are delivered concomitant with chemotherapy (i.e., surgery and radiation). However, the mechanisms associated with these toxicities are likely similar to those discussed next for the treatment of non-CNS cancer.

Possible mechanisms of cognitive impairment in non-CNS cancer include direct toxicity of chemotherapy agents to neural progenitor cells,[56] as noted previously, but research has also shown detrimental effects of other adjuvant treatments such as radiation and endocrine therapies. Other pathophysiologic factors include treatment-induced elevation of cytokine release,[57–60] estrogen/progesterone deficiency,[61,62] altered cerebral blood supply through blood vessel damage[63] and/or treatment-induced anemia,[64] oxidative stress,[65,66] and epigenetic alterations.[67] The final common biologic pathway of these mechanisms is diffuse brain injury, as indicated by multiple neuroimaging studies across various non-CNS cancers (Figure 13.2).[62,68–72]

Many of the candidate mechanisms for CRCI are closely associated with aging[67,73] and may alter or even accelerate the brain aging trajectory.[74,75] Adjuvant chemotherapy currently appears to be a primary mechanism for potentially accelerating brain aging, although studies that discriminate between various effects are limited. Older patients tend to have poorer cognitive outcome following chemotherapy.[42] The amount of gray matter atrophy following chemotherapy is analogous to approximately 4 years of aging on the brain.[76] Elevated expression of age-related molecular markers following chemotherapy corresponds to approximately 10.4 years of chronological aging.[77] As mentioned previously, a large subset of chemotherapy-treated patients demonstrate a new onset of a previously nonexistent cognitive deficit, suggesting a possible progressive cognitive phenotype.[10] Therefore, intervention approaches are needed that can prevent CRCI prior to its onset in newly diagnosed patients as well as those that can ameliorate it in long-term survivors and stop its potential progression.

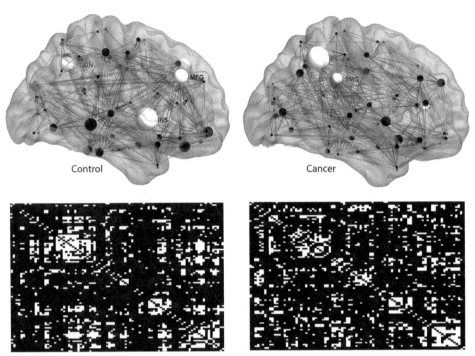

FIGURE 13.2 *Brain injury following cancer and its treatments. In this example neuroimaging study of CRCI, chemotherapy-treated breast cancer survivors demonstrated significantly reduced brain network organization compared to healthy controls. Spheres represent cortical and subcortical gray matter regions (nodes) with size indicating increasing number of connections with other regions. Nodes are notably less connected in the breast cancer group. The lighter gray spheres indicate hub regions that are highly connected (2 standard deviations above the network average) and are therefore important for interregional communication and overall brain network resilience. The breast cancer group shows fewer hub regions compared to controls. The lines represent connections (edges) between regions and illustrate a lower organizational pattern in the breast cancer group compared to controls. The connectivity matrices below the brain graphs provide further visualization of the brain network differences between the groups by illustrating divergent patterns of connectivity as well as reduced connectivity. Figure modified and reproduced from a color version[173] under the Creative Commons Attribution License (http:// creativecommons.org/licenses/by/2.0).*

INTERVENTIONS

This section describes potential interventions for CRCI that include the application of traditional approaches such as cognitive rehabilitation; considerations of very novel, untested techniques such as virtual reality; and unique potential combinations of these methods. All the interventions discussed here aim, in general, to address brain injury as the target mechanism of CRCI. The brain shows remarkable plasticity across the lifespan, and functional recovery is believed to involve reorganization of neural circuitry. Spontaneous partial or complete recovery of function can occur in some patients depending on age, health, cognitive reserve, injury severity, and other factors.[78,79] However, in many cases, neural reorganization must be supported by behavioral intervention. This may reflect the inability of the brain to re-create lost circuitry.[80,81] Reorganized neural networks cannot be expected to perform at the same level or in the same way as the original circuits, which were genetically programmed for their specific functionality and honed over varying years of development. Thus, the "new" brain network organization must often gain experience in supporting cognitive functions.

There is evidence from longitudinal neuroimaging studies of significant structural and functional brain reorganization/recovery following both CNS and non-CNS cancers.[82–84] Certain cross-sectional studies also show regions of increased brain structural and/or functional status compared to non-cancer controls, signifying a potentially compensatory reorganization.[85] In some studies, increased cognitive performance is correlated with these neurobiologic alterations, although inconsistently so and usually only moderately. In addition, despite potential compensation, cognitive performance tends to remain statistically below that of non-cancer controls. Furthermore, the interpretation of neuroimaging findings as "compensatory" is associated with several pitfalls.[86] Regardless, these findings suggest that natural neural reorganization does occur following cancer and its treatments, at least in the average patient. Recovery of acutely damaged brain regions tends to be evident by 1 year post-adjuvant chemotherapy.

Although reorganization may help preserve a certain level of cognitive performance, this level often remains below the patient's pre-existing level and/or the level of the patient's peers. This profile makes CRCI potentially very amenable to neuroplasticity-based interventions. In addition, given that CRCI tends to be mild to moderate in most non-CNS cases, a majority of affected patients would be expected to meet the somewhat intensive behavioral and motivational requirements of these interventions. On the other hand, CNS cancer is associated with a wider range of cognitive outcomes, including patients with very severe impairment who might not be able to comply with certain behavioral interventions.

Efforts to prevent cognitive dysfunction associated with surgery and radiation therapy have produced encouraging results in patients with CNS tumors. Preoperative fMRI for presurgical planning and intraoperative cognitive testing coupled with electrocortical stimulation during awake craniotomies have been used to guide surgical resection toward maximizing safe resection while minimizing cognitive morbidity.[87,88] In low-grade glioma patients, multistage serial resections have been reported in which surgical resection is stopped based on functional boundaries and subsequently further resection is conducted after documented functional reorganization has occurred.[89,90] Patients with primary brain tumor frequently require radiation therapy to extend progression-free and overall survival time.

Preliminary evidence suggests that the use of proton radiation instead of photon radiation may reduce the off-target toxicities associated with radiation.[91–93] Similarly, hippocampal-avoidance whole brain radiation therapy (HA-WBRT), which uses intensity modulated radiation therapy or volumetric arc therapy to reduce/eliminate radiation delivered to the hippocampal region including the subventricular zone, has shown great promise in terms of memory preservation after treatment compared to WBRT without hippocampal region avoidance. Both of these approaches to minimizing radiation toxicity are currently being studied in Phase III trials. Memantine, an *N*-methyl-D-aspartate (NMDA) receptor antagonist, was recently found to delay time to cognitive decline compared to placebo in patients with brain metastases who received WBRT in a double-blind, randomized, controlled Phase III trial.[94] Donepezil, a reversible acetylcholinesterase inhibitor, was tested in a double-blind, placebo-controlled trial in patients with primary brain tumor who completed radiation.[95] However, no significant differences between arms were observed, although some positive treatment effects were apparent in an exploratory subset analysis that suggested donepezil may offer benefit in patients with worse subjective cognitive complaints prior to treatment. Early uncontrolled studies reported positive effects of stimulants in the treatment and management of cognitive dysfunction and symptoms of fatigue.[96–98] However, a relatively recent randomized, placebo-controlled trial of the stimulant modafinil did not appear as promising.[99]

Cognitive Rehabilitation and Cognitive Training

Cognitive rehabilitation refers to a clinical therapeutic program aimed at improving cognitive abilities, functional capacity, and/or internal, metacognitive strategies. Some models emphasize processes (e.g., attention and memory), whereas others focus on skills to improve achievement of real-world objectives (e.g., obtaining items on a shopping list). Outcomes can be restorative, meaning that processes or skills are improved to their pre-existing status (or nearly so), and/or compensatory, such that a patient can successfully achieve particular goals using adaptive strategies (e.g., external devices for cuing, reminding, and organizing). Cognitive rehabilitation programs can include inpatients or outpatients and traditionally involve those meeting individually and/or in groups with a trained clinician one or more times per week for various durations. Some programs involve in vivo, skill-based training and practice, and many include intensive homework assignments for rehearsing and reinforcing therapeutic activities. Unfortunately, cognitive rehabilitation is not widely available, not often reimbursed by health insurance, and not feasible for some patients due to the frequent in-person appointments.

Alternatively, cognitive training is process oriented, providing adaptive practice of specific cognitive skills. Unlike cognitive rehabilitation, cognitive training tends to focus exclusively on processes without training in compensatory or metacognitive strategies and relies heavily on computerized exercises. These exercises are typically game-based, ranging from short and simple, two-dimensional casual games[100,101] to complex, immersive, three-dimensional platform games[102–104] and virtual reality environments.[105,106] Casual games available on mobile devices such as smartphones and tablets have also been used successfully in cognitive training paradigms.[107]

Cognitive training takes advantage of a fundamental aspect of game theory: The user must learn and adapt to a rule-based system in order to meet specified goals. Game theory is a mathematical field developed by John Von Neumann and Oskar Morgenstern to study strategic decision-making, particularly in the context of conflict and cooperation.[108] There are several advantages to the cognitive training approach, including standardized delivery of the intervention; algorithmic control of difficulty level to optimize the balance between challenge and motivation; automatic collection of telemetry data (e.g., performance statistics and adherence rates); the ability to practice several processes in parallel; and a structured, convenient means of mental stimulation. However, cognitive training has been criticized for lack of transfer to nontrained skills and especially to real-world skills. Some believe that cognitive training involves "training to the test" because certain cognitive exercises resemble the cognitive tests that are used to evaluate their effectiveness. Also, many studies show improvement in objective measures but less effects on subjective, patient-reported outcomes.[109,110]

Preliminary studies suggest that cognitive rehabilitation can be effective for CRCI in both CNS and non-CNS cancers. Very few studies have examined the effectiveness of cognitive rehabilitation programs in patients with brain tumor. Gehring et al.[111] conducted a randomized trial in lower grade glioma survivors who were assigned to wait-list control or an intervention that involved six weekly sessions of computer-based cognitive training (i.e., attention retraining) and compensatory skills training of attention, memory, and executive functioning sessions, as well as self-study for reinforcement and a booster session via telephone at 3 months. Compared to those placed on a waiting list, at 6 months, patients in the intervention group performed significantly better on tests of attention and verbal memory, and they reported less mental fatigue.

Regarding the validation of neuroplastic changes as the mechanism of action for these interventions, neuroimaging studies consistently demonstrate measurable brain changes following cognitive rehabilitation or cognitive training among individuals with various brain disorders.[112–117] However, such studies in CRCI have been limited to one pilot trial.[118] Cognitive rehabilitation and cognitive training studies involving CRCI are reviewed in detail elsewhere;[26,119–121] therefore, this information is not repeated here. Rather, several modifications to these interventions are proposed (e.g., combining a self-study cognitive rehabilitation patient manual with cognitive training exercises and implementing cognitive training in virtual reality environments) that may increase their effectiveness by addressing the limitations noted previously. It is hoped that these potential enhancements will guide future research toward clini cal trials of innovative intervention approaches for CRCI.

Regarding feasibility and potential for broad public health dissemination, cognitive training programs are widely available, relatively inexpensive, and allow for remote administration. Home-based cognitive training appears to have very comparable effects to those of in-person cognitive training.[100] This result was also reported from studies conducted with breast cancer survivors.[109,110] Cognitive training also shows similar effects to those of cognitive rehabilitation with respect to objective performance but poorer real-world transfer, with in-person cognitive training showing slightly better effects.[109,110] However, these studies involved small sample sizes, and direct comparison between them is difficult because they used different measures of objective and subjective performance as well as different cognitive training programs. In addition, subjective measures may not be the most optimal method for ascertaining real-world transfer given that self-ratings tend to be mediated by many confounding factors. However, the lack of transfer to patients' real-world experiences is consistent with what has been noted in the general cognitive training literature (Table 13.1).[122]

Cognitive rehabilitation tends to show much better transfer effects,[123] especially treatments that emphasize achievement of everyday objectives. This may partly reflect the fact that the majority of cognitive training trials have lacked measurements focused on meaningful daily living outcomes. In addition, traditional cognitive rehabilitation is highly individualized to the patient's specific cognitive profile of

TABLE 13.1 Effect Sizes for Cognitive Rehabilitation and Cognitive Training in Breast Cancer

Study	Intervention	Effect Size	
		Objective Tests	Subjective Tests
Von Ah et al.[119,a]	In-person CR	0.59–0.70	0.59–0.84
Von Ah et al.[119,a]	In-person CT	0.55–0.82	0.44–0.65
Kesler et al.[109]	At-home CT	0.59–0.74	0.19–0.38

[a]*Patients were randomized to cognitive rehabilitation (CR) or cognitive training (CT).*

strengths and weaknesses and also the specific life demands and interference in life activities the individual is experiencing. Cognitive training programs are adaptive to individual performance with respect to difficulty level, and many paradigms allow some level of customization in terms of task curriculum. However, some tasks might work better for some patients than others, and some patients might require a task or tasks that are not available. Nonetheless, the combination of home-based cognitive training with manualized, self-study components of cognitive rehabilitation strategies might help retain the practical, accessible elements of cognitive training while providing more clinic-based instruction.

For example, participants could be provided with a manual that contains guidelines for applying cognitive exercises to real-world tasks as well as methods for compensating for certain cognitive difficulties so that they can perform daily living tasks with success. Information such as compensatory strategies, self-regulation and stress management approaches, psychoeducational information, community resources, and other relevant reference materials could be included in patient manuals and supplemented by mobile applications, tele-health programs, and/or multimedia resources. There is some precedence for such adaptations found within clinical trials for CRCI that employ manualized cognitive rehabilitation. These studies focus on manuals that were created to help standardize the intervention implementation across providers, but many also include a patient manual or other teaching materials designed to help organize relevant treatment information, psychoeducational materials, and homework assignments.[118,124,125]

Because empirical work on cognitive training remains in its infancy, support is limited. It may be revealed in future studies that home-based approaches cannot match the ecological effects of the clinic environment. The therapeutic alliance between provider and patient, even at the minimal level of regular contact, is often a critical, non-negligible moderator of outcome in behavioral interventions. In addition, patients with more severe CRCI would not likely be good candidates for home-based intervention, so this would exclude a large number, especially among those with CNS cancer. However, further development and testing of cognitive training paradigms for CRCI, particularly with some of the enhancements discussed later, could easily provide feasible approaches for widespread use in clinic. For example, an identified best-practice CRCI program that is practical and standardized could be incorporated into a neuropsychology clinic within multiple cancer centers to provide broad access for patients.

Another potential modification to cognitive training that might enhance effect sizes as well as real-world transfer is the addition of virtual reality (VR) paradigms. VR can provide a more ecologically valid cognitive training experience that allows patients to experience in vivo skills practice. VR technology includes the use of three-dimensional, ecologically valid computer games but is rapidly developing, such that VR headsets for complete immersion into a virtual environment are now available. These headsets are approximately the size of ski goggles and track the user's head movements to provide 360 degrees of perception within the virtual environment. Such headsets are available at an affordable price, although cognitive rehabilitation/training programs for use with them are still under development.

Various forms of VR are currently being used in several programs designed to treat a variety of brain-based disorders. For example, VR is currently being used to conduct combat-related exposure therapy for veterans with post-traumatic stress disorder.[126–128] Cognitive training alone is typically done on a computer in a relatively comfortable environment. This approach is necessary to allow patients to practice cognitive skills free from distractions and other stressors that tend to increase the likelihood of cognitive failures. The addition of VR could provide a complementary exposure component that gradually increases the patient's ability to engage in cognitive tasks during realistic situational conditions.

VR is also being used to directly improve cognitive function in individuals with neurologic conditions.[129–131] One study showed that VR significantly enhanced the effects of cognitive training on cognitive performance in patients with brain tumor compared to cognitive training alone.[132] However, effects on everyday cognitive skills were not assessed. In non-interventional studies, performance within the VR environment has been successfully used as an ecological assessment of real-world cognitive function.[133–136] Therefore, VR is a very promising tool for providing both in vivo cognitive training and ecological assessment of outcome in CRCI.

Physical Exercise and Cognitive Training

Exercise is physical activity that is planned, repeated, and aimed at improving and/or preserving physical fitness.[137] Exercise is associated with improved cognitive function and increased protection from brain aging in both human and animal studies.[138–140] Significant improvements in cognitive and brain function have been noted in as little as 1 month following a regular exercise program among healthy adults.[141] Importantly, exercise is also associated with increased self-reported health-related quality of life,[142–144] physical fitness, and psychological well-being in patients with cancer.[145] In addition, regular exercise can reduce the risk of cancer-related death.[146] These effects make physical exercise an ideal potential intervention for CRCI.

Exercise is believed to improve cognitive function by increasing neurogenesis, resulting in increased neuroplasticity.[138–140] Exercise also increases the levels of neurotransmitters and neurotrophins that promote cognitive function,[138,147] increases expression of neuroprotective genes,[147] decreases chronic inflammation,[148] and stimulates positive brain vasculature changes.[138] In addition, exercise reduces the risk of chronic diseases that can have negative impacts on brain function, including stroke, diabetes, and heart disease.[140] Exercise is associated with reduction of psychiatric symptoms (depression and anxiety),[149] which may indirectly improve cognitive function. Several studies, including animal and human, suggest that certain CRCI symptoms can be improved with physical exercise.[150–154]

Both physical exercise and cognitive training increase neuroplasticity but do so through different pathways. Physical exercise increases neurogenesis, but many of these new neurons die before becoming integrated into neural networks.[155] Based on emerging animal studies, these neurons can potentially be rescued and integrated with existing neurons by including cognitive training.[155,156] Therefore, the combination of physical exercise and cognitive training may result in greater cognitive benefit compared to either approach alone. Preliminary human and animal studies provide support for this hypothesis.[140,155,157–161]

There are at least two main options for how the combination of physical exercise and cognitive training might be implemented. First, patients could be prescribed a program that simply includes both of these activities done on some regular schedule. A total of 150 minutes of moderate-intensity exercise plus 2 total hours of cognitive training per week is one example schedule that has empirical support.[109,141] Guidelines would be provided to patients to ensure they understood what moderate-intensity exercise means and how to measure and track it. In addition, patients would be instructed to distribute cognitive training and physical exercise sessions across days of the week. Computerized cognitive training would likely represent the most practical method for this aspect of the intervention in order to provide a consistent structure as well as a means for patients to track sessions and progress.

Another potential option for combining physical exercise and cognitive training would involve development of cognitively engaging and challenging physical exercise programs. Most of the research in this area derives from pediatric studies showing that aerobic games that require strategy and adaptation to changing situations have larger effects on children's cognition compared to passive exercise (i.e., treadmill walking).[162] However, aerobic games typically refer to team sports, which are not always feasible for adults. Alternatively, platform-based video games and VR-enhanced exercise equipment allow physical exercise and cognitive training to be done simultaneously. Studies suggest that these interactive "exergames" are associated with better exercise adherence and intensity as well as improved health-related and cognitive outcomes compared to traditional exercise.[163-166]

Exergames as well as traditional physical exercise interventions tend to show the greatest positive impact on executive functions compared to memory and other cognitive domains.[140,166-168] This is surprising in the context of animal studies demonstrating physical exercise-induced neurogenesis, particularly in the hippocampus, a structure critical for memory and learning.[139,140,148,155] These contradictory findings may stem partly from inadequate assessment of memory function. Most physical exercise clinical trials conducted to date on CRCI, for example, have not included neuropsychological memory measures.[26] The combination of cognitive training and physical exercise may help address this issue given that cognitive training shows positive effects on memory across various syndromes, including CRCI.[26,122]

Neurofeedback

Neurofeedback is a method that involves providing a participant with feedback regarding his or her own brain activity as a means of learning to control the up- and/or downregulation of brain activity in certain target regions. Neurofeedback studies conducted in non-cancer populations demonstrate that participants can learn to control the activation of specific brain regions related to motor function, attention, pain response, and emotion regulation, among others.[169] A relatively recent study conducted a pilot trial of neurofeedback in breast cancer survivors with CRCI and demonstrated positive preliminary effects on cognitive performance.[170]

Neurofeedback is provided via electroencephalography (EEG), functional near-infrared spectroscopy (NIRS), or real-time fMRI. Although home-based fMRI neurofeedback is currently impossible, many inexpensive, EEG and NIRS units are currently commercially available, making this a feasible endeavor. These units provide neurofeedback in natural settings, including sitting, moving, or even running. Some of these units link with smartphone applications to provide neurofeedback, an illustration of their high potential for practical implementation. Ongoing development and empirical investigation of neurofeedback paradigms for CRCI could therefore easily result in clinic or home-based programs.

One potential approach to neurofeedback that has not been extensively explored is the combination of neurofeedback with cognitive training. This would involve having patients engage in a cognitive training exercise while simultaneously receiving both behavioral feedback regarding their performance on the task and neurofeedback. One study has demonstrated the feasibility and potential effectiveness of this combined paradigm in healthy adults,[171] but its application in patients with cancer has not yet been evaluated. Being able to track changes in brain activity in addition to performance progress could be highly motivating to patients, increasing intervention adherence and engagement. For example, behavioral weight loss studies suggest that feedback and self-monitoring result in greater intervention gains.[172] The addition of neurofeedback could also improve individualization of the intervention because it relies specifically on the patient's individual profile of brain function.

CONCLUSION

Many CNS and non-CNS cancer patients experience cognitive dysfunction that impacts their scholastic, occupational, family, and/or social lives. As the lifespan of many cancer patients continues to increase, we are challenged to provide therapies that maintain or improve their "healthspan." Interventions are needed that target core and common cognitive deficits in domains of learning and memory, attention, processing speed, and executive functioning. Translational research including preclinical models and neuroimaging studies afford us a window into the mechanisms of CRCI and offer opportunities for the development of biologically rational neuroprotective therapies and effective adjuvant supportive therapies. However, far more intervention trials are required to identify behavioral and pharmacologic interventions that will decrease CRCI and enhance mood, quality of life, and functional abilities in patients with cancer.

DISCLOSURE

Dr. Wefel serves on the advisory board of Bayer, Genentech, and Roche. He is a paid consultant to AbbVie, Acerta, Angiochem, Juno, Novocure, and Roche. He receives grant support from the National Institute of Nursing Research of the National Institutes of Health (R01NR014195), the National Cancer Institute of the National Institutes of Health (T32CA009666), the National Cancer Institute of the National Institutes of Health (MH105897), the Breast Cancer Research Foundation, and MD Anderson Cancer Center.

Dr. Kesler receives grant support from the National Institute of Nursing Research of the National Institutes of Health (R01NR014195), the National Cancer Institute of the National Institutes of Health (1R01CA172145 and 1R03CA191559), and MD Anderson Cancer Center.

REFERENCES

1. Taillibert S, Voillery D, Bernard-Marty C. Chemobrain: Is systemic chemotherapy neurotoxic? *Curr Opin Oncol* 2007;19(6):623–627.

2. Boykoff N, Moieni M, Subramanian SK. Confronting chemobrain: An in-depth look at survivors' reports of impact on work, social networks, and health care response. *J Cancer Surviv* 2009;3(4):223–232.

3. Wefel JS, Lenzi R, Theriault RL, et al. The cognitive sequelae of standard-dose adjuvant chemotherapy in women with breast carcinoma: Results of a prospective, randomized, longitudinal trial. *Cancer* 2004;100(11):2292–2299.

4. Robb C, Boulware D, Overcash J, et al. Patterns of care and survival in cancer patients with cognitive impairment. *Crit Rev Oncol/Hematol* 2010;74(3):218–224.

5. Stilley CS, Bender CM, Dunbar-Jacob J, et al. The impact of cognitive function on medication management: three studies. *Health Psychol* 2010;29(1):50–55.

6. Meyers CA, Hess KR, Yung WK, et al. Cognitive function as a predictor of survival in patients with recurrent malignant glioma. *J Clin Oncol* 2000;18(3):646–650.

7. Correa DD, Ahles TA. Neurocognitive changes in cancer survivors. *Cancer J* 2008; 14(6):396–400.

8. Wefel JS, Schagen SB. Chemotherapy-related cognitive dysfunction. *Curr Neurol Neurosci Rep* 2012;12(3):267–275.

9. Janelsins MC, Kohli S, Mohile SG, et al. An update on cancer- and chemotherapy-related cognitive dysfunction: Current status. *Semin Oncol* 2011;38(3):431–438.

10. Wefel JS, Saleeba AK, Buzdar AU, et al. Acute and late onset cognitive dysfunction associated with chemotherapy in women with breast cancer. *Cancer* 2010;116(14):3348–3356.

11. Koppelmans V, Breteler MM, Boogerd W, et al. Neuropsychological performance in survivors of breast cancer more than 20 years after adjuvant chemotherapy. *J Clin Oncol* 2012;30(10):1080–1086.

12. Heck JE, Albert SM, Franco R, et al. Patterns of dementia diagnosis in surveillance, epidemiology, and end results breast cancer survivors who use chemotherapy. *J Am Geriatr Soc* 2008;56(9):1687–1692.

13. Heflin LH, Meyerowitz BE, Hall P, et al. Cancer as a risk factor for long-term cognitive deficits and dementia. *J Natl Cancer Inst* 2005;97(11):854–856.

14. Armstrong GT, Reddick WE, Petersen RC, et al. Evaluation of memory impairment in aging adult survivors of childhood acute lymphoblastic leukemia treated with cranial radiotherapy. *J Natl Cancer Inst* 2013;105(12):899–907.

15. Talacchi A, Santini B, Savazzi S, et al. Cognitive effects of tumour and surgical treatment in glioma patients. *J Neurooncol* 2011;103(3):541–549.

16. Tucha O, Smely C, Preier M, et al. Cognitive deficits before treatment among patients with brain tumors. *Neurosurgery* 2000;47(2):324—324.

17. Scheibel RS, Meyers CA, Levin VA. Cognitive dysfunction following surgery for intracerebral glioma: Influence of histopathology, lesion location, and treatment. *J Neurooncol* 1996;30(1):61–69.

18. Anderson SW, Damasio H, Tranel D. Neuropsychological impairments associated with lesions caused by tumor or stroke. *Arch Neurol* 1990;47(4):397–405.

19. Wefel JS, Noll KR, Rao G, et al. Neurocognitive function varies by IDH1 genetic mutation status in patients with malignant glioma prior to surgical resection. *Neuro-oncology* 2016;18(12):1656–1663.

20. Harris RJ, Bookheimer SY, Cloughesy TF, et al. Altered functional connectivity of the default mode network in diffuse gliomas measured with pseudo-resting state fMRI. *J Neurooncol* 2014;116(2):373–379.

21. Bosma I, Reijneveld JC, Klein M, et al. Disturbed functional brain networks and neurocognitive function in low-grade glioma patients: A graph theoretical analysis of resting-state MEG. *Nonlinear Biomed Phys* 2009;3(1):9.

22. van Dellen E, de Witt Hamer PC, Douw L, et al. Connectivity in MEG resting-state networks increases after resective surgery for low-grade glioma and correlates with improved cognitive performance. *Neuroimage Clin* 2012;2:1–7.

23. van Dellen E, Douw L, Hillebrand A, et al. MEG network differences between low- and high-grade glioma related to epilepsy and cognition. *PLoS One* 2012;7(11):e50122.

24. Kesler S, Noll KR, Cahill DP, et al. Lower brain network efficiency in IDH1 wild type (IDH1-WT) malignant astrocytoma compared to IDH1 mutant (IDH1-M). *Neuro-oncology* 2015;17(Suppl 5, v163).

25. Ahles TA, Saykin AJ, McDonald BC, et al. Cognitive function in breast cancer patients prior to adjuvant treatment. *Breast Cancer Res Treat* 2008;110(1):143–152.

26. Wefel JS, Kesler SR, Noll KR, et al. Clinical characteristics, pathophysiology, and management of noncentral nervous system cancer-related cognitive impairment in adults. *CA Cancer J Clin* 2015;65(2):123–138.

27. McGinty HL, Phillips KM, Jim HS, et al. Cognitive functioning in men receiving androgen deprivation therapy for prostate cancer: A systematic review and meta-analysis. *Support Care Cancer* 2014;22(8):2271–2280.

28. Correa DD, Hess LM. Cognitive function and quality of life in ovarian cancer. *Gynecol Oncol* 2012;124(3):404–409.

29. Correa DD, Zhou Q, Thaler HT, et al. Cognitive functions in long-term survivors of ovarian cancer. *Gynecol Oncol* 2010;119(2):366–369.

30. Hensley ML, Correa DD, Thaler H, et al. Phase I/II study of weekly paclitaxel plus carboplatin and gemcitabine as first-line treatment of advanced-stage ovarian cancer: Pathologic complete response and longitudinal assessment of impact on cognitive functioning. *Gynecol Oncol* 2006;102(2):270–277.

31. Phillips KM, McGinty HL, Cessna J, et al. A systematic review and meta-analysis of changes in cognitive functioning in adults undergoing hematopoietic cell transplantation. *Bone Marrow Transplant* 2013;48(10):1350–1357.

32. Vardy J, Dhillon HM, Pond GR, et al. Cognitive function and fatigue after diagnosis of colorectal cancer. *Ann Oncol* 2014;25(12):2404–2412.

33. Cruzado JA, Lopez-Santiago S, Martinez-Marin V, et al. Longitudinal study of cognitive dysfunctions induced by adjuvant chemotherapy in colon cancer patients. *Support Care Cancer* 2014;22(7):1815–1823.

34. Du XL, Cai Y, Symanski E. Association between chemotherapy and cognitive impairments in a large cohort of patients with colorectal cancer. *Int J Oncol* 2013;42(6):2123–2133.

35. Simo M, Root JC, Vaquero L, et al. Cognitive and brain structural changes in a lung cancer population. *J Thorac Oncol* 2015;10(1):38–45.

36. Gondi V, Paulus R, Bruner DW, et al. Decline in tested and self-reported cognitive functioning after prophylactic cranial irradiation for lung cancer: Pooled Secondary analysis of radiation therapy oncology group randomized trials 0212 and 0214. *Int J Radiat Oncol Biol Phys* 2013;86(4):656–664.

37. Krull KR, Zhang N, Santucci A, et al. Long-term decline in intelligence among adult survivors of childhood acute lymphoblastic leukemia treated with cranial radiation. *Blood* 2013;122(4):550–553.

38. Krull KR, Annett RD, Pan Z, et al. Neurocognitive functioning and health-related behaviours in adult survivors of childhood cancer: A report from the Childhood Cancer Survivor Study. *Eur J Cancer* 2011;47(9):1380–1388.

39. Dietrich J, Han R, Yang Y, et al. CNS progenitor cells and oligodendrocytes are targets of chemotherapeutic agents in vitro and in vivo. *J Biol* 2006;5(7):22.

40. Janelsins MC, Roscoe JA, Berg MJ, et al. IGF-1 partially restores chemotherapy-induced reductions in neural cell proliferation in adult C57BL/6 mice. *Cancer Invest* 2010;28(5):544–553.

41. Wefel JS, Vardy J, Ahles T, et al. International Cognition and Cancer Task Force recommendations to harmonise studies of cognitive function in patients with cancer. *Lancet Oncol* 2011;12(7):703–708.

42. Ahles TA, Saykin AJ, McDonald BC, et al. Longitudinal assessment of cognitive changes associated with adjuvant treatment for breast cancer: Impact of age and cognitive reserve. *J Clin Oncol* 2010;28(29):4434–4440.

43. Koleck TA, Bender CM, Sereika SM, et al. Apolipoprotein E genotype and cognitive function in postmenopausal women with early-stage breast cancer. *Oncol Nurs Forum* 2014;41(6):E313–E325.

44. Small BJ, Rawson KS, Walsh E, et al. Catechol-*O*-methyltransferase genotype modulates cancer treatment-related cognitive deficits in breast cancer survivors. *Cancer* 2011;117(7):1369–1376.

45. Ahles TA, Saykin AJ, Noll WW, et al. The relationship of APOE genotype to neuropsychological performance in long-term cancer survivors treated with standard dose chemotherapy. *Psycho-oncology* 2003;12(6):612–619.

46. Satoer D, Vork J, Visch-Brink E, et al. Cognitive functioning early after surgery of gliomas in eloquent areas. *J Neurosurg* 2012;117(5):831–838.

47. Gehring K, Sawyer AM, Etzel CJ, et al. Prediction of language outcomes after resection of high grade glioma. *Neuro-oncology* 2011;13(Suppl 3 (iii75)).

48. Gehring K SA, Etzel CJ, Lang FF, et al. Prediction of memory outcomes after resection of high grade glioma. *Neuro-oncology* 2011;13(Suppl 3 (iii75)).

49. Johnson DR, Sawyer AM, Meyers CA, et al. Early measures of cognitive function predict survival in patients with newly diagnosed glioblastoma. *Neuro-oncology* 2012;14(6):808–816.

50. Crossen JR, Garwood D, Glatstein E, et al. Neurobehavioral sequelae of cranial irradiation in adults: A review of radiation-induced encephalopathy. *J Clin Oncol* 1994;12(3):627–642.

51. Merchant TE, Conklin HM, Wu S, et al. Late effects of conformal radiation therapy for pediatric patients with low-grade glioma: Prospective evaluation of cognitive, endocrine, and hearing deficits. *J Clin Oncol* 2009;27(22):3691–3697.

52. Gondi V, Hermann BP, Mehta MP, et al. Hippocampal dosimetry predicts neurocognitive function impairment after fractionated stereotactic radiotherapy for benign or low-grade adult brain tumors. *Int J Radiat Oncol Biol Phys* 2012;83(4):e487–e493.

53. Tofilon PJ, Fike JR. The radioresponse of the central nervous system: A dynamic process. *Radiat Res* 2000;153(4):357–370.

54. Zhao W, Diz DI, Robbins ME. Oxidative damage pathways in relation to normal tissue injury. *Br J Radiol* 2007;80(Spec No 1):S23–S31.

55. Monje M. Cranial radiation therapy and damage to hippocampal neurogenesis. *Dev Disabil Res Rev* 2008;14(3):238–242.

56. Monje M, Dietrich J. Cognitive side effects of cancer therapy demonstrate a functional role for adult neurogenesis. *Behav Brain Res* 2012;227(2):376–379.

57. Pomykala KL, Ganz PA, Bower JE, et al. The association between pro-inflammatory cytokines, regional cerebral metabolism, and cognitive complaints following adjuvant chemotherapy for breast cancer. *Brain Imaging Behav* 2013;7(4):511–523.

58. Kesler S, Janelsins M, Koovakkattu D, et al. Reduced hippocampal volume and verbal memory performance associated with interleukin-6 and tumor necrosis factor-alpha levels in chemotherapy-treated breast cancer survivors. *Brain Behav Immun* 2013;30(Suppl):S109–S116.

59. Vardy JL, Booth C, Pond GR, et al. Cytokine levels in patients (pts) with colorectal cancer and breast cancer and their relationship to fatigue and cognitive function. *J Clin Oncol* 2007;25(18 Suppl):9070.

60. Ganz PA, Bower JE, Kwan L, et al. Does tumor necrosis factor-alpha (TNF-alpha) play a role in post-chemotherapy cerebral dysfunction? *Brain Behav Immun* 2013;30(Suppl):S99–S108.

61. Hogervorst E. Effects of gonadal hormones on cognitive behavior in elderly men and women. *J Neuroendocrinol* 2013;25(11):1182–1195.

62. Chao HH, Uchio E, Zhang S, et al. Effects of androgen deprivation on brain function in prostate cancer patients—A prospective observational cohort analysis. *BMC Cancer* 2012;12:371.

63. Seigers R, Timmermans J, van der Horn HJ, et al. Methotrexate reduces hippocampal blood vessel density and activates microglia in rats but does not elevate central cytokine release. *Behav Brain Res* 2010;207(2):265–272.

64. O'Shaughnessy JA. Chemotherapy-induced cognitive dysfunction: A clearer picture. *Clin Breast Cancer* 2003;4(Suppl 2):S89–S94.

65. Conroy SK, McDonald BC, Smith DJ, et al. Alterations in brain structure and function in breast cancer survivors: Effect of post-chemotherapy interval and relation to oxidative DNA damage. *Breast Cancer Res Treat* 2013;137(2):493–502.

66. Tangpong J, Cole MP, Sultana R, et al. Adriamycin-induced, TNF-alpha-mediated central nervous system toxicity. *Neurobiol Dis* 2006;23(1):127–139.

67. Maccormick RE. Possible acceleration of aging by adjuvant chemotherapy: A cause of early onset frailty? *Med Hypotheses* 2006;67(2):212–215.

68. Bromis K, Karanasiou IS, Matsopoulos G, et al. *Resting state and task related fMRI in small cell lung cancer patients.* Paper presented at Bioinformatics and Bioengineering (BIBE), 2013 IEEE 13th International Conference, November 10–13, 2013.

69. Correa DD, Root JC, Baser R, et al. A prospective evaluation of changes in brain structure and cognitive functions in adult stem cell transplant recipients. *Brain Imaging Behav* 2013;7(4):478–490.

70. Hsieh TC, Wu YC, Yen KY, et al. Early changes in brain FDG metabolism during anticancer therapy in patients with pharyngeal cancer. *J Neuroimaging* 2014;24(3):266–272.

71. Kesler SR, Wefel JS, Hosseini SM, et al. Default mode network connectivity distinguishes chemotherapy-treated breast cancer survivors from controls. *Proc Natl Acad Sci USA* 2013;110(28):11600–11605.

72. Deprez S, Vandenbulcke M, Peeters R, et al. Longitudinal assessment of chemotherapy-induced alterations in brain activation during multitasking and its relation with cognitive complaints. *J Clin Oncol* 2014;32(19):2031–2338.

73. Mandelblatt JS, Hurria A, McDonald BC, et al. Cognitive effects of cancer and its treatments at the intersection of aging: What do we know; What do we need to know? *Semin Oncol* 2013;40(6):709–725.

74. Ahles TA. Brain vulnerability to chemotherapy toxicities. *Psychooncology* 2012;21(11):1141–1148.

75. Koppelmans V, Breteler MM, Boogerd W, et al. Late effects of adjuvant chemotherapy for adult onset non-CNS cancer; Cognitive impairment, brain structure and risk of dementia. *Crit Rev Oncol/Hematol* 2013;88(1):87–101.

76. Koppelmans V, de Ruiter MB, van der Lijn F, et al. Global and focal brain volume in long-term breast cancer survivors exposed to adjuvant chemotherapy. *Breast Cancer Res Treat* 2012;132(3):1099–1106.

77. Sanoff HK, Deal AM, Krishnamurthy J, et al. Effect of cytotoxic chemotherapy on markers of molecular age in patients with breast cancer. *J Natl Cancer Inst* 2014;106(4):dju057.

78. Stern Y. Cognitive reserve. *Neuropsychologia* 2009;47(10):2015–2028.

79. Hukkelhoven CW, Steyerberg EW, Rampen AJ, et al. Patient age and outcome following severe traumatic brain injury: An analysis of 5600 patients. *J Neurosurg* 2003;99(4):666–673.

80. Mogensen J. Cognitive recovery and rehabilitation after brain injury: Mechanisms, challenges and support. In Agarwal A (Ed.), *Brain injury—Functional aspects, rehabilitation and prevention.* Rijeka, Croatia: InTech; 2012:121–150.

81. Mogensen J. Almost unlimited potentials of a limited neural plasticity. *J Conscious Stud* 2011;18(7–8):13–45.

82. Dumas JA, Makarewicz J, Schaubhut GJ, et al. Chemotherapy altered brain functional connectivity in women with breast cancer: A pilot study. *Brain Imaging Behav* 2013;7(4):524–532.

83. McDonald BC, Conroy SK, Ahles TA, et al. Gray matter reduction associated with systemic chemotherapy for breast cancer: A prospective MRI study. *Breast Cancer Res Treat* 2010;123(3):819–828.

84. McDonald BC, Conroy SK, Ahles TA, et al. Alterations in brain activation during working memory processing associated with breast cancer and treatment: A prospective functional magnetic resonance imaging study. *J Clin Oncol* 2012;30(20):2500–2508.

85. Hosseini SM, Kesler SR. Multivariate pattern analysis of fMRI in breast cancer survivors and healthy women. *J Int Neuropsychol Soc* 2014;20(4):391–401.

86. Poldrack RA. Interpreting developmental changes in neuroimaging signals. *Hum Brain Mapp* 2010;31(6):872–878.

87. Krivosheya D, Prabhu SS, Weinberg JS, et al. Technical principles in glioma surgery and pre-operative considerations. *J Neurooncol* 2016;130(2):243–252.

88. Mandonnet E, Sarubbo S, Duffau H. Proposal of an optimized strategy for intraoperative testing of speech and language during awake mapping. *Neurosurg Rev* 2017;40(1):29–35.

89. Duffau H. Resecting diffuse low-grade gliomas to the boundaries of brain functions: A new concept in surgical neuro-oncology. *J Neurosurg Sci* 2015;59(4):361–371.

90. Herbet G, Maheu M, Costi E, et al. Mapping neuroplastic potential in brain-damaged patients. *Brain* 2016;139(Pt 3):829–844.

91. Pulsifer MB, Sethi RV, Kuhlthau KA, et al. Early cognitive outcomes following proton radiation in pediatric patients with brain and central nervous system tumors. *Int J Radiat Oncol* 2015;93(2):400–407.

92. Yock TI, Weyman EA, Goldberg S, et al. HRQoL in medulloblastoma patients enrolled on a prospective phase II study of proton radiation. *J Clin Oncol* 2015;33(15).

93. Shih HA, Sherman JC, Nachtigall LB, et al. Proton therapy for low-grade gliomas: Results from a prospective trial. *Cancer* 2015;121(10):1712–1719.

94. Brown PD, Pugh S, Laack NN, et al. Memantine for the prevention of cognitive dysfunction in patients receiving whole-brain radiotherapy: A randomized, double-blind, placebo-controlled trial. *Neuro-oncology* 2013;15(10):1429–1437.

95. Rapp SR, Case LD, Peiffer A, et al. Donepezil for irradiated brain tumor survivors: A Phase III randomized placebo-controlled clinical trial. *J Clin Oncol* 2015;33(15):1653–1659.

96. Gehring K, Patwardhan SY, Collins R, et al. A randomized trial on the efficacy of methylphenidate and modafinil for improving cognitive functioning and symptoms in patients with a primary brain tumor. *J Neurooncol* 2012;107(1):165–174.

97. Meyers CA, Weitzner MA, Valentine AD, et al. Methylphenidate therapy improves cognition, mood, and function of brain tumor patients. *J Clin Oncol* 1998;16(7):2522–2527.

98. Weitzner MA, Meyers CA, Valentine AD. Methylphenidate in the treatment of neurobehavioral slowing associated with cancer and cancer treatment. *J Neuropsychiatry Clin Neurosci* 1995;7(3):347–350.

99. Boele FW, Douw L, de Groot M, et al. The effect of modafinil on fatigue, cognitive functioning, and mood in primary brain tumor patients: A multicenter randomized controlled trial. *Neuro-oncology* 2013;15(10):1420–1428.

100. Wolinsky FD, Vander Weg MW, Howren MB, et al. A randomized controlled trial of cognitive training using a visual speed of processing intervention in middle aged and older adults. *PLoS One* 2013;8(5):e61624.

101. Klingberg T. Training and plasticity of working memory. *Trends Cogn Sci* 2010;14(7):317–324.

102. Spence I, Feng J. Video games and spatial cognition. *Rev Gen Psychol* 2010;14(2):92–104.

103. Green CS, Sugarman MA, Medford K, et al. The effect of action video game experience on task-switching. *Computers Hum Behav* 2012;28(3):984–994.

104. Bavelier D, Green CS, Pouget A, et al. Brain plasticity through the life span: Learning to learn and action video games. *Annu Rev Neurosci* 2012;35:391–416.

105. Klinger E, Kadri A, Sorita E, et al. AGATHE: A tool for personalized rehabilitation of cognitive functions based on simulated activities of daily living. *IRBM* 2013;34(2):113–118.

106. Legault I, Allard R, Faubert J. Healthy older observers show equivalent perceptual–cognitive training benefits to young adults for multiple object tracking. *Front Psychol* 2013;4:323.

107. Oei AC, Patterson MD. Enhancing cognition with video games: A multiple game training study. *PLoS One* 2013;8(3):e58546.

108. John von N, Morgenstern O. *Theory of games and economic behavior (60th anniversary commemorative edition)*. Princeton, NJ: Princeton University Press; 2007.

109. Kesler S, Hosseini SMH, Heckler C, et al. Cognitive training for improving executive function in chemotherapy-treated breast cancer survivors. *Clin Breast Cancer* 2013;13(4):299–306.

110. Von Ah D, Carpenter JS, Saykin A, et al. Advanced cognitive training for breast cancer survivors: A randomized controlled trial. *Breast Cancer Res Treat* 2012;135(3):799–809.

111. Gehring K, Sitskoorn MM, Gundy CM, et al. Cognitive rehabilitation in patients with gliomas: A randomized, controlled trial. *J Clin Oncol* 2009;27(22):3712–3722.

112. Hampstead BM, Stringer AY, Stilla RF, et al. Mnemonic strategy training partially restores hippocampal activity in patients with mild cognitive impairment. *Hippocampus* 2012;22(8):1652–1658.

113. van Paasschen J, Clare L, Yuen KS, et al. Cognitive rehabilitation changes memory-related brain activity in people with Alzheimer disease. *Neurorehabil Neural Repair* 2013;27(5):448–459.

114. Eack SM, Hogarty GE, Cho RY, et al. Neuroprotective effects of cognitive enhancement therapy against gray matter loss in early schizophrenia: Results from a 2-year randomized controlled trial. *Arch Gen Psychiatry* 2010;67(7):674–682.

115. Takeuchi H, Taki Y, Nouchi R, et al. Effects of working memory training on functional connectivity and cerebral blood flow during rest. *Cortex* 2013;49(8):2106–2125.

116. Kirchhoff BA, Anderson BA, Smith SE, et al. Cognitive training-related changes in hippocampal activity associated with recollection in older adults. *Neuroimage* 2012;62(3):1956–1964.

117. Anguera JA, Boccanfuso J, Rintoul JL, et al. Video game training enhances cognitive control in older adults. *Nature* 2013;501(7465):97–101.

118. Ercoli LM, Castellon SA, Hunter AM, et al. Assessment of the feasibility of a rehabilitation intervention program for breast cancer survivors with cognitive complaints. *Brain Imaging Behav* 2013;7(4):543–553.

119. Von Ah D, Storey S, Jansen CE, et al. Coping strategies and interventions for cognitive changes in patients with cancer. *Semin Oncol Nurs* 2013;29(4):288–299.

120. Gehring K, Sitskoorn MM, Aaronson NK, et al. Interventions for cognitive deficits in adults with brain tumours. *Lancet Neurol* 2008;7(6):548–560.

121. Gehring K, Aaronson NK, Taphoorn MJ, et al. Interventions for cognitive deficits in patients with a brain tumor: An update. *Expert Rev Anticancer Ther* 2010;10(11):1779–1795.

122. Park DC, Bischof GN. The aging mind: Neuroplasticity in response to cognitive training. *Dialogues Clin Neurosci* 2013;15(1):109–119.

123. Bahar-Fuchs A, Clare L, Woods B. Cognitive training and cognitive rehabilitation for persons with mild to moderate dementia of the Alzheimer's or vascular type: A review. *Alzheimer's Res Ther* 2013;5(4):35.

124. Ferguson RJ, Ahles TA, Saykin AJ, et al. Cognitive–behavioral management of chemotherapy-related cognitive change. *Psychooncology* 2007;16(8):772–777.

125. Ferguson RJ, McDonald BC, Rocque MA, et al. Development of CBT for chemotherapy-related cognitive change: Results of a waitlist control trial. *Psychooncology* 2012;21(2):176–186.

126. Motraghi TE, Seim RW, Meyer EC, et al. Virtual reality exposure therapy for the treatment of posttraumatic stress disorder: A methodological review using CONSORT guidelines. *J Clin Psychol* 2014;70(3):197–208.

127. Goncalves R, Pedrozo AL, Coutinho ES, et al. Efficacy of virtual reality exposure therapy in the treatment of PTSD: A systematic review. *PLoS One* 2012;7(12):e48469.

128. Rizzo A, Parsons TD, Lange B, et al. Virtual reality goes to war: A brief review of the future of military behavioral healthcare. *J Clin Psychol Med Settings* 2011;18(2):176–187.

129. Kim BR, Chun MH, Kim LS, et al. Effect of virtual reality on cognition in stroke patients. *Ann Rehabil Med* 2011;35(4):450–459.

130. Larson EB, Feigon M, Gagliardo P, et al. Virtual reality and cognitive rehabilitation: A review of current outcome research. *NeuroRehabilitation* 2014;34(4):759–772.

131. Jacoby M, Averbuch S, Sacher Y, et al. Effectiveness of executive functions training within a virtual supermarket for adults with traumatic brain injury: A pilot study. *IEEE Trans Neural Syst Rehabil Eng* 2013;21(2):182–190.

132. Yang S, Chun MH, Son YR. Effect of virtual reality on cognitive dysfunction in patients with brain tumor. *Ann Rehabil Med* 2014;38(6):726–733.

133. Plancher G, Tirard A, Gyselinck V, et al. Using virtual reality to characterize episodic memory profiles in amnestic mild cognitive impairment and Alzheimer's disease: Influence of active and passive encoding. *Neuropsychologia* 2012;50(5):592–602.

134. Tarnanas I, Schlee W, Tsolaki M, et al. Ecological validity of virtual reality daily living activities screening for early dementia: Longitudinal study. *JMIR Serious Games* 2013;1(1):e1.

135. Weniger G, Ruhleder M, Lange C, et al. Egocentric and allocentric memory as assessed by virtual reality in individuals with amnestic mild cognitive impairment. *Neuropsychologia* 2011;49(3):518–527.

136. Widmann CN, Beinhoff U, Riepe MW. Everyday memory deficits in very mild Alzheimer's disease. *Neurobiol Aging* 2012;33(2):297–303.

137. Campbell KL, Neil SE, Winters-Stone KM. Review of exercise studies in breast cancer survivors: Attention to principles of exercise training. *Br J Sports Med* 2012;46(13):909–916.

138. Voss MW, Vivar C, Kramer AF, et al. Bridging animal and human models of exercise-induced brain plasticity. *Trends Cogn Sci* 2013;17(10):525–544.

139. Hayes SM, Hayes JP, Cadden M, et al. A review of cardiorespiratory fitness-related neuroplasticity in the aging brain. *Front Aging Neurosci* 2013;5:31.

140. Hotting K, Roder B. Beneficial effects of physical exercise on neuroplasticity and cognition. *Neurosci Biobehav Rev* 2013;37(9 Pt B):2243–2257.

141. Ahlskog JE, Geda YE, Graff-Radford NR, et al. Physical exercise as a preventive or disease-modifying treatment of dementia and brain aging. *Mayo Clin Proc* 2011;86(9):876–884.

142. Mustian KM, Sprod LK, Palesh OG, et al. Exercise for the management of side effects and quality of life among cancer survivors. *Curr Sports Med Rep* 2009;8(6):325–330.

143. Mustian KM, Sprod LK, Janelsins M, et al. Exercise recommendations for cancer-related fatigue, cognitive impairment, sleep problems, depression, pain, anxiety, and physical dysfunction: A review. *Oncol Hematol Rev* 2012;8(2):81–88.

144. Mohammadi S, Sulaiman S, Koon PB, et al. Impact of healthy eating practices and physical activity on quality of life among breast cancer survivors. *Asian Pacific J Cancer Prev* 2013;14(1):481–487.

145. Ballard-Barbash R, Friedenreich CM, Courneya KS, et al. Physical activity, biomarkers, and disease outcomes in cancer survivors: A systematic review. *J Natl Cancer Inst*2012;104(11):815–840.

146. Holmes MD, Chen WY, Feskanich D, et al. Physical activity and survival after breast cancer diagnosis. *JAMA* 2005;293(20):2479–2486.

147. Kramer AF, Erickson KI, Colcombe SJ. Exercise, cognition, and the aging brain. *J Appl Physiol* 2006;101(4):1237–1242.

148. Speisman RB, Kumar A, Rani A, et al. Daily exercise improves memory, stimulates hippocampal neurogenesis and modulates immune and neuroimmune cytokines in aging rats. *Brain Behav Immun* 2013;28:25–43.

149. Blake H. Physical activity and exercise in the treatment of depression. *Front Psychiatry* 2012;3:106.

150. Fardell JE, Vardy J, Shah JD, et al. Cognitive impairments caused by oxaliplatin and 5-fluorouracil chemotherapy are ameliorated by physical activity. *Psychopharmacology* 2012;220(1):183–193.

151. Galantino ML, Greene L, Daniels L, et al. Longitudinal impact of yoga on chemotherapy-related cognitive impairment and quality of life in women with early stage breast cancer: A case series. *Explore* 2012;8(2):127–135.

152. Janelsins M, Peppone L, Heckler C, et al. YOCAS yoga, fatigue, memory difficulty, and quality of life: Results from a URCC CCOP randomized, controlled clinical trial among 358 cancer survivors. *J Clin Oncol* 2012;30(Suppl):Abstr 9142.

153. Reid-Arndt SA, Matsuda S, Cox CR. Tai Chi effects on neuropsychological, emotional, and physical functioning following cancer treatment: A pilot study. *Complement Ther Clin Pract* 2012;18(1):26–30.

154. Oh B, Butow PN, Mullan BA, et al. Effect of medical Qigong on cognitive function, quality of life, and a biomarker of inflammation in cancer patients: A randomized controlled trial. *Support Care Cancer* 2012;20(6):1235–1242.

155. Curlik DM, 2nd, Shors TJ. Training your brain: Do mental and physical (MAP) training enhance cognition through the process of neurogenesis in the hippocampus? *Neuropharmacology* 2013;64:506–514.

156. Karr JE, Areshenkoff CN, Rast P, et al. An empirical comparison of the therapeutic benefits of physical exercise and cognitive training on the executive functions of older adults: A meta-analysis of controlled trials. *Neuropsychology* 2014;28(6):829–845.

157. Kempermann G, Fabel K, Ehninger D, et al. Why and how physical activity promotes experience-induced brain plasticity. *Front Neurosci* 2010;4:189.

158. Fabel K, Wolf SA, Ehninger D, et al. Additive effects of physical exercise and environmental enrichment on adult hippocampal neurogenesis in mice. *Front Neurosci* 2009;3:50.

159. Fabre C, Chamari K, Mucci P, et al. Improvement of cognitive function by mental and/or individualized aerobic training in healthy elderly subjects. *Int J Sports Med* 2002;23(6):415–421.

160. Holzschneider K, Wolbers T, Roder B, et al. Cardiovascular fitness modulates brain activation associated with spatial learning. *Neuroimage* 2012;59(3):3003–3014.

161. Gonzalez-Palau F, Franco M, Bamidis P, et al. The effects of a computer-based cognitive and physical training program in a healthy and mildly cognitive impaired aging sample. *Aging Mental Health* 2014;18(7):838–846.

162. Best JR. Effects of physical activity on children's executive function: Contributions of experimental research on aerobic exercise. *Dev Rev* 2010;30(4):331–351.

163. Annesi JJ, Mazas J. Effects of virtual reality-enhanced exercise equipment on adherence and exercise-induced feeling states. *Percept Mot Skills* 1997;85(3 Pt 1):835–844.

164. Lange BS, Requejo P, Flynn SM, et al. The potential of virtual reality and gaming to assist successful aging with disability. *Phys Med Rehabil Clin North Am* 2010;21(2):339–356.

165. Chuang TY, Sung WH, Chang HA, et al. Effect of a virtual reality-enhanced exercise protocol after coronary artery bypass grafting. *Phys Ther* 2006;86(10):1369–1377.

166. Anderson-Hanley C, Arciero PJ, Brickman AM, et al. Exergaming and older adult cognition: A cluster randomized clinical trial. *Am J Prev Med* 2012;42(2):109–119.

167. Colcombe S, Kramer AF. Fitness effects on the cognitive function of older adults: A meta-analytic study. *Psychol Sci* 2003;14(2):125–130.

168. Kramer AF, Erickson KI. Capitalizing on cortical plasticity: Influence of physical activity on cognition and brain function. *Trends Cogn Sci* 2007;11(8):342–348.

169. Sulzer J, Haller S, Scharnowski F, et al. Real-time fMRI neurofeedback: Progress and challenges. *Neuroimage* 2013;76:386–399.

170. Alvarez J, Meyer FL, Granoff DL, et al. The effect of EEG biofeedback on reducing postcancer cognitive impairment. *Integr Cancer Ther* 2013;12(6):475–487.

171. Hosseini SM, Pritchard-Berman M, Sosa N, et al. Task-based neurofeedback training: A novel approach toward training executive functions. *Neuroimage* 2016;134:153–159.

172. Burke LE, Wang J, Sevick MA. Self-monitoring in weight loss: A systematic review of the literature. *J Am Diet Assoc* 2011;111(1):92–102.

FOURTEEN

Current Progress and Future Potential in the Evaluation and Treatment of Age-Related Cognitive Declines

KEITH A. WESNES AND HELEN J. BROOKER

T HE TOPIC OF THIS CHAPTER WOULD BE TO MANY AN OBVIOUS AND noncontroversial issue: Mental faculties fade with age, and it would be helpful if there were readily available and reasonably safe treatments that could either slow or prevent this from occurring. Certainly, age-associated loss of mental capacity is a universally recognized phenomenon, but that is the point at which most consensus ceases. It is hoped that this chapter will shed some light upon the various controversies in this important field and help suggest a path forward.

COGNITION ENHANCEMENT

One definition of cognition enhancement proposed by Bostrom and Sandberg[1] states that cognitive enhancement is "the amplification or extension of core capacities of the mind through improvement or augmentation of internal or external information processing systems." Aspects of cognitive function that are popular targets for enhancement are attention, information processing, memory, planning, reasoning, decision making, and motor control. Bostrom and Sandberg argue that an intervention aimed at correcting a specific pathology or defect of a cognitive subsystem may be characterized as therapeutic, whereas enhancement is an intervention that improves a subsystem in some way other than repairing something that is broken or remedying a specific dysfunction. This distinction is important, and it accurately characterizes the various compounds that are being developed and studied in this rapidly growing field.

HISTORICAL PERSPECTIVE

The study of the cognition enhancing effects of drugs is entering its second century. In one early study published in 1912, Hollingworth[2] conducted a systematic investigation of the effects of caffeine on reaction time and reported that higher doses produced decreased reaction times. In 1919, the American Committee for the Study of the Tobacco Problem commissioned an investigation titled "Tobacco and Mental Efficiency."[3] This program was led by the experimental psychologist Clark L. Hull, who devised a series of automated cognitive tests to measure the effects of tobacco smoking on both smokers and non-smokers. An effective placebo was developed, together with a range of sophisticated electromechanical devices for conducting cognitive testing, including a voice key that was able to measure vocal reaction times with a precision of 0.03 seconds. Overall, this extensive research program enabled Hull to conclude, with a "fair probability," that smoking produced an improvement in speed on reading reaction time and paired-associate learning tasks.[4]

Amphetamines were the first synthetic compounds shown to improve human cognitive function; the study of the cognitive benefits of these substances started in the 1930s.[5] Weiss and Laties produced the seminal review of the field in a paper titled "Enhancement of Human Performance by Caffeine and the Amphetamines."[6] The review addressed the crucial questions that still remain in this field:

> (1) Can caffeine and the amphetamines actually produce superior performance or do they merely restore to a normal level of performance degraded by fatigue, boredom, or other influences? and (2) Are the performance-enhancing effects of these drugs counterbalanced by untoward effects to such an extent that their practical use is not feasible or desirable? (p. 2)

The previously mentioned work and other reviews of the effects of nicotine[7,8] and caffeine[9] have established these compounds as archetypal cognition enhancers whose principal action is to improve alertness and attention.

The interest of the pharmaceutical industry in drugs to improve cognitive function began with the development of hydergine, an antihypertensive, in the late 1940s. It was discovered to have pro-cognitive properties and was approved by the US Food and Drug Administration (FDA) in 1977 for persons "over sixty who manifest signs and symptoms of an idiopathic decline in mental capacity."[10] However, in the decade following prescription approval, the drug was largely abandoned due to uncertainty about its degree of clinical efficacy.[11] Nonetheless, the compound had been widely studied in patients with symptoms consistent with dementia, and a subsequent meta-analysis of 47 of a total of 151 such trials that met rigorous selection criteria identified that hydergine did indeed produce statistically reliable improvements with small to medium effect sizes in comprehensive ratings, clinical global impressions, and combined neuropsychological measures.[12] The 5 trials in patients with possible Alzheimer's disease showed an improvement in neuropsychological measures with an effect size of 0.3, which the authors described as modest. However, Rockwood[13] has shown that the anticholinesterases, the current front-line treatment for Alzheimer's disease, at the most effective doses show a median effect size of 0.28 on the cognitive subscale of the Alzheimer's Disease Assessment Scale (ADAS-Cog). Hydergine's fall from grace is difficult to understand—perhaps expectations of treatment effectiveness were too high in the 1980s—but certainly the compound compared well in terms of its efficacy as a cognition enhancer with the current anticholinesterases.

Another major stage in this field occurred in the 1960s when Corneliu Giurgea synthesized Piracetam, one of the first of such compounds for which he subsequently defined the term "nootropic."[14] The initial targets for such therapies were cognitive deficits accompanying aging, initially described as cerebral insufficiency and now recognized as various forms of dementia. Like hydergine, piracetam was extensively researched and showed modest but consistent improvements to mental ability in various elderly and impaired populations.[15] Other compounds from this class, the pyrrolidone derivatives (e.g., aniracetam, oxiracetam, and tenilsetam), have also been widely researched. However, as with hydergine, these compounds are not currently used in the treatment of severe cognitive deficits associated with aging. Other compounds widely studied in the decades preceding this millennium were vinpocetine and acetyl-L-carnitine, both of which showed evidence for improving cognitive function in the dementias[16–18] but, again, are not currently considered front-line treatments for the dementias.

METHODOLOGICAL CONSIDERATIONS

Repeated Cognitive Assessment

The basic criterion for a cognition enhancer is demonstrating that individuals perform better with the treatment than without on an established test of a major aspect of cognitive functioning. Test sensitivity is critical because improvements may be relatively small. Individuals should be tested before and a number of times after the administration of the putative compound. If the compound can improve performance relatively soon after administration, it is important to perform a number of repeated test sessions to pick up the time profile of this effect. For compounds that may take longer to show a benefit, testing needs to be repeated daily, weekly, or even monthly. This rules out tests that show marked practice effects because such effects will obscure the potential benefits of the study compound.[19]

Many traditional neuropsychological tests suffer from this limitation, which is often exacerbated by a lack of parallel forms of some tests (i.e., the same stimulus materials are used each time, and performance improves not only through practice but also by remembering the test stimuli). Clear evidence of this unwanted phenomenon was present in the healthy control cohort of the Alzheimer's Disease Neuroimaging Cohort (ADNI), in which 249 individuals (mean age, 76 years) performed the following widely used neuropsychological tests annually during a 6-year period: Rey Auditory Verbal Learning Task (RAVLT), Wechsler Logical Memory I & II, Category Fluency, Digit Symbol Substitution Test (DSST), Digit Span, Boston Naming Test, Trail Making Test A & B, Clock Copying Task, and Clock Drawing Task. Despite the fact that 11% of the population developed mild cognitive impairment during the 6 years,[20] and that there were yearly declines in cortical thickness along with a range of other physiological measures, not one of the tests used showed a pattern of decline during the 6 years.[21] In fact, Trails A & B, DSST, Boston Naming, RAVLT delayed recall, and Logical Memory I & II showed significant improvements from the start of the study, with effect sizes in the range 0.22–0.72, which for some measures lasted throughout the 6 years. This was not the first large long-term study to show year-on-year training effects in such populations with these and other neuropsychological tests.[22]

In Figure 14.1, data from a computerized test system are shown for a group of 256 nondemented elderly individuals aged 70–90 years, who were tested yearly over 5 years.[23] The data are plotted as year-by-year declines from the start of the study, and the error bars are confidence intervals. Thus, where the confidence intervals do not overlap the baseline score, the deficits are statistically reliable. As can be seen, power of attention declined year on year, and all measures showed significant declines from year 3 onward. These data indicate that certain tests that are not subject to training effects can be utilized in long-term trials and reflect more accurately changes in cognitive status over time in older populations.

COMPUTERIZED TESTING

One important advantage of computerized tests is that they can measure both accuracy and speed on tasks of cognitive function. Speed and accuracy are both important aspects

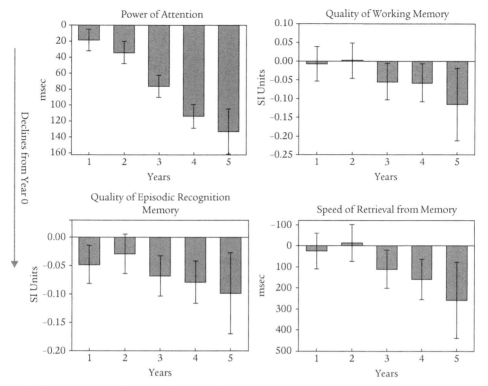

FIGURE 14.1 *Data showing declines in performance on automated cognitive tests administered yearly over 5 years in a non-demented older population aged 70–90 years.* SOURCE: WESNES ET AL. (2012).

of task efficiency, and for some cognitive measures, unless both are captured, it is difficult to determine whether performance has been favorably (or unfavorably) changed. For example, an improvement in speed at the expense of accuracy (or vice versa) cannot be interpreted unequivocally as an enhancement, and the interpretation of results thus becomes controversial.[24] An ideal result for a cognition enhancer is for both to be improved, which would thus be an unquestioned improvement of performance.

Another advantage is that it allows identifying differential benefits to performance for different tasks. For example, a compound may improve the speed of recognition in one task and accuracy in another. This potential benefit may be missed with a non-automated neuropsychological test. The relative utility of pencil-and-paper neuropsychological tests versus computerized tests has been the subject of much historical debate. Recently, the case for "equal opportunity" or "ability to get the job done" has been made, whereby tests for a particular study objective are selected solely on the basis of their proven usefulness for that objective.[25] Ultimately, researchers are responsible for the ability of their studies to adequately address the study question, and the continued use of inappropriate outcome measures in such work should become the cause of major concern.

A PROPOSED CRITERION FOR
A COGNITIVE ENHANCER

For a compound to fulfill the criteria as an enhancer, the following can be considered the minimum requirements for qualification:[26,27]

1. Improvements must be identified by well-recognized tests of cognitive function.
2. Improvements should be in one or more major domains of cognitive function—for example, attention, vigilance, information processing, spatial working memory, numeric working memory, visual episodic memory, verbal episodic memory, planning, and motor control.
3. Improvements must be seen on core measures of task performance, and any suggestions of speed–accuracy trade-offs should be interpreted with caution.
4. Improvements must not be followed by rebound declines.
5. Improvements should be of a magnitude that would be considered behaviorally or clinically relevant.
6. Improvements should not be subject to tachyphylaxis during the period in which the treatment is intended to be used.
7. Self-ratings are of interest and may be used as supportive evidence, but they are not sufficient in the absence of objective test results.

THE DECLINE OF COGNITIVE FUNCTION
WITH NORMAL AGING

The scene for the following sections is admirably set by Jelle Jolles and colleagues in their conclusions from a comprehensive review of this field:[28]

> There is a vast literature on the relationship between age and cognitive performance. It is now generally agreed that healthy individuals are characterized by a cognitive decline in the later years of adult life. The acquisition of new information becomes less efficient, which, when coupled with a diminished retention of this information, results in substantially poorer memory performance. The ability to plan new activities, solve problems, and make complex decisions is noticeably diminished. In addition, attentional processes appear to be invariably poorer in older patients than in younger ones. (p. 461)

This chapter leans heavily on the research of a group at the University of Virginia led by the renowned psychologist Timothy Salthouse. For more than three decades, he has studied the cognitive declines that accompany aging, and he has assembled a large and robust body of evidence on the topic.[29–32] The clear conclusions from his research are as follows:

1. From the early twenties onward, major aspects of cognitive function decline in a linear manner across the life span.
2. These deficits are not restricted to memory but, rather, to a range of core aspects of function, including attention, information processing, and executive control.
3. These deficits are large in magnitude.
4. They appear to occur in everybody.

Salthouse began his research against the backdrop of the summary statement of the American Psychological Association Task Force for the 1971 White House Conference on Aging: "For the most part, the observed decline in intellectual function among the aged is attributable to poor health, social isolation, economic plight, limited education, lowered motivation, or variables not intrinsically related to the aging process" (p. 33).[30] The comments of Salthouse are revealing: "Beginning with the earliest reports of age differences in cognition, researchers have considered alternative interpretations of the cognitive aging phenomenon that would minimize the negative implications of the finding that some aspects of cognitive function appear to decline with age" (p. 31).[30] During the past few decades, he has patiently and persistently gathered and reported experimental data to overcome the various "counterarguments" and misconceptions that are raised in this area. It is difficult to read his well-reasoned and data-rich book[30] and other reviews[31,32] and not be convinced of the previous conclusions.

Figure 14.2 is a summary of a core finding from Salthouse's research laboratory, neatly summarizing the data on 10 measures from a range of studies, with the number of individuals contributing to each measure ranging from 2780 to 8085. This figure makes a number of points. The first is the linear decline in ability from the twenties on eight tests that assess a wide range of important components of cognitive function. The second is that some aspects of cognitive function, notably the use of vocabulary, actually increase until approximately age 60 years and then decline thereafter. The third is the large magnitude of these deficits when expressed in standard deviations (SDs), with the smallest of the eight declines during six decades being 1 SD, which exceeds the magnitude of a large effect size in clinical research.

Figure 14.3 makes the crucial point that all of the population shows cognitive declines with aging. Taking individuals in the highest quartile, even though at

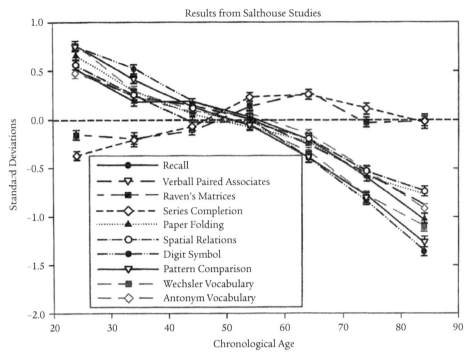

FIGURE 14.2 *Cross-sectional data for a range of tasks.* SOURCE: SALTHOUSE TA. SELECTIVE REVIEW OF COGNITIVE AGING. *J INT NEUROPSYCHOL SOC* 2010;16(5):754–760.

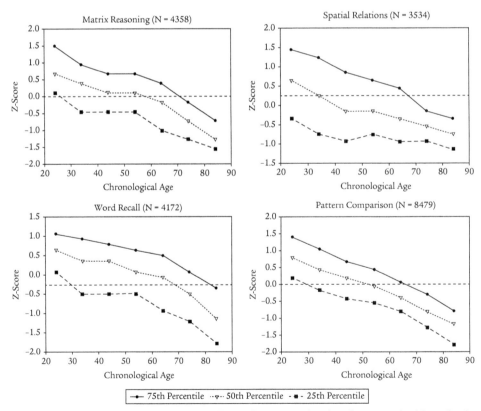

FIGURE 14.3 *Cross-sectional scores from four tasks over six decades of ageing in healthy individuals, expressed as the median scores and the upper and lower quartiles.* SOURCE: TIMOTHY SALTHOUSE. WHAT IS NORMAL COGNITIVE AGING? ALZHEIMER'S ASSOCIATION RESEARCH ROUNDTABLE: EARLY RISK ASSESSMENT FOR ALZHEIMER'S DISEASE WASHINGTON, NOVEMBER 13, 2007.

60 years they have performance levels superior or comparable to the average performance levels of people in their twenties, they still have declined by a substantial amount since they were in their twenties. There is no doubt that for many people, the accumulation of experience and life skills throughout the decades can enable them to perform at the highest levels in their fields throughout the life span, but that does not mean they could not perform at even higher levels had some core aspects of cognitive function not deteriorated throughout the years.

Figure 14.4 confirms the general findings of Salthouse, indicating that declines occur over decades on a measure of focused attention and information processing. This measure, power of attention, is a validated composite factor score from a computerized cognitive test system (the CDR system[33]). The score is the sum of the speeds of three attention tests: simple reaction time, choice reaction time, and digit vigilance. Two populations are shown, with the first (clinic) being individuals who have participated in Phase I clinical pharmacology safety and tolerability trials. The requirements for participating in such trials are for the individuals to pass stringent medical evaluations, not be taking medications or recreational drugs, to be no more than moderate users of alcohol, and to be free of medical psychiatric disorders.

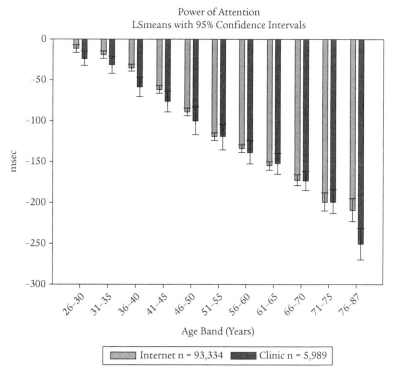

FIGURE 14.4 *Cross-sectional declines with aging compared to 18- to 25-year-olds on a measure of focused attention and information processing. The clinic population was sufficiently healthy to have taken part in early safety and tolerability trials of new medicines. The Internet population was an opportunistic sample.*

This population can thus be considered a best case for normal aging, but the linear declines for each age cohort in comparison to those individuals aged 18–25 years are clear. Furthermore, the standard deviation of a score for 18- to 25-year-olds in this population is 92 msec. It can be seen that speed declines by at least 1 SD by the late forties and by more than 2 SDs by the seventies. As Salthouse reported, the declines in healthy individuals over the age span have large effect sizes. Parallel data on more than 93,000 individuals was gathered over 18 months between 2011 and 2012 using the same tests but performed via the Internet.[34] The Internet population was purely opportunistic, with participation being open to anyone who logged onto the website. This population was thus more representative of the broader population than the particularly healthy individuals who participate in safety trials of new medicines. However, the declines in the two populations were directly comparable, which supports Salthouse's findings that the patterns of decline on various measures over the adult age span are not specific to any particular population.

In Figure 14.5, the clinic population presented in Figure 14.4 is plotted as percentiles. It can be seen as in the data from Salthouse (see Figure 14.3) that rates of decline are directly comparable in all percentiles of the population. Considering individuals in the highest 5% of the population, it is important to note that in their seventies they

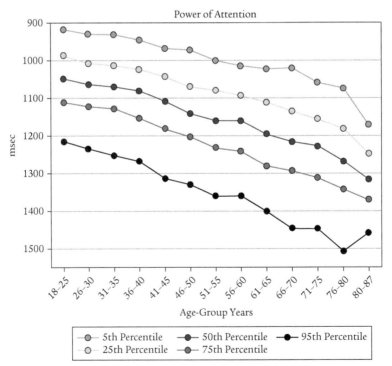

FIGURE 14.5 *Cross-sectional CDR System data from a large sample of healthy individuals showing declines by percentile over adulthood in the power of attention factor score.*

are still scoring as well as the norm for the population aged 18–25 years. However, the decline by that time from the early twenties is greater than 150 msec, which indicates that they have become more than 1.5 SD poorer on this important measure of attention over the intervening years. Possibly this is part of the problem with the acceptance of age-associated declines in some quarters; many older individuals still operate at higher levels than the average for younger individuals but possibly fail to realize the full extent to which many important aspects of their cognitive function have actually declined throughout the years.

In summary, there is little disagreement about whether cognitive function declines with age, and although the reasons for declines in cognitive function and their precise nature are the subject of debate,[35] the pattern demonstrated by Salthouse and by other researchers does present a compelling picture.

AGE-RELATED COGNITIVE DECLINE: IS IT A CLINICAL CONDITION?

Although there may be disagreement about the precise nature and causes of the declines in cognitive function, which occur with aging during adulthood, virtually everyone agrees that they happen. One important question is therefore, "If it were possible to reverse or delay this process with a pharmaceutical drug, would individuals choose to take it?" The answer for many would probably be yes, provided the cost was affordable and the side effects were not severe. One would thus imagine that the pharmaceutical industry would be heavily engaged in research in this field; but the surprising fact is that it is not. One reason is that the pharmaceutical industry operates in a regulatory environment focused on developing treatments for "established medical conditions." As discussed in the following sections, attempts to establish normal cognitive aging as a treatable condition have not been successful so far.

The most widely cited original description of age-related mental change is that of Kral,[36] who suggested a distinction between "benign" and "malignant" senescent forgetfulness. Benign senescent forgetfulness became a widely and largely uncritically accepted concept referring to the cognitive loss that accompanied normal aging, in contrast to the malignant decline that evolved into dementia. Although the word "benign" was obviously meant to discriminate the prognosis of the condition from the considerably more serious condition of dementia, the term "benign senescent forgetfulness" became synonymous with acceptable declines in memory with aging, implying an acceptability of mental loss with aging—that it "did not actually matter too much" and "that it was part of the charm of growing old." This is consistent with Salthouse's previously mentioned contention that descriptions of cognitive decline with aging generally attempt to minimize the negative nature of the effects. This point is supported by a quotation from a working group report on age-associated cognitive decline—that previous trials of medications were addressing "an inconvenient but basically benign problem" (p. 68).[37] The duality here is striking: Imagine failing eyesight being described as "a benign loss of visual acuity." Of course it has not, and society has gone ahead and dealt with the visual problems associated with aging, as it has, or has attempted to do, with the vast majority of age-related declines in aspects of health and well-being.

The first serious challenge to this dogma and inertia took place in 1986 when a National Institute of Mental Health workgroup was convened to put together diagnostic terminology and specific research diagnostic criteria "to describe the memory loss that may occur in healthy, elderly individuals in the later decades of life" (p. 262).[38] The subsequent paper was titled "Age-Associated Memory Impairment: Proposed Diagnostic Criteria and Measures of Clinical Change—Report of a National Institute of Mental Health Work Group." This milestone publication put age-associated memory impairment (AAMI) firmly on the map and was the catalyst for a large number of therapeutic clinical trials on a range of compounds in subsequent years.[39] The workgroup focused on secondary (episodic) memory, which "shows substantial age-related deficits when the memory of old and young individuals is compared" (p. 262)[38] The group also recognized the potential everyday importance of such declines:

> The effects of declining secondary memory are not trivial and may severely compromise the individual's ability to function in intellectually demanding activities and employment situations. Behavioral deficits resulting from memory impairment may extend beyond obvious everyday memory tasks such as recalling the name of an individual after introduction or remembering tasks to be performed. . . . Memory is a critical factor in fluid intelligence. . . . Remembering is an essential component of problem-solving, concept formation, and intelligent decision making. Thus the practical impact of memory loss may be far reaching and profound in some individuals. (p. 265)

The paper proposed inclusion and exclusion criteria for the condition. The aims of the inclusion criteria were to identify those individuals (aged 50 years or older) who were aware of a gradual memory loss, scoring at least 1 SD below the normal score on a widely recognized test of memory (e.g., the Benton Visual Retention Test or the Logical Memory Subtest of the Wechsler Memory Scale); showed evidence of adequate intellectual functioning (using the vocabulary subtest of the Wechsler Adult

Intelligence Scale); and showed no evidence of dementia as assessed by a Mini-Mental State Examination with a score of 24 or greater. The exclusion criteria were designed to exclude those whose poor performance could be explained in any other way—for example, as a result of depression or diabetes or from prescription medicines or recreational drugs.

The importance of this work was threefold. First, it acknowledged that cognitive declines in aging outside of those associated with dementia were neither necessarily benign nor inconsequential. Second, it highlighted that these declines were worthy of treatment. Third, it outlined clear inclusion and exclusion criteria for the identification of AAMI. However, one obvious flaw was that AAMI centered solely on memory, with no mention of the other important domains of cognitive function that also decline with age, as illustrated by the work described previously in this chapter. This was resolved in the fourth edition of the *Diagnostic and Statistical Manual of Mental Disorders* (DSM-IV)[40], which identified age-related cognitive decline (ARCD) as a condition that may be a focus of clinical attention. ARCD extended the range of impairments from simply memory to cognitive functioning in general, thus encompassing attention, information processing, and a range of other aspects now known to deteriorate with aging. ARCD was defined as a decline in cognitive functioning consequent to the aging process that is within normal limits given the person's age. It was specifically stated that "individuals with this condition may report problems remembering names or appointments or may experience difficulty in solving complex problems."

Another issue with AAMI, which subsequently became a source of contention, was the identification of the disorder in comparison to memory tests scores for the young. A working party of the International Psychogeriatric Association in collaboration with the World Health Organization met to propose guidelines for aging-associated cognitive decline (AACD).[37] As with DSM-IV, the ensuing guidelines broadened the domains of function covered to include attention and concentration, thinking, language, and visuospatial functioning. Unfortunately, the criterion for the objective decline in AACD was altered from 1 SD below that of the young to 1 SD below that of an age-matched population, which made the patients as difficult to recruit as those for trials for mild cognitive impairment (MCI); to our knowledge, no therapeutic trials were ever conducted on this condition. Other similar conditions have also since been defined, including cognitive impairment, no dementia (CIND)[41] and mild cognitive disorder.[42]

One important weakness of all three criteria is the requirement that a patient must score in the lower end of normal distributions (whether they are for the young or the aged). This must logically predispose populations identified with the criteria to not include those in the upper end of the distribution, while also independently including those who may have always resided in the lower end of the distribution (i.e., those who have perhaps shown no decline). In 1994, Levy[37] addressed this issue:

> Since we consider decline to be the cardinal feature, no definitive decision as to the characteristics of the condition can be evolved without longitudinal study. We also seek to derive an estimate of presumed baseline function which takes into account a subject's social, educational and cultural background. Until the results of longitudinal studies are available, it will not be possible to determine whether AACD represents a physiological concomitant to healthy aging or a separate pathological process.(p. 64)

As mentioned previously, the pharmaceutical industry requires a clear regulatory pathway, and despite some early interest in AAMI by the FDA,[43] no treatments have been approved. The pharmaceutical industry has now largely moved away from studying conditions such as AAMI, due in part to doubts as to whether there was a regulatory pathway and also the viewpoint typified by the following: "Overall, the merits of AAMI as a diagnosis remain unclear and some see its main purpose as a label to justify pharmacotherapy for what are essentially age-related memory changes experienced by the majority of the population."[44] This criticism that "the industry was seeking to define an illness to treat" was unfair, considering the origins of the AAMI criteria. Similarly, the viewpoint that if the majority of the population experiences symptoms, it is not a treatable condition, or a condition worthy of treatment, appears illogical and out of step with medical practice in most other age-related conditions. Although the pharmaceutical industry has largely pulled back from this field, its place has been taken by the food and nutrition industry, as well as manufacturers of herbal products. Here, the regulatory environment seems more promising. For example, the European Food Safety Authority (EFSA) has published guidelines on the scientific requirements for health claims including cognitive function.[45] EFSA clearly has no issue with the concept of products to treat normal age-related cognitive decline, as evidenced by the following:[45]

> With respect to the study population, results from studies conducted in subjects with mild cognitive decline, without clinical diagnosis of dementia or other psychological or neurological diseases which may be responsible for the impairment, could be used for the scientific substantiation of claims on cognitive function,

as long as the methods and inclusion/exclusion criteria used to characterise the study group are clearly defined. The rationale for extrapolation of the results obtained in patients with clinical diagnosis of a cognitive disease (e.g., dementia) to the target population for the claim (e.g., subjects without the disease) should be provided, and will be considered on a case-by-case basis (e.g., evidence that the mechanism by which the food constituent may exert the claimed effect on cognition in subjects with the disease is also relevant for subjects without the disease). (p. 7)

AGE-RELATED COGNITIVE DECLINES: THE ROUTE FORWARD FOR TREATMENT AND ULTIMATELY EVEN PREVENTION

For Alzheimer's disease (AD) and other dementias, there has been considerably less controversy in developing pharmacological therapies. Five products are currently registered by the FDA for AD, and one is registered for Parkinson's disease dementia. However, no new compound has been registered for any type of dementia for more than 10 years, a period that has been consistently characterized by failures of well over 100 research programs.[46,47]

Although it has long been recognized that palliative treatments for AD are required,[48] the viewpoint that treatment should start at earlier stages of AD has only gathered serious momentum in recent years.[20] The current status of research in treating AD could be characterized as the time when the field stopped waiting for the symptoms to become fully manifest before initiating treatment but instead turned its attention to intervening at the earliest stages of the disease. This change in direction was stimulated by a 2007 position paper proposing revised diagnostic criteria to capture the earlier stages of the disease, based on a clinical core of early loss of episodic memory alongside biomarker evidence of disease pathology.[49] These criteria have been further refined[50,51] with the intention of defining the symptomatic predementia phase of AD, which is also termed either mild cognitive impairment due to AD or prodromal AD. Furthermore, from the perspective of this chapter, an important landmark was the publication of the joint National Institute on Aging—Alzheimer's Association 2011 operational research criteria for preclinical AD.[52] Preclinical AD is defined as the stage of AD prior to the development of detectable cognitive impairment (MCI). Individuals who will enter preclinical AD trials will be cognitively normal for their age and thus will not experience any difficulties with performing everyday tasks. Although many may be selected on the basis of being positive on, for example, amyloid biomarkers or having genetic predispositions such as APOE4 or TOMM40 alleles, many AD patients do not show such characteristics, and thus trials will include individuals without these risk factors. It is clear that individuals in preclinical AD trials will have a considerable overlap with individuals who would satisfy the criteria for AAMI, AACD, and ARCD.

An important paradigm shift in these various recent criteria was the recognition that measured change in cognition over time would be a far more appropriate approach than any one-time assessment and that longitudinal studies of older individuals, using measures sensitive to detecting very subtle cognitive decline over time, were needed. This approach is clearly in line with Levy's previously cited suggestions for AACD.[34] As we have seen with a variety of non-automated neuropsychological tests in the ADNI study, these are not suitable instruments for the role of tracking declines in function over years in cognitively unimpaired individuals. However, automated procedures have shown just such sensitivity in a study that evaluated the effects of an angiotensin II receptor blocker on cognitive function over 5 years in a population of 257 hypertensive, but not cognitively impaired, older adults (mean age, 76 years).[53] Computerized tests of cognitive function were used together with three traditional neuropsychological tests (Trail Making test, category fluency, and verbal fluency) and administered yearly during the study period. It was found that active treatment statistically significantly reduced the rate of decline seen under placebo on computerized measures of episodic memory and attention. As may be expected based on the ADNI data, the traditional neuropsychological tests used did not show a measurable decline over time under placebo nor any benefit of active treatment. It is worth noting that the overall methodology of cognitive testing in this study, as well as the cognitive capabilities of the study population, is comparable to that which is being (and will be) used in trials of preclinical AD, suggesting that appropriate computerized testing will at a minimum be no less sensitive than traditional neuropsychological tests.

Regulatory guidance is crucial in this field, and the FDA has been proactive in this area. In February 2013, the Division of Neurology Products of the FDA issued a draft guideline for industry titled "Alzheimer's Disease: Developing Drugs for the Treatment of Early Stage Disease."[54] The document outlined the agency's thinking regarding the selection of patients with early AD, or patients who are determined to be at risk of developing AD, for enrollment into clinical trials. The guidance also addressed the selection of endpoints for clinical trials in these populations, as well as the manner in which disease modification might be demonstrated. In a subsequent publication, authored by FDA officers, the important point was acknowledged that at the earliest stages of the disease (i.e., preclinical AD), functional impairment would be difficult to assess. It was proposed that using the FDA's accelerated approval pathway, it could be feasible to approve a drug in this condition on the basis of assessment of a cognitive outcome alone.[55]

A number of preclinical AD studies have already begun,[47] including A4 and Diane, as well as an industry-sponsored therapeutic trial called the TOMMORROW study, in which more than 5700 individuals are being assessed during a 5-year period.[56] In view of the practice effects seen in the ADNI study, it is worth noting that this large long-term trial is using a range of pencil-and-paper neuropsychological tests, including several used in ADNI (e.g., trail making, digit span, clock drawing, and category fluency).

Other major regulatory bodies are also responding to the focus of research moving toward preclinical AD. The European Medicines Agency Committee for Medicinal Products for Human Use (CHMP) has published a concept paper on the need for the revision of the guidelines on medicinal products for the treatment of AD and other dementias.[57] The public consultation on the revisions concluded at the end of January 2014, with a workshop held in November 2014 and the revised guidelines expected imminently.

It is evident that the distinction between normal cognitive aging and pathological decline is becoming increasingly blurred, and it is now important to consider in more detail the concept of improving cognitive function. It is important to note that the aspects of cognitive function that decline in the dementias are not different from those that have been found to decline with normal aging.[58] Thus, the existing treatments for AD may well improve function in patients without the disorder. However, potential disease-modifying therapies under development—for example, those aimed at amyloidosis in AD—may not be in any way appropriate or safe in nondemented individuals. In contrast, any therapy that improves functioning in healthy people may have similar effects in patients with dementia.

Furthermore, because the same aspects of cognition decline in both normal and pathological aging, it has been suggested that difference are primarily quantitative. Therefore, is there a necessity to make a distinction between them in research terms? Certainly, Peter Whitehouse, one of the early researchers to identify the brain neurochemical pathology in AD, does not believe so. In his widely acclaimed book with Danny George, *The Myth of Alzheimer's Disease*, he makes a convincing case that we should be studying brain aging, as opposed to specific dementias, and that anything we can do to improve cognitive function at all stages of aging can only good in the long term.[59] In a recent paper, Whitehouse wrote, "We must essentially reverse priorities for the treatment of AD. Care must be viewed as more important than cure rather than the current message from the Alzheimer's Association and others that cure ('ending' Alzheimer's) is the answer."[60] This perspective represents a practical, realistic, and holistic approach to healthy aging. Another leading researcher in this field, Gary Small, has for many years made convincing arguments that the best way to avoid illnesses such as AD is prevention through a wide variety of achievable life-style changes, including physical exercise, nutrition, mental workouts, stress reduction, and treating various physical illnesses.[61]

As evidence accumulates that a host of factors (e.g., drugs, diet, and regular exercise) have the ability to produce improvements in cognitive function or prevent further decline, the issue becomes whether these various factors are all competing for small windows of enhancement and, when combined, whether the benefits they produce are additive or even synergistic. Such questions cannot be answered in conventional clinical trials because the costs of such trials make them impractical for studying more than one or two interventions. However, if the field is to move to the next level, this crucial question concerning additivity does need to be addressed. The solution may be Internet-based trials.

Previously, data were presented from an opportunistic sample of people who logged onto a website of a natural health product and were invited to perform a series of cognitive tests and receive general feedback on the levels of their performance. During an 18-month period, 120,171 people aged 5–102 years provided information. Of the four tests, 111,203 completed the first and 97,171 completed all four tasks, which lasted approximately 12 minutes. This example shows the potential for very large trials to be conducted. A wide range of information on drugs, diet, and lifestyle can be gathered, a range of questionnaires can be administered, and cognitive testing can be performed; these can all be repeated over an indefinite period. The "big data" that would be gathered from such trials would at a minimum enable sophisticated evaluations to determine the additivity of the wide range of factors already known or expected to promote cognitive well-being. The huge amounts of data on a wide variety of factors would also allow identifying characteristics of individuals that predispose them to cognitive decline or, for example, enable them to respond to particular lifestyle changes or interventions. It is difficult to fully imagine the massive advances in our understanding of this crucial field that could be gained from such trials, but it is also difficult to imagine the future without them.

CONCLUSION

Cognitive function declines in everyone with aging, and eventually for many this becomes marked enough to be diagnosed as dementia. There is a growing body of evidence that a wide variety of treatments, interventions, and lifestyle changes can have positive effects on cognitive function and help delay the time at which cognitive decline compromises the ability to conduct normal daily living activities. Cognitive tests necessarily play a major role in this field, and the ability to administer them via the Internet will enable a new generation of long-term global trials to be conducted with tens if not hundreds of thousands of participants. Such trials will generate the big data required to answer a host of crucial and as yet unanswered questions in this field, as well as many questions that have not yet been considered.

DISCLOSURES

Until February 2014, Keith Wesnes worked for Bracket, which provided the CDR system as a service to clinical trials. He now owns and runs a consultancy, which provides an online cognitive assessment system service and advises companies on how to best evaluate the cognitive potential of their products.

Until July 2010, Helen Brooker worked for United BioSource Corporation (now registered as Bracket), which provided the CDR system as a service to clinical trials. She currently consults for Wesnes Cognition Ltd., which provides an online cognitive assessment system service and advises companies on how to best evaluate the cognitive potential of their products.

REFERENCES

1. Bostrom N, Sandberg A. Cognitive enhancement: Methods, ethics, regulatory challenges. *Sci Eng Ethics* 2009;15:311–341.
2. Hollingworth HL. The influence of caffeine on mental and motor efficiency. *Arch Psychol* 1912;22:1–166.
3. Beach F. *Clark Leonard Hull: 1884–1952: Biographical memoirs*. Washington, DC: National Academy of Sciences; 1959:125–141.
4. Hull CL. The influence of tobacco smoking on mental and motor efficiency. *Psychol Monogr* 1924;33:1–160.
5. McNamara WJ, Miller RE. Effect of benzedrine sulphate on mental work. *Psychol Rec* 1937;1:78–84.
6. Weiss B, Laties VG. Enhancement of human performance by caffeine and the amphetamines. *Pharmacol Rev* 1962;14:1–36.
7. Wesnes KA, Warburton DM. Nicotine, smoking and human performance. *Pharmacol Ther* 1983;21:189–208.
8. Wesnes KA, Parrott A. Smoking, nicotine and human performance. In Smith A, Jones D (Eds.), *Handbook of human performance*, vol. 2. London: Academic Press; 1992:127–167.
9. Nehlig A. Is caffeine a cognitive enhancer? *J Alzheimers Dis* 2010;20:85–94.
10. McDonald R. Hydergine: A review of 26 clinical studies. *Pharmacopsychiatr Neuropsychopharm* 1979;12:407–422.

11. Ammon R, Sharma R, Gambert SR, et al. A statistical analysis of studies showing efficacy in the treatment of cognitively impaired elderly. *Age* 1995;18:5–9.
12. Schneider LS, Olin JT. Overview of clinical trials of hydergine in dementia. *Arch Neurol* 1994;51:787–798.
13. Rockwood K. Size of the treatment effect on cognition of cholinesterase inhibition in Alzheimer's disease. *J Neurol Neurosurg Psychiatry* 2004;75:677–685.
14. Giurgea C. Pharmacology of integrative activity of the brain: Attempt at nootropic concept in psychopharmacology. *Actual Pharmacol (Paris)* 1972;25:115–156.
15. Waegemans T, Wilsher CR, Danniau A, et al. Clinical efficacy of piracetam in cognitive impairment: A meta-analysis. *Dement Geriatr Cogn Disord* 2002;13:217–224.
16. Blaha L, Erzigkeit H, Adamczyk A, et al. Clinical evidence of the effectiveness of vinpocetine in the treatment of organic psychosyndrome. *Hum Psychopharmacol* 1989;4:103–111.
17. Montgomery SA, Thal LJ, Amrein R. Meta-analysis of double blind randomized controlled clinical trials of acetyl-L-carnitine versus placebo in the treatment of mild cognitive impairment and mild Alzheimer's disease. *Int Clin Psychopharmacol* 2003;18:61–71.
18. Tarnawa I, Bölcskei H, Kocsis P. Blockers of voltage-gated sodium channels for the treatment of central nervous system diseases. *Recent Pat CNS Drug Discov* 2007;2:57–78.
19. Wesnes KA, Pincock C. Practice effects on cognitive tasks: A major problem? *Lancet Neurol* 2002;1(8):473.
20. Wesnes KA, Edgar CE. The role of human cognitive neuroscience in drug discovery for the dementias. *Curr Opin Pharmacol* 2014:14:62–73.
21. Wesnes KA, Schneider LS. Are neuropsychological tests such as those used in ADNI suitable for long-term trials of cognition enhancers for preclinical Alzheimer's disease? *J Nutr Health Aging* 2012;16:810.
22. Wilson RS, Beckett LA, Barnes LL, et al. Individual differences in rates of change in cognitive abilities of older persons. *Psychol Aging* 2002;17:179–193.
23. Wesnes KA, Saxby BK, Ford G, et al. The year by year changes in cognitive function in a non-demented population aged 70 to 90 over a five year period. *J Frailty Aging* 2012;1:76.
24. Turner DC, Robbins TW, Clark L, et al. Cognitive enhancing effects of modafinil in healthy volunteers. *Psychopharmacology* 2003;165:260–269.
25. Wesnes KA. Moving beyond the pros and cons of automating cognitive testing in pathological aging and dementia: The case for equal opportunity. *Alzheimers Res Ther* 2014;6:58.
26. Wesnes KA. Cognition enhancement—Expanding opportunities in drug development: Wake-up to the MATRICS. *Int Clin Trials* 2010 June;66–72.
27. Zangara A, Wesnes KA. Herbal cognitive enhancers: New developments and challenges for therapeutic applications. In Thakur MK, Suresh IS (Eds.), *Brain aging and therapeutic interventions* New York, NY: Springer; 2012:267–289.
28. Jolles J, Verhey FRJ, Riedel WJ, et al. Cognitive impairment in elderly people—Predisposing factors and implications for experimental drug studies. *Drugs Ageing* 1995;7:459–479.
29. Salthouse TA. Selective review of cognitive aging. *J Int Neuropsychol Soc* 2010;16(5):754–760.
30. Salthouse TA. *Major issues in cognitive aging.* Oxford, UK: Oxford University Press; 2010.
31. Salthouse TA. Consequences of age-related cognitive declines. *Annu Rev Psychol* 2012;63:201–226.
32. Salthouse TA. Does the level at which cognitive change occurs change with age? *Psychol Sci* 2012;23:18–23.
33. Wesnes KA, Ward T, McGinty A, et al. The memory enhancing effects of a Ginkgo biloba/Panax ginseng combination in healthy middle-aged volunteers. *Psychopharmacology* 2000;152:353–361.
34. Wesnes KA. Internet-based cognitive function assessment. *Alzheimers Dement* 2012;8:546.
35. Ramscar M, Hendrix P, Shaoul C, et al. The myth of cognitive decline: Non-linear dynamics of lifelong learning. *Top Cogn Sci* 2014; 6: 5–42.
36. Kral VA. Senescent forgetfulness: Benign and malignant. *J Can Med Assoc* 1962;86:257–260.
37. Levy R. Ageing-associated cognitive decline—Report of the working party of the International Psychogeriatric Association in collaboration with the World Health Organisation. *Int Psychogeriatr* 1994;6:63–68.

38. Crook TH, Bartus RT, Ferris SH, et al. Age-associated memory impairment: Proposed diagnostic criteria and measures of clinical change. Report of a National Institute of Mental Health Workgroup. *Dev Neuropsychol* 1986;5:295–306.

39. Wesnes KA, Ward T. Treatment of age-associated memory impairment. In Qizilbash N, Schneider L, Chui H, et al. (Eds.), *Evidence-based dementia practice: A practical guide to diagnosis and management (with Internet updates)*. Malden, MA: Blackwell; 2000:639–653.

40. American Psychiatric Association. (1994). *Diagnostic and statistical manual of mental disorders* (4th ed.). Washington, DC: Author.

41. Tuokko HA, Frerichs RJ, Kristjansson B. Cognitive impairment, no dementia: Concepts and issues. *Int Psychogeriatr* 2001;13:183–202.

42. American Psychiatric Association. (2013). *Diagnostic and statistical manual of mental disorders* (5th ed.). Arlington, VA: American Psychiatric Publishing.

43. Leber P. Establishing the efficacy of drugs with psychogeriatric indications. In Crook T, et al. (Eds.), *Treatment development strategies for Alzheimer's disease*. Madison, CT: Mark Powley Associates; 1986:1–14.

44. O'Brien JT. Age-associated memory impairment and related disorders. *Adv Psychiatr Treat* 1999;5:279–287,

45. EFSA Panel on Dietetic Products, Nutrition and Allergies. Guidance on the scientific requirements for health claims related to functions of the nervous system, including psychological functions. *EFSA J* 2012;10(7):2816.

46. Becker RE, Greig NH, Giacobini E. Why do so many drugs for Alzheimer's disease fail in development? Time for new methods and new practices? *J Alzheimers Dis* 2008;15:303–325.

47. Mullard A. Sting of Alzheimer's failures offset by upcoming prevention trials. *Nat Rev Drug Discov* 2013;11:657–660.

48. Bartus RT. On neurodegenerative diseases, models, and treatment strategies: Lessons learned and lessons forgotten a generation following the cholinergic hypothesis. *Exp Neurol* 2000;163(2):495–529.

49. Dubois B, Feldman HH, Jacova C, et al. Research criteria for the diagnosis of Alzheimer's disease: Revising the NINCDS–ADRDA criteria. *Lancet Neurol* 2007;6:734–737

50. Dubois B, Feldman HH, Jacova C, et al. Revising the definition of Alzheimer's disease: A new lexicon. *Lancet Neurol* 2010;9:1118–1127.

51. Albert MS, Dekosky ST, Dickson D, et al. The diagnosis of mild cognitive impairment due to Alzheimer's disease: Recommendations from the National Institute on Aging–Alzheimer's Association workgroups on diagnostic guidelines for Alzheimer's disease. *Alzheimers Dement* 2011;7:270–279.

52. Sperling RA, Aisen PS, Beckett LA, et al. Toward defining the preclinical stages of Alzheimer's disease: Recommendations from the National Institute on Aging–Alzheimer's Association workgroups on diagnostic guidelines for Alzheimer's disease. *Alzheimers Dement* 2011;7:280–292.

53. Saxby BK, Harrington F, Wesnes KA, et al. Candesartan and cognitive decline in older patients with hypertension: A substudy of the SCOPE trial. *Neurology* 2008;70:1858–1866.

54. US Department of Health and Human Services, US Food and Drug Administration, Center for Drug Evaluation and Research. *Guidance for Industry: Alzheimer's disease: Developing drugs for the treatment of early stage disease*. Retrieved from https://www.fda.gov/downloads/Drugs/GuidanceComplianceRegulatoryInformation/Guidances/UCM338287.pdf; 2013. Accessed April 10, 2015.

55. Kozauer N, Katz R. Regulatory innovation and drug development for early-stage Alzheimer's disease. *N Engl J Med* 2013;368(13):1169–1171.

56. Roses AD, Welsh-Bohmer KA, Burns DK, et al. A pharmacogenetics-supported clinical trial to delay onset of mild cognitive impairment (MCI) due to Alzheimer's disease (AD). *J Nutr Health Aging* 2012;16:841.

57. European Medicines Agency. *Concept paper on need for revision of the guideline on medicinal products for the treatment of Alzheimer's disease and other dementias*. Retrieved from

http://www.ema.europa.eu/docs/en_GB/document_library/Scientific_guideline/2013/10/ WC500153464; 2013. Accessed April 10, 2015.

58. Wesnes KA, Lenderking W. The transition of cognitive decline from normal ageing to mild cognitive impairment and Alzheimer's disease. *J Nutr Health Aging* 2012;16:863.

59. Whitehouse PJ, George, D. *The myth of Alzheimer's disease.* New York, NY: St. Martin's Press; 2008.

60. Whitehouse PJ. The end of Alzheimer's disease—From biochemical pharmacology to ecopsychosociology: A personal perspective. *Biochem Pharmacol* 2014;88(4):677–681.

61. Small G, Vorgan G. *The Alzheimer's prevention program: Keep your brain healthy for the rest of your life.* New York, NY: Workman; 2012.

FIFTEEN

Ethical Considerations in Cognitive Enhancement

Clinical Responsibilities and Duties

JALAYNE J. ARIAS, BRYAN KIBBE,

AND PAUL J. FORD

INTRODUCTION

The literature addressing ethical issues associated with cognitive enhancement has an extended history. As medicine and technology have advanced, the issues have continued to morph. Yet some of the challenges and themes have persisted through time. Particularly challenging are those that impact physicians' responsibilities. Cognitive enhancement calls into question a physician's role in patient care, within the profession of medicine, and as a member of society. As this book has demonstrated in previous chapters, there is an increasing number of cognitive enhancing modalities being studied and developed. These modalities target a variety of attributes, including memory, attention, reasoning, processing speed, and affect. For the purposes of ethical analysis, the particularities of the modality—whether pharmaceutical, surgical, or physiological—are less important than the broad risk and benefits of the specific attempt. Although this chapter focuses on cognitive enhancement, many of the issues addressed here will apply generally to multiple forms of enhancement.

This chapter provides physicians a structure and tools to evaluate the ethical challenges associated with cognitive enhancement. The chapter first provides an overview of frameworks and principles that serve as the basis for ethical analysis. Next, the chapter reviews foundational concepts regarding the ethics of cognitive enhancement, including a brief review of how cognitive enhancement is defined. Following review of the foundational ethical and enhancement concepts, the chapter provides several arguments and considerations in support of the ethical permissibility of cognitive enhancement. This section includes discussion of the benefits that cognitive enhancement offers. The following section reviews several ethical challenges to cognitive enhancement that may support prohibiting enhancement or placing limitations on its use. In the final section, the chapter weighs the permissibility justifications and the challenges to provide guidance on how to incorporate this analysis in clinical practice.

The concept of enhancement is not unique to neurosciences, nor is it a new concept. Individuals and society have frequently endeavored to identify ways to better themselves.[1] As a result, differing perspectives on what it means to be human and to flourish as an individual and a society are central considerations in the ethical assessment of enhancement and particularly cognitive enhancement. Part of the difficulty in resolving what it is to be human and to flourish is due to the frequency with which we change ourselves, our tools, and our environments in pursuit of a perceived advantage (e.g., survival, efficiency, comfort, awareness and understanding, and fame). Sometimes these changes lead to momentous improvements and at other times disastrous ruin. Although present-day means of medical enhancement are undoubtedly cutting-edge, novel products, the ethical issues and questions relating to cognitive enhancement generally are not entirely new. Society has addressed various iterations of these issues and questions when pursuing educational endeavors, housing developments, transportation innovations, and communication revolutions. With each effort to alter human capabilities, similar challenges and questions arise. Does a modality for cognitive enhancement offer a genuine enhancement to its user? How do these changes alter or strain various obligations and responsibilities? Is this an acceptable way to go about achieving a particular good? Do the benefits outweigh the harms/risks? Does this violate important moral limits, standards, or guiding principles? In an effort to achieve one advantage, do we in fact lose something more important?

The questions surrounding enhancement continue to arise in real ways for the physicians. Recent data demonstrate that requests for medical means of enhancement are not uncommon. A survey of US physicians found that 61.7% of surveyed physicians ($N = 633$) receive requests for a variety of enhancements on a monthly basis or even more frequently.[2] A number of important ethical questions and considerations are prompted by requests. For example, is it ethically permissible or prohibited to prescribe a healthy patient a drug that would increase cognitive function (e.g., memory or attention)? What arguments might justify the prescription or application of a cognitive enhancement for a patient? What arguments and considerations justify prohibiting cognitive enhancements or imposing various restrictions and guidelines for use? This chapter is intended to provide health care providers with ethical resources needed to address these questions.

ETHICS AND ETHICAL ANALYSIS

An ethical dilemma involves a forced choice where all actions entail competing values with unavoidable ethical costs associated with all options. Something important is given up, even if it is not obvious what is being sacrificed and who is asked to sacrifice. These dilemmas occur in all aspects of life: personal, professional, and societal. Although many of our everyday choices have ethical aspects, they are generally well guided by habits, intuitions, and perhaps virtue. When faced with a novel situation, these everyday tools may be insufficiently systematic to justify our actions. In these circumstances, the novelty of the situation often raises new or different issues or leads to nuanced tensions or dilemmas that have not been previously resolved.

Cognitive enhancement dilemmas arise in all three aspects of life (personal, professional, and societal). An individual may need to choose whether to pursue the enhancement for him- or herself or for family members. A physician may need to choose whether to offer specific enhancements when requested. A society or health care system may need to choose whether to fund or allow groups access to a specific modality of enhancement.

Every individual owes some level of obligation to other persons, particularly when there is a relationship between the individual and another person. Professional obligations are an extension of this. A physician's obligations extend beyond those codified by licensing boards or professional organizations. The physician–patient relationship creates both a legal and an ethical fiduciary duty to the patient. As a result, when evaluating a physician's role in cognitive enhancement, we must employ a deliberative process that incorporates ethical responsibilities and duties to other persons. Allowing for transparency and promoting understanding is central to these responsibilities. Thus, to arrive at ethically justifiable choices, we should employ careful analysis that involves transparency of our premises and clear justifications. Just like in scientific research, which requires application of specific methods, we can employ methods and frameworks to reach fair and justified solutions.

A number of philosophical methods and frameworks can help identify, and highlight the ethical shortcomings of, a solution. Each philosophical method can be useful in very specific circumstances, but each method also has significant limitations. The first method centers on how to garner the greatest benefit for the most people. This can be particularly important on a policy level. A type of calculus that weighs the greatest good can be created around populations. In philosophy, this is referred to as a *utilitarian approach* and is often associated with 19th century philosophers John Stuart Mills and Jeremy Bentham. Broadly, this calculus allows, and even requires, those enhancements that would benefit the most individuals. Examples of benefits include enhancing surgeons so they can provide better health outcomes, enhancing police officers to increase the public safety, and enhancing airplane pilots to ensure safer travel. However, utilitarian approaches tend to be weak on protecting minority or individual interests, as well as fail to fully appreciate the diversity of views on which goals are judged as a benefit or as a good. The diversity of desires and values among people makes it difficult to fully justify a purely utilitarian approach. For instance, some people may believe resources should first be used to enhance soldiers, whereas others believe they should first be used to enhance artists. Each person or set of values will have a different justification for the need in terms of benefit.

A second important philosophical method, *deontology*, highlights obligation and duties as the central focus of analysis. Responsibilities and obligations associated with specific roles, including professional, should be included in an ethical analysis. These responsibilities are dependent on whether the analysis is conducted at a personal, professional, or societal level. Broadly, these theories of duty fall under the "deontology" label and are traditionally associated with the 18th-century philosopher Immanuel Kant. As a practical matter, deontology is difficult to fully apply to specific dilemmas. Two shared duties of particular importance are (1) to treat people with respect by focusing on them as the goal (or "ends") and (2) to assure a choice that will not destroy the system if everyone chooses similarly. In the first duty, we would be careful to avoid forced enhancement of surgeons, police, or pilots if it were only to use these people as a tool for the greater good and not to respect them as a person. In the second duty, as a matter of justice we can only provide free enhancement to one person if it could be assured that the system could survive offering free enhancement to all similarly positioned persons. If this is not possible, then we need to re-evaluate the choice and change some of the factors such that the action is sustainable. Although this method again allows us to identify weakness in a potential approach, there are very few details surrounding how to implement these duties or from where these duties arise.

The *principlism* method was developed as a practical approach of applying a set of overarching principles. The Principlism movement in medical ethics originated with the publication of the *Belmont Report* in the United States, which outlined three ethical principles (beneficence, respect for persons, and justice) to which we should adhere in research.[3] Subsequently, Tom Beauchamp and James Childress in their canonical text, *Principles of Biomedical Ethics*, popularized principlism and the three initial principles became four (beneficence, nonmaleficence, respect for autonomy, and justice).[4] This method provides a tool for highlighting how a specific decision might bring into conflict one or more of these overarching principles. In this way, there can be a transparent deliberation of what will be lost in each course of action. This provides an important progression in ethical evaluation. When a patient approaches a physician for an enhancement, the stakeholders can analyze what is at stake in each of the four principles and which of the principles come into conflict. The principlism method suffers from oversimplification of the stakes and potentially ignores conflicts within the principles. For instance, autonomy might need to take into account the autonomy of the patient, physician, and family that may come into conflict.

Given the complexities of daily life, an ethical analysis of a dilemma must blend approaches that depend on the specific details of the decision at hand. Intuitions and virtue are useful in self-monitoring that allows identification of problems in daily activity that need increased scrutiny and analysis. Utility and duty play important roles in our decisions, as well as a variety of other considerations. Finally, we need a specific way to sort out and balance the values' costs, which go beyond a simplified principle-based system. In this chapter, we avoid much of the philosophical and principle-based language and focus on balancing the loss and preservation of "values." These values are simply things that are held centrally important to people in their lives. Some are associated at a personal level, such as spiritual beliefs, health, pleasure, or individual goals. Some are associated with professions, such as trust, influence, or ability to practice. Some are associated with society and community, such as democracy, public health, and justice. In addressing how cognitive enhancement technologies raise specific dilemmas, we identify values that are at risk, for which stakeholders in those values are at risk, and how these value losses might reasonably be balanced.

FOUNDATIONAL IDEAS: GETTING RIGHT TO THE BASICS

There are various distinct definitions of cognitive enhancement that health care providers may encounter. One general definition states that "cognition enhancement

(CE) may be defined as the amplification or extension of core capacities of the mind, using augmentation or improvements of our information processing systems."[5] Another definition distinguishes enhancement that "would radically transform (even transcend) normal human capacities" from enhancements that "operate within the existing range of human capacities and dispositions."[6] In 2015, the Presidential Commission for the Study of Bioethical Issues evaluated cognitive enhancement within its report titled "Gray Matters." The Commission framed enhancement under the term "neural modifiers," which allowed the Commission to broaden the application of its recommendations on the topic beyond pharmacological and technical interventions.[7] In doing so, the Commission explicitly considered any neural modifier as an "enhancement" of function, even if it is to promote proper development or to ameliorate an illness. Last, and perhaps most narrow, the American Academy of Neurology's Ethics, Law and Humanities Committee defined "neuroenhancement" as "prescribing medications to normal adults for the purpose of augmenting their normal cognitive or affective function."[8] These definitions are similar in their emphasis on the augmentation of human cognitive processing systems. However, they differ in terms of the modalities of enhancement, the medical/nonmedical nature of enhancement, the impact of enhancement on affect in addition to cognitive processing, the presence or absence of illness, and addressing specifically adults. In this chapter, cognitive enhancement is defined as the provision of medical means unrelated to disease pathology or injury to optimize or improve the existing cognitive performance (e.g., memory, attention, and reasoning) of individuals.[a] Implicit in this definition is a contentious distinction between treatment for a disease or injury and enhancement.

The ethical dilemma surrounding cognitive enhancement should not, as Kass[1] points out, be resolved simply by labeling some uses of devices, drugs, or procedures as medical treatments and others as enhancements. However, this distinction can be useful for descriptive purposes in focusing discussion on particular drugs and technologies and their intended uses. Medical treatment can be understood as a type of repair work, directed at identifiable damage (e.g., disease or injury) that impairs or hinders the use of a particular object (e.g., the human body) and aims to make the object ready for reliable use again.[9] Enhancement, by contrast, is characterized by the effort to overcome, improve, or go beyond the current functions or capabilities of an object.[5] Significantly, an individual seeking enhancement (or a society supporting it) may recognize various limitations in cognitive ability but does not necessarily regard these limitations as damage. This chapter focuses on healthy individuals who request drugs,

---

[a] Notably, we are focused on the improvement or augmentation of existing cognitive processing capabilities and not on the invention or conferral of new cognitive processing capabilities (e.g., mind reading).

devices, or procedures that may optimize or improve their cognitive performance in the absence of a pathology interfering with cognition. Throughout the chapter, the ethical analysis draws from the distinction between cognitive enhancement of healthy individuals and the treatment of patients with disease or injury.[b]

Apart from definitions and distinctions, a foundational concept in this chapter is the proper role of a physician. In order to effectively evaluate whether it is ethically permissible to provide a cognitive enhancement drug, device, or procedure to a healthy individual, it is necessary to clearly define the physician's proper role and resulting duties. The consideration of a physician's role and duties and responsibilities owed to patients and society is rich with debate. One view of the physician's role is that a physician is limited to treating sickness and injury in patients. A contrasting view of the physician's role is that a physician not only treats the sick and the injured but also strives to optimize a patient's sense of health and well-being. On this latter view, the physician is not only focused on treating disease and injury but also endeavors to help the patient to be and to feel healthier than he or she is currently.

Using these foundational ideas (the definition of enhancement, the distinction between enhancement and treatment, and the role of physicians), this chapter next provides insight on factors and considerations that support resolving the ethical dilemma for a particular modality of cognitive enhancement or when considering cognitive enhancement for a specific individual.

JUSTIFICATION FOR PERMISSIBILITY

This section considers arguments that justify a physician providing cognitive enhancement for healthy individuals. At the outset, it must be stated that the safety and efficacy of any given form of cognitive enhancement are vital ethical concerns based on a health care provider's commitment to not harming patients, to provide benefit, and to tell individuals the truth about the medical interventions they receive. Such considerations, embedded in the various medical codes of ethics, are core professional commitments.[10] Much of the following discussion assumes that a drug or technology has been approved as a safe and effective use of the modality. However, this is not sufficient to determine the ethical permissibility of providing the cognitive enhancement to a patient. There are more ethical values and commitments to consider beyond safety and efficacy. This section addresses the physician's role,

---

[b] We acknowledge that the term "healthy," like the term "normal," is not a fixed standard and is open to debate and revision as population characteristics change and medical knowledge is advanced. Moreover, what is considered healthy will vary with respect to age due to the changing characteristics of the human body as it ages.

compares nonmedical enhancements, evaluates the importance of individual autonomy, and considers the role of enhancement in public safety.

A Physician's Role

A growing shift in medical focus on preventative medicine and wellness supports the
perspective that a physician's role is to optimize the well-being of a patient. If the
proper role of a physician is to optimize a patient's sense of health and well-being,
and not merely to treat disease and injury, then a physician might have justification
providing a safe and effective cognitive enhancement drug or technology to a healthy
patient. Cognitive enhancement is not the first form of enhancement that seeks to
improve an individual's well-being in the absence of disease or injury. Cosmetic surgery, which is generally considered an ethically permissible extension of traditional
medicine, also aims to promote and optimize patient well-being.

Nonmedical Means of Cognitive Enhancement

Medical means of cognitive enhancement do not serve as the only modality of providing enhancement to an individual. There are also nonmedical means of cognitive enhancement.[5] Considering the nonmedical means associated with enhancement
provides a different perspective on the ethics of the medical provision of a prescription drug or medical technology for cognitive enhancement.

In recent years, a body of literature has developed around what is broadly
termed "situated cognition."[11] One of the general insights of this literature is that
human beings appear to frequently utilize an array of objects and technologies in
order to carry out cognitive processing in a faster, more efficient, and/or more reliable manner.[12–17] Humans utilize objects and technologies to augment and extend
their brain's cognitive processing capabilities. An everyday example of this behavior can be observed in the ways that many individuals use cellular phones to store
large collections of phone numbers instead of trying to memorize the numbers.[14]
To the extent that the cell phone allows a person to retain more phone numbers
or to utilize phone numbers more quickly and reliably, the cell phone serves to
enhance some of a person's memory processing capabilities. Unless an individual
is using the technology to cheat or otherwise cause harm, we generally regard
these nonmedical, technological augmentations of cognitive processing capabilities as ethically permissible and even sometimes as commendable examples of
ingenuity and creativity to overcome some biological limitations (e.g., a limited
biological memory).

Although nonmedical means of cognitive enhancement (e.g., the cell phone) often work in very different ways to achieve cognitive benefits versus medical means of cognitive enhancement (e.g., prescription drugs), it is possible that in some cases the nonmedical and the medical means of cognitive enhancement could each achieve the same or closely similar cognitive benefits (e.g., improved memory performance). The similarity of goals between nonmedical and medical means of enhancement supports similar ethical conclusions for both[18]—that is, unless the means of enhancement (e.g., a cell phone vs. a prescription drug) are different in ethically important ways (we return to this concern later).

Respect for Personal Choices

An individual's capacity to make free and informed medical decisions for him- or herself (patient autonomy) is a basic and vital ethical commitment of modern medicine. As such, physicians are called upon to respect free and informed patient decisions. Physicians respect patient decision-making, in part, by soliciting patient preferences, values, and requests and then incorporating those preferences, values, and requests into a plan of care that is in keeping with medical standards and professional roles and responsibilities. Therefore, if an informed adult patient freely asks for what a physician would consider is a reasonably safe and effective cognitive enhancing drug, there is a presumption in favor of honoring that patient's request out of a respect for patient autonomy. However, a patient request is the beginning of a conversation and not the end of a conversation. Patient autonomy, although important, is not decisive in determining whether to offer cognitive enhancement. As discussed later, there are a number of ethical considerations to weigh and consider upon any given patient's autonomous request for cognitive enhancement.

Promoting Public Safety

Cognitive enhancements might offer a means of providing a social good, such as increased public safety. The potential societal benefits associated with cognitive enhancement are well described within the literature. Common examples include improving the performance of individuals who are responsible for the public's safety in some capacity and who are exposed to cognitively challenging circumstances, including long stretches of performance.[19] Therefore, it is possible that a patient might direct enhanced cognitive capabilities to morally good and praiseworthy ends. For example, commercial airline pilots may collectively determine that in the interest of public safety, it would be best if the attention spans of all pilots were medically enhanced. The generally accepted good of promoting public safety might then justify providing some forms of cognitive enhancement that can safely provide the benefits sought for that population of patients.

Summary

The ethical considerations and arguments previously discussed do not offer decisive justification of the ethical permissibility of providing even safe and effective medical cognitive enhancements to patients. Instead, each consideration provides support and justification when examining a specific modality. However, each justification faces an objection or exception that forces an evaluation of the specific nature of the cognitive enhancement modality under consideration, the means of enhancement, the patient, and the larger picture with competing and complimentary ethical values and commitments. The justification suggests that cognitive enhancement may be permissible. The next section examines more closely some of the ethical concerns about cognitive enhancement.

IMPERMISSIBILITY, BOUNDARIES, AND LIMITATIONS

Ethical considerations that call into question support for cognitive enhancement relate to a physician's professional duties, the potential risks and safety concerns for individuals, and the potential social impact of enhancement. This section addresses these consequences to provide guidance when evaluating the ethical support for or against cognitive enhancement.

A Counterperspective of a Physician's Role

A central consideration of cognitive enhancement focuses on physicians' role within medicine and their professional duties. Ethical codes and law establish duties first and foremost to patients, but also to society, to the profession, and to themselves.[10] The American Academy of Neurology Ethics, Law and Humanities Committee's framework for determining whether a clinical practice is obligatory, permissible, or prohibited relies on whether the practice is within the core domain of medical practices or is socially useful.[8] Traditionally, the goals of medicine, or the core domain of practices, have been centered on preventing, diagnosing, and treating illness or disease. Cognitive enhancement thus extends beyond the boundaries of the traditional goals of medicine. Therefore, adopting a conservative understanding of the physician's role, cognitive enhancement would not be ethically justified on this basis.

The fact that a practice would not fall within the traditional goals of medicine does not alone make the practice unethical or support absolute prohibition. The result of determining that enhancement is not within the traditional goals of medicine is an increased scrutiny on other factors central to an ethical analysis. The overarching question to consider remains: Does cognitive enhancement impede a physician's duties to patients, society, the profession, or him- or herself?

Is This an Enhancement?

A central concern with cognitive enhancement is that what is labeled and marketed as cognitive enhancement may not actually be experienced as an enhancement within an individual's life over time.[20] The concern here is not whether a particular drug or technology provides the physiological effects that it promises (e.g., improved memory and attention performance) but, rather, whether the effects of a successful drug or technology will actually be experienced as genuine improvements or enhancements within an individual's life over time. For example, improved memory and attention performance that helps in one area of a patient's life may be harmful in another area. A student might benefit from improved memory retention in an academic setting, but in the context of everyday social relationships, this improved memory retention may lead to more acute memories of painful and upsetting experiences. There can be a measure of grace in being able to forget some experiences or at least to not remember them as vividly. Therefore, to the extent that a physician's role is to optimize a patient's health and well-being, it is important that a physician provides not only medications or technologies that are physiologically effective but also those that are actually experienced as increasing a patient's sense of health and well-being. This is in keeping with a physician's duty to seek to do genuine good for the patient.

Patient Autonomy Revisited

As discussed previously, physicians are called upon to respect patients' values and wishes. This assumes that the patient's requests and decisions are informed and free of coercion. Although coercion can include direct threats to an individual, there are subtle forms of coercion as well. With respect to cognitive enhancements, an individual might feel unduly pressured to request medical cognitive enhancements if there is tremendous social pressure to excel in various activities that require intensive cognitive processing (e.g., academic research and test-taking).[21] As a number of commentators on the ethics of enhancement have observed, the pressure to seek out enhancements is likely to increase as more people obtain those enhancements and the gap widens between those who benefit from cognitive enhancement and those who do not.[1,21,22]Although this social pressure to excel and/or compete effectively with one's peers does not automatically rule out the possibility of making a free and informed decision, it does call such decisions more frequently into question. Sometimes patients may not be making a free decision to obtain medical means of cognitive enhancement because of intense pressure from family, friends, peers, or other social forces that force or constrain a patient's behaviors and requests. (Although the focus is on adult patients in this brief discussion of cognitive enhancement, the issue of patient freedom is especially significant and complex in the case of children and young adults). Therefore, although physicians may receive patient requests for various forms of cognitive enhancement, it may not be ethically permissible to honor those requests because the requests are not sufficiently free.

Even if a patient makes a free request for medical, cognitive enhancement, this will not be decisive in determining whether or not it is ethically permissible to honor this request. Patient autonomy, although important, is not the only ethical value and commitment to be respected and promoted in various situations. For example, as Mill[23] argued, a patient's ability to make free choices and to act on those choices is justifiably limited to choices and behaviors that do not cause direct harm to other persons. In the case of cognitive enhancement, sometimes it may be relevant to consider the ends or goals to which a patient intends to use his or her enhanced cognitive capabilities. For example, if a physician inadvertently learned that a patient intended to use his enhanced cognitive capabilities to better remember and calculate the shipping details of his human trafficking business, the physician would have strong moral grounds, based on a concern for the safety and well-being of other human beings, for refusing to facilitate a potentially free and informed patient request for medical, cognitive enhancement. The ends or goals to which a patient might direct her cognitively enhanced capabilities are important. It is an open question as to whether a physician should actively seek out this information, but when the physician learns credible information about a patient's goals, it may be an important source of insight into the permissibility or impermissibility of providing cognitive enhancement.

Efficacy and Informed Consent

Efficacy considerations regarding cognitive enhancement modalities again raise the distinction between treatment of a disease or injury and enhancement. Whereas treatment may offer disease-modifying or symptom relief, enhancement is associated with a particular and often personal goal. The issues of efficacy correlate with those discussed previously, but they are distinctly focused on the evidence proven through clinical studies. Many of these studies evaluate the effectiveness of drugs that have been approved and marketed for other purposes ("off-label"). Given the purpose, or at least a justification, of cognitive enhancement is to optimize well-being, it is important that the modality of enhancement be demonstrated as efficacious for meeting that goal. For practices that are not treatment, and thus not a core domain of medicine, the threshold of effectiveness is higher to justify the potential risks associated with a pharmacological or other modality for enhancement.

Methylphenidate (MPH) and modafinil, two of the most popular cognitive enhancing drugs, serve as examples of some of the limitations related to proven efficacy of enhancement in healthy individuals. These medications alter neurotransmitters in the dopaminergic areas of the brain and are used to treat attention deficit hyperactivity disorder (ADHD) and narcolepsy, respectively.[24,25] Modafinil and MPH promote wakefulness and alertness in ADHD and narcoleptic patients, but they have also been speculated to provide cognitive enhancement in healthy adults. Several studies have tested the efficacy of each drug in healthy adults. The results of these studies vary and are conflicting. Most studies of MPH and modafinil have small samples and use different tools to measure cognition. As a result, outcomes reported by individual studies are difficult to either confirm or challenge by other studies' outcomes.

Several research studies have indicated that MPH enhances cognition in the realms of working memory and speed of processing.[26–28] Linssen and colleagues found that healthy volunteers who experienced increased declarative memory consolidation did not experience effects in spatial working memory or planning.[29] Linssen and colleagues[30] also found that MPH failed to enhance retention of words after 30 minutes in healthy participants, but more participants remembered more words after a 24-hour delay. Mixed findings regarding MPH inspired a literature review of 59 studies that tested methylphenidate in healthy individuals. The review reported two main domains that the drug enhances most. Working memory improved in 65% of the studies, and processing speed improved in 48% of the studies. Other domains, such as verbal learning memory, attention, and reasoning, were somewhat enhanced but not significantly. This review also found that the effects of methylphenidate are very dose dependent. Importantly, higher doses seem to hinder cognitive enhancement in certain areas, such as working memory.[31]

Studies on the efficacy of modafinil use in healthy populations have also yielded mixed results. A systemic review that included modafinil indicated that modafinil enhanced attention but had no effect on memory, mood, or motivation in non-sleep-deprived individuals.[12] However, this outcome conflicts with those of several studies that report modafinil enhances memory, learning, visual–spatial memory, attention, planning, and so on.[32–34] Additional factors may impact the efficacy of enhancers.

For example, there is evidence that the effect depends on a participant's baseline performance. It has been reported that low-preforming participants will benefit more from the drug compared to than a high performers. High baseline performers may actually experience impairment of cognition with higher doses. This is presumed to be because low performers have a lower baseline of dopamine and noradrenaline.[35]

Due to the challenges related to efficacy and the actual functional outcomes of enhancers, consideration of whether it is ethical to prescribe medications for enhancement purposes supports limitations. Managing patient expectations during the informed consent process is central to resolving challenges relevant to limitations of enhancement efficacy. During the consent conversation, inquiring into the rationale for requesting access to enhancement, the expected outcomes of enhancement, and identifying an outcome or endpoint for use will be critical. The informed consent process is not merely a review of the potential harms; it should also serve as an opportunity for the physician to evaluate whether the patient understands and appreciates the consequences of using enhancement with realistic goals. An articulation of goals serves as a critical element of analyzing the benefits and risks for a particular patient.

Safety Concerns

The "do no harm" principle is a widely accepted foundation of medical practice.[36] As a result, the potential for harm or adverse consequences must be evaluated prior to determining whether cognitive enhancement is widely permissible or even permissible for an individual circumstance. Prior literature highlights safety concerns as paramount to physicians when considering ethical challenges relevant to cognitive enhancement.[2] The overarching concern about risk may be founded on a number of factors inherent to enhancement (vs. other nontreatment practices), including the complexity of cognition and the neurologic system.[37] The nuanced distinctions between modalities that may offer enhancement benefits warrant an independent evaluation of each related to safety. Two general themes, adverse effects and addiction, can provide a starting point for considering safety within the ethical assessment of enhancement.

An initial consideration is the potential adverse effects (or side effects) of a given drug or technology for a healthy individual. It is well understood that every drug and technology has potential adverse effects associated with it. When treating an illness or condition, such risks can be weighed against the consequences of not treating the illness. For some patients, the potential adverse consequences can outweigh the potential benefits associated with the treatment. For example, donepezil, also known as Aricept, is used in Alzheimer's disease and has been shown to mitigate cognitive symptoms. It has also been considered as a cognitive enhancing drug.[19] However, the drug is also associated with sleep disturbances (nightmares) that have deterred patients from continuing its use.[38] Patients and their families can weigh the potential impact of nightmares versus the symptoms they suffer associated with Alzheimer's disease. In contrast, evaluating the potential risks for enhancement exposes healthy individuals to risks for an outcome beyond the traditional goal of medicine to treat an illness.[39] In addition, little is known about the adverse effects of various cognitive enhancement modalities, which are currently off-label uses, for healthy adults.[40] Even less is known about the consequences of long-term versus short-term use. Physicians should incorporate the distinction between known adverse effects in the targeted population and the unknown effects for a healthy population when educating individuals about cognitive enhancement options.

The potential risk of dependence and addiction associated with pharmaceuticals raises a second safety concern related to cognitive enhancement. Some pharmaceuticals, including stimulants, carry a heightened risk of dependence. In a 2006 study, Kroutil and colleagues[41] reported a significant correlation between the nonmedical use of stimulants and abuse or dependence. The risk of dependence is particularly prevalent in those younger than age 25 years. Although an individual may initially seek enhancement for a specified purpose or goal (improving focus while studying), the risk of dependence cannot be ignored.

The potential risks associated with cognitive enhancement may fall on a spectrum for any given modality relative to the expected goal or outcome. Whereas some modalities may expose an individual to a risk significant enough to warrant prohibiting their use, other modalities may be permissible with appropriate safeguards and boundaries. When an individual requests some form of medical, cognitive enhancement, it is vital that the individual is properly informed about the risks and benefits of the specific drug, device, or procedure. If an individual does not demonstrate sufficient understanding and appreciation of the risks and benefits of a specific cognitive enhancement drug, device, or procedure, it would not be ethically permissible to provide the patient with the cognitive enhancement. Informational barriers, however, can sometimes be overcome with educational efforts.

Distinguishing Nonmedical Means of Cognitive Enhancement

One of the arguments discussed previously considered the ethical comparison between medical and nonmedical means of cognitive enhancement. However, a false analogy may be at play in this line of reasoning. The previous permissibility argument focused exclusively on the outcomes of using various forms of cognitive enhancement and did not adequately account for ethically relevant differences between cognitive enhancement found in either medical or nonmedical means. The analogy breaks down as follows: Using a nonmedical technology such as a sophisticated cellular phone to enhance memory capabilities is a different experience than taking a prescription drug. For example, an individual can more readily control and understand the technology of a cellular phone than a prescription drug. In addition, an individual can simply choose to stop using a cellular phone for enhanced memory capabilities, unlike an individual taking a prescription drug, who might need to taper use before stopping the drug completely and therefore cannot readily choose those activities in which the drug will and will not be effective. Because of the potentially important differences between at least some nonmedical and medical means of cognitive enhancement, they should not be automatically treated as ethically equivalent.

Societal Factors

Societal factors extend the ethical considerations of cognitive enhancement to include physicians' responsibilities to not only their patients but also to society as a whole. As discussed previously, the use of a drug or technology may be permissible if it is socially useful. The implied contradiction to this is that enhancement may be impermissible or limited if it has adverse social consequences. The literature surrounding cognitive enhancement is rich with philosophical debates about whether cognitive enhancement improves or harms society. Some argue that enhancement betters society by "leveling the playing field" and improving the performance of those with socially relevant duties (military). However, cognitive enhancement may cause further injustice if access to a modality is not equitable or the use of it creates unfair employment and academic environments. This section focuses on adverse social consequences, including fairness and unequal access.

Cognitive enhancement creates an opportunity for some to access a resource that may provide an "upper hand" in employment and academic settings. Another way to interpret this concern is that enhancement constitutes cheating. Consider, for example, law students who are graded on a curve. The potential outcome of allowing a student access to enhancement that improves performance not only leads to a higher grade for that student but also impacts the curve for other students. Certainly, society has recognized other "enhancements" as cheating, particularly with regard to steroids or other banned supplements in professional and collegiate sports. What, then, of the use of cognitive enhancement to gain an edge on exams or other cognitive performances? Certainly, this will be an issue for different regulatory bodies to take into consideration, including academic institutions. Physicians challenged with responding to requests by individuals for cognitive enhancement will need to be aware of any prohibitive uses. However, physicians will also be challenged when considering whether an individual's motivation and expectation for requesting enhancement are consistent with the physician's responsibilities and duties.

Injustice and unequal access (or distribution) are an overarching concern associated with cognitive enhancement. One part of the justice consideration concerns issues of distribution and access. Many scholars argue that only those in upper socioeconomic classes will be financially able to access enhancement. It is unlikely that insurers would cover access to cognitive enhancement without a medical indication.[40] Such limitations on access may exacerbate the influence of the technology related to disparities.

A second aspect of the justice consideration concerns issues of discrimination and prejudice. There is considerable risk in justifying the provision of medical means of enhancement based on the social goods that might be brought about by the enhancement. In particular, it quickly becomes problematic if it is left to individual health care providers to determine the moral goodness or praiseworthiness of patients' descriptions of the ends/goals to which they will apply their enhanced, cognitive capabilities. Different evaluations among health care providers could lead to inconsistent and unjust (i.e., discriminatory or prejudicial) treatment of individuals and groups of people. The initial effort to promote certain goods (e.g., public safety) would be offset by the gross evils of social injustice.

Summary

An evaluation of whether it is impermissible to provide medical means of cognitive enhancement to a patient may result in determining either that a modality is impermissible or that a modality is permissible, but safeguards and restrictions are necessary. Like those considerations that support the permissibility of cognitive enhancement, the considerations provided in this section are not alone conclusive. A determination that a modality is unsafe and would expose an individual to risks that far outweigh any perceived benefits may lead to a finding that the modality is ethically impermissible. However, such a finding will be rare. In a majority of circumstances, the modality will be evaluated using factors that justify and also those factors that challenge ethical support for a particular analysis. The following section provides guidance on weighing these factors.

NAVIGATING BETWEEN PERMISSIBLE
AND IMPERMISSIBLE

A physician may face a dilemma in which his or her obligation affects many levels of responsibility (personal, professional, and societal). In this situation, a physician must consider the short- and long-term implications as well as the implications to an individual, a profession, and a larger community. Even when an enhancement appears to be ethically justified and preferable for an individual, when applied to all individuals it may create an unsustainable environment. For instance, current social circumstances could not sustain all people receiving expensive brain implants. Alternatively, to focus only on the societal needs puts social justice at risk if there is a failure to consider disparities and unjust distribution. Furthermore, a system that permits all individuals access to any technology they can afford could result in community harms. Societal safeguards can guide good practice through careful deliberations. System safeguards include ethical review of research, safety and approval processes for new treatment modalities, professionalization, and truth-in-advertising regulations. A further safeguard is the legal system injury law; however, this system only self-corrects after injuries have occurred and is not a preventative measure except to provide an incentive for manufacturers to make safe products. Physicians should consider societal safeguards when assessing a provision of cognitive enhancement, but safeguards create a floor and not a ceiling for ethical consideration. That floor only gives the minimum responsibility and not what is ethically preferable. In general, those mechanisms aim to provide protection from harm rather than allow access to technologies for broader populations.

There is also a gap in safeguards when technologies are unproven and are not part of formal research. This scenario is discussed as "off-label" or "innovative" therapy and pushes the boundaries of safety and efficacy. Society gives professionals a broad opportunity to use judgment in exceptional cases requiring creative solutions. A physician can have a particularly difficult dilemma in deciding when to place a patient at risk of cognitive enhancement when insufficient evidence exists regarding risks and efficacy. The patient may be demanding a drug for an unproven use, be fully cognizant of the unknown nature of harms and benefits, but believe it is necessary for advancement in his or her life goals (e.g., a musician asking for a novel anxiolytic for improved performance). Declining the request may be the conservative and "safe" choice, but it also denies the individual the prospect of optimizing his or her well-being and challenges the patient's autonomy. In addition, the choice of whether to prescribe may be subject to legal or licensure boundaries or safeguards due to the lack of governmental approval or "labeling" for that indication. There are explicit choices made between erring on the side of safety and efficacy based on knowledge or based on clinical judgment.

Most of this chapter has considered the ethically permissible, preferable, and impermissible. It is important to consider whether there might be circumstances in which enhancement might be considered ethically obligatory for physicians to offer or even for physicians to use for themselves. This potential obligation is most clear when considering safety. If a community's safety depends on a the wakefulness of a guard to warn of impending danger, then the use of a drug such as modafinil to promote wakefulness could be thought of as an obligation for the guard to use and the for the physician to provide. A similar argument could be generated when considering a sleep-deprived surgeon. As with every choice, an assessment of potential options with an analysis of the possible consequences is necessary. In particular, referring to the example above, does the use of modafinil properly balance the individuals' free choice in the least restrictive manner to liberty while still considering the needs of the community? Even if the guard is willing to take on this obligation, the physician's obligation to provide the modafinil to the patient may still pose challenges to the prescribing physician. If the physician has a conscientious objection to providing the guard this drug because the physician believes it is outside of his or her role as a healer, this creates a potential values conflict between obligation to self and obligation to the patient. If there are other physicians in the community that could provide the modafinil than the conflict has only implications to the personal values of the conscientious objector. However, if there are no other professionals available to provide the modafinil except the one whose conscience is at stake, then that professional might be compelled to provide the drug by threat of loss of licensure. However, in a community with few physicians, the loss of a licensed physician might impact the health of the community in worse ways than if a guard has poor wakefulness. When considering the values at stake with an obligation to provide cognitive enhancement, there needs to be transparency regarding whose values are being sacrificed and who is benefiting. Whenever navigating between the permissible and impermissible, a deliberative approach is needed with full understanding of the values at stake for all stakeholders.

CONCLUSION

Ethical dilemmas are characterized as a conflict between values or beliefs, and they often lack a clear "right" answer. Although from the outset it seems that there are only two potential responses to a request for cognitive enhancement—yes or no—there are other avenues to resolve the dilemma. Even if a particular medical means of cognitive enhancement is determined to be ethically permissible, it may still be the case that medical means of cognitive enhancement are not the best way to engage in cognitive enhancement efforts. In addition to considering the potential use of medical means of enhancement, physicians can also discuss other options to help their patients or the requesting individual meet the same or similar goal or objective. It is important to not only determine whether it is ethically permissible but also consider whether the particular medical means of enhancement is ethically better or worse than other nonmedical means of accomplishing the goal.

In 2015, the Presidential Commission for the Study of Bioethical Issues emphasized exploring other means of modification, including nutrition and lifestyle, before considering the use of pharmaceuticals.[7] As discussed, faced with finite biological memory capacities, human beings have developed some tremendously creative, nonmedical external mechanisms to better remember information. In such cases, the biological limitations of memory persist, but an individual's capability to remember information expands through the use of creative, nonmedical external mechanisms that also introduce other valuable goods. The comparison of medical to nonmedical means of enhancement builds on a familiar skill to health care providers and researchers, who often evaluate whether a particular drug or treatment is better or worse than alternative drugs and treatments. However, here the consideration is not simply between one medical means of cognitive enhancement and another but, rather, between various medical means of cognitive enhancement and a range of nonmedical means of cognitive enhancement.

Physicians who are challenged by requests for enhancement must weigh the nuances of the circumstances, the requested drug or technology, and their responsibilities and duties to patients, society, and themselves. In some circumstances, this assessment will be intuitive, and the resolution will be easily identified. However, as is common with innovative practices, the evaluation will often be complicated by tension and competing interests and values specific to a patient (and his or her motivation for requesting enhancement) and the modality requested. This chapter focused on providing frameworks to help weigh the ethical issues related to cognitive enhancement. Although not exhaustive, this is a starting point.

REFERENCES

1. Kass L. *Beyond therapy: Biotechnology and the pursuit of human improvement.* The President's Council on Bioethics. Retrieved from https://bioethicsarchive.georgetown.edu/pcbe/background/kasspaper.html. Published January 2003. Accessed March 31, 2015.

2. Hotze TD, Shah K, Anderson E, et al. "Doctor would you prescribe a pill to help me . . .?" A national survey of physicians on using medicine for human enhancement. *Am J Bioethics* 2011;11(1):3–13.

3. The National Commission for the Protection of Human Subjects of Biomedical and Behavioral Research. *The Belmont report: Ethical principles and guidelines for the protection of human subjects of research.* National Institutes of Health Office of Human Subjects Research; 1979. Retrieved from https://www.hhs.gov/ohrp/humansubjects/guidance/belmont.html. Accessed March 31, 2015.

4. Beauchamp TL, Childress JF. *Principles of biomedical ethics* (7th ed.). New York, NY: Oxford University Press; 2012.

5. Sandberg A. Cognition enhancement: Upgrading the brain. In Savalescu J, ter Meulen R, Kahane G (Eds.), *Enhancing human capacities.* Malden, MA: Wiley–Blackwell; 2011:71.

6. Kahane G, Savulescu J. Normal human variation: Refocussing the enhancement debate. *Bioethics* 2015;29(2):133–143.

7. Presidential Commission for the Study of Bioethical Issues. *Gray matters: Topics at the intersection of neuroscience, ethics, and society* (Vol. 2). Retrieved from http://bioethics.gov/sites/default/files/GrayMatter_V2_508.pdf. Published March 26, 2015. Accessed March 31, 2015.

8. Larriviere D, Williams MA, Rizzo M, et al. Responding to requests from adult patients for neuroenhancements: Guidance of the Ethics, Law and Humanities Committee. *Neurology* 2009;73:2.

9. Kibbe B. *Mindful mending: The repair of thought and action amidst technologies* [Dissertation]. Chicago, IL: Loyola University Chicago; 2014:5–6.

10. American Medical Association. *Principles of medical ethics.* . Retrieved from https://www.ama-assn.org/sites/default/files/media-browser/public/ethics/principles-of-medical-ethics-20160627.pdf. Accessed March 31, 2015.

11. Robbins P, Murat A (Eds.). *The Cambridge handbook of situated cognition.* New York, NY: Cambridge University Press; 2008.

12. Clark A, Chalmers D. The extended mind. *Analysis* 1998;58(1):7–19.

13. Clark A. *Natural-born cyborgs: Minds, technologies, and the future of human intelligence.* New York, NY: Oxford University Press; 2004.

14. Clark A. *Supersizing the mind: Embodiment, action, and cognitive extension.* New York, NY: Oxford University Press; 2008.

15. Sterelny K. Minds: Extended or scaffolded? *Phenomenol Cogn Sci* 2010;9:465–481.

16. Kirsh D, Maglio P. On distinguishing epistemic from pragmatic action. *Cogn Sci* 1994;18:513–549.

17. Hutchins E. How a cockpit remembers its speeds. *Cogn Sci* 1995;19:265–288.

18. Levy N. *Neuroethics: Challenges for the 21st century.* New York, NY: Cambridge University Press; 2007.

19. Yesavage JA, Mumenthaler MS, Taylor JL, et al. Donepezil and flight simulator performance: Effects on retention of complex skills. *Neurology* 2002;59(1):123–125.

20. Kass L. *Beyond therapy: Biotechnology and the pursuit of human improvement.* The President's Council on Bioethics. Retrieved from https://bioethicsarchive.georgetown.edu/pcbe/background/kasspaper.html. Published January 2003. Accessed March 31, 2015.

21. Hamilton R, Messing S, Chatterjee A. Rethinking the thinking cap: Ethics of neural enhancement using noninvasive brain stimulation. *Neurology* 2011;76:187–193.

22. Chatterjee A. Cosmetic neurology: The controversy over enhancing movement, mentation, and mood. *Neurology* 2004;63:968–974.

23. Mill JS. *On Liberty.* New York, NY: Barnes & Noble; 2004.

24. Challman TD, Lipsky JJ. Methylphenidate: Its pharmacology and uses. *Mayo Clin Proc* 2000;75(7):711–721.

25. Gerrard P, Malcolm R. Mechanisms of modafinil: A review of current research. *Neuropsychiatr Dis Treat* 2007;3(3):349–364.
26. Mehta MA, Owen AM, Sahakian BJ, et al. Methylphenidate enhances working memory by modulating discrete frontal and parietal lobe regions in the human brain. *J Neurosci* 2000;20(6):RC65.
27. Elliott R, Sahakian BJ, Matthews K, et al. Effects of methylphenidate on spatial working memory and planning in healthy young adults. *Psychopharmacology (Berl)* 1997;131(2):196–206.
28. Agay N, Yechiam E, Carmel Z, et al. Non-specific effects of methylphenidate (Ritalin) on cognitive ability and decision-making of ADHD and healthy adults. *Psychopharmacology (Berl)* 2010; 210(4):511–519.
29. Linssen AM, Vuurman EF, Sambeth A, et al. Methylphenidate produces selective enhancement of declarative memory consolidation in healthy volunteers. *Psychopharmacology (Berl)* 2012; 221(4):611–619.
30. Linssen AM, Sambeth A, Vuurman EF, et al. Cognitive effects of methylphenidate and levodopa in healthy volunteers. *Eur Neuropsychopharmacol* 2014;24(2):200–206.
31. Linssen AM, Sambeth A, Vuurman EF, et al. Cognitive effects of methylphenidate in healthy volunteers: A review of single dose studies. *Int J Neuropsychopharmacol* 2014;17(6):961–77.
32. Müller U, Rowe JB, Rittman T, et al. Effects of modafinil on non-verbal cognition, task enjoyment and creative thinking in healthy volunteers. *Neuropharmacology* 2013;64:490–495.
33. Esposito R, Cilli F, Pieramico V, et al. Acute effects of modafinil on brain resting state networks in young healthy subjects. *PLoS One* 2013;8(7):e69224.
34. Gilleen J, Michalopoulou PG, Reichenberg A, et al. Modafinil combined with cognitive training is associated with improved learning in healthy volunteers—A randomised controlled trial. *Eur Neuropsychopharmacol* 2014;24(4):529–539.
35. Finke K, Dodds CM, Bublak P, et al. Effects of modafinil and methylphenidate on visual attention capacity: A TVA-based study. *Psychopharmacology (Berl)* 2010;210(3):317–329.
36. National Library of Medicine, National Institutes of Health. *Greek medicine: Hippocratic Oath*. Retrieved from https://www.nlm.nih.gov/hmd/greek/greek_oath.html. Accessed April 2, 2015.
37. Farah MJ, Illes J, Cook-Deegan R, et al. Neurocognitive enhancement: What can we do and what should we do? *Nat Rev Neurosci* 2004;5(5):421–425.
38. Repantis D. Psychopharmacological neuroenhancement: Evidence on safety and efficacy. In Hildt E, Franke AG (Eds.), *Cognitive enhancement*. Dordrecht, the Netherlands: Springer; 2013:29–38.
39. Delaney JJ, Martin DP. The role of physician opinion in human enhancement. *Am J Bioethics* 2011;11(9):19–20.
40. Forlini C, Gauthier S, Racine E. Should physicians prescribe cognitive enhancers to healthy individuals? *CMAJ.* 2013;185(12):1047–1045.
41. Kroutil LA, Van Brunt DL, Herman-Stahl MA, et al. Nonmedical use of prescription stimulants in the United States. *Drug Alcohol Depend* 2006;84(2):135–143.

SIXTEEN

Regulatory Issues in Cognitive Enhancement Treatment Development

NICHOLAS KOZAUER

AND KARL BROICH

Cogito Ergo Sum. (I think, therefore I am.)

Rene Descartes (1637)

PERHAPS NO OTHER QUOTATION REGARDING COGNITION SO SUCCINCTLY describes the relationship that exists between our ability to think and our very nature as human beings. It is precisely for this reason that the myriad of diseases that can degrade our cognitive capacities represent such important targets for pharmaceutical intervention. As the previous chapters have already discussed, attempts to develop more effective treatments for a wide range of conditions that impact cognition continue to progress. However, it is also essential that a well-described regulatory framework exists that can guide the development of these compounds as well as ultimately accurately evaluate their suitability for marketing approval.

A range of conditions, most notably the dementias, are defined by the presence of cognitive dysfunction. However, there are a range of other illnesses (e.g., schizophrenia and depression) in which cognitive impairment, although still frequently disabling, is generally viewed as a secondary symptom of the disorder. Because the key regulatory considerations differ somewhat between these situations, this chapter addresses each area separately.

Both the US Food and Drug Administration (FDA) and the European Medicines Agency (EMA) have relatively recently published documents that outline their current thinking regarding a number of the pertinent topics discussed in this chapter. Although the majority of this chapter therefore focuses on advice given by both agencies for that reason, it is also clear that many other world regulatory bodies are working to address these issues as well. Finally, regulatory guidance in drug development is most often provided directly and individually to sponsors of drug development programs. As a result, although this chapter attempts to outline the current regulatory thinking in a number of critical areas, it is important to remember that drug developers should continue to discuss the specific circumstances of their respective programs with the relevant regulatory agencies.

ASSESSING COGNITION IN ALZHEIMER'S DISEASE AND OTHER DEMENTIAS

Alzheimer's Disease

In 2011, the National Alzheimer's Project Act (NAPA) was signed into law in the United States. A critical component of NAPA was to create a National Alzheimer's Plan intended to provide a framework for how the US federal government would begin to address Alzheimer's disease (AD) and other dementias on a number of fronts. The first iteration of the plan was finalized in May 2012. Although broad in its focus, a prominent emphasis was to explicitly "accelerate the development of treatments that would prevent, halt, or reverse the course of Alzheimer's disease." The activities of federal agencies such as the National Institutes of Health (NIH) were directly affected by this provision. In addition, the FDA was also charged with examining and re-evaluating the manner in which drugs for dementias are regulated. Beyond the United States, the increasing emphasis by world governments on dementia is evidenced by the first World Dementia Summit of the G8 nations held in December 2013 in London.

One of the most important steps that regulators can take in facilitating drug development is to provide transparency regarding the approval requirements in a given disease area. In addition, there is a clear benefit for all stakeholders when regulators actively engage in discussions with the researcher community and industry along with patients, caregivers, and advocacy groups in the process of developing their guidelines. There are a handful of drugs approved and marketed to treat the overt dementia stage of AD, including several cholinesterase inhibitors (i.e., donepezil, rivastigmine, and galantamine) and memantine. These drugs are all largely believed to confer symptomatic benefits and are not thought to have a persisting effect on the underlying disease process or on the patient's ultimate clinical course. However, the landscape of drug development in AD is shifting dramatically to focus increasingly on the stages of the disease spectrum that occur prior to the onset of dementia. The ability to detect the presence of biological evidence of key AD pathology in vivo has enabled the potential identification of individuals prior to the onset of dementia who are at the greatest risk of disease progression. In addition, many of the drugs that are currently under investigation are now targeting the underlying disease pathophysiology. Therefore, the nature of the clinical trials that are being used to evaluate these novel agents in earlier stage patients diverges in some important ways from historical convention. It is precisely for this reason that ongoing engagement and guidance from drug regulatory agencies are crucial.

Fortunately, the increased focus of international governments on the growing dementia crisis has led to just that sort of interaction. Moreover, both the FDA and the EMA have recently released preliminary publications that detail their recommendations regarding how drugs for AD and other dementias might be developed. In February 2013, the FDA released its *Draft Guidance for Industry: Alzheimer's Disease: Developing Drugs for the Treatment of Early Stage Disease.*[1] The focus of the document was to provide initial recommendations regarding how drugs targeting the pre-dementia stages of AD might be developed. This draft guidance received a large number of public comments during an open comment period, and it is currently in the process of being finalized. In addition, in the process of updating its 2008 AD guidelines, the EMA released its *Discussion Paper on the Clinical Investigation of Medicines for the Treatment of Alzheimer's Disease and Other Dementias* in October 2014.[2] This paper was intended to serve as a foundation for ongoing discussions with the field related to a broad range of drug development issues in AD across the entire disease spectrum. Other dementias were also briefly addressed. Subsequently, the EMA sponsored a conference to discuss these guidelines in November 2014 that was attended by a large number of stakeholders, including representatives from the FDA and the Pharmaceuticals and Medical Devices Agency of Japan. Based on careful consideration of the feedback received, in January 2016 the EMA issued a draft guidance document for external consultation. As the most recent description of the current thinking on a range of regulatory topics in AD trials, these two publications are referenced frequently in the subsequent sections.

It must be stressed that just as the understanding of how best to develop drugs for AD continues to rapidly evolve, so does the understanding of how best to regulate these programs. As such, it is important to remember that both FDA and EMA guidelines are currently in a preliminary form. The following sections highlight the most salient aspects of their recommendations with the understanding that they will very likely continue to evolve in parallel with the scientific understanding in this area. In addition, this chapter focuses exclusively on the regulatory requirements for drugs being developed to treat the core cognitive symptoms of AD and does not cover the regulatory requirements for other aspects of the condition (e.g., neuropsychiatric symptoms). Finally, the chapter focuses primarily on the current regulatory guidelines as they relate to the design of registration trials that could support a marketing approval, and it avoids a discussion of earlier phase and nonclinical requirements, which are generally not specific to AD.

Diagnostic Criteria

Until recently, the vast majority of trials in AD were conducted in patients who suffered from overt clinical dementia. This disease state is defined as the presence of cognitive impairment sufficiently severe that it disrupts patients' ability to function normally in their daily activities. However, it is widely accepted that the underlying biological changes in AD begin many years prior to the onset of clinical symptoms. In addition, one of the prevailing theories behind the high failure rate of AD development programs, particularly for drugs intended to modify pathophysiology, is that these interventions may have been tested too late in the disease process to have a meaningful impact. For these reasons, the research community has sought to develop improved diagnostic guidelines across the entire spectrum of the AD continuum. A primary goal of these efforts is to allow for the more efficient conduct of clinical trials; therefore, regulatory guidance as to their ultimate acceptability for this purpose is critical.

Historically, clinical trials conducted in patients with dementia utilized the National Institute for Communicative Disorders and Stroke–Alzheimer's Disease and Related Disorders Association's (NINCDS-ADRDA) diagnostic criteria, established in 1984, as the basis for enrollment.[3] However, recent clinical data from the development of solanezumab, a monoclonal antibody targeting β-amyloid, suggest that a substantial number of subjects identified using these criteria lack the presence of β-amyloid as detected by positron emission tomography (PET) imaging using an amyloid binding agent (26% of those tested in that program).[4] The correct identification of individuals with the biological hallmarks of AD is especially critical in the development of drugs that are designed to target a specific aspect of this pathology.

In addition to developing core clinical criteria for the pre-dementia disease stages, these newly proposed criteria have also incorporated the use of biomarkers in an attempt to increase diagnostic sensitivity in all phases. Leading examples of these new diagnostic frameworks include criteria developed by the National Institutes of Health–Alzheimer's Association (NIH-AA) as well as the International Working Group's (IWG) new research criteria for the diagnosis of AD.[5–8]

In addition to the NIH-AA and IWG criteria, the most recent edition of the *Diagnostic and Statistical Manual of Mental Disorders* (DSM-5) also includes criteria for the diagnosis of major and mild neurocognitive disorder due to Alzheimer's disease.[9] Regulatory guidance has most directly addressed the NIA-AA and IWG criteria because they are more granular and more commonly used for trial enrollment, although the relevant principles are expected to be the same. Both the FDA and the EMA have expressed openness to these revised diagnostic criteria in their recent publications. However, both agencies also comment that the need for their further validation precludes the formal regulatory endorsement of any specific framework at this time. The EMA further stresses the importance of the harmonization of these criteria, which it states would allow for a greater ability to carry out global development programs. The EMA guidance notes that the

> selection of patients with early AD for long term disease modification trials is complex and should not be unnecessarily subdivided in clinical trials if not justified from a clinical viewpoint. Following this approach, subjects with prodromal AD/MCI due to AD and mild AD may be studied together.[2]

Furthermore, the EMA perspective includes the notion that efficacy should be demonstrated at two different stages along the AD continuum. This approach can include two separate trials or a single trial whereby patients are studied for a sufficient amount of time to inform the effect of treatment in subsequent stages.[2]

Multiple development sponsors have already begun enrolling subjects using inclusion/exclusion criteria based on the NIH-AA and IWG proposals following discussions with regulatory bodies regarding their individual programs. In other words, novel diagnostic criteria do not need to receive a formal regulatory "endorsement" before they can be used in a registration study because some of the evidence that will eventually support their validity may actually come from these trials. Ultimately, if a clinically meaningful benefit can be demonstrated in a reliably identifiable patient population, this is generally viewed as sufficient to support a marketing approval. It is true, however, that regulators' willingness to accept the risk of a given intervention, particularly in asymptotic at-risk subjects identified based largely on biomarker evidence of disease pathology, will be dependent on the existence of a plausible rationale and proof of concept of the proposed treatment.

Distinct from the research community's ongoing validation attempts, the EMA has also accepted, via its formal biomarker qualification process, cerebrospinal fluid markers as well as magnetic resonance imaging and amyloid PET imaging for the enrichment of pre-dementia populations.[10,11]

Finally, in successful development programs that enroll patients using biomarker-based diagnostic criteria, regulators will be faced with the question of whether the specific biomarkers that are utilized during the conduct of the trial will be necessary for the safe and effective use of the therapy in clinical practice. If so, these biomarkers may then be considered as companion diagnostic agents, and their performance characteristics (e.g., specificity and sensitivity) would also then be evaluated as part of the development program's approval process because they would be a required component of the final product label.[12]

ENDPOINTS

This section begins with a discussion of regulatory recommendations regarding clinical endpoints in AD trials, as well as the role that biomarkers might play as outcome measures in these investigations. Recent regulatory guidelines indicate that the most appropriate approach to endpoint selection will vary based on the stage of the disease continuum in which a trial is conducted. Specifically, endpoint recommendations are largely dependent on a trial's baseline enrollment criteria.

Clinical Endpoints

Dementia Trials

Regulators are tasked with approving safe and effective medical treatments that provide clinically meaningful benefits to patients. However, cognitive assessment tools tend to evaluate a range of cognitive domains through the use of relatively sensitive performance measures. Although the accurate understanding of a drug's effect on these domains is important, it does not necessarily follow that a statistically significant treatment effect on such a measure will translate into a clinically meaningful difference in patients' abilities to function in their daily lives.

To address the issue of demonstrating a clinically meaningful response in dementia trials, regulators have had the long-standing expectation that in addition to demonstrating an effect on cognition, a drug must also show a benefit on a measure designed to evaluate the impact of that cognitive benefit in patients' daily lives. Although they fundamentally share similar views, the FDA and the EMA differ somewhat in how this recommendation is operationalized as outlined in their recent publications. The FDA indicates that a co-primary outcome measure that is either a global rating scale or a functional assessment should be utilized in addition to a cognitive assessment. The EMA states that both a functional measures and a global assessment should be evaluated and that the functional scale should be prioritized as the co-primary endpoint, with the global scale as a secondary endpoint. In addition, the EMA also asks that a responder analysis be illustrated in terms of the overall benefit (response) in individual patients with the proportion of patients who achieve a clinically meaningful benefit (response) based on a consideration of the natural progression of the disease. The EMA also comments that in severe dementia, functional and global domains may be more appropriate as the primary endpoints as cognitive changes become more difficult to quantify. Conversely, the FDA still recommends an assessment of cognition as a co-primary endpoint in all stages of dementia.

Prodromal Alzheimer's Disease/Mild Cognitive Impairment Due to Alzheimer's Disease

The clinical progression of AD exists on a continuum that includes a period in which patients begin to manifest detectable cognitive deficits that do not yet sufficiently impact their daily functioning to warrant a dementia diagnosis. As previously discussed, the current research nomenclature refers to these subjects as having either prodromal AD or mild cognitive impairment (MCI) due to AD. However, it is also generally acknowledged that these subjects experience increasingly present levels of subtle functional impairments prior to the onset of dementia.

Regulators have proposed a number of possible approaches to demonstrating a clinically meaningful treatment effect in this population. In their recent publications, both the FDA and the EMA acknowledge the current lack of appropriate measures of daily function for these patients. However, they also indicate that should such a scale be developed, the use of co-primary outcome measures that evaluate both cognition and function, as is the expectation in dementia trials, would remain a valid means of establishing clinical efficacy.

In the absence of a suitable functional scale, however, the FDA has indicated that it would also be acceptable to use a composite scale that assesses both cognition and function. In the FDA's draft guidance on early AD, the Clinical Dementia Rating–Sum of Boxes (CDR-CB) score is proposed strictly as an example of such a suitable tool. The EMA has also suggested that the CDR-SB might be an example of a suitable outcome measure. Several authors have addressed the psychometric performance characteristics of the CDR-SB as an outcome measure for interventional trials (sensitivity to treatment effects, interrater reliability, etc.), with varying conclusions, and other novel composite measures are currently under development.[13–15] It is also worth noting that, somewhat uniquely, the CDR scale is a Clinician Rated Outcome (CRO) measure consisting of scores in six subdomains (i.e., boxes) that can combine to yield a total score (i.e., the Sum of Boxes).[16] The scale is designed to allow a qualified and trained clinician to utilize his or her clinical judgment in assigning scores based on input from both the patient and a caregiver. This approach, in essence, allows an evaluation of functional status to be factored into the process of assigning a score on one or more of the scale's cognitive domains (e.g., memory). Therefore, a score change in one of the test's cognitive domains cannot be driven solely by sensitive changes in cognition that lack face-valid clinical importance.

In contrast, the use of a more standard composite scale that simply combines separate measures of cognition and function in deriving a total score poses important regulatory questions with regard to what the standard for approval might be in terms of demonstrating an effect on each of the subdomains. In general, composite outcome measures typically include components that are all obviously clinically meaningful in their own right but perhaps occur so infrequently that combining them into a single endpoint makes sense.[17] An example of a well-accepted composite measure is the Major Adverse Cardiac Events (MACE) endpoint in cardiovascular drug trials. The applicability of such an instrument for prodromal AD might not be sufficient in the case of a combined assessment of cognition and function, in which the cognitive components alone may be too sensitive to have face-valid clinical significance. Further work needs to be done to inform how the clinical meaningfulness of a result on this sort of composite can be best supported.

A relatively recent approach has been to consider performance-based functional outcomes.[18,19] Among these tests are the UCSD Performance-Based Skills Assessment (UPSA)[20] and the Virtual Reality Functional Capacity Assessment Tool (VRFCAT).[21,22] The UPSA uses household props to challenge patients in the clinic to demonstrate their ability to perform skills related to communication, transportation, and shopping. Success on the items of the measure is driven primarily by cognitive ability, and deficits on the measure are related to performance on standard measures of cognition in prodromal AD or MCI.[18] The VRFCAT has similar challenges, but it is administered in a computerized format with realistic interactions involving preparing a shopping list, searching a kitchen for items required to fulfill a recipe, paying for transportation, and shopping in a supermarket. Validity studies in patients with serious mental illness have been completed,[22] and they suggest strong psychometrics for clinical trials. The UPSA has been shown to be sensitive to change over time in patients with MCI or prodromal AD,[18] although its capacity to predict conversion to AD has not been demonstrated.

Alternatively, regulators have also indicated that a time-to-event survival analysis approach (e.g., time to a consensus diagnosis of dementia) would also be an appropriate endpoint in early AD trials. However, several authors have expressed concern that an approach that dichotomizes a continuous disease process, in contrast to an event-based-outcome such as myocardial infarction in cardiovascular disease trials, risks losing information that could be better gleaned from a continuous endpoint.[23] The use of a suitable continuous endpoint would also presumably have a favorable impact on design characteristics such as sample size and trial duration.

Preclinical Disease

As previously discussed, research criteria now exist that attempt to identify individuals very early on in the AD continuum, even prior to the prodromal AD/MCI due to AD stage. By necessity, these subjects are determined to be at risk for progression based largely on biomarker evidence that indicates they have the underlying pathologic hallmarks of AD and/or are genetically at a high risk. Many of these subjects, although they may appear clinically intact, may have detectable deficits on highly sensitive neuropsychological measures of cognitive performance. By definition, however, these impairments are unlikely to manifest in any demonstrable way in their daily functioning.

If a drug were shown to be able to alter the biological progression of AD, the greatest theoretical benefit would presumably be in these earliest stage patients. The challenge for regulators is that it would be extremely difficult to demonstrate a clinically meaningful effect of treatment in patients whose cognitive deficits may only be detectable on sensitive neuropsychological measures. Fortunately, recent regulatory publications have discussed possible pathways forward in this population.

Regulatory agencies have the ability to approve a drug based on an effect on what is known as a biological surrogate endpoint. Surrogate endpoints have been typically defined as a biomarker intended to substitute for a clinical endpoint (i.e., a measure reflecting how a patient feels, functions, or survives).[24] Fully validated biological surrogate outcome measures are able to support full regulatory approvals because there is a well-accepted understanding of the link between a drug's effect on the biomarker and the ultimate clinical benefit to patients. Examples of validated surrogates include blood pressure readings in hypertension and CD4 count or viral load in HIV.

The FDA also has the ability to approve drugs using the accelerated approval mechanism based on an effect on an outcome measure that is *reasonably likely* to predict the ultimate clinical benefit of interest (e.g., persistent improvement in cognition and function).[25] Under this pathway, following the initial approval, a drug sponsor would then be required to demonstrate in adequate and well-controlled studies or continuation of the initial studies that the observed benefit persists and positively affects the overall course of a patient's condition. This approval pathway is frequently associated with oncology approvals in which a drug may be provisionally approved based on a biomarker effect such as tumor size and the clinical meaningfulness of that effect is subsequently confirmed in the post-approval setting. The EMA also has an accelerated approval mechanism (conditional approval and accelerated assessment) similar to the FDA. A new initiative by EMA is the so-called Priority Medicines Initiative (PRIME).[26] This mechanism was launched to enhance support for the development of medicines that offer a major therapeutic advantage or target an unmet medical need. It is voluntary, and it enables enhanced interaction and very early dialogue between EMA representatives and developers of promising medicines in order to optimize development plans and expedite evaluation of medicines that are deemed to be particularly valuable to patients. PRIME builds on the existing regulatory framework and tools already available, such as scientific advice and accelerated assessment. PRIME aims to improve clinical trial designs so that the data generated are suitable for evaluating a marketing-authorization application.

Although these regulatory processes offer the potential for accelerated approval, regulators have made clear that in the case of AD they do not believe that reliable evidence currently exists that a drug's effect on an AD biomarker can serve as a validated surrogate endpoint. The FDA has also indicated that the current lack of a clear understanding between a drug's effect on an AD biomarker and a future potential clinical effect also precludes it from concluding that such a marker would be reasonably likely to predict clinical benefit (and therefore as the basis for an accelerated approval).

In its draft guidance on early AD, the FDA recognizes the importance of demonstrating efficacy as early on in the illness course as possible. To address this issue, the FDA notes that the accelerated approval pathway also allows for a provisional approval based on an effect on an intermediate clinical endpoint, as opposed to a biomarker, that is reasonably likely to predict future clinical benefit. The FDA goes on to suggest that assuming that these earliest stage patients can be reliably identified, a valid, reliable, and sensitive cognitive assessment could serve as the basis for such an approval under this approach. There has yet to be agreement, however, regarding the manner in which a development program could then provide the post-marketing confirmation of benefit. In addition, recent draft AD guidance from the EMA observes that validation efforts for tools that are designed to detect and monitor the earliest signs of cognitive impairment are currently underway, although they are not yet validated and cannot be solely endorsed as primary endpoints in this population. Trials should be undertaken in a biomarker-enriched population.

As with patients in the prodromal AD/MCI due to AD stage, regulators have expressed openness to the use of a time-to-event approach utilizing the time to onset of cognitive impairment (e.g., an MCI diagnosis) as a primary endpoint. However, these trials would present many logistical challenges given the large sample sizes and long durations that are necessary in these very early stage populations.

Autosomal Dominant Alzheimer's Disease

Studies on the rare autosomal dominant Alzheimer's disease (ADAD) populations are currently underway.[27,28] These trials are of great scientific interest because they arguably provide the most suitable clinical setting in which to test some of the major mechanistic hypotheses of AD drug development. Regulatory guidance regarding outcome measures that has been provided in the context of at-risk subjects would also appear to be most relevant for trials in ADAD. An important question is the extent to which a clinical effect in ADAD could be extrapolated to sporadic AD. The EMA draft guideline is not clear on this point. Because the extent to which the pathophysiology of autosomal dominant AD overlaps with sporadic AD remains to be established, such data could be viewed as supportive, but immediate extrapolation would not be possible. To date, the FDA has not provided any formal guidance in this respect.

Disease Modification

Many of the drugs that are currently under development for the treatment of AD attempt to target elements of the underlying disease biology (e.g., β-amyloid or tau). The expectation is that these therapies may ultimately be able to slow the long-term course of the disease process, as opposed to treating symptoms in the short term, and they are often referred to as purported "disease-modifying" agents.

Regulators have offered some preliminary guidance regarding how a presumed disease-modifying drug effect may be more definitely established in a manner that could support such a labeling claim. Notably, no currently approved drugs for any CNS indications have any language related to disease modification in their label. Conversely, although it is generally accepted that these approved agents have effects that are largely symptomatic in nature, their labeling indications state only that they are approved for a given stage of AD and are silent to whether that effect is exclusively symptomatic.

In its early AD draft guidance, the FDA indicated that it might be appealing to interpret the demonstration of a divergence of slopes between treatment arms on a clinical outcome measure as evidence of disease modification in AD. However, the FDA also considered the fact that a pharmacologically reversible effect that increases over time could also lead to a similar outcome. The guidance goes on to state that a claim of disease modification may be supported by evidence of a meaningful effect on a biomarker, in combination with a clinical benefit. The FDA is careful to note that there is currently a lack of consensus in the research community regarding what sort of biomarker effect would be most suitable for this purpose. Furthermore, the FDA suggests that a randomized start or randomized withdrawal design (using clinical outcome measures) could theoretically be a more convincing means of establishing disease modification. The FDA's draft on early AD guidance states that for ethical reasons, a randomized start design would be most appropriate for use in AD. The FDA explains that in this study design, patients are randomized to drug and placebo, and at some point, placebo patients are crossed over to active treatment. If patients in the trial who were initially on placebo and then assigned to active treatment fail to *catch up* (after a reasonable period of time) to patients who received active treatment for the entire duration of the trial, a disease-modifying effect of treatment would have been shown. Recent attempts at using this approach, however, have served to highlight its inherent challenges, and the FDA is explicit in stating that it is unaware of any instances to date in which this design has been successfully employed to establish a disease-modifying effect.

The EMA's comments on the subject of disease modification in its AD draft guidance, although largely consistent with the FDA's guidance, also carry a number of somewhat nuanced but important distinctions. The EMA begins by suggesting that

> a medicinal product can be considered to be disease modifying, if the progression of the disease as measured by assessment tools addressing both cognition and function is reduced or slowed down and if these results are linked to a significant effect on adequately qualified and validated biomarkers.[1]

Similar to the FDA, the EMA states that a true disease-modifying effect cannot be conclusively based on clinical outcome data alone and that biomarker support is necessary.

The critical difference in the EMA's discussion paper compared to the FDA's view on this subject is that if the correlation with relevant biomarkers is unclear, evidence of change in the disease course supported by an innovative study design such as those suggested previously, together with suitable analyses, could be acceptable as an alternative treatment goal such as "delay or slowing in rate of decline" if efficacy in cognition and function is demonstrated. The first step of this pathway involves establishing an improvement in the rate of decline of clinical signs and symptoms that could lead to a more limited claim (e.g., delay of disability). The FDA has not expressed a willingness to consider granting such a claim. Although both the FDA and the EMA note that the demonstration of a clinical effect in both the cognitive and functional domains may be more difficult to establish in patients who are earlier on in the disease process, depending on how ongoing research evolves, the EMA indicates that it is possible that an effect on a sensitive cognitive outcome measure alone in a biomarker-enriched population could serve as a primary outcome measure, as indicated previously. This clinical effect, in combination with the demonstration of a delay in the progression of brain neurodegeneration, could support a full claim of disease modification. Another important divergence between the FDA and the EMA in this area is that the EMA explicitly states that in the absence of a demonstrated meaningful biomarker effect, the absence of reversibility in randomized withdrawal studies is insufficient to merit a disease-modifying claim.

There is currently a lack of consensus among researchers and regulators regarding the most appropriate approach to convincingly demonstrate that a drug's effect goes beyond treating symptoms alone. Clinical trial designs based only on clinical endpoints (e.g., randomized start and randomized withdrawal designs) for this purpose are fraught with a variety of operational and analytical challenges. The use of biomarkers, although inherently more appealing, also requires additional research to address unresolved issues, including the best marker(s) to use and the sort of effect that would be required. In light of these challenges, it is important to observe that although a claim of disease modification is attractive for pharmaceutical companies, it is in no way a regulatory requirement for approval. In addition, drugs that convey a small clinical effect that is shown to be disease modifying could conceivably be ultimately less meaningful overall to patients than one that led to a large symptomatic effect. Therefore, although discussion on this topic should persist, undue attention on the support needed for what is ultimately a labeling claim should not detract from the more important focus on developing drugs that have large and important benefits to patients.

Combination Therapies

Alzheimer's disease has multiple biological abnormalities that are both intrinsic to the disease (e.g., amyloid plaques) and extrinsic comorbidities (e.g., hypertension and diabetes). The complex interactions among these various elements potentially argue for the development of combination therapies that target multiple aspects of disease simultaneously. The FDA has published a guidance document titled *Codevelopment of Two or More New Investigational Drugs for Use in Combination* that discusses both the nonclinical and clinical regulatory recommendations for these programs.[29] Although this guidance is not specific to AD, its principles would still apply. The EMA also addresses the issue of combination therapy development in AD in its draft guidance.

The standard approach to demonstrating the clinical efficacy of a combination drug product involves providing evidence that each of the component drugs makes a contribution to the claimed effect. This is usually accomplished through the use of a full-factorial design in which the combination (a two-drug combination product in this example) is compared to both of the individual components and placebo. However, regulators also acknowledge that these full-factorial trials are more difficult in situations in which a long-duration trial is required with large sample sizes. This would be expected to be the case for disease-modifying drugs in AD. The FDA guidance states that

> if findings from in vivo or in vitro models and/or Phase 2 trials adequately demonstrate the contribution of each new investigational drug to the combination, Phase 3 trials comparing the effectiveness to standard of care or placebo generally will be sufficient to establish effectiveness.[29]

The EMA also makes a similar comment in its AD draft guidance, stating that the exclusion of monotherapy arms needs to be scientifically justified and the appropriateness of the approach will be evaluated case by case. Because these strategies are new, scientific advice is encouraged.

The AD research community is beginning to discuss the possibility of conducting combination drug trials, although the scientific basis for choosing a given combination continues to require further study. It is encouraging that regulators appear open to helping facilitate these trials and have provided guidance regarding how this may be accomplished. It is important to note, however, that the specific requirements for any such development program will require detailed conversations between its sponsor and the appropriate regulatory bodies.

Non-Alzheimer's Disease Dementias

Although AD is by far the most prevalent dementia, there are a significant number of other etiologies of dementia that also lack adequate medical therapies. The FDA has not provided formal public guidance with respect to regulatory considerations specific to these disorders. However, the principles discussed in the context of AD would largely be expected to apply to other neurodegenerative dementias as well. For example, rivastigmine has been approved for the treatment of mild to moderately severe dementia due to Parkinson's disease.[30] The clinical trial that supported this approval utilized co-primary endpoints that assessed cognition and function, as is the expectation in AD. However, some considerations will also be unique to specific dementias. For example, in the case of dementia due to Parkinson's disease, it would also be important to understand the effect of the intervention on the core symptoms (e.g., motor function) of the disorder.

The EMA draft guidance on AD briefly addressed a number of other dementias in addition to AD, while noting that a detailed discussion was beyond the scope of the document. The EMA acknowledges the prevalence of "mixed" dementias that involve more than one co-occurring pathological finding. The recommendation, however, is that given the added complexity that studying such states would cause, development programs should begin with as "pure" a disease state as possible before expanding to the mixed forms. As with the FDA, the EMA reaffirms that similar principles to the study of drugs for AD would generally apply. It advises drug developers to seek more formal scientific advice in the context of their individual programs.

ASSESSING COGNITION IN DISORDERS NOT PRIMARILY DEFINED BY COGNITIVE IMPAIRMENT

In addition to neurodegenerative dementias, which are fundamentally defined as disorders of cognition, cognitive impairment is also a prevalent and troubling aspect of a number of other conditions, as described in detail in other chapters of this volume. However, the consideration of a marketing claim specific to the improvement of cognitive symptoms in these disorders presents a set of interesting regulatory challenges. Regulatory agencies have discussed these issues most in the context of the cognitive impairments associated with schizophrenia (CIAS), an area that is addressed in detail next. However, somewhat similar principles may also apply to a range of neuropsychiatric conditions in which cognitive deficits are observed. Current regulatory thinking regarding the conduct of clinical trials intended to address cognition in schizophrenia and depression is also addressed next.

Schizophrenia

Among the neuropsychiatric conditions that can affect cognition but are not primarily defined by those impairments, schizophrenia has received the greatest attention from both drug developers and regulators alike. In April 2004, investigators from the Measurement and Treatment Research to Improve Cognition in Schizophrenia (MATRICS) project convened a consensus meeting to include representatives from the FDA and the National Institute of Mental Health (NIMH), academic researchers, and industry representatives to develop guidelines for the design of clinical trials of cognitive enhancing drugs for patients with schizophrenia.[31] This meeting helped to springboard a complex and still ongoing discussion regarding a number of key challenges in this area in the intervening decade. In addition, regulators have both published on this topic and engaged in a number of related public meetings and working groups.

Regulators have endorsed the construct of cognitive impairment in schizophrenia as a legitimate target for drug development.[32,33] Furthermore, it is clear from their level of engagement and dialogue that regulators recognize the importance to the public health of advancing effecting therapies in this area. However, despite this degree of interest, no products have been approved to date for this indication. The following sections highlight the current regulatory positions related to the development of treatments for CIAS by topic area. Note that in many, if not most, cases, regulators have expressed receptiveness to data-driven recommendations that support other alternative approaches.

Population

The 2004 FDA–NIMH–MATRICS guidelines recommend that only subjects with schizophrenia, and not those with schizoaffective disorder, be enrolled in cognitive enhancement trials. The rationale behind this position is that although both conditions share similar patterns of cognitive deficits (which differ from those in mood disorders), the FDA preferred to have the greatest possible diagnostic specificity of the target population in the product label.

The guidelines further suggest that trials include subjects who (1) have been clinically stable and in the residual (non-acute) phase of their illness for a specified period of time (e.g., 8–12 weeks); (2) have been maintained on current antipsychotic and other concomitant psychotropic medications for a specified period of time sufficient to minimize potential complications of assessment of cognitive status (e.g., 6–8 weeks) and on current dose for a specified time period (e.g., 2–4 weeks); (3) have no more than a "moderate" severity rating on hallucinations and delusions (e.g., Brief Psychiatric Rating Scale (BPRS) Hallucinatory Behavior or Unusual Thought Content item score #4); (4) have no more than a "moderate" severity rating on positive formal thought disorder (e.g., BPRS Conceptual Disorganization item score #4); (5) have no more than "moderate" severity rating on negative symptoms (e.g., all Scale for the Assessment of Negative Symptoms global items #3 or Positive and

Negative Syndrome Scale–Negative Syndrome total score #15); and (6) have a minimal level of extrapyramidal symptoms (e.g., Simpson–Angus Scale total score #6) and depressive symptoms (e.g., Calgary Depression Scale total score #10). These suggested guidelines apply to studies of either adjunctive/co-treatment or broad-spectrum agents.

In addition, the guidelines recommend excluding subjects taking more than one antipsychotic because this would pose an unnecessary complication. With respect to the level of cognitive impairment that should be studies, the guidelines suggest excluding subjects only if their cognitive impairment severity (as assessed by clinical judgment and objective data) compromises the validity of the cognitive outcome assessment. On the higher end of cognitive functioning, the recommendation is to exclude subjects who are functioning so well that it would be unlikely that they could demonstrate any improvement during a trial, which is very rare. Finally, the guidelines indicate that a screening assessment, if used, should be different from any proposed primary outcome measure in order to avoid complications such as practice effects, novelty effects, and regression to the mean.

A more recent publication written by many of the original FDA–NIH–MATRICS authors, although supporting most of the original FDA–NIH–MATRICS guidelines, has made several recommendations for their revision based on evolving research.[34] Specifically, the authors suggest the use of a greater maximum allowable score for hallucinations and delusions while eliminating the negative symptom criteria from Phase II trials. They also recommend allowing first-generation antipsychotics in a trial's inclusion criteria if a subject is not co-prescribed an anticholinergic agent and has minimal extrapyramidal symptoms. In addition, it is argued that antipsychotic polypharmacy should be permitted in the absence of pertinent pharmacokinetic or pharmacodynamic considerations. Finally, the authors indicate that although illicit substance use should still be excluded from early phase trials, it should be permitted in Phase IIB and Phase III studies to allow for greater generalizability of the findings. It is noteworthy that these decisions were made in the absence of large clinical trials for CIAS. As new data continually emerge from ongoing studies, these guidelines may benefit from refinement.

Endpoints
COGNITIVE
Stemming from the 2004 FDA–NIMH–MATRICS conference, the MATRICS cognitive assessment battery was developed to serve as a cognitive outcome measure in trials of treatment for CIAS. This effort was largely due to the fact that at that time, no such standard neuropsychological test was available for this purpose. The test,

known as the MATRICS Consensus Cognitive Battery (MCCB), assesses the following seven domains: attention/vigilance, reasoning and problem-solving, speed of processing, social cognition, verbal learning and memory, visual learning and memory, and working memory. An analysis by Buchanan et al.[34] that was based on the use of the MCCB in two large multisite cognition trials suggests that the scale has proven reliability for such studies and clinical relevance for real-world functioning. Largely for these reasons, regulators have preferred the MCCB as the cognitive outcome measure for trials in CIAS. However, they are open to alternative measures provided that these measures cover the same domains as the MCCB and can be shown to be valid for assessing these domains. Perhaps the most unsettled concern about the MCCB lies in the uncertainty regarding its sensitivity to detect treatment effects. This issue is, of course, further complicated by the lack of any successful development programs in this area.

An additional consideration lies in whether the MCCB (or a similar measure) must be used only in its complete form or whether components of the scale can be used as outcome measures in their own right if a drug is believed to have a more targeted effect. This approach would likely require evaluation of a deleterious impact on any of the key cognitive domains not a part of the primary outcome measure. It has been suggested that a data-driven argument in favor of either approach could support a case to regulators.[35] However, the clinical meaningfulness of any cognitive effect (broad or targeted) would also need to be established, as discussed later.

FUNCTIONAL

A perennial concern to drug regulators lies in the establishment of a clinically meaningful treatment effect beyond the demonstration of statistical significance alone. This is particularly true in an area such as cognition, in which the demonstration of a drug's effect on a sensitive cognitive battery does not necessarily have clearly interpretable implications for how a patient feels, functions, or survives. As a result, as for drugs being developed for primary cognitive disorders, the FDA has required the use of a co-primary assessment of functional improvement in addition to the cognitive scale. Similarly, the EMA, while allowing such a measure to serve as a mandatory key secondary assessment, in essence follows a similar paradigm.

Unlike the MCCB for cognition, however, there is not yet a widely accepted tool for assessing the functional effects of a therapy in CIAS. Nutt et al.[36] rightly observe that regulators have not mandated a requirement that a drug for CIAS necessarily demonstrate an effect on real-world functioning because this might be challenging to assess in the context of a 6-month clinical trial. They also observe that a variety of possible co-primary measures are worth exploring, including interview-based measures as well as laboratory-based measures of functional capacity, which is defined as a clinical demonstration that a patient has the capacity to demonstrate changes in functioning in the community.

As Nutt et al.[36] also note, an empirical comparison of a variety of potential co-primary measures, sponsored by NIMH and executed by the MATRICS group, compared six different measures. Of the outcomes evaluated, the UPSA had the best psychometric characteristics, with test–retest interclass correlations of 0.74 and a strong correlation with cognitive performance at $r = 0.67$. The UPSA also received high ratings for practicality and tolerability. Potential drawbacks include the fact that it was designed for elderly patients with schizophrenia and that the international version (the UPSA-Brief) consisted of only two domains. However, Nutt et al. also note that the UPSA does appear to be sensitive to treatment-related improvements.

It is clear that additional work is needed before any consensus in support of a co-primary outcome measure can be established.

Trial Designs
ADJUNCTIVE AGENTS

In addition to the considerations regarding outcome measures, regulators have also weighed in on several other critical aspects of trial designs for drugs targeting CIAS. One such debate concerns the choice of comparator, which differs between adjunctive agents and so-called "broad-spectrum" drugs. For adjunctive or co-treatment products, a relatively straightforward comparison with placebo is warranted and supported by the FDA. In such a design, one group would be randomized to continue to receive the baseline antipsychotic agent plus the new adjunctive drug, whereas the comparator group would also continue to receive the baseline antipsychotic agent with the addition of placebo.

As Laughren and Levin[37] note, the necessary comparison in this context would be a function of the baseline antipsychotic agents allowed in the trial. For example, if all patients were enrolled on the same antipsychotic drug, this would presumably require that the FDA's combination drug policy be met, which would necessitate a comparison that the combination drug was superior to each of its individual components (i.e., in a full-factorial design). However, if patients were allowed to be enrolled on a range of different antipsychotic agents at baseline, the FDA would then allow a two-arm trial comparing the combination agent to placebo. This approach would also permit greater generalizability of the results.

BROAD-SPECTRUM AGENTS

The case of a broad-spectrum agent, which would be thought to target cognition in addition to other aspects of the condition (e.g., positive symptoms), requires more thoughtful consideration. The FDA–NIMH–MATRICS guidelines note that the evaluation of a drug's effects on cognition should be assessed separately from its effects on other symptomatology. In contrast to the stable population being studied in the case of adjunctive agents, a broad-spectrum agent would need to be tested in an acutely ill patient population in order to determine its efficacy as an antipsychotic.

Three potential comparator options exist: placebo, a conventional antipsychotic, or a second-generation antipsychotic. The FDA–NIMH–MATRICS guidelines discuss the relative advantages and disadvantages of these approaches, including the potential for symptom exacerbation with a placebo comparison (which is viewed as ethically unacceptable given the trial durations that would be required) and the potential confound of extrapyramidal symptoms and other neurologic adverse events with a conventional agent. In addition, conventional agents are often used with anticholinergics, which have well-described negative effects on cognition. However, although a second-generation antipsychotic may pose fewer challenges than either placebo or a conventional agent, it is not without complications. Most notably, the lack of a placebo control (which also applies to studies of conventional agents) allows for multiple possible interpretations of an observed treatment effect between study arms. Of course, the desired interpretation would be that the broad-spectrum agent improves cognition to a greater degree than the comparator. However, as Laughren and Levin[37] also observe, an alternative interpretation could be that the broad-spectrum agent actually has no effect while the comparator is impairing cognition. Similarly, it is also possible that both agents are ultimately impairing cognition, albeit that the broad-spectrum agent is doing so to a lesser degree. As Laughren and Levin further comment, because of these possible confounds, the FDA–NIMH–MATRICS guidelines conclude that any claim related to cognition for a broad-spectrum agent studied in such a manner would not likely be appropriate to include in the Indications and Usage section of a product label because that placement would imply that an effect on cognition has clearly been established when, in fact, that might ultimately not be the case. Rather, the guidelines suggest that the effects could instead be described in the Adverse Reactions section of the label, noting that although the absolute effect of the broad-spectrum agent on cognition cannot be determined, it appears to have significantly less cognitive liability than the studied comparator agents.

A subsequent FDA commentary on the possible trial designs for broad-spectrum agents addresses the proposal by Marder et al.[38] to conduct a trial using a run-in period during which patients would be stabilized on a standard antipsychotic agent (either conventional or atypical) followed by a double-blind phase during which they would be randomized to either continue on the standard agent or be switched to the new broad-spectrum agent. Although in agreement that this may be the only feasible design for this circumstance, the FDA authors disagree with how this trial may be interpreted. Specifically, they state that without the presence of a placebo arm in such a study, the same confounding interpretations that have been previously discussed will continue to exist. They do acknowledge that in the highly unexpected case in which the new agent returned subjects to an entirely normal state with no negative symptoms, the interpretation would become more straightforward.

Trial Duration

The FDA has indicated that trials of at least 6 months' duration would be required to support an approval for CIAS. Similarly, the EMA also requires trials of a minimum of 6 months' duration as well as a maintenance study of an additional 6–12 months. The FDA–NIMH–MATRICS guidelines further state that the primary outcome should be measured multiple times during the course of the trial (either in the original or through the use of alternative forms) and that the statistical procedures to be used must be capable of accommodating data from multiple time assessments. As with all trials in theory, the guidelines also encourage following all subjects who drop out through the duration of the trial—an approach that is presumably more feasible in a stable baseline population.

OVERLAP WITH NEGATIVE SYMPTOMS

Although, as previously noted, regulators have endorsed the construct of cognitive impairment associated with schizophrenia as a suitable drug target, they also recognize that there is a possible overlap with the negative symptoms of schizophrenia. Therefore, the FDA, as discussed by Laughren and Levin,[37] currently recommends that trials that target either the negative or the cognitive symptoms of schizophrenia should collect data on both domains. By doing so, the FDA suggests that if both domains consistently demonstrate similar benefits, the separation of the two constructs for the purposes of product labeling becomes less attractive. The FDA also suggests the possibility that such a circumstance may merit a more general claim such as "residual phase schizophrenia," although the FDA is clear to comment that this area remains an unanswered question in the absence of additional data.

Major Depressive Disorder

Pseudospecificity

The regulatory considerations that relate to the construct of the cognitive impairments associated with major depressive disorder (MDD) can in many ways be discussed in contrast to those in CIAS. As has already been described, regulators have endorsed the construct of CIAS as a suitable target for drug development. The rationale behind this decision lies in the fact that they have been convinced that these deficits are distinct from the positive symptoms of the disorder. The same may hold true for the negative symptoms, although their concerns and potential remedy for any potential overlap with cognitive deficits have also been addressed. In contrast, although the cognitive impairments that are observed in MDD are unquestionably disruptive to patients, it becomes much more challenging to disentangle them from the core syndrome itself.

For regulators, the most pressing concern in this circumstance relates to the desire to avoid granting a "pseudospecific" labeling claim. Such a claim is defined as being artificially narrow. As described by Laughren and Levin,[37] in the absence of data that support the distinct nature of the target of investigation from other aspects of a condition, these claims serve only promotional purposes and are potentially misleading, in the sense that they imply advantages over other drugs in a class. In 2016, an FDA panel concluded that cognition is a legitimate endpoint for clinical trials in MDD.[39] An EMA concept paper released in 2017 indicates that cognitive impairment in MDD may be a separate indication disentangled from the overall depressive symptoms. A guideline is expected to be released at the end of 2017, and EMA will host a multi-stakeholder workshop on this topic in 2018. Furthermore, it is worth noting that in addition to cognition and negative symptoms in schizophrenia, the FDA has accepted other subdomains as valid indications, including suicidal ideation and agitation in schizophrenia, bipolar disorder, irritability of autism, impulsive aggression in attention deficit hyperactivity disorder, and agitation/aggression and psychosis in dementia.

Endpoints

Although a few studies have evaluated treatments for cognition in depression, there is currently no clear scientific or regulatory consensus regarding the most suitable cognitive assessment tool for this purpose. The FDA briefing document was indecisive on which cognitive domains are essential to include in a cognitive endpoint and which methods are best to assess the affected cognitive domain. Furthermore, as with dementia and CIAS, a small effect on a sensitive cognitive measure will not necessarily translate into a clinically meaningful benefit for patients. Therefore, regulators are expected to continue to mandate that a co-primary (or key secondary) assessment of function, or a functional proxy, be a necessary element of any trial targeting cognitive impairment in depression. Currently, however, there are no widely accepted and validated scales for this purpose.

Trial Designs

Several trial designs have been proposed as possible approaches for studying treatments targeting cognition in MDD. The first is an adjunctive design that targets cognition in residual phase depression. The key aspect in this scenario would be that the added therapy must only treat depression. If, instead, depression also improved overall, this may likely be considered as an adjunctive antidepressant. The relatively recent publication of a placebo-controlled trial with the antidepressant lisdexamfetamine to augment adult patients with persistent executive dysfunction after partial or full remission of MDD yielded such results.[40] Whereas the primary cognitive endpoint (the Behavior Rating Inventory of Executive Function–Adult Version (BRIEF-A)) demonstrated an effect of treatment ($p = 0.0009$), the depression scale (the Montgomery–Asberg Depression Rating Scale (MADRS)) also favored lisdexamfetamine ($p = 0.0465$). These findings complicate the interpretation of the study with respect to the demonstration of an isolated effect on cognition apart from the drug's broader antidepressant properties.

A second possibility would be to conduct an acute phase study comparing two antidepressants on cognitive impairment. In this situation, the new antidepressant would need to be superior to the standard agent on cognition alone, with both drugs being superior to placebo on a broad depression scale. The question of what the comparison would need to be from a regulatory standpoint is not completely clear, however. Specifically, would it be sufficient for the new drug to beat placebo on cognition while the active control does not? Or, instead, would the new drug need to show head-to-head superiority over the active control on cognition? A recent illustration of such a circumstance derives from the results of a trial comparing the antidepressant vortioxetine to both the antidepressant duloxetine and placebo.[41] Whereas vortioxetine was shown to be statistically superior to placebo ($p < 0.05$) on the Digit Symbol Substitution Test (DSST), duloxetine was not. The study authors note that the study was not powered for a comparison of the relative benefits on cognition of the two active agents. Based on the results of this trial, the EMA issued a positive opinion for a label update to reflect vortioxetine's effect on certain aspects of cognitive function in patients with depression.[42]

A third approach that has also been suggested is to conduct a switching study in residual phase depression that would seek to demonstrate a benefit on cognition in switching to another antidepressant. Obviously, such a study would need to enroll subjects in the residual phase of depression who have clinically important residual cognitive impairment—a construct that has not been clearly defined. The desired outcome for such a trial would be that the initial antidepressant response is sustained during the switch, but cognition improves in subjects who are switched to the new agent. However, the same concerns that were raised when this design was considered for broad-spectrum agents in CIAS remain valid here. Primarily, an interpretation of superiority on cognition is confounded by the fact that the new drug may theoretically simply have a lesser effect on impairing cognition.

Cognition in Other Central Nervous System Disorders

Cognitive dysfunction is also a disabling symptom in a number of other CNS disorders that have not been discussed in this chapter given the lack of specific public regulatory guidance in these areas. However, as with the non-AD dementias, the principles outlined in this chapter would also be expected to apply with the caveat that drug developers should always discuss disease-specific circumstances with the appropriate regulatory agencies.

REFERENCES

1. Center for Drug Evaluation and Research. *Alzheimer's disease: Developing drugs for the treatment of early stage disease—Guidance for industry.* Washington, DC: US Food and Drug Administration; 2013.
2. European Medicines Agency. *Discussion paper on the clinical investigations of medicines for the treatment of Alzheimer's disease and other dementias.* EMA/CHMP/539931/2014, October 23, 2014.
3. McKhann G, Drachman D, Folstein M, et al. Clinical diagnosis of Alzheimer's disease: Report of the NINCDS-ADRDA work group under the auspices of the Department of Health and Human Services Task Force on Alzheimer's Disease. *Neurology* 1984;34:939–944.
4. Doody RS, Thomas RG, Farlow M, et al; Alzheimer's Disease Cooperative Study Steering Committee; Solanezumab Study Group. Phase 3 trials of solanezumab for mild-to-moderate Alzheimer's disease. *N Engl J Med* 2014;370(4):311–321.
5. Albert MS, DeKosky ST, Dickson D, et al. The diagnosis of mild cognitive impairment due to Alzheimer's disease: Recommendations from the National Institute on Aging–Alzheimer's Association workgroups on diagnostic guidelines for Alzheimer's disease. *Alzheimers Dement* 2011;7(3):270–279.
6. McKhann GM, Knopman DS, Chertkow H, et al. The diagnosis of dementia due to Alzheimer's disease: Recommendations from the National Institute on Aging and the Alzheimer's Association workgroup. *Alzheimers Dement* 2011;7:263–269.
7. Sperling RA, Aisen PS, Beckett LA, et al. Toward defining the preclinical stages of Alzheimer's disease: Recommendations from the National Institute on Aging–Alzheimer's

Association workgroups on diagnostic guidelines for Alzheimer's disease. *Alzheimers Dement* 2011;7:280–292.

8. Dubois B, Feldman HH, Jacova C, et al. Advancing research diagnostic criteria for Alzheimer's disease: The IWG-2 criteria. *Lancet Neurol* 2014;13(6):614–629.

9. American Psychiatric Association. *Diagnostic and statistical manual of mental disorders*. 5 ed. Arlington, VA: American Psychiatric Publishing; 2013.

10. Hill DL, Schwarz AJ, Isaac M, et al. Coalition Against Major Diseases/European Medicines Agency biomarker qualification of hippocampal volume for enrichment of clinical trials in pre-dementia stages of Alzheimer's disease. *Alzheimers Dement* 2014;10(4):421–429.

11. Isaac M, Vamvakas S, Abadie E, et al; European Medicines Agency. Qualification opinion of Alzheimer's disease novel methodologies/biomarkers for the use of CSF AB 1-42 and t-tau signature and/or PET-amyloid imaging (positive/negative) as biomarkers for enrichment, for use in regulatory clinical trials in mild cognitive impairment. *Eur Neuropsychopharmacol* 2011;21(11):781–788.

12. Center for Drug Evaluation and Research, Center for Biologics Evaluation and Research, and Center for Devices and Radiological Health. *In vitro companion diagnostics: Guidance for industry*. Washington, DC. US Food and Drug Administration; 2014.

13. Rockwood, K., Strang, D., MacKnight, C., et al. Interrater reliability of the Clinical Dementia Rating in a multicenter trial. *J Am Geriatr Soc* 2000;48:558–559.

14. Cedarbaum JM, Jaros M, Hernandez C, et al; Alzheimer's Disease Neuroimaging Initiative. Rationale for use of the Clinical Dementia Rating Sum of Boxes as a primary outcome measure for Alzheimer's disease clinical trials. *Alzheimers Dement* 2013;9(1 Suppl):S45–S55.

15. Donohue MC, Sperling RA, Salmon DP, et al; Australian Imaging, Biomarkers, and Lifestyle Flagship Study of Ageing; Alzheimer's Disease Neuroimaging Initiative; Alzheimer's Disease Cooperative Study. The preclinical Alzheimer cognitive composite: Measuring amyloid-related decline. *JAMA Neurol* 2014;77(4):961–970.

16. Hughes CP, Berg L, Danziger WL, et al. A new clinical scale for the staging of dementia. *Br J Psychiatry* 1982;140:566–572.

17. Freemantle N, Calvert M, Wood J, et al. Composite outcomes in randomized trials: Greater precision but with greater uncertainty? *JAMA* 2003;289:2554–2559.

18. Gomar JJ, Harvey PD, Bobes-Bascaran MT, et al. Development and cross-validation of the UPSA short form for the performance-based functional assessment of patients with mild cognitive impairment and Alzheimer disease. *Am J Geriatr Psychiatry* 2011;19(11):915–922.

19. Atkins AS, Stroescu I, Spagnola NB, et al. Assessment of age-related differences in functional capacity using the Virtual Reality Functional Capacity Assessment Tool (VRFCAT). *J Prev Alzheimers Dis* 2015;2(2):121–127.

20. Patterson TL, Goldman S, McKibbin CL, et al. UCSD performance-based skills assessment: Development of a new measure of everyday functioning for severely mentally ill adults. *Schizophr Bull* 2001;27(2):235–245.

21. Ruse SA, Davis VG, Atkins AS, et al. Development of virtual reality assessment of everyday living skills. *J Vis Exp* 2014;86:1–8.

22. Keefe RSE, Davis VG, Atkins A, et al. Validation of a computerized test of functional capacity. *Schizophr Res* 2016;175(1–3):90–96.

23. Vellas B, Aisen PS, Sampaio C, et al. Prevention trials in Alzheimer's disease: An EU–US task force report. *Prog Neurobiol* 2011;95(4):594–600.

24. NIH Definitions Working Group. Biomarkers and surrogate endpoints in clinical research: Definitions and conceptual model. In Downing GJ (Ed.), *Biomarkers and surrogate endpoints*. Amsterdam: Elsevier, 2000:1–9.

25. Accelerated Approval, 21 CFR part 314, subpart H and 21 CFR part 601, subpart E. (1992).

26. European Medicines Agency. *Enhanced early dialogue to facilitate accelerated assessment of PRIority MEdicines (PRIME)*. February 25, 2016. Retrieved from http://www.ema.europa.eu/docs/en_GB/document_library/Regulatory_and_procedural_guideline/2016/03/WC500202636.pdf

27. Morris JC, Aisen PS, Bateman RJ, et al. Developing an international network for Alzheimer research: The Dominantly Inherited Alzheimer Network. *Clin Invest* 2012;5:975–984.
28. Reiman EM, Langbaum JB, Fleisher AS, et al. Alzheimer's Prevention Initiative: A plan to accelerate the evaluation of presymptomatic treatments. *J Alzheimers Dis* 2011;5:321–329.
29. Center for Drug Evaluation and Research. *Codevelopment of two or more new investigational drugs for use in combination: Guidance for industry.* Washington, DC: US Food and Drug Administration; 2013.
30. Emre M, Aarsland D, Albanese A, et al. Rivastigmine for dementia associated with Parkinson's disease. *N Engl J Med* 2004;351(24):2509–2518.
31. Buchanan RW, Davis M, Goff D, et al. A summary of the FDA–NIMH–MATRICS workshop on clinical trial design for neuro-cognitive drugs for schizophrenia. *Schizophr Bull* 2005;31:5–19.
32. Laughren T, Levin R. Food and Drug Administration perspective on negative symptoms in schizophrenia as a target for a drug treatment claim. *Schizophr Bull* 2006;32:220–222.
33. European Medicines Administration. *Guideline on clinical investigation of medicinal products, including depot preparations, in the treatment of schizophrenia.* EMA/CHMP/40072/2010 Revision 1, September 20, 2012.
34. Buchanan RW, Keefe RS, Umbricht D, et al. The FDA–NIMH–MATRICS guidelines for clinical trial design of cognitive-enhancing drugs: What do we know 5 years later? *Schizophr Bull* 2011;37:1209–1217.
35. Laughren T. Commentary on "Regulatory issues in drug development programs targeting cognitive impairment in schizophrenia." *Eur Neuropsychopharmacol* 2013;23:784–785.
36. Nutt D, Gispen-de Wied CC, Arango C, et al. Cognition in schizophrenia: Summary Nice Consultation Meeting. *Eur Neuropsychopharmacol* 2012;23(8):769–778.
37. Laughren T, Levin R. Food and Drug Administration commentary on methodological issues in negative symptom trials. *Schizophr Bull* 2011;37:255–256.
38. Marder SR, Daniel DG, Alphs L, et al. Methodological issues in negative symptoms trials. *Schizophr Bull* 2011;37:250–254.
39. US Food and Drug Administration. *FDA briefing document Psychopharmacologic Drugs Advisory Committee (PDAC) meeting, February 3, 2016. Topic: Cognitive dysfunction in major depressive disorder.*
40. Madhoo M, Keefe RS, Roth RM, et al. Lisdexamfetamine dimesylate augmentation in adults with persistent executive dysfunction after partial or full remission of major depressive disorder. *Neuropsychopharmacology* 2014;39(6):1388–1398.
41. McIntyre RS, Lophaven S, Olsen CK. A randomized, double-blind, placebo-controlled study of vortioxetine on cognitive dysfunction in depressed adults. *Int J Neuropsychopharmacol* 2014;17:1557–1567.
42. H. Lundbeck, A/S. *European CHMP issues positive opinion for a label update of Brintellix (vortioxetine) to reflect its effect on certain aspects of cognitive function in patients with depression* [Press release]. Retrieved from https://globenewswire.com/news-release/2015/03/05/712567/0/en/European-CHMP-issues-positive-opinion-for-a-label-update-of-Brintellix-vortioxetine-to-reflect-its-effect-on-certain-aspects-of-cognitive-function-in-patients-with-depression.html

Index

.